Introduction
to Person-Centered Nursing

Introduction to Person-Centered Nursing

Janice B. Lindberg, R.N., M.A., Ph.D.

Former Area Chairperson, Fundamentals
Associate Professor
The University of Michigan, School of Nursing
Ann Arbor, Michigan

Mary Love Hunter, R.N., M.S.

Clinical Nursing Specialist
University of Michigan Hospitals
Coordinator, Fundamentals
Assistant Professor
The University of Michigan, School of Nursing
Ann Arbor, Michigan

Ann Z. Kruszewski, R.N., M.S.N.

Assistant Professor, Fundamentals
The University of Michigan, School of Nursing
Ann Arbor, Michigan

 J. B. Lippincott Company Philadelphia

London   Mexico City   New York   St. Louis   São Paulo   Sydney

Sponsoring Editor: Diana Intenzo
Manuscript Editor: Rachel Bedard
Indexer: Ann Cassar
Art Director and Designer: Tracy Baldwin
Production Supervisor: Carol Kerr
Production Assistant: Corey Gray
Compositor: Monotype Composition Company, Inc.
Printer/Binder: The Murray Printing Company

6 5 4 3 2 1

Library of Congress Cataloging in Publication Data

Lindberg, Janice B.
  Introduction to person-centered nursing.

  Bibliography: p.
  Includes index.
  1. Nursing—Psychological aspects. 2. Nursing.
I. Hunter, Mary Love. II. Kruszewski, Ann Z.
III. Title. [DNLM: 1. Philosophy, Nursing.
2. Nurse-patient relations. 3. Nursing care.
WY 87 L742i]
RT86.L54 1983   610.73   82-14929
ISBN O-397-54345-X

The authors and publisher have exerted every effort to ensure that drug selection and dosage set forth in this text are in accord with current recommendations and practice at the time of publication. However, in view of ongoing
research, changes in government regulations, and the constant flow of information relating to drug therapy and drug reactions, the reader is urged to check the
package insert for each drug for any change in indications and dosage and for
added warnings and precautions. This is particularly important when the recommended agent is a new or infrequently employed drug.

Contributors

Margaret A. Banning, R.N., M.N.
Clinical Nurse Specialist, Rehabilitation
Adjunct Assistant Professor, Montana State University
Bozeman, Montana

Bobbie Bloch, R.N., M.S.N.
Educational Specialist in Community Health Nursing
The University of Michigan, University Hospitals
Ann Arbor, Michigan

Martha Keehner Engelke, B.S.N., M.P.H., C.S. (Medical-Surgical)
Assistant Professor
East Carolina University, School of Nursing
Greenville, North Carolina

Sue V. Fink, R.N., M.S.
Specialist in Gerontology Certificate, Institute of Gerontology
The University of Michigan
Assistant Professor, Fundamentals
The University of Michigan, School of Nursing
Ann Arbor, Michigan

Marguerite Babaian Harms, R.N., M.S.
Associate Professor, Fundamentals
The University of Michigan, School of Nursing
Ann Arbor, Michigan

Sharon Hein Jette, R.N., M.S.N., M.P.H.
Gerontologic Nurse Practitioner
Boston, Massachusetts

Evelyn Malcolm Tomlin, R.N., M.S., C.C.R.N.
Assistant Professor, Fundamentals
The University of Michigan, School of Nursing
Generalist Nurse in Private Practice
Ann Arbor, Michigan

Terry M. Vanden Bosch, R.N., M.S.
Assistant Professor, Fundamentals
The University of Michigan, School of Nursing
Clinical Nursing Specialist
University of Michigan Hospitals
Ann Arbor, Michigan

Preface

The authors of this text believe that introductory level nursing courses ought to reflect a broad perspective of nursing care on which advanced nursing courses can build. We believe that person-centered nursing care is the foundation basic to all clinical specialties and levels of nursing practice. All professional nursing practice evolves from care of the person.

This text builds on the basic human needs approach, which is commonly used in nursing practice and educational programs at all levels. Further, the text extends this approach by adding a person-centered focus. Although it has long been recognized that the person is the object of nursing care, this conceptualization is often not developed in such a way that both beginners and experienced practitioners can make the necessary application to their own practice situations. From experience, the authors recognize that purposeful and consistent attention to person-centered care, coupled with a human needs approach, has several positive consequences:

- Theory is more easily incorporated into practice because real-life experiences reinforce theory application in such a way that they are vividly remembered.

- The person-centered approach enhances recognition and utilization of individual client strengths to meet human needs.

- Students learn intervention strategies that are congruent with the most sophisticated level of nursing practice, thereby encouraging personal and professional development to a level of maximum potential.

The authors believe that nurses deliver care using the same concepts, regardless of the care setting or particular health concern expressed by the person seeking care. The text is organized around seven concepts that are fundamental to nursing practice: person, health and adaptation, health care, professionalism, communication, nursing process, and teaching/learning. Sections 1 through 6 address these concepts individually. Section 7 describes their application in two specific situations: persons experiencing loss and persons experiencing surgery. The purpose of Section 7 is to help students synthesize a variety of principles while caring for persons with special needs. Although the text is focused primarily on the individual, we expect that students, as developing professional nurses, will build on basic principles when learning to work with families, groups, communities, and persons with more complex health problems.

The authors believe that health is promoted, maintained, and restored to the person who has control over his life and who takes care of himself with the assistance of others as he needs them. Some persons may be very dependent, either physically or psychologically. They may need almost constant help and support from the nurse and other members of the health team. This text shows, however, that the goal of nursing is to assist persons in all states of dependency to achieve health to the greatest extent possible.

The idea of functioning at an optimal level assumes man is a unique adaptive being with an inherent striving to achieve his fullest potential. Therefore, the concepts of adaptation and a holistic perspective of man provide the unifying themes of the text. We use the nursing process framework to develop approaches to the delivery of care. We will not focus on the process itself but rather on the use of it as a tool to assist the nurses as they provide person-centered care.

Although a review of literature reveals variations in the way that nurses conceptualize nursing process, there are four elements that are common to all: assessment, planning, implementation, and evaluation. This text discusses nursing process in three phases (assessment, therapy, and aggregation) that include these four elements. The assessment phase involves assessing the person, analyzing data, and establishing nursing diagnoses; the therapeutic phase includes planning, implementing, and evaluating nursing care. The aggregation phase, which is not usually found in nursing literature, involves synthesizing the results of nursing interventions from a variety of situations to make predictions about the most effective approach for persons of a given age, sex, cultural background, and so forth. This phase has the potential for yielding researchable problems and developing a theoretical basis for nursing.

Specific content related to nursing process has been divided according to the functional abilities of the person, for example, circulatory status or mobility status. These functional abilities or statuses reflect the level at which the person is meeting his human needs, such as oxygen or activity. We have attempted to help the reader focus on the total person with a certain highlighting of the particular status being addressed at the moment. For example, if the person is having difficulty breathing, we have attempted to describe the respiratory system and how the nurse may assist the person with dyspnea. We have then suggested what it is like for the person to have difficulty breathing: how this affects his ability to eat, sleep, move about, honor his work commitments, and generally enjoy life. How do the changes that can occur because of dyspnea affect the person's view of himself; how do others, especially those he cares about, see him? We also wish to give the student a sense, not only of what the nurse can do, but of what the nurse can assist the person to do so that he may function at an optimal level within the constraints of the respiratory difficulties.

As we teach students to provide care focused on the person they are committed to assist, we hope to offer that same person focus for the students themselves. That is, we wish this text to function as a means of support for students as they build their cognitive and technical skills. We hope to help them become aware of their feelings and assist them to function more comfortably. The text is not intended to be either prescriptive or inclusive. Most basic nursing interventions are presented as general principles of care rather than as explicit procedures. If, as we believe, nursing is nursing wherever it happens, then students can apply general principles and adapt these to fit both the local circumstances and available equipment. This approach is consistent with our belief that nurses as students and practicing professionals must expect to consult a wide variety of current references and resources in their practice. Similarly, students who use this book are expected to have knowledge in basic sciences such as anatomy, physiology, and social sciences. We expect to provide students with both a knowledge foundation and encouragement to develop as professional nurses. We hope to help them develop confidence in their observations, problem solving, and judgments so that they will see their role as essential for the promotion of health and as collegial with other health professionals.

This approach to health care and nursing focuses on persons as unique beings. Persons, whether seekers or providers of nursing, have health and strengths as well as needs. These strengths, the best in us, will help us rise to the highest level of our capabilities.

Janice B. Lindberg
Mary L. Hunter
Ann Z. Kruszewski

Note, when referring to persons in general the authors have chosen to use the male pronoun. This was done for the sake of simplicity and clarity and should not imply failure to recognize the needs of female clients.

Acknowledgments

Any text of this nature reflects the inspiration and diligence of many persons. The authors of *Introduction to Person-Centered Nursing* gratefully acknowledge the faithful peers who offered support, encouragement, and validation, especially members of the Fundamentals Area of Instruction of the baccalaureate program at The University of Michigan School of Nursing. These colleagues know that from the richness of their clinical practice, research, and teaching came many of the ideas and thoughts that stimulated our own. We indeed appreciate their incentive. Some of these persons also shared their expertise as contributors to the text. The authors, however, accept full responsibility for any inadvertent alterations in the contributors' intent that may have occurred in the process of achieving consistent terminology and a cohesive conceptual approach.

Karen Hoxeng, former acquisitions editor, nursing department, J. B. Lippincott Company, initiated the project and encouraged our commitment to a person-centered text. Jon Martin persuaded us to write the person-centered laboratory manual that accompanies the text. A special debt of gratitude is owed to Diana Intenzo, our faithful editor, who adapted to the idiosyncrasies of the three authors and several contributors.

Unless otherwise acknowledged, photographs were furnished by The University of Michigan Information Services. Among these, some are credited to photographer Bob Kalmbach, whose artistry so often reflects the essence of the person.

Virginia Hinderer, Nancy Crisp, and Diane Craven provided the typing assistance.

The authors gratefully express appreciation to certain individuals who offered objective critique and special expertise. These include the following:

Teresa Bruggeman, R.N., Ph.D.
Assistant Professor of Nursing, University of Michigan

Beverly Linde, R.N., M.S.N.
Lecturer, University of Michigan School of Nursing

Susan Muscarella Parsonage, R.N., M.S.N.
Clinical Specialist with expertise in respiratory nursing care

Nancy Reame, R.N., M.S.N., Ph.D.
Associate Professor of Nursing, University of Michigan

Finally, we offer a special thank you to our family members, who endured steadfastly and then gave an extra measure to enable us to complete the project.

Contents

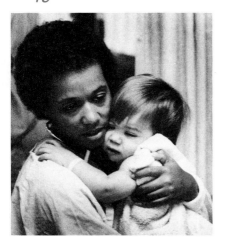

II
Health and Adaptation

61

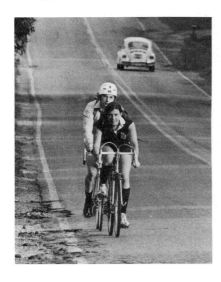

III
Health Care
105

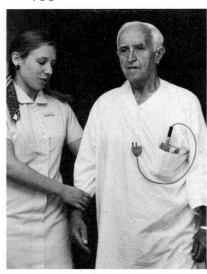

IV
Professionalism
145

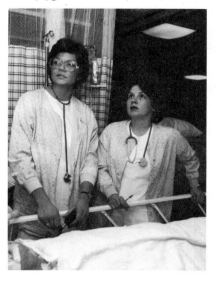

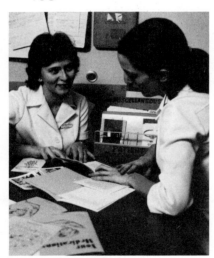

VI
Nursing
Process

225

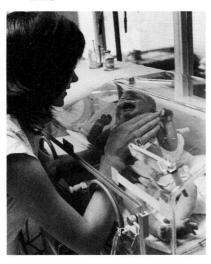

VII
Learning and Teaching

611

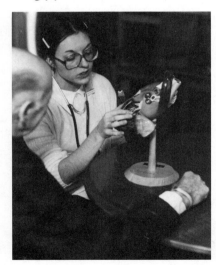

VIII
Synthesis of Concepts

635

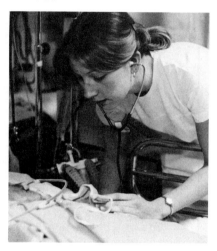

Introduction to Nursing Concepts

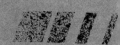

Ann Z. Kruszewski, Mary L. Hunter, Janice B. Lindberg

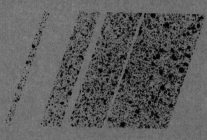

1

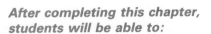

After completing this chapter, students will be able to:

● Identify the expertise of the profession of nursing.

● Identify common elements of several leaders' definitions of nursing.

● Explain the concept of caring in relation to nursing practice.

● Identify the elements of person-centered nursing care.

● Describe the connotations of the terms "patient" and "client."

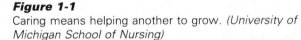

This text is an introduction to the practice of nursing. It is organized around the following seven concepts, which are basic to nursing in any setting or specialty:

● Person
● Health and adaptation
● Health care
● Professionalism
● Communication
● Nursing process
● Learning and teaching

Before beginning a detailed discussion of the individual concepts, it is important that we have a clear understanding of how these concepts relate to nursing. In order to do this, we must first have a firm understanding of what *nursing* is. Beginning nursing students may now be saying to themselves, "But I know what nursing is. I learned that from my aunt who is a nurse (or from books, television, volunteer work in hospitals, guidance counsellors . . .)." When asked to define nursing, most beginning students respond that it involves helping people. The authors' own concept of nursing is similar, for we believe that the essence of nursing is caring for **persons.** This is the approach to nursing that inspires this textbook. This chapter discusses what we mean by person-centered nursing practice and presents the concepts that we believe are essential to this practice. We hope to provide our readers with an appreciation of the philosophy that underlies this text.

Figure 1-1
Caring means helping another to grow. *(University of Michigan School of Nursing)*

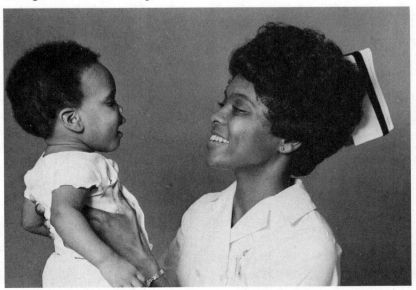

Person-Centered Nursing Care

There are many professions in today's society. In this wide array, nursing is viewed as one of the health professions. Although the term "profession" has many common meanings, some writers have tried to ascribe a tighter definition to it. Schein and Kommers have identified certain criteria of a true profession, including a body of knowledge on which expert skills and services are based (1972, p. 8). In Table 1-1 we list some of the groups that are considered professions and identify their expertise.

Nursing is an emerging profession trying to fulfill the criteria that define a profession. What is the expertise that nursing claims? The authors believe that it is *caring for persons.*

Caring as a Basis for Nursing

Nurses constantly use the term "caring": "I'm caring for seven patients today," "Mr. Jones needs complete care," "Mrs. Smith doesn't require much care." When this text uses the term "caring," it does so with a specific meaning in mind. Caring should involve more than just carrying out nursing procedures such as bedmaking and treatments. True caring is based on an attitude of nurturing, of helping another to grow. Mayeroff, a philosopher who explores the nature of caring, states, "To care for another person, in the most significant sense, is to help him grow and actualize himself" (1971, p. 1). He continues, "In caring, I experience the other as having potentialities and the need to grow" (p. 6).

Caring nurses recognize that persons have strengths as well as needs and that they possess worth and potential to grow. Rather than seeing the person as helpless because he needs care, caring nurses respect him as independent in his own right (Fig. 1-1). Caring nurses assist this person out of a desire to foster growth and independence. They want to enhance their clients' ability to manage their own health needs as a result of the care received. As Mayeroff says, "To help another person grow ... is to help that other person come to care for himself" (p. 10).

We hope that you are now thinking, "Yes, I want to be a caring person. This is what brought me to nursing." You will be interested to learn that these same thoughts are reflected in many of the definitions of nursing put forth by nursing leaders such as Harmer, Henderson, Rogers, Levine, and Mitchell. Table 1-2 summarizes these definitions and shows that a common element in each of them is caring

(Text continues on page 6)

Table 1-1
Professions and Their Expertise

Profession	Expertise
Lawyer	Law
Pastor or minister	Spirituality
Physician or doctor	Illness, disease
Psychologist	Mind/behavior
Social worker	Societal support systems

Table 1-2
Nursing Definitions: Thoughts on Caring and Related Nursing Concepts

Definition	*Thoughts on Caring*	*Related Nursing Concepts*
Harmer Nursing is rooted in the needs of humanity and is founded on the ideal of service. Its object is not only to cure the sick and heal the wounded but to bring health and ease, rest and comfort to mind and body, to shelter, nourish, and protect and to minister to all those who are helpless or handicapped, young, aged, or immature. Its object is to prevent disease and to preserve health. Nursing is, therefore, linked with every other social agency that strives for the prevention of disease and the preservation of health. The nurse finds herself not only concerned with the care of the individual but with the health of a people (Harmer, 1924, p. 3).	Caring is bringing rest and comfort to the mind and body, in sickness and in health.	Nurses are concerned with the health of people. Nursing is linked with other professions in *health-care delivery* that preserve health and prevent disease.
Frederick and Northam Modern nursing is by no means limited to the giving of expert physical care to the sick, important as this is. It is more far reaching, including as it does helping the patient to adjust to unalterable situations, such as personal, family, and economic conditions; teaching him and others in the home and in the community to care for themselves; guiding him in the prevention of illness through hygienic living; and helping him to use the available community resources to these ends (Frederick and Northam, 1938, p. 3).	Caring is helping persons adjust to unalterable situations.	Nurses *teach* persons to care for themselves.
Henderson Nursing is primarily assisting the individual (sick or well) in the performance of those activities contributing to health or its recovery (or to a peaceful death) that he would perform unaided if he had the necessary strength, will, or knowledge. It is likewise the unique contribution of nursing to help the individual to be independent of such assistance as soon as possible (Henderson, 1955, p. 4).	Caring is assisting persons in performance of activities they would accomplish unaided if they had the necessary resources.	The *person* is a unique individual. Nursing as a *profession* makes a unique contribution to society.

Definition	Thoughts on Caring	Related Nursing Concepts
Rogers		
Nursing aims to assist people in achieving their maximum health potential. Maintenance and promotion of health, prevention of disease, nursing diagnosis, intervention, and rehabilitation encompass the scope of nursing's goals (Rogers, 1970, p. 19).	Caring is assisting persons to achieve their maximum health potential.	Nursing activities involve diagnosis, intervention, and rehabilitation *(nursing process).*
Levine		
The nurse participates actively in every patient's environment, and much of what she does supports his adaptations as he struggles in the predicament of illness. Nursing intervention means that the nurse interposes her skill and knowledge into the course of events, which affects the patient. Thus, nursing intervention must be founded not only on scientific knowledge but specifically on recognition of the individual's organismic response, which indicates the nature of the adaptation taking place (Levine, 1973, p. 13).	Caring is using nursing knowledge and skill to support persons' adaptations.	Nursing care supports or maintains persons' *adaptations.*
Nursing is a human interaction. It is a discipline rooted in the organic dependency of the individual human being on his relationships with other human beings. An "interaction" by its very nature presupposes a system of exchange between individuals; it can occur only if communication can occur (p. 1).		*Communication* is essential to nursing, since nursing is an interpersonal process.
Mitchell		
Nursing is a means to help people whose actual or potential deviations from health have impaired their ability to cope with some aspects of daily living. Nursing care may be aimed at preventing the initial or further deviations from health, at restoring or enhancing the ability to cope with daily activity, and at maintaining or sustaining the person's capacities through a health problem (Michell, 1973, p. vii).	Caring is helping persons with their actual or potential deviations from health.	Nurses assist persons who have difficulty coping with some aspect of daily living (*i.e., adaptation*).

for or helping persons with their health needs. Each of the concepts in the text is also addressed in these definitions. Since nursing is a profession that is experiencing growth of its own, we feel there is no single definition of nursing. You might develop a new definition of your own while reading this text. Whatever your definition, we hope that the element of caring for or nurturing persons is the goal that directs your nursing efforts.

None of these thoughts is new. Nurses have always valued the idea of caring for persons; this is what attracts many nurses to the profession. Unfortunately nurses sometimes lose sight of this goal in the reality of practice. For example, as a beginning student you may find at times that you are so concerned about your own nursing skills that you forget that the person for whom you are caring may have anxieties. Even experienced nurses may become so overwhelmed by the complex technology involved in nursing care or by institutional demands that they lose sight of the person who is the object of their activities. Nursing texts frequently focus on concepts or techniques without considering how they will relate to the persons who will benefit from them. For this reason, this text uses the term "person-centered nursing" as a reminder that caring for persons is the organizing focus for all aspects of nursing. Each of the concepts in the text is presented within this context. We have attempted to emphasize the person in each of our discussions, whether this means the nurse or the client.

Elements of Person-Centered Care

What is person-centered care? Carl Rogers provides us with many thoughts that can be applied to nursing. Rogers is a psychotherapist who challenges the manner in which traditional psychology is concerned with human behavior, particularly behavior that is considered abnormal. Rogers feels that rather than emphasizing what is wrong with a person, psychotherapists would do better to concentrate on strengths, in order to facilitate personal growth toward one's highest potential. He feels that all persons are in the process of "becoming" (*i.e.,* moving toward their potential) rather than representing finished products. He also believes that persons move in a basically positive direction toward growth. Related to this belief is an appreciation of the value or worth of each person. Rogers stresses that facilitating optimal growth requires a strong interpersonal relationship between the therapist and client. Through his experiences in psychotherapy he came to believe "that it is the *client* who knows what hurts, what directions to go, what problems are crucial, what experiences have been deeply buried. It began to occur to me that ... I would do better to rely upon the client for the direction of movement in the process." Thus, his "client-centered" approach to psychotherapy began.

Some attributes of the therapist's use of a client-centered approach include the following (Rogers 1961, pp. 11–55):

- Trustworthiness
- Ability to communicate unambiguously (verbal behavior matches nonverbal behavior)
- A positive attitude toward the client built on a respect for his worth
- Ability to convey empathic understanding
- Acceptance of the client's feelings
- Ability to remain separate from the client (avoiding sympathy)
- Ability to allow the client to remain a separate person (avoiding taking over for the client)
- Acceptance of the client as a person in the process of becoming rather than as a fixed product or psychiatric diagnosis

Abraham Maslow, a psychologist who shares this humanistic view of persons, defined categories of basic needs ranging from the most fundamental (food, oxygen, shelter) to the highest level (self-actualization or the desire for self-fulfillment). His approach is also person-centered since it focuses on assisting people to meet basic needs, thereby freeing them to grow and achieve their potential (1970).

Attributes of the Person-Centered Nurse

Many of the beliefs about nursing presented in this text evolved from Rogers's and Maslow's philosophies. Since nursing is an interpersonal process, much of their work is applicable to our profession. We believe that nurses who give person-centered care will act as follows:

- Appreciate that each person is a unique product of heredity, environment, and culture. This means that we must interact with our clients on an individual basis even though their health-care needs may appear to be similar.
- Believe that persons strive for their highest potential. Nursing's function is to assist persons to achieve growth in relation to their health needs.

- Respect the worth of each individual. We appreciate each person's potential no matter how impoverished or ill he appears to be. We recognize that even the sickest or poorest of people have strengths that can be mobilized to meet their needs and achieve their potential.

- Recognize one's own humanity. Nurses are persons, too, with unique strengths and needs. To care effectively for others, nurses must have self-awareness in order to recognize what they can offer another and what their own personal limitations are.

- Be genuine. Rogers uses the term *congruence* to describe a condition in which a person is "without 'front' or facade; that ... feelings ... are available to his awareness and he is able to communicate them if appropriate." A nurse cannot be truly genuine without the self-awareness just described. Rogers feels that congruence is essential to an effective helping relationship (p. 61).

- Allow control to remain with the client. Nurses who are truly genuine as well as comfortable with and aware of their own feelings will be able to let clients be themselves. These nurses will not need to feel authority over their clients; rather they will view clients as partners in the helping relationship. They will see the process of nursing as facilitating clients to meet their

own needs. They will feel comfortable allowing the clients to express their needs freely and set their own goals for nursing care.

- Recognize that persons have basic needs and are motivated to fulfill these needs. For this reason a person's behavior is the result of his needs. This is an important idea, for it implies that each person's behavior has meaning, no matter how different or "wrong" this behavior may appear.

- Since all behavior has meaning, nurses should appreciate that a person's actions communicate messages about his feelings, beliefs, or physical functioning. The nurse should respect the meaning of a person's behavior and avoid such labels as "wrong," "bad," or "weird," even though the behavioral manifestations may be perplexing or difficult to deal with.

These attributes (Table 1-3) are important for nurses practicing in any setting, whether it be the hospital, the client's home, or a community agency. Person-centered care can be given to any age group from infancy through old age, from birth through death (Fig. 1-2). This kind of caring is nursing's unique contribution to the health professions.

Figure 1-2
Person-centered care is given in any setting and to people of any age. (*University of Michigan School of Nursing*)

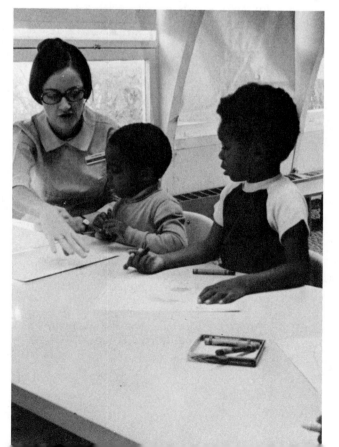

Table 1-3
Attributes of a Person-Centered Nurse

- Appreciates that each person is a unique product of heredity, environment, and culture
- Believes that each person strives for his or her highest potential
- Respects the worth of each individual
- Behaves in a genuine manner
- Enables control to remain with the person
- Recognizes that each person has basic needs and is motivated to fulfill these needs
- Appreciates that each person's behavior communicates information about his feelings, beliefs, and physical and mental state.

The Person as a Recipient of Care

Patient versus Client

You will note that throughout this book the word "person" is used when referring to anyone for whom nursing care is provided. On occasion the word "client" may also be used and, even more rarely, "patient." There are some very important distinctions to be made among these words, as indicated by their definitions.

The "Patient"

The dictionary defines a **patient** (noun) as "an individual awaiting or under medical care and treatment; the recipient of any of various person services." We are also informed that to be **patient** (adjective) is to "bear pains or trials calmly and without complaint; to be steadfast despite opposition, or adversity; to be able or willing to bear."

Looking at the definition of patient may help us realize that while a person receiving health care and treatment may not behave in the manner described, that description represents what we, as health-care providers, often expect. We wish for our patients to be cooperative, to behave themselves, to do as they are told, and generally to provide us with little trouble in this cumbersome business of getting them well. As you progress through the book, you may recognize that health-care providers become distressed when their patients do not behave patiently. It is with this idea in mind that the authors have attempted to underscore the notion that the person receiving care is more healthy than ill and more capable of strength than weakness. Persons who seek health care remain unique human beings who, although sharing some characteristics with other persons, nonetheless have their own individual thoughts, feelings, and ways of responding. That some people may be patient during an illness is more a characteristic of their individual personalities than their role as ill persons.

P. D. James, in her novel *The Black Tower*, describes this point quite clearly (1975, pp. 9–10). The scene is a patient's hospital bedside. The people present are the patient himself, a consultant physician, a nurse, and several medical students. The physician is speaking:

> "We've had the most recent path. report and I think we can be certain now that we've got it right . . . It isn't acute leukemia, it isn't any type

of leukemia. What you're recovering from—happily—is an atypical mononucleosis. I congratulate you, Commander. You had us worried."

> "I had you interested; you had me worried. When can I leave here?" The great man laughed and smiled at his retinue, inviting them to share his indulgence at yet one more example of the ingratitude of convalescence.

Although this attitude is expressed by a physician, it should be recognized that nurses are capable of similar responses to persons seeking their help. This example provides us with several interesting insights. We note that the patient is called Commander, indicating that he has some level of personal achievement. We can assume that he is intelligent, probably educated, and has been given a great deal of responsibility in some organization or other. Even if we did not have the name "Commander" to give us an idea of the character, we could see his individuality clearly in the response he gives. The last statement points out that the provider of services, in this case, the physician, does not think his patient is behaving very well.

The "Client"

At this point we should examine the word "client." The dictionary defines a **client** as "a person who engages the professional advice or services of another; a person served by or utilizing the services of an agency."

A client is a person who has contracted for services from another who is qualified to provide those services. There is an assumption that this kind of relationship is a negotiated partnership and that the client is capable of taking the information provided and utilizing it in some fashion or other. Should he decide that it is not useful, he generally feels free to take his business and go elsewhere. Although some people approach health care with the same sense of independence, most simply do what they are told, including going into the hospital when so directed. They may feel incapable of physically "taking their business and moving elsewhere." The fact that we, as health-care providers, are well aware of this passive type of response is reflected in the name we have so frequently given these people, "patients," and the way in which we have often assumed control over so many facets of their lives.

As beginning students of nursing, you may not be aware that this inequitable relationship often exists between a person and the provider of health services. We suggest that you accept a challenge to note this inequality as you go out into the world of health-care delivery. You are challenged, moreover, to look first at yourselves to become aware of the degree to which you share these attitudes, many of which are rooted in our history as a people and in our cultural value systems. Indeed, the receiver of health-care services may be as likely to expect (and even want) control from the provider as the provider is likely to exert it.

It is the belief of the authors of this book, however, that if nurses are to provide care that encourages each person to grow, then we must view those who seek our services as primarily unique beings. We must appreciate their worth, recognize their strengths, and offer a caring relationship in which they may truly be partners in this growth process.

Concepts Basic to Person-Centered Care

As noted earlier, this text identifies seven concepts that are essential to person-centered nursing. They are: the person, health and adaptation, health care, professionalism, communication, nursing process, and learning and teaching. The concepts have been identified not only by the authors but by nursing theorists as well. Elements of most of these concepts can be found in the definitions of nursing presented in Table 1-2. Nurses who truly give person-centered care use these concepts in a unique way. Their goal is always to facilitate growth in their clients.

Person

Since persons are the ultimate focus of nursing care, professional nurses need to be "person experts." Persons are composed of biological, psychological, social, and spiritual subsystems, each interacting with the others. Thus, nurses not only need to be knowledgeable in areas such as biochemistry, physiology, psychology, and sociology, they also need an awareness of how physical and psychosocial aspects interact. For instance, anxiety may be expressed by stomach pain; refusal to interact with others may be a culturally learned expression of the physical sensation of pain. A nurse who gives person-centered care will attempt to discover the meaning behind any such behavior and will assist the person to meet the basic need (*i.e.,* pain relief) that this behavior represents.

Nurses must not only have knowledge of a person's basic needs but they must also be aware of how differently individuals express their needs. This may be as simple as asking a diabetic client what unique symptoms he experiences when his blood glucose level falls below normal. Or it may be as complex as assisting a mother who views food as an expression of her nurturing to work with a diet for her overweight child.

Health and Adaptation

In nursing we are concerned with persons' health. Health represents optimal biological, psychological, and social functioning. The concepts of health and adaptation are closely related. Adaptation is the process of changing in response to the environment; successful adaptation leads to health and growth. For instance, when we feel the sensation of thirst we adapt by drinking. Were we to ignore this stimulus, we would soon die of dehydration. Since the environment is constantly changing we are all in a continuous process of adaptation. By our constant adaptations, we move toward attaining our potential; that is, we continue to grow as individuals. The goal of person-centered nursing is to assist individuals to adapt to changes in their environments. Through our nursing care, we hope to promote optimal functioning and growth (biological and psychosocial) for each person.

Health Care

Nurses do not practice their profession in a void; rather, we are members of complex health-care delivery systems. Our current systems for delivering health care in the United States are diverse and complicated, involving many settings and professionals. Frequently, the health care delivered results from poor coordination between settings and providers. In many instances, the health-care system functions to meet its own needs at the expense of the consumer. Since nurses contribute an essential service to the health-care system, we need to be aware of its complexities and its current problems.

Person-centered nurses recognize the needs of clients who are the consumers of health care and act as their advocates. This may mean helping clients make informed choices about health care, assisting them through the maze of the health-care system itself, and ensuring that the client's rights are respected.

Nurses face another problem within our current system. Much effort continues to be directed toward illness care rather than health care (*i.e.,* health promotion and maintenance). If nursing's goal is the promotion of personal growth through optimal biopsychosocial adaptation, we are in potential conflict with the goals of most health-care systems. Today we need caring nurses who are concerned about wellness and who are willing to work on influencing health-care delivery so that it meets the *health* needs of consumers.

Professionalism

Professionalism is the concern and activity of practitioners on behalf of their chosen profession. Nursing considers itself a profession whose purpose is assisting persons to achieve optimal biopsychosocial health or adaptation. In order to achieve this goal, nurses must recognize their own "personhood," that is, they must be aware of their own feelings, values, beliefs, strengths, and weaknesses. As nurse persons, we must be responsible for facilitating our own personal growth and that of our profession, if we are to achieve our goal of nurturing growth in others. To attain this end, we must commit ourselves to professional involvement and lifelong learning. Professional involvement is not only appropriate but also mandatory if nursing is to remain an acknowledged profession. Only nurses know how nursing ought to grow and develop; we cannot leave this decision to others. Students are asked from the start to assume responsibility for nurturing their profession as well as their clients. Nurses must also appreciate that learning does not end with a degree. As professional persons we are maximizing not only our clients' potential but our own as well. You must care well for your profession; who else will be concerned about nursing if nurses are not?

Communication

Communication is the complex process in which meanings are exchanged between or among persons. Because interaction between persons is the heart of nursing, nurses need a sound knowledge of the principles of communication. Communication assists nurses to build trusting relationships between themselves and their clients (Fig. 1-3). Listening to our clients is often a way of showing we care. Communication is also used to assist persons to adapt to stressors, whether these affect physical, psychological, or social functioning. Nurses who deliver person-centered care value the rights of others to control their own health. Therapeutic communication is one way to achieve this end. For instance, a nurse might use this skill to help a client

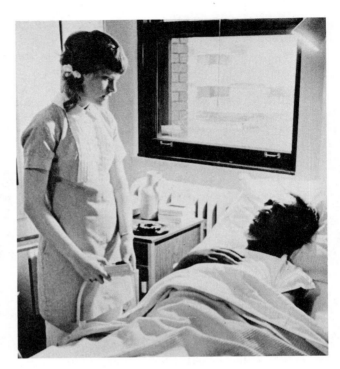

Figure 1-3
Communication is the heart of nursing and assists in building trusting relationships.

reduce anxiety about a heart problem and concentrate on learning about diet as one facet of self-care. Nurses who believe that persons have inherent ability to achieve optimal health will value communication as a skill that assists their clients to attain this goal.

Nursing Process

Nursing process may be a mysterious term to beginning students, yet it is nothing more than the problem-solving process by which nurses meet a person's needs. It has its roots in the scientific method with which you are already familiar. You probably remember science projects in which you first used the scientific method. You began to study a problem by finding out all you could about its nature, proposing possible solutions, then trying out one or more solutions to see if these were successful. Nursing process is quite similar, but the problems we deal with are persons' health-care needs. We work with our clients to identify all we can about their needs, we devise possible solutions with them, and then we assist them to try out approaches to meeting their needs. Nursing process is our professional method of assisting persons to achieve their highest level of functioning.

Nurses who give person-centered care view nursing process as a tool to help meet a client's needs. At the same time, it is important to identify a client's strengths as well as his needs, for we draw upon strengths to assist each person to regain health. Nursing process, by focusing on the person who needs care, enables that person to express his own perceptions of his needs and determine his own goals for health care to the level of his ability.

Since nurses care for persons (rather than working with scientific problems), we must work *with* our clients rather than do nursing activities *to* them. Caring nurses are less concerned with what clients should or ought to do than with supporting them to attain their goals. By providing the framework for respecting our clients' health and strengths and their worth and individuality, the nursing process becomes not only our professional method but truly a caring process as well.

Learning and Teaching

Learning can be defined as a change in behavior in response to a stimulus. Nurses use their teaching skills to assist persons who have learning needs related to their health. Person-centered care recognizes that teaching is significant only insofar as it facilitates learning for clients. This is important, for persons only learn that which they perceive as having meaning for themselves, no matter how earnestly the nurse teaches them.

Nurses who give person-focused care are concerned with the concept of learning, because many clients need new skills or knowledge in order to adapt to their health needs. Teaching is valued as a nursing activity since it assists persons to achieve control over their health and enables them to take better care of themselves. Since person-centered nurses recognize that each client is unique, they vary their teaching approaches to meet individual learners' needs.

Conclusion

You may now be feeling overwhelmed by all the concepts presented here. You are probably wondering how you could ever put all of this into practice. The best example of person-centered nursing that we can present comes from a beginning nursing student. She describes her relationship with a client whom she has been visiting for 12 weeks. This client is an elderly woman who has severely impaired vision due to cataracts. The student has been working with this woman in her home.

Example ☐ I began by developing a trusting relationship with E.B. I worked to maintain an open atmosphere and encouraged E.B. to discuss her visual impairment and the problems that had arisen due to her condition. This led to a significant exchange, by both parties, of personal feelings and opinions concerning E.B.'s problem. A trusting and open relationship such as this helped E.B. to air out any ill feelings of confusion, dismay, loneliness, or good feelings of happiness, contentment, and relief to a person who could lend support and understanding.

In the course of our relationship, E.B. revealed many of her strengths to me. It is these strengths that I picked out and reinforced to help her adapt. I accomplished this by making E.B. aware of her many positive attributes. I let her know how I admired her ability to learn to do such things as cooking, crossing streets, and becoming involved in outside activities in a different way than she had before.

From the very beginning, E.B. revealed a self-esteem need. Self-esteem is extremely important to adaptation. Self-esteem provides motivation to change, makes a person feel worthwhile, gives them a reason to be. Therefore, I found it extremely important to incorporate an intervention to satisfy E.B.'s self-esteem need. I allowed E.B. to give me advice and use her "nurturing" qualities to help me in any way she could. In this way, E.B. could feel that she was needed, accomplishing something worthwhile. Secondly, I let E.B. know the "helping" relationship was mutual. For even though I was assigned to her as the Student Nurse to spend time with her and help her in any way, I made it clear that I got just as much help out of the relationship by talking with her and learning from her. In addition, I periodically spoke highly of E.B., for example, gave her a compliment or a pat on the back, and encouraged a positive response from her. In this way, I could bring out in the open E.B.'s many good traits and reinforce them in an attempt to make E.B. feel more important and valuable. Finally, I was a good listener and let E.B. know that I was interested in her and what she had to say. I did all of these things in an attempt to boost E.B.'s morale and to make her feel better about herself as a whole.

Finally, I set goals with E.B. leading to change and optimal adaptation. I encouraged E.B. to do new things, such as exercising with barbells, taking walks in front of her house, and listening to tapes specially made to entertain the visually impaired. I also determined the degree of independency E.B. would like to be functioning at, and encouraged her to attain it. At the present, E.B. is adapting and is working to become adapted. By setting goals, E.B. has something to strive for, to work harder for, to live for. Such a healthy attitude can only promote adaptation to its fullest.* ☐

* O'Shea K: *Adaptation to visual impairment.* Unpublished manuscript, 1980

As you read this example, you can probably identify many of the components of care presented in this chapter. You will notice that the student nurse was able to identify many strengths in her client even though this woman had impaired vision, which created many problems for her. You can identify how the student used most of the seven basic concepts presented in this text, such as adaptation, communication, nursing process, and learning and teaching. We hope that this example will serve as an inspiration and a challenge to you, for as caring nurse persons you all have the potential to practice nursing in this manner. As you read through the text we encourage you to read this student's work again for it shows how you can "put it all together" to give person-centered nursing care to each of your clients.

Study Questions

1. What is your own definition of nursing? Are there common elements between your definitions and those in Table 1-3?

2. How do you define "caring for persons?" Think of a nurse you know who exemplifies this definition. What attributes does he or she have?

3. How can you incorporate Roger's philosophy of client-centered therapy into your nursing care?

4. Consider any of your family members who have received health care. Were they treated as "clients?" As "patients?" As "persons?"

Glossary

Client: a person who engages the professional advice or services of another; a person served by or utilizing the services of an agency; a person who has contracted for services from another who is qualified to provide those services.

Patient: (noun) An individual awaiting or under medical care and treatment; the recipient of any of various person services.

Patient: (adjective) To bear pains or trials calmly and without complaint; to be steadfast despite opposition or adversity; to be able or willing to bear.

Person: A unique human being who has some characteristics in common with others as well as his own individual thoughts, feelings, and ways of responding.

Bibliography

Ashley JA: Nurses in American history: Nursing and early feminism. Am J Nurs 75:1465–1467, Sept 1975

Binger JL, Jensen LM: Lippincott's Guide to Nursing Literature. Philadelphia, JB Lippincott, 1980

Bullough V, Bullough B: The Care of the Sick: The Emergence of Modern Nursing. New York, Prodist, 1978

Chaska, NL (ed): The Nursing Profession: Views Through the Mist. New York, McGraw-Hill, 1978

Ehrenreich B, English D: Witches, Midwives, and Nurses: A History of Women Healers, 2nd ed. Old Westbury, New York, Feminist Press, 1973

Ellis JR, Hartley CL: Nursing in Today's World: Challenges, Issues, and Trends. Philadelphia, JB Lippincott, 1980

Frederick HK, Northam A: A Textbook of Nursing Practice 2nd ed. New York, Macmillan, 1938

Harmer B: Textbook of the Principles and Practice of Nursing. New York, Macmillan, 1924

Harmer B (revised by Henderson V): Textbook of Principles and Practice of Nursing, 5th ed. New York, Macmillan, 1955

James PD: The Black Tower. New York, Scribner, 1975

Kalisch B, Kalisch P: The Advance of American Nursing. Boston, Little, Brown & Co, 1978

Kelly LY: Dimensions of Professional Nursing, 4th ed. New York, Macmillan, 1981

Levine M: Introduction to Clinical Nursing 2nd ed. Philadelphia, FA Davis, 1973

Maslow A: Motivation and Personality, 2nd ed. New York, Harper & Row, 1970

Mayeroff M: On Caring. New York, Harper & Row, 1971

Mitchell P: Concepts Basic to Nursing. New York, McGraw-Hill, 1973

Nightingale F: Notes on Nursing: What It Is and What It Is Not, 1st ed. London, Harrison, 1860. Facsimile edition New York, Appleton-Century Company, 1938

Palmer I: Florence Nightingale: Reformer, reactionary, researcher. Nurs Res 26:84–89, Mar–Apr, 1977

Rogers C: On Becoming a Person. Boston, Houghton Mifflin, 1961

Rogers M: An Introduction to the Theoretical Basis of Nursing. Philadelphia, FA Davis, 1970

Schein EH, Kommers DW: Professional Education. New York, McGraw-Hill, 1972

Simms LM, Lindberg JB: The Nurse Person: Developing Perspectives for Contemporary Nursing. New York, Harper & Row, 1978

The Person

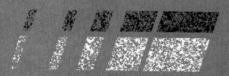

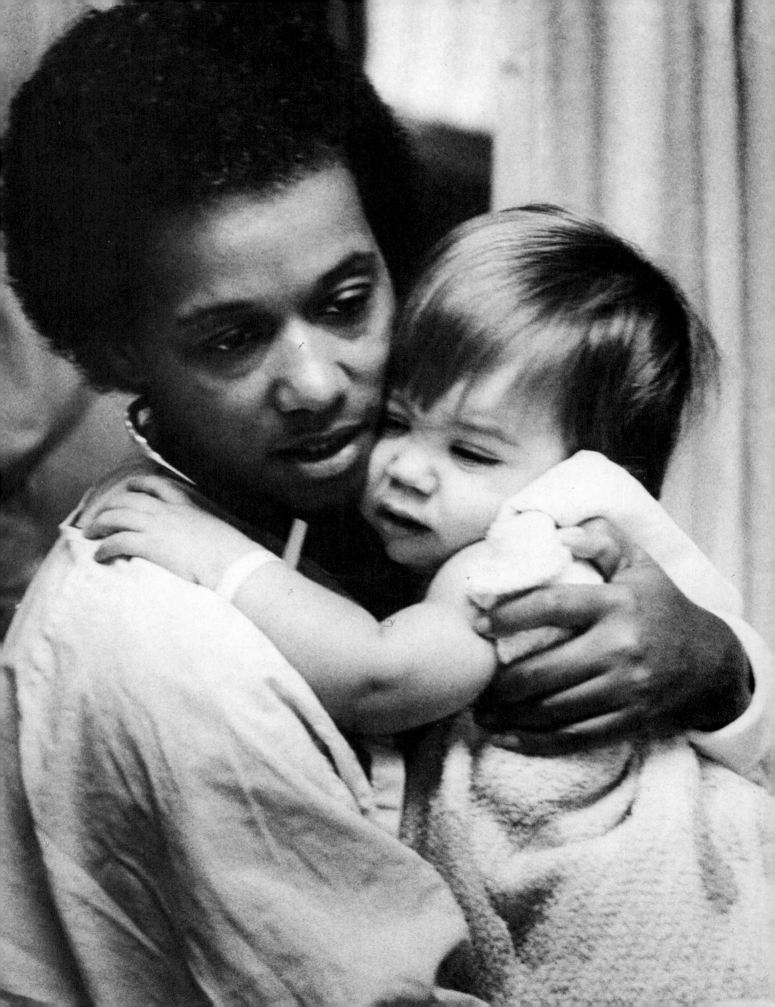

I

The Person

(Photo by Bob Kalmbach; University of Michigan Information Services)

The section called "The Person" is presented first in this book, to emphasize that the person is the center of health and nursing care. Although this might seem a statement of the obvious, students will not be involved long in health-care delivery before realizing that person-centered care is not frequently provided. Health-care agencies and providers become involved with their own policies and needs, forgetting their purpose for being. We hope that our discussion, which presents exciting components of the person, will set a tone for your entire career in nursing.

This section describes persons as holistic beings who, while sharing characteristics with all other persons, nonetheless are unique. For example, all persons interact and exchange energy with the environment, and yet each has his own unique response to that environment. All persons have basic needs, but the ways in which these needs are expressed and satisfied may vary greatly from one person to another. All persons proceed through phases of growth and development, and yet the rate at which they progress and the extent to which they succeed is a very individual matter.

Persons have strengths and knowledge that enable them to take care of themselves and accept the help of a care giver when needed. As nurses, we can help persons use these individual strengths to continue on a course of growth and self-actualization, no matter how great their needs are. We can help persons recognize the control they have in achieving their potential. If we learn truly to value the uniqueness of each person and provide person-centered care, we will achieve a difference in the health, not only of individuals, but also of many groups of people across this nation.

The Holistic Person

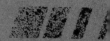

Mary L. Hunter

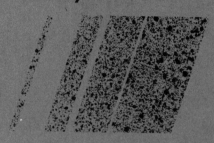

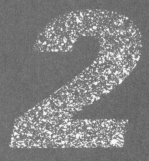

Each person is a unique and complex human being consisting of biological, psychological, and sociological components. These components include many unique characteristics and many characteristics held in common with other persons. As an open system, the person is in constant interaction with both his internal and external environments. Inherent in this interaction is a unifying element, called the spirit. This component is not necessarily religious in nature, although some may view it as such. Rather, it is the inspiring or animating principle that pervades thought, feeling, and action. As nurses, we view the person as a complete, holistic being who is greater than the sum of his individual parts, with a spirit that makes him unique from his fellow creatures.

The Person as a System

Holism

The words holistic and **holism** are derived from the Greek word meaning whole. Holism is basically a theory that the universe, and especially living nature, is seen in terms of interacting wholes that are more than the mere sum of their parts. Smuts has indicated that holism is a theory that describes the parts of a person as dependent upon each other and coordinated in a systematic fashion (1926). According to this theory, if we study one part of a person we must also consider how that part interrelates with all other parts of the person. As we learn to appreciate the total of the parts as a whole, we begin to understand why any part functions as it does. The interrelationships also contribute to making the whole greater than the sum of its parts. This further increases the complexity of each of us as unique individuals. Figure 2-1 is a typical representation of the holistic person.

General Systems Theory

A discussion of general systems theory might be helpful at this point. We have already stated that man is an open system. Let us first consider the meaning of **system.** Abbey describes a system as an "organized unit with a set of components that mutually react. The system acts as a whole; the dysfunction of a part causes a system disturbance rather than the loss of a single function" (1978, pp. 20–21). Looking around us we can find systems everywhere. A car, for example, is a mechanical system with many parts, all of which must function with reasonable precision for the car to move. In biology, a plant is a living system with interacting parts consisting of its leaves, stems, and roots, as well as many smaller structures. All of these parts function together to promote life and growth. These two systems—car and plant—have definite boundaries that are readily apparent.

Other systems within our social structure have boundaries that are less apparent. The public-school system, as a social system, might exemplify this idea. Certainly each individual school has visible boundaries in the form of its building, teachers, students, books, media, and desks. However, each school district has its own school board, and the states have certain kinds of legislation relating to their own school systems. Financial support comes from a

Figure 2-1
A model of the components of the holistic person.

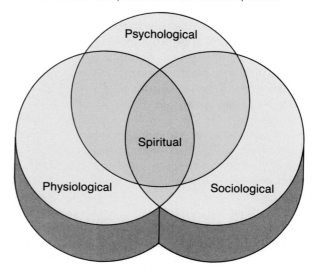

21

variety of sources. Philosophies of education, which may vary considerably across the nation, permeate each component of the system. With such a large and unwieldly system, it is often difficult to grasp how one component interrelates with another. If we imagine each individual school and its parts as a system, then the functioning of the larger system becomes more understandable. We can now say that the public-school system is made up of thousands of smaller systems. We can also call the smaller systems *subsystems*. A subsystem has the same characteristics as a system but is considered a part of the larger system as well.

General systems theory is a formalized means of describing the interplay of many systems. The idea of general systems theory was proposed by Ludwig von Bertalanffy in the 1950s. He wrote, "General systems theory then consists of the scientific exploration of 'wholes and wholeness' ... the interdisciplinary nature of concepts, models, and principles applying to 'systems' provides a possible approach toward the unification of science" (1968, p. 30). Klir suggested the following definition, "General Systems Theory in the broadest sense refers to a collection of general concepts, principles, tools, problems, methods, and techniques associated with systems" (1972, p. 1). Ashby states, "Systems Theory is essentially a demand that we treat systems as wholes composed of related parts, between which interaction occurs to a major degree" (1972, p. 95).

Open and Closed Systems

There are essentially two types of systems: open systems and closed systems. The distinguishing difference is the extent to which a system can exchange matter, energy, and information with its environment. The environment of the system has been defined by Hall and Fagan as all factors that affect the system and also all factors that are affected by the system (1968). The system that can exchange matter, energy, and information with its environment is termed an **open system;** one that cannot is termed a **closed system.** Because nearly all systems contain many subsystems, it is possible to have an open system that contains several closed subsystems. Systems that are essentially open include living, social, behavioral, and environmental systems. All of these contain closed subsystems.

Persons are examples of open systems. As persons, we constantly exchange matter, energy, and information with our environment. We hear, see, and process information that is given us, and then disseminate information to others. We respond to the weather by changing clothes to adapt to it. We absorb energy from the sun, from food, and from other sources. As living systems, we are capable of self-regulation and growth.

Chemical reactions are examples of closed systems. Some compounds, when dissolved in water, dissociate reversibly to produce negatively charged ions (anions) and hydrogen ions, for example:

$$\text{Lactic acid} \longleftrightarrow H^+ + \text{lactate}$$
$$\text{Carbonic acid} \longleftrightarrow H^+ + \text{bicarbonate}$$

These systems will remain the same forever and be unaffected by their environments unless new variables are added. Persons have closed systems within them; for instance, the chemical reaction above occurs continuously within the body and helps to maintain a stable internal environment. Another example of a closed system is the withdrawal reflex that protects a person from painful stimuli.

Systems Theory Applied to the Person

Man contains many systems and subsystems that interrelate in an integrated fashion to become one total system. We have already mentioned the biological, psychological, social, and spiritual components that constitute this interaction. Each of these could be considered a system having subsystems. For instance, the biological system contains subsystems such as the neurological, circulatory, and gastrointestinal systems, to name a few. The neurological system in turn consists of the brain, the spinal cord, and the peripheral nerves throughout the body. Each of these parts is a subsystem in itself. The circulatory system consists of the heart and the blood vessels. The two systems interrelate as the brain sends messages to the heart that signal it to pump. The heart, however, must pump in order to keep the brain functioning so that it can send those signals.

The psychological system contains subsystems that include thinking and feeling. Our feeling states also affect the autonomic nervous system, which signals the heart to beat faster or slower.

It was mentioned earlier that systems were open when they exchange energy with other systems. Consider the systems of the person and the constant exchange of energy that occurs among these internal systems as well as with the outside environment.

Each system contains many **variables.** Wandelt defined a variable as "... a measurable or potentially measurable component of an object or event that may fluctuate in quantity or quality, or that may be different in quantity or quality from one individual object or event to another object or event of the same general class" (1970, p. 101). Systems and variables are both components of a large whole. In many instances, both terms apply to the same object or event. Table 2-1 lists some of the variables that are part of the complex biopsychosocial system called the person.

It is important to note that many of these variables, while primarily associated with the above classification, may also fall under another heading in certain circumstances. The concept of role, for example, is generally thought of as sociological. However, there are many psychological components to this notion, and some might consider it as classified with those variables.

Exchanges of Energy Among the Subsystems of a Person

Systems have a certain amount of energy that can be exchanged within the subsystems and with the environment. If the person, a being greater than the whole of his combined parts, uses coping mecha-

nisms that help achieve a successful growth and development throughout his life, then each subsystem will retain its maximum potential health. However, if one component, such as the psychological subsystem, becomes stressed, the person may be unable to cope effectively. At that point energy may be drawn from another subsystem, which in turn may become less healthy.

In order to apply this idea to everyday situations, let us look at two kinds of examples: one that represents a temporary breakdown in a system, and another that reflects more far-reaching implications for one person and those around her.

A bad cold is perhaps a good example of a temporary problem, but one that affects the person severely, even for a short period of time. One nursing student described her situation this way:

Example 1 ☐ "The day I was to have two exams I woke up with a cold. I hadn't had enough sleep as it was and now I felt chilled and achy all over, as well as tired. By the time I went to breakfast I was blowing my nose constantly and everything tasted like paper.

Table 2-1
Selected Variables of the Person

Biological	Psychological	Sociological	Spiritual
Age	Attitudes	Basic needs	Beliefs
Genetic structure	Basic needs	Culture	Philosophy of life
Sex	Body image	Family	Religion
Race	Communication	Group membership	Values
Biological rhythms	Coping mechanisms	Language	
Basic needs	Defense mechanisms	Life-style	
Growth	Feeling states	Relationships with others	
Acid–base balance	Level of developmental task resolution	Roles	
Circulation	Perception	Role prescriptions	
Digestion	Self-concept	School systems	
Electrolyte balance	Values		
Immune response	Cognition		
Mobility	Consciousness		
Reproduction	Knowledge		
Respiration	Memory		
Temperature regulation	Thought process		
Physical health			
Past illnesses			

I took my exams and decided I had done poorly on both. My head was all stuffed up and I could hardly think. By the time I got back to the dorm my nose was raw from blowing and I was really feeling sorry for myself. I tried calling some friends but no one was home. I felt like crying but could hardly breathe as it was.

I lay around indulging in self-pity. I felt rotten, I seemed to be failing everything and no one even cared! I finally fell asleep and slept right through till the next morning! When I awoke my cold wasn't gone, but I was rested and felt much better. Remembering my thoughts of the day before, I had to be amused. How had I gotten into such a state?'' □

This example demonstrates the many physical effects that a "simple cold" can have. Although it most specifically affects the upper part of the respiratory system, it also affects how we eat and sleep; it affects our sense of heat and cold, our muscles, and the skin on our nose. When our physical system is so weakened, we begin to extract energy from our psychological system. That too, however, becomes stressed, as in our example, with having to take exams, and with being unable to find someone to show a little concern. So much energy is used trying to cope with the physical effects and then with the psychological stress that we begin to feel exhausted and finally helpless. It is possible, also, that the stress of two exams really began the chain of events in the first place. Undoubtedly, the exams contributed to the inadequate sleep that the student mentions early in her description.

When a person is generally healthy and happy and the physical problem is transitory, natural recuperative powers can work quickly after some rest. Consider, however, the person who has engaged in a lifetime of ineffective coping behavior and then has one component or subsystem severely stressed. How might this person respond? Consider the following example.

Example 2 □ Mrs. Thomas described her health history as one long series of problems. The trouble began with the development of diabetes during her third pregnancy. It continued over the years with several surgeries, decreasing vision, aggravating skin disruptions, obesity, hypertension, and a chronic heart condition that was likely to require surgery.

Severely uncontrolled diabetes was always present. She recalled also that the pregnancy that occurred at the time of the onset of diabetes was unrecognized by her until a doctor diagnosed her "trouble" as pregnancy in the fifth month. Both the onset of diabetes and the pregnancy occurred close in time to the death of her younger brother in an automobile accident. At the same time that she was

trying to help her parents cope with their grief over the death of their son, she herself became ill.

For the next 10 years her health was interrupted by episodes of illness and difficulty in controlling the diabetes. However, she was not seriously ill nor incapacitated until the death of her own son in an automobile accident. She stated, "My blood sugar went way up (900 mg%) and I had to go to the hospital. It stayed up and I couldn't get well. I knew I wouldn't get well until I finally gave Billy up. At first I thought I could never give him up, but finally I did and then I began to get better." She did recover from that episode of illness, but the following 10 years were fraught with increasingly severe health problems. About her son's death she now has this to say: "There is nothing we can do about it, so I just don't think about it. There's no sense thinking about what you can't change."* □

This example suggests severe psychological stress with which Mrs. Thomas has attempted to cope. Although research is not conclusive enough at this point to state that the physical illness was a result of the inability to cope effectively with the psychological stress, we can certainly note the proximity of the physical problems to the time of stress. We also have Mrs. Thomas's own belief that she wouldn't get well until she gave Billy up. If this is indeed the case, then we become aware of the physical energy that was channeled into coping with the psychological problem of grief and the severe physical illnesses that followed. For further discussion of the person's response to loss, see the discussion of grief and loss in Chapter 29. The important point to consider is the effect that one component has on the person as a whole.

Basic Needs of Persons

Maslow's Hierarchy of Needs

The extensive work of Abraham Maslow on the theory of motivation and the basic needs of man has provided a framework for nursing through which we can learn to understand both ourselves as persons and the persons for whom we provide care. Maslow's basic belief was that each person wants to be the most self-actualized person he possibly can be. In

---

* Hunter ML, Swain MN, Erickson H: Physical illness and psychosocial adaptation: Nursing observations in support of the link. Manuscript submitted for publication, 1980

other words, the person wishes to reach his fullest potential and to become all he is capable of becoming.

This notion led Maslow to study how and why some persons become self-actualized and others do not. He states, "If I had had to condense the thesis of this book (*Motivation and Personality*) into a single sentence, I would have said that, in *addition* to what the psychologies of the time had to say about human nature, man also had a higher nature and that this was instinctoid, i.e., part of his essence. And if I could have had a second sentence I would have stressed the profoundly holistic nature of human nature. . . ." (1970, p. ix).

Maslow points out that if we are truly to understand persons we must consider their highest aspirations: growth, self-actualization, the striving toward health, the quest for identity and autonomy, and the yearning for excellence. He believes that the "instinctoid nature of basic needs" constitutes a system of intrinsic human values that are not only wanted and desired by all human beings but also needed, in the sense that they are necessary to avoid illness and psychopathology (p. xiii).

Figure 2-2 is a representation of the hierarchy of human needs as identified by Maslow, beginning with the basic physiological needs and progressing to the need for safety and security, the need for love and belonging, the need for self-esteem, and, finally, the need for self-actualization.

The following ideas are extracted and adapted from Maslow (1970). They may assist you to apply concepts from basic-need theory to your practice:

Figure 2-2
Maslow's hierarchy of human needs. *(From Maslow A: Motivation and Personality, pp 80–106. New York, Harper & Row, 1954)*

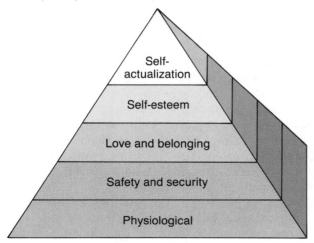

- The basic needs of a person can be regarded as rights as well as needs.
- As one group of needs is gratified, another of a higher order will appear.
- All human beings have the same needs, but the means by which they gratify those needs and the extent to which they must be gratified varies considerably among individuals.
- The gratification of needs is not an absolute state. Rather, one level of needs may be partially gratified before another group begins to appear. However, this second group of needs may be less intense due to the fact that the lower needs were not completely gratified.
- The physiological needs serve as channels for all sorts of other needs as well. The person who thinks he is hungry may actually be seeking comfort or dependence rather than nutrition.
- A conscious desire or motivated behavior may serve as a kind of channel through which other purposes may express themselves. The person who seeks sexual encounters may be searching for a way to feel a sense of belonging.
- Although a person may be quite capable of meeting his basic needs and be generally physically healthy, safe, loving, and self-actualized, stress may occur in his life and cause a reappearance of a basic need, which he will again strive to gratify.
- Needs are sometimes conscious and sometimes unconscious.
- The gratification of needs may be determined in some measure by one's cultural expression.
- There are multiple motivations for behavior and multiple determinants of behavior. Thus, to say that a person would respond in any exact manner to this hierarchy of needs would be to oversimplify human nature.

If, as nurses, we accept the premise that all human beings strive for health and excellence, then it makes sense for us to plan care accordingly. This seems a reasonable statement when we consider the many persons we encounter who certainly behave as if they are striving as suggested. However, it may not seem so reasonable when we are faced with a person in a state of helpless–hopelessness, or, even more difficult, a person whose behavior is antisocial or criminal. Let us consider the basic needs to see if they help us to understand the meaning of certain kinds of behavior.

Physiological Needs

A list of basic physiological needs might include oxygen and gas exchange, fluids, food, elimination, rest, avoidance of pain, and sexual fulfillment.

We can all remember times when we were somewhat hungry, tired, or had a slight headache and yet could continue with our usual activities. As the need became greater, however, the urgency to gratify it became stronger. Our other activities were carried out less effectively because the need began to dominate our thoughts. For most of us it is a simple matter to obtain food, to lie down, or to do whatever one normally does to cope with a headache.

Persons on strict diets, however, who feel quite hungry much of the time, report that they have such a heightened awareness to food that they notice every picture of it, smell every aroma, and generally think about it constantly. One woman reported dreaming about it much of the time. She said, "I dreamed about mountains of mashed potatoes with loads of rich gravy streaming over them. The most interesting part of all is that I really don't care much for mashed potatoes and gravy and would probably not choose them if another kind of potato were available." As food is denied to a greater and greater extent, all other wishes and desires may be lost and the quest for food will dominate totally.

If the person is extremely fatigued, the need for rest may dominate even though he has not eaten recently. Generally we respond to basic needs according to a number of variables. These may include our life-style, cultural values, general health, and that which we have come to know is attainable. It is also interesting to consider several other responses to the hunger state. For example, consider the need to create, as expressed by the artist or the poet. Sometimes these people will not take a steady paying job but will endure hunger just so they can continue to gratify their self-actualization needs. The philosopher may even have the means by which to take care of his physiological needs, but his thought processes and his work are so important that they dominate his whole being. As long as life can be sustained, these persons will give little attention to further gratification of the physiological needs.

We occasionally read about situations like the following:

☐ One nurse told of an elderly gentleman who was brought to the emergency room by concerned neighbors. He was obviously starving, was inadequately clothed for the freezing winter weather, and was apparently confused. The neighbors said that there had been no food or heat in the house and that the oil tank for fuel was empty. The nurse was horrified and immediately thought he was extremely poor. As she began to help him out of his clothes, which were filthy and stiff from urine, she noted his bulging pockets. On examining them, she found wads of money. Later, when authorities went to this man's home, they found piles of money in drawers and cannisters. ☐

What prevents such a person from using his money or from accepting the assistance of neighbors is not clear. But as we look at the next level of basic needs we may be able to hypothesize from them.

Safety and Security Needs

These needs might be listed as follows: security, stability, dependence, protection, freedom from fear, freedom from anxiety and chaos, the need for structure, order, law, limits, strength in the protector, and so forth (Maslow, 1970, p. 39).

We frequently see these needs demonstrated in small children who "test" their parents to learn whether limits will be set on their behavior. If children are allowed to throw temper tantrums, they may begin to feel very unsafe. They may feel that no one will make them stop behaving badly and thereby protect them from themselves. When safety and security needs are met in childhood, they are less likely to surface in usual daily adult life, according to Maslow. However, when a severe stress occurs, an adult may feel very unsafe. If the stress is great enough, and if safety seems severely threatened, as may have been the case with the elderly man in the emergency room, the safety needs will dominate even the physiological ones.

We see the safety of a relatively secure adult threatened when illness and hospitalization are experienced. At times, the safety need may be conscious and the person can express his fears. However, if the need is unconscious and fears are not expressed, we often see what is termed the "difficult patient." This is the person who submits to medications and treatments only with a struggle or, in some cases, actually refuses to cooperate at all. He may exhibit anger and hostility toward the nurse yet call her constantly with requests. As nurses, we might consider what factors underlie such behavior, instead of feeling threatened or exasperated ourselves. With this approach, we can more readily assist this person to cope with the stress he feels.

Maslow states that the relatively healthy adult in our society is generally able to meet his needs for safety and security, because the United States is stable and runs fairly smoothly. The affluent can buy various kinds of insurance and seek the health care they desire to feel safe. Those who are less fortunate have had some of their more urgent needs supplied through government funding. Although this assistance may be distressing for many of those persons, it nevertheless provides them with some means of security.

Love and Belonging Needs

Needs for love and belonging might include affectionate relationships; a place in the family and in other social groups; the need for a spouse, sweetheart, lover, children, friends; the need for roots in a particular neighborhood or place. Maslow clearly points out that this need includes the need to give as well as to receive love, warmth, affection, and friendship. Persons who cannot meet these needs will feel rejected, lonely, friendless, and without roots. As they feel more and more that no one cares about them, they will develop a sense of helpless–hopelessness and diminished feelings of self-esteem (p. 43).

The desire for sexual gratification should be considered for a moment. The sexual drive, mentioned earlier as a physiological need, can be considered as a purely biological need. Beyond that, sexual expression may be a channel through which love and belonging needs are met. A woman who had engaged in what she felt to be promiscuous sexual behavior after a divorce put it this way, "I did it because I kept thinking that it made me belong to someone, It wasn't true, of course, but somehow it helped for a little while."

As nurses, we often discover that as we provide care, those who respond most readily to our help and who can most easily mobilize their health resources are the ones whose love and belonging needs are being met. They have a support system of family and friends in which they feel both a sense of belonging and a sense of security.

Esteem Needs

Esteem needs include a high evaluation of the self, self-respect, self-esteem, and the esteem of others. Maslow suggests that these needs can be divided into two subsets: those related to self-esteem (desire for strength, achievement, adequacy, mastery, competence, and independence) and those related to respect and esteem from others (reputation, prestige, status, fame, glory, dominance, recognition, attention, importance, dignity, and appreciation).

Those who can meet their needs for self-esteem will face the world with confidence, feelings of self-worth, capability, adequacy, and usefulness or purpose in the scheme of things. Those whose needs are thwarted will often demonstrate helplessness, inferiority, and weakness. They will be discouraged and nonassertive, demonstrating a diminished sense of the confidence they need to face their daily activities. Maslow also points out the danger that people face if they gratify their esteem needs primarily from the opinions of others. To have the deserved respect of others is rewarding, but true esteem comes from within (pp. 45–46).

Self-Actualization Needs

The need for self-actualization essentially describes the need to reach one's fullest potential, the need to become that which one is capable of becoming, the desire for self-fulfillment (p. 46). This need will emerge when the physiological, safety, love, and esteem needs have been basically met.

Maslow describes the self-actualized person as having a variety of characteristics, some of which are spontaneity, centering on problems rather than self, enjoying solitude and privacy, autonomy (independence from culture and environment), continued fresh appreciation for the basic goods of life, creativity, and the ability to develop deep and profound interpersonal relationships. These people are not perfect, however; Maslow also describes some of their shortcomings. They can be silly, wasteful, thoughtless, boring, stubborn, and irritating. They may be somewhat vain and given to outbursts of temper (p. 175).

Other Needs

Maslow also describes two other higher levels of basic needs: The desire to know and understand, which is satisfied through the acquiring of knowledge through curiosity, learning, philosophizing, and experimenting; and the aesthetic needs, the need for beauty and specifically for beauty in one's environment.

Spiritual Needs

These last two levels of needs, added to the prior five levels, will help us understand another notion of needs, those of the spiritual aspect of the person. If we state that we are biopsychosocial–spiritual beings and we can identify basic needs that flow from the biopsychosocial spheres, it follows that there are needs associated with the spiritual sphere. Although Maslow himself does not deal directly with this issue, some authors have attempted to describe the notion. It might be suggested that spiritual needs include the following: the need to believe in a Supreme Being or in a special order for the universe, the need to believe that one has a place in that Being or order and that there is some meaning in life, and the need to feel hopeful about one's destiny.

It is not clear where on the hierarchy one should place spiritual needs. Some might consider them a higher order of need that arises after all others have been somewhat gratified. Others might suggest that they surface far sooner, indeed perhaps even earlier than some of the physiological needs defined by Maslow. We might also consider that the spiritual needs are inherent in all the other needs and therefore are not appropriately defined as a separate category. However we choose to look at this notion, we will want to be aware that most persons have a philosophy of life or a system of faith that directs their lives or serves as a refuge in times of need.

Freedom Needs

Maslow indicates that, in order to meet any of the basic needs, certain conditions must exist. He lists those conditions as a series of freedoms: freedom to speak, to do what one wishes so long as it does not harm others, to express oneself, to investigate and seek information, to defend oneself, to seek justice, to find fairness, honesty, and orderliness in the group (p. 47).

It is interesting for us, as nurses, to speculate on these freedoms as they apply to the persons for whom we provide care. For example, do these freedoms exist in a doctor's office or a hospital setting? Do we as nurses recognize these freedoms as the rights of our clients as well as the rights of persons who are not currently seeking health care? Hospitals have been compared with prisons by some authors. Whether that is a fair description need not be answered here. Rather, the student may want to consider these questions during the reading of the self-care section of this chapter, as well as of Chapter 8, Health-Care Delivery.

The following example demonstrates the basic needs in various stages of being met.

Example □ Mrs. Brown is a 78-year-old woman who lives alone in a mobile home. She has many neighbors but knows only a few and generally feels very lonely. Her daughter and grandchildren live several miles away and visit occasionally. Her daughter brings groceries every few weeks; this is helpful to Mrs. Brown because walking to the store makes her feel dizzy and weak. She would like to do her shopping with her daughter or grandchildren but her slowness aggravates them.

Mrs. Brown has diabetes and needs to manage her diet properly. Her daughter's inconsistent shopping schedule often leaves her short of the foods she needs. This worries her because she is well aware that eating improperly can affect her blood sugar. Other worries and fears she has are associated with dying alone and lying unfound for days. She believes that when she dies she would no longer be with her body but with God. However, it offends her sense of dignity and worth to imagine her body lying in a degraded state.

Mrs. Brown also feels unsafe in her environment. She lives in a mobile-home community that is quite transient. She describes loud parties, motorcycle races, and what she believes to be drug traffic. She says there have been fires and even a murder there, and she worries that because she is elderly, someone in the neighborhood might harm her, as she has sometimes read in the paper. She is often so nervous and fearful that she can neither eat nor sleep.

Although at this particular time she is feeling cast off by those who are supposed to care about her, she is able to talk fondly about happier days. She had a happy marriage before her husband died, and together they raised their own children and several others. She remembers all of them with love and pleasure. She becomes very sad and sometimes feels acute grief when she thinks about her husband and the several children who have died. At these times she is also unable to eat.

Mrs. Brown has a love of plants, animals, and needlework. She likes talking about her things and always introduces her pets to visitors. She spends hours with her plants and needlework and feels satisfaction in being able to create something beautiful. She receives the affection and companionship from her pets that she often feels is missing from her family. □

This woman demonstrates a mixture of met and unmet needs. She has many strengths: knowledge of her diet and concern for following it, ability to feel love and affection for the people in her past life, a strong religious faith. She finds pleasure in creating beauty; she has a strong sense of self-esteem, which is violated by her fear of dying alone. On the other hand, when she feels a loss of love or fear for her safety she is unable to eat or rest properly.

If, as nurses, we are aware of a person's needs and how they may be met, we can often be of great assistance in helping to make their days more comfortable.*

* Hunter ML, Swain MA, Erickson H: Physical illness and psychosocial adaptation: Nursing observations in support of the link. Manuscript submitted for publication, 1980

Person's Perception of Self

View of Self

As we work with our clients to meet their basic needs, we will become aware of how the person views himself. One's **self-concept** is a collection of notions, feelings, and beliefs about one's self with which one identifies and through which one relates and communicates with others and interacts with the environment. The ideas of self-concept are developed from many of the variables inherent in the biopsychosocial systems of the person (Table 2-1). Persons generally have a **self-ideal** that might be considered the superego. The self-ideal refers to how one believes one ought to function and behave given a personal value system and a set of personal standards. One develops this ideal with influences from family structure, cultural values, teachers, and one's own talents. strengths, and goals for the future.

Self-Esteem and Body Image

An important aspect of self-concept is one's sense of **self-esteem**—the personal judgment one makes about one's own self-worth. A person may arrive at this perception by considering how well he measures up to his self-ideal and how often the goals he sets for himself are attained. The ability to set and attain goals provides the person with a sense of power and control over his life as well as with a hopeful feeling about the future.

Another component of the self-concept is one's **body image.** The body is the structural, functional, substantiative, and visible part of the self. It is the packaging in which the self is enclosed and through which one interacts with other people and the environment. The body image is how one views or thinks of that physical part of one's self (Fig. 2-3). Research studies have often demonstrated that persons who are comfortable with their bodies and like how they look and feel generally have a high sense of self-esteem. Tolstoy said, "I am convinced that

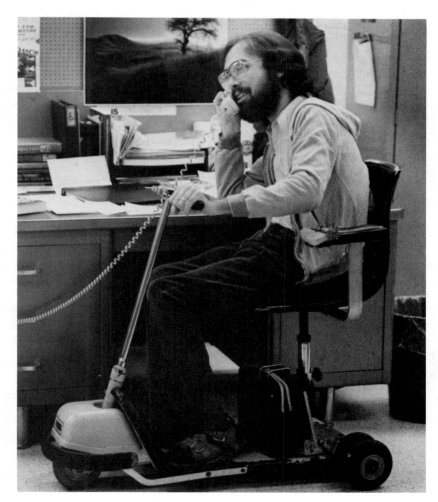

Figure 2-3
Body image is the way one views or thinks of one's physical self. *(Photo by Bob Kalmbach; University of Michigan Information Services)*

nothing has so marked an influence on the direction of a man's mind as his appearance, and not his appearance in itself so much as his conviction that it is attractive or unattractive'' (1904). A satirical play, *The Apollo of Bellac* by Jean Giraudoux, depicts a young man instructing a young woman, who is unsophisticated in the ways of the world, how to make a man do anything she wants. He explains that she must tell the man he is very handsome and that if she says this to every man she meets she will receive all she wants in the world. As the play progresses the young woman first obtains a job from one man and finally a large diamond ring and proposal of marriage from a millionaire, all because, Giraudoux would have us believe, she tells them how handsome they are. Of course the play is all in fun, but as in any sort of caricature, there is a basic truth in the matter.

When one's view of the self does not correspond with what one actually sees, it often results in a decrease of self-esteem. This has been noted in persons who have had surgery, whether or not the surgical alteration is visible to others. Some theorists believe that phantom pain, the pain that occurs in an absent body part such as an amputated limb, is the result of certain nerve activity. Others, however, would suggest that the pain is as much a result of the severe alteration in one's body image or view of the physical self as it is related to unusual nerve activity.

Some persons feel a disruption in their body image when they must wear glasses or a hearing aid. Others will describe difficulty in communicating or in projecting themselves effectively when, in their view, their hair is dirty or too long, or when they are not pleased with the clothes they are wearing. Daphne du Maurier describes the feelings of her hero in *Scapegoat* when he first notices the man who resembles him exactly (1957). "The resemblance made me slightly sick, reminding me of moments when, passing a shop window, I had suddenly seen my reflection, and the man in the mirror had been a grotesque caricature of what, conceitedly, I had believed myself to be. Such incidents left me chastened, sore, with ego deflated . . ." (p. 17).

Inner versus *Outward Feelings*

Our total self-concept consists not only of how we believe we appear but also of the expectations we have of how we ought to behave and what we should achieve. Sometimes we are not sure what or who that self is and how that person ought to be expressed. The expression "identity crisis" is common in our current Western culture, and refers to the difficulty we sometimes have in grasping the meaning of our inner workings (thinking) or our outward behavior. As with basic needs or developmental tasks, one may function well until stress occurs. At that point, however, it becomes difficult to meet our needs, resolve our tasks, and understand the meaning of our behavior. What we present of ourselves to others may be vastly different from what we actually feel about ourselves.

Again we turn to du Maurier's hero as he talks of his struggle to understand his real self as opposed to the self he presents to others. He appears to be a quiet, law-abiding professor, aged 38, but he wonders about the self, the man within.

> Who he was and whence he sprang, what urges and what longings he might possess, I could not tell. I was so used to denying him expression that his ways were unknown to me; but he might have had a mocking laugh, a casual heart, a swift-roused temper and a ribald tongue . . . Perhaps, if I had not kept him locked within me, he might have laughed, roistered, fought and lied. Perhaps he suffered, perhaps he hated, perhaps he lived by cruelty alone. He might have murdered, stolen or spent himself in lost causes, loved humanity, embraced a faith that believed in the divinity of both God and Man. Whatever his nature, he always hovered beneath the insignificant facade of that pale self who now sat in the church . . . The question was, how to unlock the door? What lever would set the other free? (pp. 14, 15)

As nurse persons, it is important that we understand ourselves, or at least that we are aware of the questions we have about ourselves. As we become more comfortable with our own self-concept, we are better able to understand the strivings of those for whom we provide care. As we are aware of our own inner workings, we can more readily accept the inner workings of others as well as the facade they present to the world in general. This will enable us to find the uniqueness of each person and to use that uniqueness to facilitate growth.

Values

The particular value system a person espouses is another way in which he is unique and yet shares features in common with others. Our values help us to view ourselves in relation to others.

A **value** is a belief or a custom that frequently arises from cultural or ethnic backgrounds, from family tradition, from peer group ideas and practices, from political philosophies in one's country, and from educational and religious philosophies with which one identifies. Some values are unique to the individual; other values are more readily identified as arising from a particular group, philosophy, or culture.

Because we all form values and value systems, we also engage in a practice called **value judgment.** This practice refers to a personal decision about whether something is right or wrong. The decision is usually affected by the society we live in, the culture or subculture in which we function, and the period of history in which we live. We generally hold these decisions to be true and right and find support for them from others around us who agree and will support our claim to righteousness.

Since we are nurses as well as persons, we also have another set of values under which we operate. We will be expected to provide care for others who often feel or believe very differently from ourselves. Our professional value system, as well as our personal one, often dictates that we must proceed and not abandon the person who has sought our care and assistance. We can handle this situation in two different ways. First, we may decide to continue with the person and assist him with the plans he wishes to make. In order to maintain our own integrity, however, we do not have to become involved in the process but may merely stand by and support the person to carry through the plan himself. The notion of empathy and techniques in problem solving are discussed in succeeding chapters and will be of use to the nurse involved in this kind of situation. Second, if our values are seriously threatened, we may decide not to assist the person. Nurses making this kind of decision would want to find another person or agency to assist the client.

We might consider the example of a person who wishes to stop his chemotherapy for cancer. The nurse may know, given the statistics concerning the chemotherapy, that the person has a strong chance for long-term survival if he continues the therapy. On the other hand, he may live only a year or so if he stops the therapy. The nurse may feel uncomfortable and may believe that stopping therapy is an inappropriate decision for the person to make. The nurse can remain objective and simply act as a listener so that the person can talk out his ideas. However, the nurse whose values are seriously threatened and who believes that the person is behaving in a suicidal manner may want to leave the situation. The nurse then will want to engage another nurse who does not feel threatened by the person's decision, to assist him with his planning and problem solving.

Conclusion

This chapter has presented a holistic perspective of the person, based on the Maslovian hierarchy of basic human needs. Each person shares basic needs and aspirations with other persons but is also unique in heritage, particular needs, and strivings. Values and perceptions of self contribute another dimension to a person. The self-actualizing tendency of man motivates the person to fulfill individual potential. Using this holistic perspective, the nurse considers clients' strengths and needs, not in isolation but in relation to other needs and strengths. The holistic person is the object of nursing. Person-centered care is the essence of professional nursing.

Study Questions

1. You are caring for a 45-year-old man who is recovering from a severe heart attack. His wife divorced him a year ago, leaving their three teenage children in his care. The children are alone while he is in the hospital. Consider the biopsychosocial needs of this man and discuss how you would use the concept of holism in this situation.

2. Explain the terms *open* and *closed systems* and discuss how they occur within the person.

3. Describe the notion of energy movement between systems and subsystems.

4. Discuss the categories of basic needs on Maslow's hierarchy and give a clinical example of each.

5. Consider yourself as a person. How do such terms as self-concept, self-ideal, self-esteem and body image apply to you?

6. Consider the following situation. You are caring for a 45-year-old woman who has had a radical mastectomy (removal of the breast). Throughout her recovery period in the hospital she wears a large heavy robe, even though it is summer. She is aloof to the female nurses and openly rude to her male doctor. She stares out the window when her husband visits and doesn't even show much interest in the activities of her children. Analyze this woman's response using the concepts discussed in *The Person's View of Self*.

7. Discuss the notions of *value* and *value judgment*. What kinds of experiences influence how we develop value systems? How would you feel about the person who refuses chemotherapy for cancer? If you were unable to assist him, how would you feel about yourself?

Glossary

Body image: How one views or thinks of the physical part of the self.

Closed system: A system that cannot exchange matter, energy, and information with its environment.

Holism: A theory that the universe, and especially living nature, is correctly seen as interacting wholes that are more than the mere sum of elementary particles; a theory that describes the parts of a person as dependent upon each other and coordinated in a systematic fashion (Smuts, 1926).

Open system: A system that can exchange matter, energy, and information with its environment.

Self-concept: A collection of notions, feelings, and beliefs about the self with which one identifies and through which one relates and communicates with others and interacts with the environment.

Self-esteem: One's personal judgment of one's own self-worth.

Self-ideal: How one believes he ought to function and behave given his personal value system and set of personal standards.

System: "An organized unit with a set of components that mutually react" (Abbey, 1978).

Value: A belief or a custom that frequently arises from cultural or ethnic backgrounds, from family tradition, from peer group ideas and practices, from political philosophies in one's country, and from educational and religious philosophies with which one identifies.

Value judgment: A personal decision about whether something is right or wrong.

Variable: "A measurable or potentially measurable component of an object or event that may fluctuate in quantity or quality or that may be different in quantity or quality from an individual object or event (when compared) to another object or event of the same general class" (Wandelt, 1970).

Bibliography

Abbey JC: General systems theory: A framework for nursing. In Putt, A: General Systems Theory Applied to Nursing. Boston, Little, Brown & Co., 1978

Ashby WR: Systems and their informational measures. In Klir GL (ed): Trends in General Systems Theory. New York, John Wiley & Sons, 1972

Blaesing S, Brockhaus J: The development of body image in the child. Nurs Clin North Am 7, No. 4: 594–607, 1972

Cooper RH: Concentration camp survivors: A challenge for geriatric nursing. Nurs Clin North Am 14, No. 4: 621–627, 1979

Daly KM: Don't wave good-bye. Am J Nurs 74, No. 9: 1641, 1974

Dempsey MO: The development of body image in the adolescent. Nurs Clin North Am 7, No. 4: 609–615, 1972

Dubree M, Vogelpohl R: When hope dies—So might the patient. Am J Nurs 80, No. 11: 2046–2049, 1980

du Maurier D: The Scapegoat. Garden City, New York, Doubleday, 1957

Erikson E: Childhood and Society, 2nd ed. New York, WW Norton, 1963

Giraudoux J: The Apollo of Bellac. In Four Plays, adapted, with an introduction by Maurice Valency. New York, Hill & Wang, 1958

Hall AD, Fagen RE: Definitions of Systems. In Buckley W (ed): Modern Systems Research for the Behavioral Scientist. Chicago, Aldine, 1968

Hazzard ME: An overview of systems theory. Nurs Clin North Am 6, No. 3: 385–393, 1971

Joseph LS: Self care and the nursing process. Nurs Clin North Am 15, No. 1: 131–143, 1980

Klir GJ: Preview: The polyphonic general systems theory. In Klir GJ (ed): Trends in General Systems Theory. New York, John Wiley & Sons, 1972

Levine ME: The pursuit of Wholeness. Am J Nurs 69, No. 1: 93–98, 1969

Maslow AH: Motivation and Personality, 2nd ed. New York, Harper & Row, 1970

Menninger K: The Vital Balance. New York, Viking, 1963

Murray RLE: Body image development in adulthood. Nurs Clin North Am 7, No. 4: 617–630, 1972

Otto, HA: The human potentialities of nurses and patients. Nurs Outlook 13, No. 8: 32–35, 1965

Orem DE: Nursing: Concepts of Practice, 2nd ed. New York, McGraw-Hill, 1980

Putt AM: General Systems Theory Applied to Nursing. Boston, Little, Brown & Co, 1978

Rawnsley, MM: Toward a conceptual base for affective nursing. Nurs Outlook 28, No. 4: 244–247, 1980

Riffee DM: Self-esteem changes in hospitalized school-age children. Nurs Res 30, No. 2: 94–97, 1981

Simms LM, Lindberg JB: The Nurse Person: Developing Perspectives for Contemporary Nursing. New York, Harper & Row, 1978

Smith JJT, Selye H: Reducing the negative effects of stress. Am J Nurs 79, No. 11: 1953–1964, 1979

Smuts JC: Holism and Evolution. New York, Macmillan, 1926

Stoll RI: Guidelines for spiritual assessment. Am J Nurs 79, No. 9: 1574–1577, 1979

Summers A: Billy was totally unresponsive, Am J Nurs 79, No. 7: 1262–1263, 1979

Sutterly, DC, Donnelly GF: Perspectives in Human Development. Philadelphia, JB Lippincott, 1973

Tolstoy L: Childhood. In Tolstoy L: The Complete Works of Count Tolstoy, Vol I. Dana Estes, 1904. Reissued by Colonial Press. Electrotyped and printed by CH Simon, Boston

von Bertalanffy L: General systems theory: A critical review. In Buckley W (ed): Modern Systems Research for the Behavioral Scientist. Chicago, Aldine, 1968

Wandelt M: Guide for the Beginning Researcher. New York, Appleton-Century-Crofts, 1970

Growth and Development

Mary L. Hunter

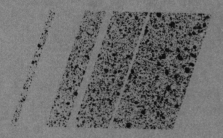

Objectives

Introduction

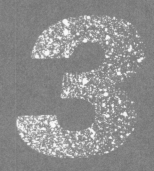

3

The purpose of this chapter is to underscore the application of growth and development theories to the delivery of relevant and effective nursing care. Growth and development are variables in the biopsychosocial functioning of the person. We wish to acquaint students with several prominent theorists to provide background and resource material for skills the nurse will practice later. For example, understanding how people think may assist with health teaching, and being aware of psychosocial development may provide the nurse with guidelines for doing counseling. An appreciation of the physical growth patterns that occur in people at different ages and stages helps the nurse concentrate on pertinent areas when doing physical assessment.

This knowledge will make the nurse aware of the need to look at the concept of the total person. For example, knowledge about psychosocial development can help the nurse work with the teenager whose lagging physical development may contribute to his failing school work. The most exciting reason for considering growth and development, however, is that it demonstrates the unending potential of the human being throughout life.

The subject and theories of growth and development fill many books and supply the content for total courses. A brief discussion of growth and development is included in this text for the purposes stated above. We expect that students will use the ideas presented here to understand aspects that are both common and unique to their clients. For a more thorough examination of the subject, students are referred to the publications cited at the end of this chapter.

General Principles of Growth and Development

Growth

The term **growth** refers to an actual biological or quantitative increase in physical size, that is, the enlargement of any body components by an increase in the number of cells. **Maturation** means development of those cells until they can be completely utilized by the organism (Turner and Helms, 1979, p. 7).

Some key ideas related to growth are as follows:

- Physical growth occurs at different rates among individuals.

- Growth of the body parts and systems of a person occurs at different rates; for example, a child may be within normal height and weight ranges for age 5 but may have a less mature urinary elimination system that causes him to wet the bed at night. During adolescence a person's features may appear too large for his face but will fit nicely as the size of the head increases.

- There is a wide range of normal values for height, weight, muscle development, and physical abilities at all ages and stages of development. Charts that describe physical characteristics of different ages should be used as guidelines only.

Development

"**Development** is the patterned, orderly, lifelong changes in structure, thought, or behavior that evolve as a result of the maturation of physical and mental capacity, experiences, and learning and result in a new level of maturity and integration" (Murray and Zentner, 1979, p. 2). A **developmental task** is a growth responsibility that arises at a certain time in the course of development. If resolution of the task occurs, satisfaction and success with later tasks will likely result. Failure to resolve the tasks in a satisfactory manner leads to unhappiness, disapproval by society, and difficulty with later developmental tasks and functions.

Some principles of development to consider are listed here:

- Development that occurs in childhood provides a base for the rest of life.

- Development proceeds in a predictable and sequential way throughout life.

- The developing person acquires competency in four major areas across the life span:
    - Physical—Gaining motor and neurological capacities
    - Cognitive—Learning how to perceive, think, and communicate thoughts and feelings
    - Emotion—Developing awareness and acceptance of self as a unique individual, reacting to the environment, coping with stresses, assuming responsibility for personal behavior
    - Social—Learning to interrelate first with the family and later with different persons in many situations (Murray and Zentner, pp. 2–5).

We have not attempted to describe physical development for the various ages and stages of growth because of the vastness of the subject. We suggest, however, that the student use the references at the end of this chapter for more information on all areas of growth and development and on the physical aspects in particular.

When doing a nursing assessment (see discussion of nursing process in Section 6), it is especially useful to consider those aspects of physical development that are most pertinent to the client's age. For example, the 6-year-old child will be learning to write in school. Thus an assessment of his fine motor development would be useful. The adolescent person who is struggling with identity and changes in body image may benefit most from assessment and care planning related to secondary sex characteristics and the condition of the skin. Older adults who are experiencing changes in body structure will be helped if planning centers on their motor ability.

The remainder of the discussion in this section of the chapter will describe the theories of Erik

Figure 3-1
The infant learns trust by having basic needs met. *(Photo by Bob Kalmbach; University of Michigan Information Services)*

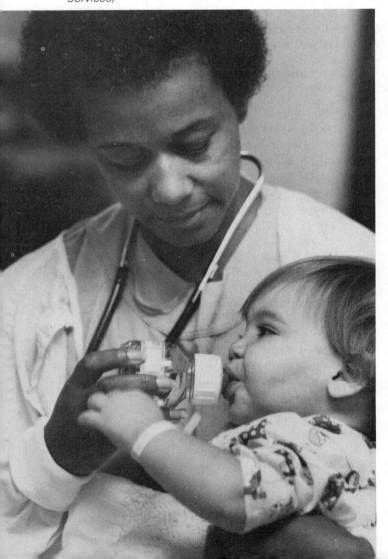

Erikson, a major theorist in psychosocial development, and Jean Piaget, a major theorist in cognitive development. These two men are well known and accepted in their fields. Their work provides nurses with a base for understanding the development of the psychological and social components of the person.

Psychosocial Development: Erikson

Our discussion of Erikson begins with his developmental tasks as outlined in Table 3-1.

The following ideas from Erikson can be used by the nurse to apply concepts from psychosocial development theory to practice (1963).

- Developmental levels are not achieved, they are resolved.

- The negative senses (mistrust, shame, guilt, *etc.*) of each stage are the dynamic counterparts of the positive ones throughout life. Some aspects of these counterparts are present in all of us at one time or another.

- At each stage of development, a ratio, hopefully a favorable one, develops between the positive and negative senses such that skills are formed that can be used throughout life for coping with stress. For example, trust is learned in infancy through satisfaction of basic needs (Fig. 3-1).

- Stressors impact on our lives and new inner conflicts develop during the life span. Our ability to cope may be closely associated with the ratio of resolution that has occurred during work on previous tasks.

- At some level, all the developmental tasks are present in us at all ages.

- Each task exists from birth in some form before its critical time for resolution normally arrives.

- Theorists have suggested that the first two tasks (trust *vs* mistrust and autonomy *vs* shame and doubt) may be the most important tasks of all. These tasks lay the groundwork, and many of the conflicts that occur in later life may well be a reflection of the ratio of resolution that has occurred in those early tasks. For example, Erikson believes that in society at large, the resolution of basic trust is reflected in religious faith or faith in social action or scientific pursuit. The resolution of autonomy is reflected in the principles of law and order.

(Text continues on page 42)

Table 3-1
Developmental Tasks According to Erikson

Age	Task	Favorable Outcome	Unfavorable Outcome
Birth to 1 year	Basic trust *vs* mistrust	Lets mother out of sight without undue anxiety or rage.	Senses an inner division; feels deprived or divided: feels abandoned.
		Learns that mother has become an inner certainty and an outer predictability.	Develops defense mechanisms, projection and introjection against anticipated loss or disappointment. Projection: "Attributing one's own thoughts or impulses to another person" (Stuart, 1979, p. 84). Introjection: "Intense type of identification in which a person incorporates qualities or values of another person or group into his own ego structure" (p. 84).
		Correlates inner remembrances and anticipation of sensation with outer sameness of experience; this leads to familiarity and prediction. Engages in constant testing of relationships both inside and outside.	
		Begins not only to trust the outer provider but also to trust oneself and the capacity of one's own organs to cope with urges.	
1 to 3 years	Autonomy *vs* shame and doubt	Develops a set of social modalities associated with holding on and letting go.	Develops a set of social modalities associated with holding on and letting go.
		Benign expectations: letting go (to let be); holding on (to have and to hold).	Hostile expectations: letting go (letting loose of destructive forces); holding on (destructive or cruel restraining forces).
		Experiences definite wish to have a choice, begins to stand on own two feet, begins to develop a sense of self-control without loss of self-esteem; this can develop into a lasting sense of good will and pride.	Shame: becomes conscious of being upright and exposed; tries to get away with things unseen; could become defiant and shameless.
			Doubt: senses that one is dominated by the will of others; senses a loss of control and of foreign overcontrol; develops a lasting propensity for doubt and shame.

(Continued)

Table 3-1
Developmental Tasks According to Erikson (Continued)

Age	Task	Favorable Outcome	Unfavorable Outcome
		Develops basic faith in existence. Autonomy fostered in childhood helps develop a sense of justice later in life.	
4 to 5 years	Initiative *vs* guilt	Senses hope and new responsibility; a vigorous unfolding. Learns quickly and avidly.	Superego becomes cruel and uncompromising, causing repressionism in some persons (who become inhibited or impotent) and exhibitionism ("showing off") in others.
		Develops judgment; is active, energetic; develops direction; can undertake, plan, and attack a task.	
		Cooperates, works with other children for a purpose, constructs and plans cooperatively.	
		Establishes a moral sense that restricts the horizon of the permissible.	Submerges rage, which causes self-righteousness. Often psychosomatic disease is noted in the adult who fails to resolve this developmental task.
6 to 11 years	Industry *vs* inferiority	Wins recognition by producing things, because this is the age of formal and systematic instruction, whether the school is the classroom, field, or jungle.	
		Begins readiness to move beyond or outside the family.	Remains unsure of status with peers and partners.
		Begins to handle tools and develops skills with them.	
		Applies self to skills and tasks.	Feels unsure of skills and tools.
		Directs attention and perseveres; goes beyond desire to plan and develop a sense of satisfaction in work completion.	
		Senses a division of labor and differential opportunity.	Restricts self and horizons to include only his own work; becomes a conformist and thoughtless slave of his technology.
		Senses the characteristics of the culture.	Begins to feel the color of skin and background of parents and to feel judged by it.

Age	Task	Favorable Outcome	Unfavorable Outcome
12 to 20 years	Identity vs role confusion	Questions continuity and sameness from past; searches for a new continuity and sameness.	Confuses sex roles because of doubt regarding sexual identity.
		Concerns self with appearance to others vs what one feels oneself to be.	Overidentifies with heroes, cliques, and crowds (to the loss of individual identity). Behaves in a clanish and cruel manner to all those who are different (a defense against a sense of identity confusion).
		Develops a confidence that the inner sameness and continuity prepared in the past are matched by the sameness and continuity of one's meaning for others, as evidenced in the tangible promise of a career.	
		Senses an ideology and a commitment to it; finds self in the stage between the morality learned by the child and the ethics developed by the adult.	Becomes an easy prey to cruel totalitarian doctrines and ideology.
20 to 40 years, early adulthood	Intimacy vs isolation	Becomes eager and willing to fuse one's identity with others; ready for intimacy; has capacity to commit oneself to concrete affiliations and partnerships.	Avoids intimate relationships and commitment for fear of ego loss. This leads to a deep sense of isolation and self-absorption.
		Develops the ethical strength to abide by one's commitments.	Develops prejudice.
		Welcomes situations that require self-abandonment: solidarity of close affiliations, sexual unions, close friendships, physical combat, and experiences of inspiration from teachers, institutions, and the recesses of the self.	Fears others' encroachment on one's territory.
41 to 60, middle adulthood.	Generativity vs stagnation	Concerns self with establishing and guiding the next generation. Mature persons need to be needed.	Experiences a pervasive sense of stagnation and personal impoverishment; needs pseudointimacy.
		Produces and creates.	
		Believes in and has faith in the species, sees the child or the younger generation as a welcome trust.	Indulges self; early invalidism, physical or psychological disorders become a vehicle of self-concern.

(Continued)

Table 3-1
Developmental Tasks According to Erikson *(Continued)*

Age	Task	Favorable Outcome	Unfavorable Outcome
64 years and on, late adulthood	Ego integrity *vs* despair	Sees self as the originator of others or a generator of products and ideas. In this person the fruits of other stages of development gradually ripen: hope, willpower, purpose, competence, fidelity, love, care, and wisdom.	Feels despair: time is too short to start over.
		Senses an assurance that there is order and meaning, in the sense of the world and in a spiritual sense.	
		Accepts one's own life cycle as the way it had to be. Experiences a sense of comradeship with the past.	Does not accept one's only life cycle as the ultimate of life.
		Defends the dignity of one's own lifestyle.	
		Experiences a final consolation and emotional integration.	Behaves with disgust, which hides despair and the fear of death.
		Acceptance of death.	

Adapted from Erikson E: Childhood and Society, 2nd ed, pp. 247–274. New York, WW Norton, 1963

- There is evidence to suggest that persons may become ill physically as well as psychologically if the impact of stressors is great enough. This can be influenced by the person's development of skills for coping through the resolution of developmental tasks.

- Erikson believes these stages of development are present in all of the human species. The realization and demonstration of resolution may be reflected in the particular customs and style of many different ethnic, cultural, and national groups. The essence of development, however, is the same for us all.

- The strength acquired at any stage is tested by the necessity to transcend it in such a way that the individual can take chances in the next stage with what was most vulnerably precious in the previous one.

We continue to work on resolution of all the tasks throughout life. Erikson describes the outcome potential of the favorable ratios of each stage of development, calling the words italicized below the "basic virtues." He points out that these basic virtues are those that reemerge from generation to generation and constitute the spirit and relevance of human systems.

> Basic trust *versus* mistrust: drive and *hope*
>
> Autonomy *versus* shame and doubt: self-control and *willpower*
>
> Initiative *versus* guilt: direction and *purpose*
>
> Industry *versus* inferiority: method and *competence*
>
> Identity *versus* role confusion: devotion and *fidelity*
>
> Intimacy *versus* isolation: affiliation and *love*
>
> Generativity *versus* stagnation: production and *care*
>
> Ego integrity *versus* despair: renunciation and *wisdom*

The following anecdotes are entries from the logs of two sophomore nursing students. Both students have recorded their experiences with persons representing two of the age groups discussed by Erikson. They have described these persons appropriately and with insight.

Example 1 □ According to Erikson, these children are working on the task of initiative *versus* guilt. Today the children were working with sponge painting—making pumpkin faces. Julie was acting silly like 4-year-olds do and she just colored the whole piece of paper (pumpkin) while watching others make eyes, nose, and mouth. Christopher was soaking up lots of paint in his sponge, then pressing it down hard so it made a big pool of paint. Even after he was told not to press so hard he went ahead and did it anyway. Sometimes (probably a lot of the time) children of this age don't listen very well; they just go ahead with what they are doing. The rest of the children, from what I observed, did a good job making two eyes, a nose, and a mouth on their pumpkins, showing their ability to be creative. Kevin did better in this aspect than some of the others but he observed for a while before he started to draw.

When the children were having their snack they were acting silly, which is normal for this age group. They were grabbing each others' arms and shaking them. Kevin would do this to Carey, but he wouldn't let her do it to him. Maybe this was Kevin's way of protecting his body, which children of this age are now learning to do.* □

Example 2 □ According to Erikson, E.B. is facing integrity *versus* disgust and despair. I feel E.B. has resolved this task. She was telling me about the "old Ann Arbor," the way it was when she was young. Some of what she liked then included such things as no cars on campus. She explained how things have changed so much, especially for women (*i.e.*, athletics, females in the band, cheerleading). Even so, as she looks at it, she always has had the philosophy that she was only young once and that it was her opportune time to have fun, and she did. Granted, things maybe did not turn out exactly the way she had planned (she didn't get into medical school), yet she became a med. tech. and worked in that field for many years. She also became a teacher. E.B. adjusted to her life as she went along and had fun in the process. Now, when she looks back, she doesn't regret any of it or hopelessly long for the past. She accepts it as a good part of her life, which she enjoys remembering and talking about with people like me.

E.B. has pursued new interests in order to gain status, recognition, and a feeling of being needed. She also uses her nurturing qualities to help others (myself, her friends) and, in so doing feels needed and feels good about herself.† □

* Keskey A: Personal communication, November, 1980
† O'Shea K: Personal Communication, November, 1980

The theories of Maslow and Erikson blend well together. One might note that a person's ability to meet his basic needs may be reflected by the degree to which he has resolved his developmental tasks of trust and autonomy. When stress seriously affects one's sense of safety, adaptive coping can occur if the person has a sense of trust, self-control, direction, purpose, and competence. In other words, the ability to meet our basic needs on a daily basis may be directly related to the amount of skill we have developed through resolution of the developmental tasks.

Maslow emphasizes that the basic needs are satisfied not only by receiving, but also by giving. In fact, giving is essential to satisfaction. We provide a safe atmosphere and protect the safety needs of small children and others who are unable to do this for themselves. We wish to give love and friendship, as well as to receive it. Erikson points out the need to be trusted as well as to trust, to develop a sense of devotion and intimacy toward others, and to produce or care for the next generation. He states that the mature man needs to be needed, and that the older adult develops wisdom that he wishes to pass on to the younger generation.

If, as persons ourselves, or as persons who are nurses, we consider our own development and our own ability to meet our basic needs, we can be more effective in helping others move toward the basic virtues and self-actualization.

Cognitive Development: Piaget

Piaget describes cognitive development as a continuous progression from the spontaneous movements and reflexes of the newborn, to acquired habits of the infant, to the beginning of the development of intelligence which becomes apparent toward the end of the first year of life (Fig. 3-2). Cognitive development is cumulative; understanding of new experiences evolves what was learned from earlier ones. Piaget identifies four major levels in the development of cognition or growth of thought, listed below (1973).

Sensorimotor Level: Birth to 2 Years

The following discussion describes the mechanism of progression towards the development of intelligence.

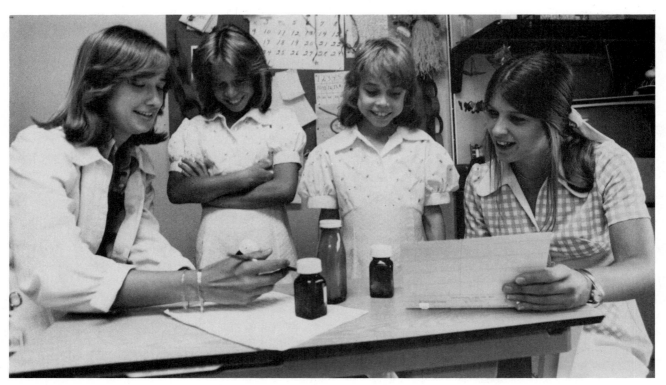

Figure 3-2
Piaget's theory of cognitive development can be useful.
(Photo by Bob Kalmbach; University of Michigan Information Services)

Assimilation

Reality data (*i.e.*, input from the real world) are treated or modified in such a way as to become incorporated into the **structure** of the person. Piaget uses structure to describe how information is organized within the person to make a simple mental image or pattern of action. Although the necessary mental structures are genetically destined, these structures mature with age. The organizing activity of the person is as important as the relationships inherent in the external stimuli. This idea might be represented in the following way:

$$\text{S (stimulus)} \underset{\text{Person}}{\longleftrightarrow} \text{R (response)}$$

The input stimulus is filtered through a person who develops action-schemes or, at a higher level, the operations of thought. These in turn are modified and enriched when the person's behavioral repertoire increases to the demands of reality. **Assimilation,** then, is the process of taking novel information and making it fit a preconceived notion about objects or the world. Later, the child will be able to find new ways of looking at things.

Accommodation

Accommodation is the alteration of internal schemes to fit reality; reconciling new experiences or objects by revising the old plan to fit the new input. Singer and Revenson provide us with an example of this process in the infant (1978). Initially the child attempts to understand something new by using old solutions, that is, by assimilation. When this does not work the youngster is forced to modify his existing view of the world to interpret the experience. The baby who attempts to drink milk from his rattle (assimilation) quickly learns that rattles make noise but do not yield milk. The rattle no longer substitutes for feeding (accommodation).

This dual process of assimilation–accommodation leads to **adaptation,** which is a continuing process of learning from the environment and learning to adjust to alterations in the environment. Adaptation allows the child to form a **schema,** a more complex mental image, an action organization that a person uses to explain what he sees and hears (Singer and Revenson, pp. 13–15).

During this period from birth to 2 years, the infant relies on his senses and his motor activity for information about the world. Reflex actions occur during this period. The infant recognizes these as successful actions but has no knowledge about them. The infant's understanding of the world involves only perceptions and objects with which he has direct experience. As language appears, usually at about 1½ to 2 years, the development of symbolic or preconceptual thought begins. Toward the end of the sensorimotor phase, the child begins to understand the concept of **object permanence.** He begins to realize that objects can exist apart from himself. When he cannot see an object, he begins to understand that it is still there. He can accept his mother leaving his sight because he knows she is near and will return.

Preoperational Level: Age 2 Through 7 Years

This is the period of curiosity, questioning, and investigation. The child is taking an interest in his environment but is still interpreting it according to his own point of view. This approach is called egocentrism. The child uses explanations of the world that he knows and makes up others to answer his questions.

Concrete Operations Level: Age 7 Through 11 Years

Piaget defines an **operation** as an interiorized action or an action performed in the mind (Singer, 1978, p. 20). There are several characteristics of this level:

- *Reversibility*—The direction of thought can be reversed mentally. The child understands that if he can add figures he can also subtract them. He knows how to find his way to school or to the store and how to turn around and find his way home again.
- *Seriation*—The child has the ability to arrange objects mentally according to a quantitative dimension such as size or weight.
- *Conservation*—The person has the ability to see that objects or quantities remain the same despite a change in their physical appearance. The child understands such quantities as number, substance (mass), area, weight, volume. He can understand that a quantity of liquid is the same whether it fills a short, fat container, or a tall, thin one.

The child still applies his concrete operations to objects that are physically present.

Formal Operations Level: Age 11 Through 16 Years

The child can now consider objects that are not present and perform formal operations by considering the future and the abstract. As he reaches adolescence he can do problem solving using more rational and scientific processes. His thinking is more flexible, and he can consider several possible ways to solve a problem or to view an experience. He can make relationships between several pieces of information and draw rational conclusions. Piaget hypothesized that we do not develop any new mental structures after the stage of formal operations. He believed that intellectual development from this point on consists of an increase of knowledge and depth of understanding.

Nursing Implications

The theory of cognitive development as described for us by Piaget can be very useful to nursing. It becomes apparent, as we examine how children learn to think and how they develop intelligence, that certain approaches to teaching are more effective at different times. As we consider our adult clients, we may also recognize that stress affects how they think and learn. Moreover, the response to learning under stress may vary according to the individual. Some may learn when they are alarmed or aroused because of a great need for information, whereas others will be unable to concentrate on the task at hand. The nurse will want to assess how stress affects the ability of the person to learn.

Piaget describes intelligence as the indispensable instrument for interaction between the subject and the universe. Feeling directs behavior by assigning a value to its end; feeling provides the energy necessary for action, and knowledge gives a structure to it. He states that every action involves an energetic or affective aspect and a structural or cognitive aspect (Piaget, 1973, pp. 4–5).

It is wise to take note of the fact that the ages as stated for each level are somewhat arbitrary. That is, a child may be either slower or faster than suggested in reaching a new level; the range of normal is very broad.

Nurses may also want to consider that adults demonstrate great variance in the ability to engage in the formal operations of thought. This may become more apparent when we assist adult clients to learn about their health needs. Those who are more comfortable with concrete thought operations may take longer to understand and apply new information, and those who have been able to think formally may understand more quickly.

Nurses will need to be aware not only of the age level of their clients but also of their abilities to grasp and apply information when receiving health teaching or attempting to participate in health-care planning.

In summary, we might reconsider how we as nurses can use the theories of Erikson, Piaget, and Maslow together when planning nursing care. For example, we know that persons use their intelligence as well as their feeling states to solve problems and to develop skills toward the resolution of developmental tasks. The infant learns to trust, in part, because he uses his beginning cognitive skills of recognition and memory to know who mother is. The adolescent or young adult uses his ability to think conceptually and to make relationships among the pieces of information he receives. This assists him in making good decisions about how to take care of himself and how to plan the direction he wishes his life to take. If we consider Maslow's theories, we know that a person's ability to meet his basic needs may also influence the decisions he makes about himself and his life.

From Developmental Theory to Clinical Application

We have drawn on Maslow and Erikson to talk about the control persons have in achieving their potential. Nursing views persons as individuals with the potential to take care of themselves and achieve a high level of health. Carl Rogers has provided us with several important "learnings," as he calls them, which give support to the concept of person-centered nursing care and the self-care discussion that follows (1961). He has developed a person-centered therapy throughout his many years as a counselor and psychotherapist. He states, "... it is the *client* who knows what hurts, what directions to go, what problems are crucial, what experiences have been deeply buried. It began to occur to me that unless I had a need to demonstrate my own cleverness and learning, I would do better to rely upon the client for the direction of movement in the process" (pp. 11–12).

Rogers describes how he has learned to listen to and accept himself and his own feelings about a person he is helping or a situation he is in. He believes that to act one way on the surface while feeling another way underneath becomes more of a hindrance than a help in developing a therapeutic relationship. It is important for him not to try to be something he is not.

Although Rogers does not use the word "empathy," which the student will find in the chapter on Communication, he nevertheless describes it when he gives us another of his learnings, "I have found it of enormous value when I can permit myself to understand another person" (p. 18). He uses the word "permit" because he believes that too often we respond immediately to another person's ideas as right or wrong, good or bad, moral or immoral. We respond because of our own value system and out of fear that if we really understand the person, this might somehow change us or our way of thinking. This can be very distressing. We do not want to lose a part of ourselves in response to another person. He goes on to point out, however, that rather than changing, we become enriched and can grow when we truly understand the ideas and feelings of others.

Rogers believes strongly in learning from his own experience and in trusting what he learns. He states, "I can only try to live by *my* interpretation of the current meaning of *my* experience, and try to give others the permission and freedom to develop their own inward freedom and thus their own meaningful interpretation of their own experience. If there is such a thing as truth, this free individual process of search should, I believe, converge toward it" (p. 27). These words provide for us the very essence of the person-centered approach to nursing care and can, if we return to them again and again, assist us in developing and delivering effective and relevant care to the persons we seek to help toward the healthy state.

This Incredible Being: The Person

And so what is this incredible being called a person, with all of his systems that interrelate, integrate, and produce a being greater than the sum of those total parts? What causes him to be strong in the face of weakness, healthy in the face of illness, brave in the face of grief? How is it that he can continue to grow and flourish through a lifetime, even during periods of social, emotional, and physical diminishment? We have some answers to those questions and many theories, but we are missing large pieces of the puzzle. In the book *Heart Sounds*, Lear describes her husband, who lived through a cardiac crisis despite the expectations of all his physicians (1980).

An intern recalled, "we got a guy with an infiltrated intravenous. So he wasn't getting dopamine, the drug to maintain blood pressure. He had no palpable blood pressure and yet he was able to talk to us. This in itself was unusual. He was in cardiac shock: blood pressure too low to maintain life; no urine; decreased mentation; clammy extremities. I would have thought his chances of coming through were very, very small."

And after he had improved the cardiologist came out to tell his family. "He's better. He wants to know every detail of treatment. He's driving them all crazy in there. It's unbelievable. It's something spiritual, that fight, that fight that keeps him alive."

When Mrs. Lear goes in to see her husband she describes it like this:

> ... he lay still panting, his eyes closed, his face remote behind the [oxygen] mask, and I wondered *Better?* but surely they are wrong. How can anyone who looks like this be *better?* And I bent down again ... and whispered, "Darling.

You're *much better*. You've got to *fight*. You're going to *make it*. You're going to *make it*...."

And with one sudden swift move he ripped the mask off his face and turned to confront me directly. His eyes consumed me. *"I've already made it"* he said (pp. 338–339).

Conclusion

This chapter has introduced some of the basic understandings of growth and development that apply to person-centered nursing care. The resolution of developmental tasks is a lifelong process, as is self-actualization. Both illustrate that life itself is a dynamic process of becoming. The cognitive skills that are uniquely human cannot be separated from other aspects of the holistic person. If a person experiences an alteration in any component of the holistic system, it may be reflected in functioning that is characteristic of an earlier stage of growth and development.

Study Questions

1. Discuss how the terms *growth*, *maturation*, and *development* are pertinent to each person.

2. State the age, the developmental task, and the basic virtue of each age of man according to Erikson. Describe how these factors would influence the nursing care of a variety of persons.

3. Consider several persons in different stages and assess their resolution of the developmental tasks. Consider the balance they have attained between the favorable and unfavorable outcomes for their particular level.

4. Define the terms associated with Piaget's theory of cognitive development. Describe how you would use the theory when teaching nutrition to a group of sixth-grade children.

5. Identify three "learnings" according to Rogers and suggest a clinical application for each of these ideas.

Glossary

Accommodation: The alternation of internal schemes to fit reality; reconciling new experiences or objects by revising the old plan to fit the new input (Piaget).

Adaptation: The dual process of assimilation–accommodation (which leads to adaptation) is a continuing process of learning from the environment and learning to adjust to alterations in the environment (Piaget).

Assimilation: Reality data or input from the real world are treated or modified in such a way as to become incorporated into the structure of the person (Piaget).

Development: The patterned, orderly, lifelong changes in structure, thought, or behavior that evolve as a result of the maturation of physical and mental capacity, experiences, and learning and that result in a new level of maturity and integration.

Developmental task: A growth responsibility that arises at a certain time in the course of development.

Growth: An actual biological or quantitative increase in physical size, that is, the enlargement of any body component by an increase in the number of cells.

Maturation: Development of cells until they can be completely utilized by the organism.

Object permanence: Realization by the child that objects can exist apart from himself; understanding that though he may not see the object, it still exists.

Operation: An interiorized action or an action performed in the mind (Piaget).

Schema: A more complex mental image, an action organization that a person uses to explain what he sees and hears (Piaget).

Structure: The way in which information is organized within the person to make a simple mental image or pattern of action (Piaget).

Bibliography

Bancroft A: Integrity and despair: A contrast of two lives. In Burnside I (ed): Psychosocial Nursing Care of the Aged. New York, McGraw-Hill, 1973

Betz CL: Faith development in children. Pediatr Nurs 7, No. 2: 22–25, March-April 1981

Boesky D: Introduction: Symposium on object relations theory and love. Psychoanal Q 49: 48–55, 1980

Bowlby J: Attachment, Vol I. New York, Basic Books, 1969

Bowlby J: Separation, Vol II. New York, Basic Books, 1969

Bowlby J: Child Care and the Growth of Love, 2nd ed. Harmondsworth, Middlesex, England; Penguin Books, 1965

Box M: Development assessment. Health Visit 53, No. 11: 461–463, 1980

Burnside IM: Nursing and the Aged. New York, McGraw-Hill, 1976

Burnside I, Ebersole P, Monea H: Psychosocial Caring Throughout The Life Span. New York, McGraw-Hill, 1979

Butler R: Successful aging and the role of the life review. J Geriatrics Society 12: 529–535, 1974

Cooper S: Accidents and the older adult. Geriatric Nurs 2, No. 4: 287–290, 1981

Dashiff CJ: Coaching developmental differentiation. Top Clin Nurs 3: 11–20, 1979

Diekelmann NL: The young adult: The choice is health or illness. Am J Nurs 76, No. 8: 1272–1289, 1976

Ebersole P: Reminiscing. Am J Nurs 76, No. 8: 1304–1305, 1976

Erikson EH: Childhood and Society, 2nd ed. New York, WW Norton, 1963

Fraiberg SH: The Magic Years: Understanding and Handling the Problems of Early Childhood. New York, Charles Scribner's Sons, 1959

Hrobsky DM: Transition to parenthood: A balancing of needs. Nurs Clin North Am 12, No. 3: 457–468, 1977

Huges CB: An eclectic approach to parent group education. Nurs Clin North Am 12, No. 3: 469–479, 1977

Kalish RA: Late Adulthood: Perspective on Human Development. Belmont, California, Wadsworth, 1975

Klein M, Overholser M, Rynbergen H: Putting down roots in retirement. Geriatric Nurs 1, No. 2: 114–119, 1980

Lear MW: Heartsounds. New York, Simon & Schuster, 1980

Lidz T: The Person: His and Her Development Throughout the Life Cycle, rev. ed. New York, Basic Books, 1976

Lowrey GH: Growth and Development of Children, 7th ed. Chicago, Year Book Medical Publishers, 1978

Maclay E: Green Winter: Celebrations of Old Age. New York, Reader's Digest Press, distribution by Thomas Y. Crowell, 1977

Maier HW: Three Theories of Child Development: The Contributions of Erik H. Erikson, Jean Piaget and Robert R. Sears and Their Applications, rev. ed. New York, Harper & Row, 1978

Michael MM, Sewall KS: Use of the adolescent peer group to increase the self-care agency of adolescent alcohol abusers. Nurs Clin North Am 15, No. 1: 157–176, 1980

Murray R, Huelskoetter M, O'Driscoll D: The Nursing Process in Later Maturity. Englewood Cliffs, New Jersey, Prentice-Hall, 1980

Murray RB, Zentner JP: Nursing Assessment and Health Promotion Through the Life Span, 2nd ed. Englewood Cliffs, New Jersey, Prentice-Hall, 1979

Phillips JL Jr: The Origins of Intellect: Piaget's Theory, 2nd ed. San Francisco, WH Freeman, 1975

Piaget J: The Psychology of Intelligence. Totowa, New Jersey, Littlefield, Adams & Co, 1973

Pontious SL: Practical Piaget: Helping children understand. Am J Nurs 82, No. 1: 114–117, 1982

Rogers CR: On Becoming a Person. Boston, Houghton Mifflin, 1961

Schroell MM: Holistic Assessment of the Healthy Aged. New York, John Wiley & Sons, 1980

Singer DG, Revenson TA: A Piaget Primer: How a Child Thinks. New York, The New American Library, 1978

Smoyale SA: Symposium on parenting: Introduction. Nurs Clin North Am 12, No. 3: 447–455, 1977

Stokes S, Rauckhorst L, Mezey, M: Health assessment considerations for the older individual. J Gerontol Nurs 6, No. 6: 328–337, 1980

Stuart GW, Sundeen SJ: Principles and Practice of Psychiatric Nursing. St. Louis, CV Mosby, 1979

Turner JS, Helms DB: Life Span Development. Philadelphia, WB Saunders, 1979

Webster-Stratton C, Kogan K: Helping parents parent. Am J Nurs 80, No. 2: 240–244, 1980

Zaichkowsky D, Zaichkowsky LB, Martinek TJ: Growth and Development: The Child and Physical Activity. St. Louis, CV Mosby, 1980

Self-Care

Evelyn Tomlin

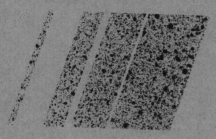

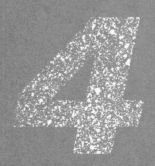

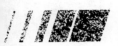

After completing this chapter, students will be able to:

● Describe the concept of self-care

● Describe consumers who are "rejectors" and "modifiers" of traditional health care.

● Identify three nurses who have demonstrated the self-care concept in their professional practice.

● Describe the relationship of self-care to each of the following: an acute-care situation, an unconscious person, infants, and caregivers.

Many definitions of nursing imply that the nurse assists others with health-care practices and activities of daily living when they are unable to care for themselves. Persons may have valuable information about both the meaning of self-care and how they wish to have others assist them or intervene on their behalf. Carl Rogers speaks of the need for clients to experience permission and freedom "... and thus their own meaningful interpretation of their experience" (1961, p. 27). It is in this context that the idea of self-care is introduced.

This chapter briefly mentions consumers who are "rejectors" or "modifiers" of traditional health care. It speaks primarily to three nursing concepts of self-care, espoused by Dorothea Orem, M. Lucille Kinlein, and Helen Erickson.

Addressed within this section are the following:

• The importance of client-identified needs and goals
• The indications that suggest that "doing for" is appropriate
• The inherent-health principle or capacity of the client
• The nurse's self-awareness.

Although self-care is frequently viewed as relating primarily to health maintenance and promotion, the concept of self-care can apply wherever persons receive nursing care. Therefore, the chapter concludes with sections illustrating self-care in an acute-care situation, with an unconscious person and infants, and with caregivers themselves.

The term **self-care** enjoys wide attention in our contemporary society, among lay persons and health-care professionals alike. Yet you will not find the expression defined in most dictionaries published before 1961. Webster defines self-care simply as "care for oneself."

A related term, **self-help,** is defined by Random House as "the act of providing for or the ability to provide for or help oneself without assistance from others."

Any widely used expression that is not clearly defined in the average dictionary is bound to command many connotations or nuances of meaning. Inevitably, our individual understandings of the term self-care will differ. As we join related ideas to form more complete concepts, our differences emerge even more clearly.

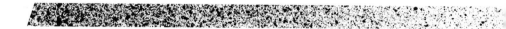

Consumer Concepts of Self-Care

"The Rejectors"

For some lay persons, self-care has connotations closer to the aforementioned dictionary definition of self-help. They envision a care of self that does not include any assistance at all from traditional health-care providers. These persons might be called the "rejectors" of traditional medical and health care. They gravitate to the idea of self-help drawn by several root concerns: professional health care is not readily available to all segments of our society; medical costs mount alarmingly; people object to impersonal treatment; the mass media disperses information to lay persons that raises their questions and increases their sophistication. Some persons adopt a critical view of contemporary medical and health-care delivery systems. Some simply decide to medicate themselves or feel they have no time to get sick. Others use folk medicine and beliefs when their health needs clamor for attention.

Self-care and self-help classes and groups and a vast popular literature have sprung up. During the 1960s, the feminist movement gave impetus to many self-help innovations. One example is a radical change in childbirth practices in the United States, with lay midwives helping woman deliver their babies at home. This is not altogether a new phenomenon, because women gave birth at home before hospital care became the traditional mode for childbirth. Alcoholics Anonymous and Recover, Inc. (for former "mental" patients) are older more established self-help groups. These have been joined by newer ones, such as Overeaters Anonymous.

"The Modifiers"

Persons who are not wholly disillusioned with the existing health-care delivery system have defined self-care in terms of more active participation in decisions made about their health. These persons might be called the "modifiers" of traditional health care. Driven by the escalating costs, fragmented care, and unequal distribution of caregiving personnel and facilities, they are beginning to take more responsibility and control over their health states. Many are eager to learn more. They realize that because of our exploding knowledge, the increasing variety of caregivers, and the complexity of care and treatment modalities, the one person best equipped to remain "in charge" of his or her own care is the client contracting for professional service. They know that they themselves are ultimately accountable for goal-setting, achievement of outcomes, and the coordination of various facets of their own care.

These people realize that only they can make the life-style changes needed to prevent or forestall calamities associated with the "diseases" of adaptation or stress-induced disorders. They demand that power and control, reserved in the past for professionals, be placed actively in the hand of the person seeking care. They cite our society's greater geographic mobility as one compelling reason for this approach.

This connotation of self-care opposes the obsolescing notion that diseases and discomforts somehow attack from outside the person and in a manner largely outside of an individual's control. A great number of people are learning how very much power they do have to alter the undesirable aspects and conditions of their lives when they receive the help they need to reach their own goal of improved wellness.

All this makes explicit a phenomenon that is well known to experienced health-care practitioners. We have long known that unless persons are significantly involved in their own care and invited and encouraged to participate in the fullest possible way in decisions concerning themselves, they will not achieve the "best-laid plans" imposed on them by well-intentioned caregivers.

Nursing Concepts of Self-Care

Nurses, too, vary in their ideas of self-care. Beyond our peripheral differences, we agree that self-care is and has been an integral, consistent part of nursing's long history. All nurses have observed that some degree of **self-care agency** (ability, power, or control) resides in every living person regardless of the health state in which they may be when they first require nursing assistance. Most people have more control and power over their health states than they or others realize. Many will take that control and responsibility when they are invited and encouraged to do so.

Dorothea Orem's Concept of Self-Care

The term "self-care" first appeared explicitly in the nursing literature in 1959 in a publication by Dorothea Orem. As Orem developed her theory of nursing, she built a complete concept of self-care suitable for nursing practice. Her notions include self-care assets and self-care deficits, self-care agency (power) and therapeutic self-care demand. These ideas lend themselves particularly well to providing nursing care for persons who are ill. Practitioners who use Orem's concept to organize and govern their nursing actions have elaborated on its application in various situations of nursing, especially in acute-care units of hospitals. Since Orem places emphasis on biophysical aspects of care of acutely and chronically ill persons, her concept stresses problem solving in nursing situations and places a heavy emphasis on patient or client education. We note that this concept is often used in actual practice to individualize an essentially standard form of care prescribed, recommended, and often imposed upon a person by members of the health team.

M. Lucille Kinlein's Self-Care Concept

M. Lucille Kinlein, a former student and colleague of Orem, set forth her own self-care concept, modified from that of Orem, whom she credits as her original inspiration (1977). Kinlein's concept applies particularly well to nursing persons who are essentially healthy but want to maintain or enhance their present state. Kinlein's 9 years in a private practice of nursing showed that people want verification and expansion of their own knowledge and self-care practices. She expected her clients to express their particular need or desire for her care through their verbalization as she gave them her undivided attention. Nurses violate Kinlein's self-care concept when they introduce, either by consciousness raising or by direct statement, a problem or potential problem that was not first suggested by the client.

Helen Erickson's Concept of Self-Care

Just as Kinlein modified Orem's concept in her private practice, in which she nursed essentially healthy or well persons, others have naturally and inevitably adapted the concept of self-care to their experiences. Helen Erickson's concept of self-care incorporates ideas common to many nurse experts, including Orem and Kinlein, into her own special perspectives. Erickson's concept of self-care, when applied from her comprehensive conceptual framework or model for nursing, is equally useful with persons who are ill or well, young or old, in whatever place they may be receiving or needing nursing.

Client-Identified Goals

At the heart of Erickson's concept of self-care is the notion of client-identified needs and goals. Each individual knows the kind of help he needs to mobilize his own strengths and resources. Erickson has said that those who are ill know what has made them ill and what will make them well. According to Erickson, if a person does not know this at a conscious level, he knows it subconsciously and may need expert nursing to identify the particular help he wants and needs.

This type of nursing respects an individual's personal timing and readiness for action. It takes heed of the system(s) within which a person lives, the effect of change in a single member, and the speed of that change upon the system as a whole. When one member of a family or group changes, others are also affected in some significant way. Such nursing requires skillful listening and observing. Subsequent nursing actions or interventions are based on judgments made of the individual's coping or adjusting potential. These judgments enable the nurse to offer confidently either of two services:

- Supportive nursing consisting of information, support for emotional self-expression, or assistance with desired behavior changes

- More assertive nursing agency designed to anticipate basic biophysical and psychosocial needs, reduce stressors, reinforce available resources, or replenish depleted ones

Interdependency and Autonomy

Erickson teaches that a person never reaches a state of life in which he does not at some time want or need the help of another. Healthy, happy persons, particularly those who live up to their fullest health potential, enjoy interdependency, a state of freely giving and receiving help in a continuous interactive flow or process. Caring (well) for oneself, taking (good) care of oneself, and that which some call "self-care for health" involve learning to know and exercise one's power to choose and creating conditions within one's relationships with persons and one's environment wherein personal growth and development toward an ever-healthier state occur (Fig. 4-1).

The nurturance or *nursing* of these self-care powers is the ultimate goal of nursing judgments and action. Some would call this the nurturance of autonomy—a state of knowing and freely exercising persons' actual, reality-based choices. The choices are either to do alone what persons are perfectly capable of doing for themselves or to ask their associates or support systems openly, directly, and kindly for what they want or need from them. They do this to attain, maintain, or increase a state of health.

Nursing Implications

Nurses help people do those things they would do unaided if they had the necessary strength, will, or knowledge. As we help them cope with their life circumstances and events, it is important that we do not unthinkingly do for people what they have power to do for themselves. Our ultimate purpose will be to help them become truly independent of us, no longer needing the assistance of a professional. This includes deciding for themselves when and if that point is reached.

In gaining that goal, however, there are times

Figure 4-1
Self-care for health is many things. *(Photo by Bob Kalmbach; University of Michigan Information Services)*

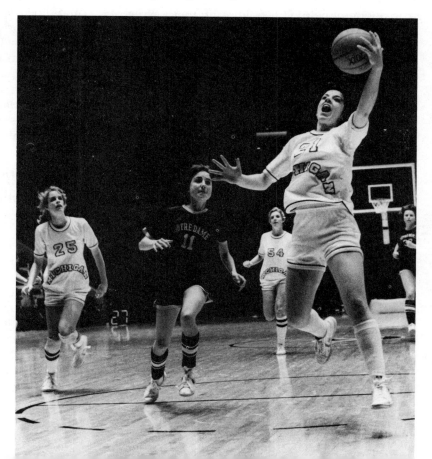

when a nurse will choose to do for the person something he or she may have the physical capacity to do. There are times when "doing for" is indicated because the nurse has identified the person to be in an impoverished coping state in which a more immediate emotional need for someone to "take over" temporarily exists. A nurse practicing from Erickson's framework will purposefully meet that need. Using the guideline of such a framework helps to ensure that the nurse will not add extra debilitating stressors upon a person. The nurse will not, therefore, insist that he attain a state of independence prematurely, given his individual readiness and timing, or hold him back by an uncritical application of "nursing routines" or traditions.

If a client learns that doing for himself invariably leads to a loss of contact with someone who cares, the exercise of self-care power may be undermined. In such instances, the person may come to equate independence with a loss of important caring relationships or attachment figures. Nurses need to convey that caring will be extended even when active physical assistance or problem solving is no longer needed. Persons need to know that they may contact their nurses to share satisfactions, gains, and achievements without receiving a brush-off or perfunctory attention.

Self-Care Goals

The notion of helping people reach their own goals is vitally linked to Erickson's central self-care assumption. A capacity for healing and movement toward health and wholeness exist at both conscious and unconscious levels of individuals whom she describes as multisystem persons. Quality nursing is not doing activities for, to, or at a person. Rather, it provides care a person values at important levels of his being. It is given through an interactive process, in which the person perceives himself to be deeply respected as a participant–executor to the fullest possible extent in the decisions that affect his care. For example, acting on the assumption that someone is capable of understanding often gives a person strength to concentrate so that he does indeed understand. It may seem more efficient at times to tell someone what to do or to skip the explanations. But in the long run, it can be the least efficient means to achieve a desired outcome. It can cause setbacks in a person who uses precious energy in a struggle to meet demands made by caregivers who believe he is capable of something he actually cannot do or does not currently believe himself ready to do. Patients under such pressure sometimes achieve a

pseudoindependence that is subject to relapse with the first additional stressor that reactivates old beliefs and convictions of helplessness and hopelessness.

To be sure that we do not impose our personal goals upon patients and clients and to guard against exercising any personal need to control or have inordinate authority over others, each nursing student needs to develop self-awareness about his or her own continuous personal growth and development. Whenever students or graduate nurses find themselves labeling patients, calling them "stubborn," "uncooperative," or "noncompliant," it is instructive for them to take stock of their own expectations and behaviors. These are common warning signals that a power struggle may be developing. These situations are particularly out of place when nursing is practiced from a self-care concept. To regain a professional perspective, it is often helpful to share one's feelings, thoughts, and perceptions about a particular nursing situation with a trusted instructor or other colleague. As we continue to grow along with our clients and patients, we receive multiple benefits—personal as well as professional.

At times, persons may refuse or decline suggestions, recommendations, and assistance offered by health-care providers. From a nursing perspective, we may personally desire a client to have different understanding, attitudes, and behaviors. Yet we must take care not to withdraw our professional support and concern for the client as a whole person, however misguided, misbehaved, or maladaptive portions of his behavior may seem to us. Occasionally a client asks a nurse to do something that would violate the nurse's own values. It is essential to communicate one's personal position along with any supportive information and then to continue interacting or gracefully standing by until the individual either changes his requirements of the nurse or ends the professional relationship on his own initiative.

Setting Priorities

Erickson ordinarily ranks interventions designed to meet unmet basic needs according to the client's own priorities. She invites clients to share the worry, question, or concern that most immediately engages his attention. His immediate priorities may not match the nurse's own. Erickson comfortably accepts a gradual uncovering of unmet needs as mutual trust between nurse and client is established and allowed to develop. It is imperative to Erickson that the client perceive no further losses through the action of a caregiver. The nurse helps either by adding to existing strengths or resources or by substituting new thoughts, feelings, and actions that the client prefers. It has been Erickson's and others common experience that a "ripple-out" effect occurs as a result of a fulfilled need. That is, the client himself often takes over caring for other aspects of his health that also need attention. Sometimes he does this through newly learned or reinforced skills of asking directly for specific help he desires and choosing to follow through with alacrity. Often he simply takes care of these matters by himself with the help of his personal support system, vividly illustrating the phenomenon that success breeds success. In these instances he has, indeed, made the common sense of nursing operational for himself.

Self-Care Concept Illustrated

Erickson and Tomlin, in their association with M. A. Swain, have collected significant research data in support of key elements of the Erickson conceptual model.

Acute-Care Situation

The following example from Tomlin's practice illustrates this perspective.

Example □ A woman in her sixties was being treated medically with radiation and chemotherapy following surgery for removal of a cancer that had subsequently spread widely throughout her body. Her physicians judged that she was not responding as they expected to their current treatment.

Her white blood count and resistance to infection were dangerously low. She had no appetite, had developed pneumonia, and was plagued with intense pain on moving in bed and especially when getting out of bed to attend to toileting needs. She requested help from the nurse, to talk in order to prepare herself for what her doctors had concluded would be her soon and certain death.

When first seen by the nurse, she complained of deep fatigue, her color was gray, she was short of breath and lying stiffly in bed with lines in her forehead and lackluster eyes. She spoke slowly and softly with many short sighs interspersed.

As the nurse sat beside her bed ready to carry out their explicit contract to deal with her death concern, the nurse noted that her client ranged in random fashion from topic to topic, none of which touched on the subject of dying. She spoke of her extreme weakness and fatigue, of her sadness seeing her husband's emotional response to

her deteriorating condition, of the excruciating nature of her pain when getting out of bed, her terror of its inevitable recurrence because using a bedpan was "even worse." She lamented her inability to believe her doctors when they spoke of their findings and their earlier expressed hope for her favorable response to therapy. She felt exhausted from her visitors but would not ask any of them to shorten or postpone their stays. She would sacrifice any mention of her particular wants or needs to a preeminent need to be liked and approved of by the nurses as an undemanding "good patient." There were others on the acute-care hospital unit "who need the nurses' care more than I."

She had spent precious energy giving gifts to and "entertaining" many nurses who, with genuine personal affection and sympathy, stopped by her bedside frequently to say a cheery word to this "incredible lady" who had so many friends, whose condition and prognosis (or medical prediction) was so "helpless and tragic."

After establishing through active listening that the patient's main concern now was her pain on getting up out of bed, the nurse contracted to set a time together to exchange information, feelings, knowledge, and skills in an effort to find a way to work with or reduce that pain to a tolerable level. The setting of this simple goal in itself required much reassurance of the nurse's willingness to spend the necessary time and effort to carry out the plan. Clearly Mrs. A. suffered a severe loss of self-esteem and found it hard to believe that she could be "worth so much time and attention." Hesitantly, she gave the nurse the very essential data she alone knew about her past efforts and experiences in attempts to get up.

The 15-minute interval spent working together on this problem required continuous attention to Mrs. A.'s sense of safety and security: her fear of encountering a pain over which she would have no control, her repeatedly verbalized reluctance to bother the busy nurse by taking her time in this manner. At first, she believed herself helpless and lacking the ability to make any contribution to the project—even discounting the usefulness of describing her anticipated fears and present-moment sensations—until she was reassured by a variety of means, including gentle yet confident voice tones, thoughtfully placed touches, soft smiles, and a bit of humor.

The time the nurse took to deal with her escalated fear, as well as the control the nurse repeatedly gave back to her over the "what if's" she raised, finally paid off. As Mrs. A. accepted the particular suggestions of the nurse which she felt she could handle, she built on each successful step of an incremental process to bring herself to a sitting position on the side of the bed through her own power entirely.

Sitting on the side of the bed, shaking her head in disbelief at having raised herself up without a twinge of pain, she gave a deep sigh of relief, "For the first time, I have hope." She promptly launched into an animated description of how she would be able to get up to the bathroom freely where she would assume "the only sitting position" that would enable her to deep breathe and cough without aggravating her pain. Although she knew how important this was to combat the pneumonia, she had been reporting falsely to the nurses her compliance with these doctor's orders because of the extreme pain and her fear of displeasing her caregivers. She also volunteered that she had been limiting her own fluid intake to reduce the number of times she needed to get up out of bed and would now no longer risk giving herself a urinary-tract infection through that practice. She requested a favorite sandwich for dinner, affirming that she knew she would be able to "keep it down" now. And she capped her remarks by announcing her intention to live at least "till Christmas" (6 months away) to fulfill a special dream she had earlier abandoned.

She did indeed follow through on every one of her own decisions. Within a few days, she amazed her physicians, who asked her, "Just what did that nurse *do* to turn you around?" She laughed merrily when she reported that they wanted to learn the particular method by which she had brought herself up to the side of the bed. She herself knew that although she had indeed taken advantage of some important principles of body mechanics, what had really happened was a reactivation and resumption of her self-care powers through an integrative nursing process that had restored her hope and belief in herself as a worthwhile person. She herself had accepted the invitation given her to actively take her strengths and the power she still had—to choose to live! □

Situation with an Unconscious Person

Recent studies have shown that unconscious persons actually hear and retain remarks made in their presence. We propose that "not dying" is an expression of a desire to live. As the nurse provides holistic care, the person will hear inspiriting, encouraging remarks. He will also tactilely sense or experience the respect with which his body is handled. To whatever extent the tissues are capable of regaining a former healthy state, the person will be facilitated by the nurse's "invitation to live." Relatives and significant others need the nurse's support to supplement and reinforce those "invitations" while receiving support as necessary from nurses for their own whole-person needs.

Erickson tells of a 34-year-old patient in her experience who was unconscious following surgery for an inoperable tumor of the brain that had begun

a dreaded spread. A deeply concerned husband repeated his communications of caring in her ears, reminding her of her worth and importance to him and their children. He spoke of feelings he presumed her to have about her current total dependency on others for every physical need. He expressed his hope for her recovery and plans for their continuing life together. Despite predictions of a fatal outcome with the best medical treatment, the patient recovered and two years later showed a completely normal brain scan.

Situation with Infants

Fascinating studies involving the newborn are increasing our understanding of the indivduality and differing preferences of the youngest of infants. Although without verbal language skills during their earliest months, even the youngest infants know how to make their wants and needs known—as most mothers and fathers will readily confirm. This is indeed a very real self-care capacity and can be nurtured ever more deliberately as we continue to learn more of children and their deep need for attachment to a primary caregiver.

Situation with Care Givers

A discussion on self-care is incomplete without mention of the principle that as nurses engage increasingly in more effective caring for themselves as whole persons, they provide a powerful model for clients to reach ever healthier levels of self-caring. It is still true that "what you *are* speaks so loudly, I cannot hear what you say." From a purely practical perspective, nurses who do not take necessary steps to see that their own real needs are met will become less and less able to lend their strengths and skills to others.

Conclusion

Although ideas about self-care may vary among nurses and lay persons, the term is widely used. Caring for self may be a reaction to the confusion and complexity of health-care delivery. Clients' desires to practice self-care are also a statement of belief about controlling individual destiny and potential.

Self-care is a contemporary value held in common by differing segments of our society. The notion that each individual has a right and responsibilty to choose, to create, and to care for himself or herself is deeply rooted in Judeo–Christian teaching. These religions value each individual because he has been created in God's image (and is thus creative) and has been given a divine imperative to love God and others as he loves or cares for himself. Naturalistic humanists find the self-care concept compatible with their belief in the centrality of human values, welfare, and dignity, which is linked to their belief that individuals create and develop their own futures. Eastern religious teachings, including those of the mystical systems, emphasize certain humanist values that are consistent with self-care practices.

Nurses who seek to give person-centered care will recognize that their clients are the source of much valuable information about themselves and their own self-care. Nurses will use the person's knowledge, strengths, and goals to provide meaningful individualized care. The challenge of self-care is one of collaboration between nurse and client. The subject is a broad and engrossing one, and we encourage you to take advantage of the readings listed at the end of this chapter.

Study Questions

1. What are your own self-care practices?

2. How will you discover your client's self-care potential?

3. How do the ideas of self-care relate to Maslow's hierarchy of needs?

4. How do self-care abilities relate to Erik Erikson's developmental tasks and change with age?

Glossary

Self-care: Caring for oneself (Webster).

Self-care agency: Ability, power, or control over one's health state.

Self-help: The act of providing for or the ability to provide for or help oneself without assistance from others (Random House).

Bibliography

Cheek DB, LeGron LM: Clinical Hypnotherapy. New York, Grune & Stratton, 1968

Erickson HC, Tomlin EM, Swain MAP: Modeling and Role Modeling: A Theory and Paradigm for Nursing. Englewood Cliffs, New Jersey, Prentice-Hall, 1983

James D, Jongeward D: Born to Win: Transactional Analysis with Gestalt Experiments. Reading, Massachusetts, Addison-Wesley, 1971

Joseph L: Self care and the nursing process. Nurs Clin North Am 15, No. 1: 131–143, 1980

Jourard SM: The Transparent Self. Princeton, Van Nostrand, Reinhold, 1964

Kinlein ML: Independent Nursing Care with Clients. Philadelphia, JB Lippincott, 1977

Levin LS, Katz AH, Holst E: Self Care: Lay Initiatives in Health. New York, Prodist, a Division of Neale Watson Academic Publications, 1976

Mullins V: Implementing the self care concept in the acute care setting. Nurs Clin North Am 3:177–190, 1980

Norris CM: Self Care. Am J Nurs 79, No. 3: 486–489, Mar 1979

Orem DE: Nursing: Concepts of Practice. New York, McGraw-Hill, 1971

Orem D (ed): Concept Formalization in Nursing: Process and Product. Boston, Little Brown & Co, 1979

Orem DE: Guides for Developing Curricula for the Education of Practical Nurses. Washington, DC, Government Printing Office, 1959

Powell J: Why Am I Afraid to Tell You Who I Am? Chicago, Argus Communications, 1969

Rogers C: On Becoming a Person. Boston, Houghton Mifflin, 1961

Satir V: Making Contact. Milbane, California, Celestial Arts, 1976

Simonton OC, Matthews-Simonton S: Getting Well Again. Los Angeles, Tarcher, 1978

Steckel S: Patient Contracting. New York, Appleton-Century-Crofts, 1982

Swain MA, Steckel SB: Influencing adherence among hypertensives. Res Nurs Health 4: 213–222, 1981

Williamson J: Mutual interaction: A model of nursing practice. Nurs Outlook 29:104–107, 1981

Williamson JD, Dancher K: Self-Care in Health. New York, Neale Watson Academic, 1978

Health
and Adaptation

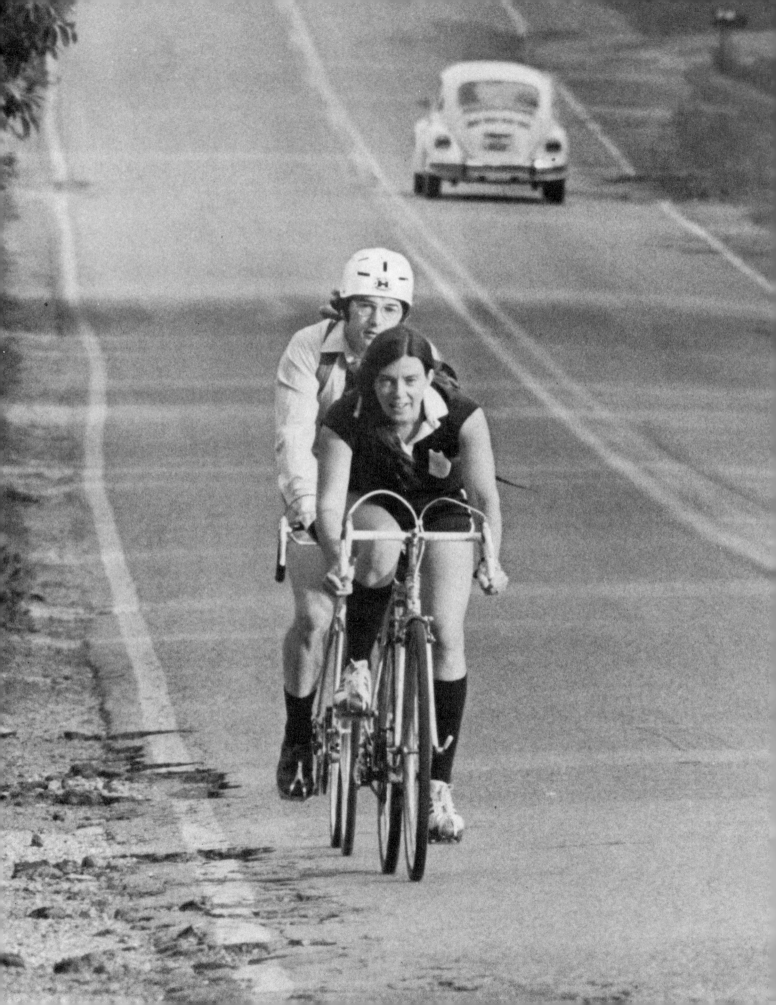

II

Health and Adaptation

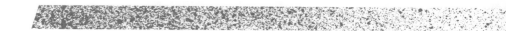

The purpose of this section is to present the concepts of health and adaptation that underlie person-centered nursing practice. Discussion in the previous section dealt partly with the nature of the person. This section focuses on how persons adapt to their world.

A goal of nursing is to help people maintain optimal biopsychosocial functioning by coping with a changing environment and functional alterations or deviations from health. To accomplish this goal, nurses need to understand the interaction of persons and their environment, as well as the evolution of the concepts of health and adaptation.

The concepts of health and adaptation are of necessity interwoven, although we have separated them for purposes of discussion. Evolving definitions of health recognize and mention the holistic nature of persons and the complexity of interaction between persons and their environment. The process of adaptation that contributes to health is concerned not only with environment but with what happens within the person as he copes.

A major premise of this section is that, because each person is unique, nurses must develop unique ways to help each person adapt. This section, therefore, presents several theories of adaptation and several approaches to the person-environment interaction. This will enable nurses to assist clients in adapting to their unique life experiences. Within nursing, students will encounter many experts who believe that the concept of adaptation is an important key to establishing a unique body of knowledge or a unifying theory base for nursing. The section concludes with a particular consideration: adaptation of the older person.

Health

Marguerite B. Harms

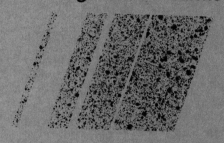

Objectives

Introduction

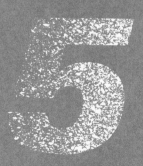

After completing this chapter, students will be able to:

● Develop a nursing perspective of health.

● Identify environmental variables.

● Describe reciprocal interactions between persons and the environment as systems.

● Relate own nursing practice to knowledge of biopsychosocial variables of persons in their interactions with the environment.

● Recognize various definitions of health.

● Contrast the primitive, medical–physiologic, ecologic, equilibrium, and social models of illness.

● Identify ways the professional nurse promotes health.

As a nurse you are in a unique position to learn how to help yourself at the same time you learn how to help others. You are privileged to assist persons in dealing with some of their most difficult, intimate life experiences. As a health professional, you make life and death decisions in collaboration with clients, their families, and other health professionals. Nurses need to know a great deal about life and people and health.

Currently, we are learning more and more about human health and survival, stress, crisis, coping, prevention, biofeedback, fitness, and wellness. Research findings support the belief that many illnesses and health problems are stress related and preventable. Many psychophysiological disorders—often labeled psychosomatic illnesses—are now recognized as stress related, occurring when people do not cope effectively with change. Certain disorders, such as asthma, ulcers, hypertension, some cancers, depression, phobias, alcoholism, drug abuse, periodic attacks of epilepsy, and migraine headaches, are also considered by some authorities to be linked to stress.

With so many health problems apparently associated with ineffective coping, every individual is presented with the opportunity and the challenge to learn how to stay well. Before we address this opportunity and challenge through the process of adaptation in Chapter 6, we must look at the environment within which the person lives and interacts. Next, we must consider how the concept of health has evolved over time.

Persons, Environment, and Their Interaction

Environment

The person was described in Chapter 2 as an open system composed of biological, psychological, and social variables. The **environment** also can be considered an open system composed of subsystems and their variables, whether they be social, natural, or man-made. The *social environment* consists of other human beings with whom persons interact in the family, in the community, and in society. The *natural environment* includes those aspects of the environment that exist independently of humans, such as climate or topography. The *man-made environment* includes human achievements in service to others, as well as undesired consequences of man's creativity. All are essential to the study of persons.

Examples of environmental variables are presented in Table 5-1. These examples point out how complex each subsystem is. Consequently, the survival and health of each of us is dependent upon our own strengths and resourcefulness in dealing with forces to which we are subject.

Both people and environments are living, dynamic systems with porous boundaries capable of exchanging matter, energy, and information. The person, for example, receives internal information from his body indicating hunger. His response is to take food from the environment. The same food becomes a source of energy for the person's body.

Picture the interaction between living systems such as would occur with a man lost on a rainy day in a noisy, crowded city in a foreign country whose language he does not speak. Figure 5-1 shows the reciprocal interaction between these two systems—person and environment. Note the multiple complex systems and subsystems within the environment that each person with his or her multiple subsystem is likely to encounter. Considering the amount of matter, energy, and information that is exchanged between these systems, it is remarkable that we complex persons are able to maintain equilibrium in an equally complex environment.

Homeodynamics

When living systems operate in an effective or healthy state, they interact to produce a balance within each system and a balance among the various systems (Fig. 5-2). This reciprocal interaction to maintain equilibrium is called **homeodynamics.** When change occurs in either the person or the environment, disequilibrium or disorganization may result. This disequilibrium requires an adjustment. For example, a person responds to a change in the weather by altering the amount of clothing worn for protection. Such a response maintains health against the threat of heat or cold.

If the person and his environment do not interact in an effective, healthy way, regaining the homeodynamic state becomes difficult. For example, a man who smokes heavily may eventually develop respiratory disease. If he also lives in an area with high concentrations of air pollutants, this likelihood becomes even greater. Health, then, is linked to the effective interaction of persons with their environ-

Table 5-1
Examples of Environmental Variables

Social Variables	Natural Variables	Man-Made Variables
Human relationships	Water	Tools and machines
Interpersonal communications	Air	Buildings
Community groups	Land	Towns and cities
Family groups	Plants	Business and industry
Interest groups	Animals	Transportation
Culture	Microorganisms	Technology
Societal norms	Minerals	Pollution
Life-style	Space	Chemical
Philosophy	Solar systems	Noise
Social roles	Natural laws of physics	Accidents
Societal institutions	Energy	Overcrowding
Education	Weather	Privacy
Marriage	Heat	Urban decay
Government	Cold	Drugs
Economy	Light	Violence
Religion	Sound	Conservation
		Art
		Music
		Architecture
		Books

ments. As stated in *Healthy People: The Surgeon General's Report on Health Promotion and Disease Prevention:* (DHEW, 1979, pp. 1–12, 13)

> For decision makers in the public and private sector, a recognition of the relationship between health and the physical environment can lead to actions that can greatly reduce the morbidity and mortality caused by accidents, air, water, and food contamination, radiation exposure, excessive noise, occupational hazards, dangerous consumer products and unsafe highway design.

As informed decision makers, nurses ought to influence health-promoting action both in their private lives as citizens and in their professional lives as nurses concerned with person-centered care. For example, with a knowledge of both the community environment and local health practices, the community-health nurse may alert citizens to hazards they have not recognized. The mechanism by which persons adjust to their environment is the process of adaptation.

What Is Health?

Nurses promote health by helping the person to preserve and strengthen adaptation and to develop new strategies to regain homeodynamics. Therefore, it is essential that we understand the concept of health and the process of adaptation.

Health means different things to different people; nevertheless, the term is a familiar one. It is easy to relate the concept of health to ourselves by recalling past experiences of illness as well as those activities performed to keep well. Some consider health the opposite of illness. Others view health as something one has or does not have, as shown in these statements:

- When you have your health, you have everything.
- My health is good.
- I lost my health when. . . .
- I have a health problem.
- How's your health?

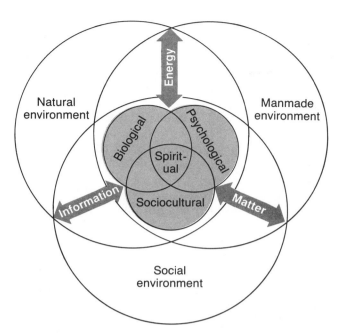

Figure 5-1
There is a reciprocal interaction between person and environment.

Figure 5-2
Persons and environments are open systems that interact with each other. *(Photo by Bob Kalmbach; University of Michigan Information Services)*

Control over one's health may be implied when persons refer to various activities or substances:

- It is healthy to exercise and eat well.
- Smoking may be hazardous to your health.

These examples illustrate a variety of perspectives about the concept of health. Definitions developed over the past several years will demonstrate the effort being made by the scientific community to define health more precisely.

Definitions of Health

Absence of Disease

For many years the phrase "absence of disease" was the criterion for defining health. It reflected the medical model of health. Over the years, other definitions evolved, such as the one issued by the World Health Organization.

World Health Organization

The World Health Organization was hailed for recognizing the whole person when, in 1947, it stated a new, very broad definition of health in its constitution. This definition was unique because it introduced a more humanistic perspective than previously accepted. The definition of health was as follows:

> . . . a state of complete physical, mental, and social well-being, not merely the absence of disease or infirmity.

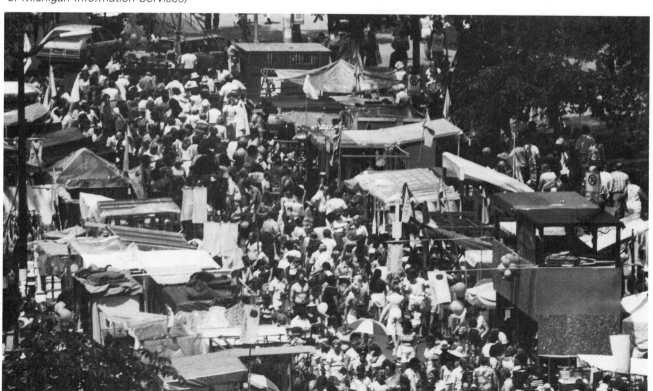

Health–Illness Continuum

Another definition, the health–illness continuum, perpetuated the medical model by equating health with absence of illness. This model pictured a horizontal scale with health at one pole and illness at the other. Health was viewed as the opposite of illness. Many found the health–illness continuum model unsatisfactory because most people are neither totally healthy nor totally ill. It was difficult to accept a model that placed persons at one particular point of the continuum. Jahoda rejected the health–illness continuum in reference to mental health. She wrote, "As with every other typological classification, pure types do not exist. Every human being has simultaneously healthy and sick aspects, with one or the other predominating" (1958, p. 75).

Humanistic Perspective

In the 1950s, some psychologists began to question the emphasis that traditional psychology placed on human continuity with the animal world. This continuity is seen in both Freud's perception of man as dominated by base instincts and Skinner's perception of man as responding mechanically to stimulation. Through these approaches, specific scientific methods were applied to the study of human beings, in an attempt to organize human characteristics into categories and subsequently to predict behavioral outcomes. However, neither the psychoanalytical model (identified with Freud and called "first-force psychology") nor the behavioral-modification model (identified with Skinner and called "second-force psychology") addressed variables that contributed to the uniqueness of humans or the humanism of persons.

The humanistic psychologists who emerged in the 1950s became identified with "third-force psychology." They did recognize the uniqueness and wholeness of persons and pointed to significant human qualities that were previously overlooked—qualities such as growth, individuality, autonomy, self-actualization, self-development, productivity, and self-realization. Among these new psychologists was Abraham Maslow, whose work is described in Chapter 2. Humanistic philosophy forms a basis for person-centered psychology and, by extension, for person-centered nursing. Maslow wrote (1968, p. 27):

> . . . The psychological life of the person, in many of its aspects, is lived out differently when he is deficiency–need–gratification-bent and when he is growth-dominated or "meta-motivated" or growth motivated or self-actualizing."

Maslow and others such as Carl Rogers recognized that striving and growing are essential to human life and health. Their work challenged both Freudian beliefs about the pleasure principle and Skinnerian behaviorist principles, and a holistic view of persons evolved.

As a result of this humanistic movement, perspectives on health began to broaden; perceptions of human potential expanded. The previously dependent patient emerged as a liberated, rational, creative, free-thinking person capable of self-realization, self-development, and autonomy. Informed persons began to take responsibility for their own health care; nurses and other health professionals helped clients to achieve self-care.

By the 1950s, for example, Yale–New Haven Hospital in Connecticut had instituted the humanistic practice of childbirth education classes. Expectant parents, both wives and husbands, were invited to learn natural childbirth, relaxation techniques, and new options for labor and delivery. Husbands were taught how to support their wives during labor. The choice of breast-feeding *versus* bottle-feeding was encouraged, as were rooming-in for mother and baby and expanded visiting privileges for fathers. These innovative practices gradually became the norm. Today's movement toward homelike birthing represents an extension of humanistic and consumer-oriented choice.

Dubos and King

Dubos, a 20th-century biologist and philosopher, wrote that health or disease is the expression of the success or failure by people in their efforts to respond adaptively to environmental challenges (1965, p. xvii). This description postulates a relationship between health, adaptation, and environment. Imogene King, a nurse educator, wrote a working definition of health that elaborates on Dubos' premise (1971, p. 72):

> Health is a dynamic state in the life cycle of an organism which implies continuous adaptation to stresses in the internal and external environment through optimum use of one's resources to achieve maximum potential for daily living.

Her reference to health as a dynamic state supports the contention that illness is not the opposite pole of health but rather an interruption of or interference with a healthy state.

Murray and Zentner

More recently, Murray and Zentner developed working definitions of health and illness for their text,

Nursing Concepts for Health Promotion. They wrote (1979, pp. 5–6):

> Health is a purposeful, adaptive response, physically, mentally, emotionally, and socially, to internal and external stimuli in order to maintain stability and comfort; and illness is a disturbed adaptive response to internal and external stimuli resulting in disequilibrium and inability to utilize the usual health-promoting resources.

High-Level Wellness

Another view on health favors the concept of wellness. H.L. Dunn contrasted "wellness" with "good health" (1959, p. 447):

> Good health can exist as a relatively passive state of freedom from illness in which the individual is at peace with his environment—a condition of relative homeostasis. Wellness is conceptualized as dynamic—a condition of change in which the individual moves forward, climbing toward a higher potential of functioning.

He defined **high-level wellness** as "an integrated method of functioning which is oriented toward maximizing the potential of which the individual is capable within the environment where he is functioning" (p. 447). High-level wellness involves the following:

- A continuing improvement in the way we function
- Continuing progress in our ability to respond to life's challenges
- Increasing oneness of our whole being—mind, body, and spirit—in the way we function

Dunn's views reflected the humanism of third-force psychologists; moreover, his role as a physician in the U.S. Public Health Service gave him the opportunity to influence a vast number of health professionals. For generations health care has been illness care in the United States and throughout many parts of the world. Both health-care providers and recipients often expect health-care professionals to treat illnesses and infirmities, not to deliver health maintenance and prevention of illness.

For many years, nurses in public health, industry, schools, and maternity hospitals have been engaged in efforts to promote health, prevent illness, and maintain wellness (Fig. 5-3). Recently, the impact of Dunn's thinking has begun to reach beyond the community of those health professionals who have been promoting the philosophy of health–wellness and self-care. Today, consumers are actively engaged

Figure 5-3
Nurses have traditionally been engaged in efforts to promote health and maintain wellness. *(Photo by Bob Kalmbach; University of Michigan Information Services)*

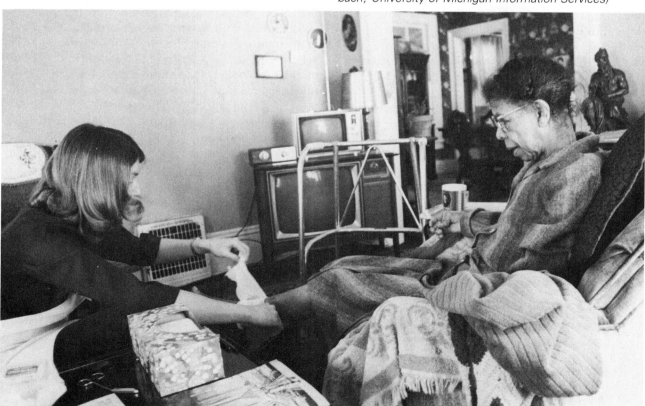

in health promotion by taking fitness classes, jogging, eating more natural foods, attending weight-reduction clinics voluntarily, and so on. Health educators are also joining the effort. Hospital administrators, personnel directors, and health-insurance firms that are concerned about the rising costs of illness care are encouraging the development of health–wellness programs to reduce their costs and to educate the public.

Related to the concepts of health maintenance and self-care is the important concept of a person's strengths. When the nurse assists people in situations of wellness, it is important to assess their strengths by learning about their past as well as their present abilities, skills, interests, coping capacities, and general life experiences. The nurse needs to recognize and mobilize the person's unique strengths. Otto states that those strengths "relate both to the self-concept and to feelings of self-esteem and self-worth which the patient has, and they can be an aid in mobilizing health and regenerative processes" (1965, p. 32). Otto also wrote (p. 33):

> By recognizing the potentialities which are present in every human being, the element of hope is extended and this in turn functions as a dynamic force in the struggle for restoration of health and well-being."

Holistic Health

The term "holistic," introduced in Chapter 2, refers to the concept of each person as a separate whole being. Holistic health, also spelled "wholistic," is a contemporary term for the humanistic movement in health-care delivery whereby the health-care provider and client examine together every aspect of the client's life-style to promote wellness. By learning skills for coping and by changing life-styles and attitudes, an individual may achieve a high level of wellness.

Some refer to holistic health care as a specific treatment modality and an alternative to the medical model of treatment. The medical model of care assumes that, after medical diagnosis of a specific illness or dysfunction, a specified medical treatment (such as a drug, surgery, therapeutic diet, or exercise) will be prescribed as an external cure for the diagnosed condition. On the other hand, the holistic approach to health-care delivery includes all helping professions working in concert on behalf of the whole person.

The East–West Academy of Healing Arts, located in San Francisco, has described holistic health as "the teachings and traditions of ethnic cultural groups who have brought forth a functional theory of an existing energy system which is basic to all living forms." In addition they say that "... the mind and the will play important roles in the individual's capability to assume responsibility for his/her role as the ultimate resource for assessing and coping with the stressors of life" (East–West Academy of Healing Arts). Healing arts of East and West include accumassage, accupressure, relaxation techniques, exercises, and meditation.

Today we see persons with high blood pressure responding to the techniques of relaxation and biofeedback as a method for controlling and lowering blood pressure. Another innovation is relaxation response, which is a specific treatment modality using meditation for stress reduction that has been promoted by Herbert Benson, a physician at Harvard. Conventional therapy and adjunctive interventions, such as imagery and reinforcement of strong spiritual belief systems, also have contributed to rallying the immune system of responsive individuals with cancer, either to delay or to overcome the expected progression of metastasis and ultimate death (e.g. the work of the Simontons). Therapeutic touch is a form of touch healing practiced by Krieger, a nurse. All of these more recent therapeutic modalities, of course, are subject to further study.

Health and Illness

Certain life experiences that interfere with an individual's health have been called illness. As perspectives about health have changed, so have perspectives about illness. A cursory review of five different models of the nature of illness illustrates various perspectives on humans. Table 5-2 presents the key points of five models of illness. The primitive model, the medical–physiological model, the ecological model, the equilibrium model, and the social model.

Key concepts within the description of each model have been underscored. These concepts point out the relevance of all models to our present understanding of humans and the phenomenon of illness. The overlapping of concepts among models supports the view that illness is the result of multiple physiological, ecological, and social causes.

The key concepts also pose questions about health. If we believed that persons were defenseless victims of disease as described in the primitive model, we could do little to prevent or treat those who are affected. Of course, we recognize the fallacy of this belief because we have seen persons recover from many serious afflictions. Yet some depressed persons

Table 5-2
Models of Illness

Model	Description
Primitive	Views illness as an autonomous, amorphous being that attacks and kills *defenseless persons*. Also sees it as a punishment for sins.
Medical–physiological	Views illness according to directly observable aberration; *i.e., presence of microorganisms, toxic germs, bacteria,* or *trauma*. Aberrations fit into certain static or divisional lines, which are classified (clinical syndromes).
Ecological	Views illness according to directly observable aberrations, in which interaction between *poor* or *unhealthy environment* and virulent *disease* or injury-producing agent meet *susceptible individual*.
Equilibrium	Views illness as a dynamic process, a *disturbance in equilibrium between humans and their environment*. Illness is a *reaction of the whole organism*, a consequence of factors in a reaction—internal and external stimuli as well as predisposition of the individual.
Social	Views illness as incapacity to perform social roles and tasks based upon feelings of not being well. (Cause not identified.)

who are grieving and guilt-ridden over their past behaviors (which they may view as sins) may be operating according to this model.

On close examination, the other models also exhibit shortcomings. Using the medical–physiological model, how do we explain the variety of responses we see among persons exposed to the same organisms or traumas? Not everyone becomes ill when exposed to the same environment. The ecological model describes the susceptibility of individuals to illness. Yet how do we evaluate who is susceptible and who is not when all other factors are present, as in the ecological and medical–physiological model? The equilibrium model reflects the concept of adaptation. This model includes concepts from the four previous ones and focuses on the organism as a whole.

The social model has long been in existence among many societies and cultures. Persons who give complaints of illness are excused from their social roles and responsibilities. However, subjective feelings alone are not always considered sufficient determinants of illness. For many, such illnesses are seen as avoidance behavior. Consider how many years women were excused from physical exertion and other activities during menstruation. For many others, such as the combat soldier or migrant farmer, the excuse of "not feeling well" would be scorned.

These five models suggest a number of perspectives about health. Today, nurses encounter a variety of views about health held by persons from different cultures in the United States and other parts of the world. Actually, wellness and illness are culturally determined; what is healthy, normal behavior in one culture may be considered unhealthy, abnormal behavior in another. Therefore, the nurse is challenged to understand the biological, psychological, social-cultural, and environmental facets of persons who may be patients or clients.

Health Behavior and Illness Behavior

Efforts by others to define health have been directed toward objective criteria, namely behavior. The term **behavior** is defined as an emitted response (action or reaction); it is overt, observable, and measurable. Consequently, scientists in the health-care field have begun research to define and clarify behavior as outcomes of health that can be measured and evaluated.

The concept of health behavior is quite complex and extensive, as evidenced by the literature on the subject. However, Wu's definition is one of the most succinct and serves the nurse and consumer well. Wu wrote that **health behavior** is ". . . any activity undertaken by an individual who believes himself to be well to avoid an encounter with illness." Behaviors such as regular hygienic practices and participation in "well-balanced programs of rest, exercise, diet, and elimination," may be considered health behaviors (1973, p. 112). Health-wellness, Wu writes, is a behavioral manifestation characterized by "a feeling of well-being, a capacity to perform to the best of one's ability; it is evidenced by an ability to adjust to and adapt actively to varying situations, to perceive correctly, free from need distortions, complemented with a wholesome outlook on life" (p. 86).

Illness behavior, on the other hand, is defined as follows (Wu, pp. 136–137):

> ... behavior that is triggered by such cues as pain, discomfort, signs of malfunction, and/or by confirmation by word of mouth that the individual is experiencing illness. (It) is the initial response of the person to aberrations of the body and psyche which he perceives as incapacitating and therefore as a sign of illness.

In the growing field of health behavior, health-care professionals join with behavioral and social scientists to study the effectiveness and the results of health care.

Conclusion

The concept of health has been discussed from the perspective of changing perceptions of humankind.

Health has been described from different points of view without reaching a conclusive definition. Nevertheless, ideas about health may be summarized in the following statements:

- Health is a dynamic process.
- Health is determined subjectively and objectively.
- Health is a goal.
- Health is being able to take care of yourself.
- Health is optimal functioning in body, mind, and spirit.
- Health is integrity of self.
- Health is a sense of wholeness.
- Health is coping adaptively.
- Health is growing and becoming.
- Health is a broad concept.

Health is a complex concept. Persons and their interactions with the environment form the basis for many views about health. These views show how the ideas of health have evolved over time. Nurses have been instrumental in developing and encouraging holistic notions of health. One may or may not accept the viewpoints espoused by the Wholistic Health Movement. Nevertheless, the idea of the individual person as the primary resource for his own health is an idea that is basic to person-centered nursing care. To understand how persons use their strengths to achieve health, nurses need to understand the process of adaptation.

Study Questions

1. Explain environment and its variables as a system.
2. What impact has humanistic psychology had upon health care?
3. Describe the major thrust of holistic health.
4. What are the common elements of the five models of illness: primitive, medical–physiological, ecological, equilibrium, and social?
5. What is your definition of health?
6. What is your definition of illness?

Glossary

Behavior: An emitted response (action or reaction); it is overt, observable, and measurable.

Environment: An open system composed of the social, natural, and man-made subsystems and their variables; the external system.

Health behavior: Actions by persons who believe they are well to avoid an encounter with illness.

High-level wellness: An integrated method of functioning that is oriented toward maximizing the potential of which the individual is capable within the environment in which he is functioning (Dunn).

Homeodynamics: A reciprocal interaction of living systems that maintains a balance within each system and a balance among them.

Illness behavior: The initial response of the person to psychological and somatic cues that are perceived as incapacitating, therefore, signs of illness.

Bibliography

Auger JR: Behavioral Systems and Nursing. Englewood Cliffs, New Jersey, Prentice-Hall, 1976

Bennett H, Samuels M: The Well Body Book. New York, Random House, 1973

Benson H: The Relaxation Response. New York, William Morrow, 1975

Bergerson BS: Adaptation as a unifying theory. In Murphy JF (ed): Theoretical Issues in Professional Nursing, pp 45–60. New York, Appleton-Century-Crofts, 1971

Burgess AW: Nursing: Levels of Health Intervention. Englewood Cliffs, New Jersey, Prentice-Hall, 1978

Byrne M, Thompson LF: Key Concepts for the Study and Practice of Nursing. St. Louis, CV Mosby, 1972

Department of Health, Education, and Welfare: Healthy People: The Surgeon General's Report on Health Promotion and Disease Prevention. Washington, Office of the Assistant Secretary for Health, 1979

Dubos R: Mirage of Health. New York, Harper & Row, 1959

Dubos R: Man Adapting. New Haven, Yale University Press, 1965

Dunn HL: What high level wellness means. Can J Public Health 50:447–457, 1959

East–West Academy of Healing Arts. Mimeographed handout distributed by Ann Arbor Nurses for Wholistic Health at conference on Holistic Health: Its Place in Health Care, sponsored by University of Michigan School of Nursing–Continuing Education Services, Dearborn, Michigan, May 5, 1980

Flynn PAR: Holistic Health: The Art and Science of Care.

Bowie, Maryland, Robert J Brady, 1980

Garfield CA (ed): Stress and Survival: The Emotional Realities of Life-Threatening Illness. St. Louis, CV Mosby, 1979

Goble F: The Third Force. New York, Pocket Books, 1971

Jahoda M: Current Concepts of Positive Mental Health. New York, Basic Books, 1958

King IM: Toward a Theory for Nursing: General Concepts of Human Behavior. New York, John Wiley & Sons, 1971

Krieger D: The Therapeutic Touch: How to Use Your Hands to Help or to Heal. Englewood Cliffs, New Jersey, Prentice-Hall, 1979

Otto H: The human potentialities of nurses and patients. Nurs Outlook 8:32–35, 1965

Maslow AH: Toward a Psychology of Being, 2nd ed. New York, Van Nostrand Reinhold, 1968

Murray AB, Zentner JP: Nursing Concepts for Health Promotion, 2nd ed. Englewood Cliffs, New Jersey, Prentice-Hall, 1979

Roberts SL: Behavioral Concepts and the Critically Ill Patient. Englewood Cliffs, New Jersey, Prentice-Hall, 1976

Roberts SL: Behavioral Concepts and Nursing Throughout the Life Span. Englewood Cliffs, New Jersey, Prentice-Hall, 1978

Simonton OC, Mathews-Simonton S, Creighton J: Getting Well Again. Los Angeles, JP Tarcher, 1978

Sutterly DC, Donnelly GF: Perspectives in Human Development: Nursing Throughout the Life Cycle. Philadelphia, JB Lippincott, 1973

Thoms H, Roth LG, Linton D: Understanding Natural Childbirth: A Book for the Expectant Mother. New York, McGraw-Hill, 1950

Totman R: Social Causes of Illness. New York, Pantheon Books, 1979

World Health Organization Interim Commission: Constitution of the World Health Organization. Chronicle of the World Health Organization 1:29, 1947

Wu R: Behavior and Illness. Englewood Cliffs, New Jersey, Prentice-Hall, 1973

Adaptation

Marguerite B. Harms

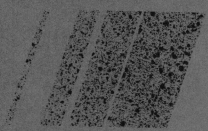

Objectives

Introduction

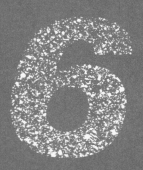

After completing this chapter, students will be able to:

- Develop a nursing perspective of adaptation.

- Discuss the relationship between health and adaptation.

- Describe the phenomena of change, stress, crisis, anxiety, and coping, and their effects upon persons.

- Identify theories of adaptation as they relate to persons and their environment.

- Identify ways the professional nurse facilitates adaptation of persons.

Do you think you are too young to die? You and death, a gloomy thought? Perhaps! Then do something about your life. You are not a helpless soul tossed in the sea of life. You have knowledge available to you to keep yourself well; you have freedom to live the life-style that will enhance your well-being; you can learn to cope with life experiences to improve your well-being. Essentially, you can change. The challenge that all persons must face in this process of change is called "adaptation."

The goal of nursing, as stated earlier, is to help persons maintain optimum biological, psychological, and social functioning by adapting to a changing environment and functional alterations or deviations from health. In order to accomplish this goal, nurses need to understand the interaction between persons and their environment.

This chapter will explore the processes by which persons adapt to their world. Several theories of adaptation will be discussed, as well as related concepts of crisis, coping, anxiety, and stress. Applications to nursing practice will also be explored.

What is Adaptation?

A definition of **adaptation** includes the concepts of persons as biopsychosocial beings, the interaction or process of exchange with the environment, change or transformation, and health (the goal of adaptation). A working definition reads as follows:

> Adaptation is the process of changing throughout life by persons faced with new, different, or threatening experiences without loss of health, a sense of wholeness, or integrity of self.

The essence of adaptation is change; it is a process of dynamic equilibrium that is vital for survival. In broad terms, adaptation consists of biological, psychological, social, and spriritual facets. The concept of health, discussed in the previous chapter, is closely related to adaptation. Adaptation moves a person toward health and growth. **Maladaptation,** on the other hand, occurs when a person uses inadequate ways of dealing with stress in an attempt to maintain equilibrium.

In Chapter 2, persons were described as open systems who are constantly interacting and exchanging energy with their environment. When change occurs in the environment, the person must adapt. This process requires energy. Rapid change may require more energy than the person has available. When the rate or amount of change exceeds our capacity to adapt, illness may occur. Yet, successful adaptation may strengthen integrity of self or lead to an even higher level of functioning.

Adaptation Theories

Historical Development

The concept of adaptation, as developed over the past century, is outlined in Table 6-1 and summarized below.

Bernard (Steady State). Claude Bernard, a French physiologist, was one of the pioneers in the study of the body's attempts to achieve a steady state while dealing with change. He pointed out that the internal environment of all organisms remains fairly constant even though the external environment changes. For example, the body maintains a stable core temperature despite changes in the weather.

Cannon (Homeostasis). In the early part of this century, Walter B. Cannon, an American physiologist, introduced the concept of homeostasis (1939). *Homeostasis* means the maintenance of equilibrium or a steady state of the body. For instance, the oxygen concentration within arteries remains fairly constant, even though carbon dioxide is continually given off by cells and oxygen is taken in by the lungs. Cannon recognized that this steady state was not completely fixed; rather, it varied within certain limits.

The term "homeostasis" has been replaced by **homeodynamics** in current usage, indicating that processes are continually taking place to maintain a steady state. Consider the expected changes that occur to cells and organs from conception through

Table 6-1
Perspectives on Adaptation

Scientist	Country	Profession	Theory
Claude Bernard	France	Physiologist	The internal environment of all organisms remains fairly constant even though the external environment changes.
Walter B. Cannon	United States	Physiologist	Homeostasis is the ability of living organisms to maintain their own equilibrium.
Hans Selye	Austria and Canada	Endocrinologist	General adaptation syndrome (G.A.S.). The body's response to stress of any kind occurs as a unified defense mechanism with specific structural and chemical changes. The reaction elicits resistance by the body to stressful agents and protects against disease. When the reaction is too long or faulty, disease or death may occur.
Rene Dubos	France and United States	Biologist	Health or disease is the expression of the success or failure by persons in their efforts to respond adaptively to environmental challenges.
Alvin Toffler	United States	Experimental psychologist and author of *Future Shock*	The faster the rate of change in a given time span, the more difficult it becomes for persons to adapt.
T.H. Holmes and R.H. Rahe	United States	Psychiatrists	Use of the Social Readjustment Rating Scale demonstrates a correlation between life events and illness and may be a predictor of illness.

aging. We know that certain changes are likely to occur at specific times in our lives. There is relative constancy in the growth and developmental processes, yet at the same time these are self-regulated. "The wonder increases," Cannon wrote, "when we realize that the system is open, engaging in free exchange with the outer world, and that the structure itself is not permanent but is continuously being broken down by the wear and tear of action, and is continuously built up again by processes of repair" (Cannon, 1939, p. 20).

Selye (Stress). More recently, the work of Hans Selye has stimulated great interest in the concepts of stress and adaptation (1956). Selye is a Canadian endocrinologist, originally from Austria, who explained **stress** as the normal wear and tear of daily living and defined a **stressor** as anything that induces stress. He described the body's response to stress as a unified defense mechanism with specific

structural and chemical changes and called this the *general adaptation syndrome (G.A.S.).* The G.A.S. response elicits resistance by the body to stressful agents, enhancing its ability to ward off these stressors. However, if this reaction is faulty or prolonged, disease or death may result.

The G.A.S. has three phases: alarm reaction, resistance, and exhaustion. The responses in each stage are as follows:

- Alarm—Defenses mobilize to respond to stressor.
- Resistance—Body tries to adapt to stressor.
- Exhaustion—If stressor persists or is severe, or if the person has limited adaptive capacity, the body loses ability to adapt; exhaustion and death follow.

Selye's early work concentrated on the physiological response to stress. He now recognizes the role of psychological stress in the adaptation syndrome. However, the relationship between psychological stress and physiological response is still under study.

Dubos.   Another perspective is that of Rene Dubos, an American biologist originally from France. He wrote, "Health or disease is the expression of success or failure by persons in their efforts to respond adaptively to environmental challenges" (1965, p. xvii).

Toffler (Culture Shock).   Alvin Toffler, an experimental psychologist from the United States, described adaptation in his famous work, *Future Shock* (1970). In it he discussed what happens to persons who encounter change of any kind. Toffler pointed out that the faster the rate of change in a given time span, the more difficult it becomes for persons to adapt. The term **culture shock** has become a byword to convey "profound disorientation suffered by the traveler who has plunged without adequate preparation into an alien culture" (p. 308). Today we recognize that the ability of persons to adapt in our rapidly changing world is being tested as never before.

Holmes and Rahe.   Research on the relationship of adaptation to wellness has increased in recent years. Holmes and Rahe stimulated well-known research in this area (1967). They developed the *Social Readjustment Rating Scale* to demonstrate the correlation between stressful life events and serious illness. The ranking of life events was the result of perceived changes in life-style following the events. The life events identified were not necessarily undesirable; rather they included any experience that required some degree of adaptation (Table 6-2).

Studies showed that the number of life changes and subsequent alterations in the life-styles of persons did have an effect on physiological adaptation. That is, persons who experienced a number of stressful events within 1 year were more likely to develop illness. Later studies by Holmes, Rahe, and others supported this belief. Therefore, it is reasonable to expect that persons experiencing too many life changes (multiple stressors) in a short span of time may be suitable candidates for intervention to prevent serious illness.

Development of the Adaptation Concept in Nursing

The concept of adaptation has been the focus of studies by professional nurses in education, research, and practice. Since adaptation is essential in order to maintain health, this concept is important to nursing as a profession. Florence Nightingale, Myra Levine, Imogene King, Martha Rogers, and Sister Callista Roy are among those nurses who have contributed to the development of a nursing perspective on adaptation.

Nightingale.   Florence Nightingale, often called the founder of modern nursing, was the first to consider the concept of adaptation (1859). Nightingale felt that the condition of the environment affected a person's ability to adapt. Although she did not specifically use the term "adaptation," her writings about the importance of the environment have affected all of the nursing theorists who followed her. A poor environment requires that a sick person use much of his energy to deal with these conditions rather than to recover from illness. Nightingale felt that a nurse's function was to provide a favorable environment (adequate ventilation, water, cleanliness, and warmth) so that the person would be in the best possible position for the natural healing processes to occur.

Although many of the housekeeping activities that once were performed by nurses have been delegated to non-nursing personnel today, nurses still are concerned with environmental factors that affect health. For instance, a nurse in the hospital tries to provide adequate stimulus in the environment to prevent boredom or withdrawal. In the community, a nurse might recognize that an overcrowded apartment potentially affects a family's health and might assist them to find a more suitable living space.

Levine.   Like Nightingale, Myra Levine believed that nursing is based on the person's response to the environment. She wrote, "The nurse participates actively in every patient's environment and much of what she does supports his adaptations as he struggles in the predicament of illness" (Levine, 1973, p. 13). Levine defined adaptation as a process of change to meet the realities of the environment, enabling the person to retain integrity or wholeness of self. Nursing involves recognizing the adaptive behavior or changes in functioning of the body and taking appropriate actions.

Levine defines two types of nursing actions: supportive (those actions that help the person adapt to an altered level of health, such as with dying persons) and therapeutic (those that promote healing and restoration of health). Note that both Nightingale and Levine considered only the nurse's role with ill persons; today we recognize that nurses assist persons in any state of health.

King. Imogene King also considered the environment and its relationship to adaptation and to health (1971). She believes that persons are constantly in the process of using energy to change so that they can meet the requirements of the environment. She states that to remain healthy, persons must continually adapt to stress in the environment through the best possible use of their resources. Maintaining health is a dynamic process.

The goal of nursing, according to King, is to help persons cope with health problems or adjust to interference in their health state. In other words, nurses help human beings cope with health and illness.

Rogers. Martha Rogers explained adaptation as the change resulting from the interaction of a person and the environment (1970). Change is an ongoing, irreversible process that prevents a person from going back to what he was before. Rogers uses systems

---

Table 6-2
Social Readjustment Rating Scale

Rank	Life Event	Mean Value*	Rank	Life Event	Mean Value*
1	Death of spouse	100	23	Son or daughter leaving home	29
2	Divorce	73	24	Trouble with in-laws	29
3	Marital separation	65	25	Outstanding personal achievement	28
4	Jail term	63	26	Wife begin or stop work	26
5	Death of close family member	63	27	Begin or end school	26
6	Personal injury or illness	53	28	Change in living conditions	25
7	Marriage	50	29	Revision of personal habits	24
8	Fired at work	47	30	Trouble with boss	23
9	Marital reconciliation	45	31	Change in work hours or conditions	20
10	Retirement	45	32	Change in residence	20
11	Change in health of family member	44	33	Change in schools	20
12	Pregnancy	40	34	Change in recreation	19
13	Sex difficulties	39	35	Change in church activities	19
14	Gain of new family member	39	36	Change in social activities	18
15	Business adjustment	39	37	Mortgage or loan less than $10,000	17
16	Change in financial state	38	38	Change in sleeping habits	16
17	Death of close friend	37	39	Change in number of family get-togethers	15
18	Change to different line of work	36	40	Change in eating habits	15
19	Change in number of arguments with spouse	35	41	Vacation	13
20	Mortgage over $10,000	31	42	Christmas	12
21	Foreclosure of mortgage or loan	30	43	Minor violations of the law	11
22	Change in responsibilities at work	29			

* Values were assigned to life events according to the degree of change in life-style they require. (Holmes TH, Rahe RH: J Psychosom Res 2:214, August 1967).

theory (discussed in Chapter 2) to describe the relationship between persons and the environment. She believes that a person and his environment need to be considered as a single system, because energy is being exchanged constantly between them and each is affecting the other continually. Rogers sees the nurse as a part of the person's environment; the nurse's goal is to promote a harmonious interaction between persons and environment. Rogers's theory has the limitation of being complex and difficult to understand.

Roy. Sister Callista Roy defines adaptation as a positive response to the demands made on a person by the changing environment (1976). Persons use biological, psychological, and social mechanisms to cope with their world. The goal of nursing is to promote adaptation in four modes:

- Physiological needs (elimination, nutrition, etc.)
- Self-concept (sense of who we are)
- Role function (socially expected behaviors)
- Interdependence (balance between independence and dependence in our relationships with others).

A person needs nursing care when his adaptive responses are inadequate.

Overview

There are several common themes in each of these discussions. They are as follows:

- Persons continually interact with their environment.
- Adaptation is the person's response to a change in the environment.
- Environmental changes occur constantly, so adaptation is a continuous process.
- The goal of nursing is to promote adaptation.
- As we help persons to adapt, we are helping them to maintain or achieve health.

From this summary it is easy to recognize why adaptation is such an important concept in nursing. Health depends on using our powers to respond to the environment effectively. It is true that all nurses do not practice using adaptation theory as a base. Yet each of us, whether we realize it or not, is actively helping our clients to adapt.

Rogers, Erikson, and Maslow, whose theories have been represented earlier, also use the concept of adaptation even though they are not nurses. They refer to adaptation indirectly when they state that persons have the power within themselves to achieve their potential. In other words, each of us has the power to adapt. So adaptation is a key concept for any professional who assists persons with their health.

Process of Adaptation

In order to understand the process of adaptation, nurses must be familiar with several of its subconcepts:

- **Stress** and **stressor**
- **Anxiety**
- Adaptive and maladaptive **coping behavior**
- **Crisis**

None of the subconcepts is a synonym for the others; yet, each is related to the others as indicated in the following statement (subconcepts in italics):

> Wear and tear of a *stress*ful event may produce disequilibrium, especially if persons are unprepared or unskilled to deal (*cope*) with the event. The failure to regain equilibrium will lead to *anxiety*, and excessive anxiety that remains unrelieved may lead to a *crisis*.

Stress

Stress has been defined as both a state and a response by various authors. Selye defines stress as "the nonspecific response of the body to any demand made upon it" (Selye, 1975, p. 14). Selye emphasized that stress is a normal part of life. Freedom from stress occurs only with death (Selye, 1956). Any stressful event produces disequilibrium; however, each person's perceptions of an event are unique.

The term stressor is often used in lieu of stress. The stressor (stimulus) places demands on persons to prepare for change, for instance, pain, cold, a test. Stressors such as those identified in the Social Readjustment Rating Scale by Holmes and Rahe may or may not be happy events. **Eustress** is a state induced by pleasant stimuli, whereas **distress** is a state induced by unpleasant stimuli. Persons themselves define whether stimuli are pleasant or unpleasant, because perceptions of such events are an individual matter. For this reason, how persons respond to stressful events is critical to health.

Nurses need to obtain information about their client's strengths, risk-taking behaviors, past successes, and present abilities to change and adapt.

Anxiety

Any threatening situation may produce anxiety. **Anxiety** is defined as a diffuse, unpleasant, vague feeling of apprehension, nervousness, or dread expressed both somatically and psychically. Like fear, it is a reaction to a threat; however, unlike fear (which is a response to a known, definite, external and immediate danger), anxiety is felt as a threat from something unknown, vague, internal, and in the future (Henderson and Nite, 1978, p. 1617).

Anxiety is a normal response to a stressful event; everyone experiences it. Caplan describes anxiety in a crisis situation: "When the individual's usual problem solving methods fail, and the problem persists, he or she experiences a rise in inner tension, unpleasant emotional feelings, and disorganized functioning" (1964, pp. 38–39).

Because the discomfort (anxiety) of a stressful situation needs to be relieved, the individual will utilize **coping behavior** to protect against disorganization or an unstable state of physical and emotional health. Therefore, some kind of adaptation or reorganization takes place; the result may be either growth or regression.

Nurses need to understand the phenomenon of anxiety when working with persons in crisis. Individuals who are experiencing a high level of anxiety often have limited ability to solve problems and, therefore, to adapt. These persons need assistance to lower their anxiety to a functional level. A mild degree of anxiety may be beneficial because it motivates persons to make needed changes in their behavior. Determining the level of anxiety is essential for choosing successful nursing actions.

Coping

The term "coping" refers to the way we deal with our life experiences. It means "to fulfill our needs, to find safety and love and self-respect, freedom from worry, opportunities for growth, and , ultimately, a satisfying meaning for our existence" (Allport, 1965, p. 262). As defined by Allport (p. 243), coping is characteristically

- Purposive
- Determined by the needs of the moment and situation
- Formally elicited rather than spontaneously emitted
- More readily controlled
- Aiming to change the environment

To cope implies action in response to our environment; effective coping leads to health. Coping behaviors consist of use of the cognitive functions (perception, memory, speech, judgment, reality testing), motor activity, affect, and psychological defenses (Mattsson, 1979, p. 257).

Coping behavior may involve muscle activity, such as withdrawing one's hand from a hot stove, or it may require the use of knowledge, skills, recall from past experiences, and judgment. Sometimes effective coping behavior may be to ignore certain stimuli in favor of other stimuli that have meaning in one's life. For instance, most students can remember studying for an examination in spite of fatigue or a headache. The importance of getting a passing grade exceeded the need for sleep or comfort and was reflected by the choice of coping behaviors. Whatever form they take, successful coping behaviors result in adaptation.

Adaptive versus *Maladaptive Coping*

Coping behaviors may be either adaptive or maladaptive. Adaptive behaviors lead persons toward effective biopsychosocial functioning within their environment; maladaptive behaviors deter achievement of or move persons away from health and growth. Maladaptive behavior does achieve some goal for the persons at the time it is used, however. Roy writes, "An adaptive response in general is behavior that maintains the integrity of the individual. A maladaptive response is one that does not maintain integrity and is disruptive of the person" (1976, p. 13). Therefore, adaptation is successful when the person responds to stressful events in a way that maintains or enhances integrity.

Maladaptation occurs when inadequate or ineffective methods of coping are used to maintain equilibrium. Illness may be considered the result of maladaptive coping. It should be noted, though, that maladaptive coping is not to be considered a fault. A person is never prepared for all the contingencies

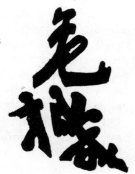

Figure 6-1
An Oriental ideogram for crisis combines the symbols for danger and opportunity.

of change. On occasion he finds himself in new situations for which previous coping methods may not be effective, and his attempts to survive in the situation may fail. Under such circumstances he may need to seek help and learn coping methods. Unfortunately, many times persons who cope maladaptively with changes in their environment may not be aware that they need help. Some persons may find it extremely difficult to seek help even when they recognize their problems. For instance, a woman who discovers a breast lump may delay seeking help because she cannot cope with the possibility of having cancer. If persons reach the state of exhaustion, as in a serious illness, help may be imposed on them. However, the need for action will be perceived differently by each person. As an example, many of us can recall delaying health care because other needs took priority.

When circumstances warrant help, nurses, as well as other professionals, become resources in the environment. Nurses assist persons to cope adaptively. It should be remembered that behaviors considered maladaptive in one culture may be adaptive in another. Consequently, nurses need to understand the person's sociocultural beliefs before making plans to intervene.

Crisis

The phenomenon of crisis is universal. No one escapes crisis because no one escapes change. The term **crisis,** like the term stress, has been used frequently to imply that which is positive and desirable as well as that which is negative or undesirable. Also, stress and crisis have been used interchangeably by some. Sheehy writes, "Our culture's interpretation of the Greek word *Krisis* is pejorative, implying personal failure, weakness, and inability to bear up against stressful outside events" (1974, p. 16). Erikson, however, uses the term crisis to describe a turning point, a crucial period of increased vulnerability and heightened potential (1963). Both interpretations have merit.

The period of crisis is temporary and usually lasts no longer than 4 to 6 weeks. Because a person's usual coping mechanisms do not work, this period may be both a time of danger and an opportunity for learning new coping patterns. Whereas crisis may be overwhelming to some (e.g., a woman who considers suicide after the death of her husband), others may use this time as a period of growth. Figure 6-1 illustrates the Chinese ideogram for crisis, which combines the symbols of danger and opportunity.

Figure 6-2
Birth is an example of a maturational crisis. *(Photo by Bob Kalmbach; University of Michigan Information Services)*

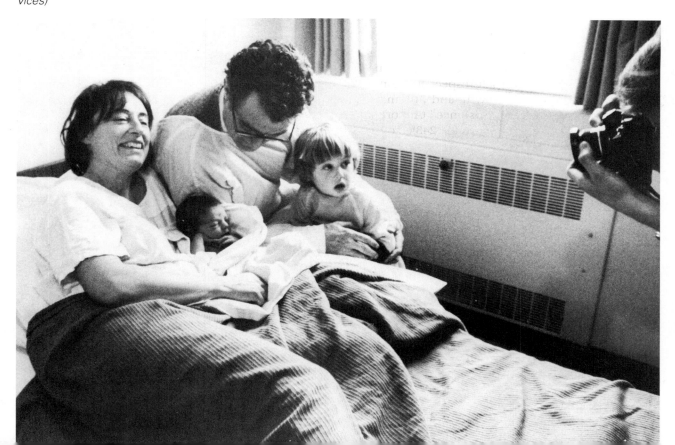

Whether a crisis has a positive or negative outcome depends on its nature and the person's adaptive abilities and resources.

Situational versus Developmental Crises

Crises may occur as the result of a sudden and significant change in a person's life. During crisis a person may be helpless and less able to find a solution. His functioning becomes disorganized.

Crises are of two types: **situational** or **accidental;** and **maturational, normative,** or **developmental.** A situational or accidental crisis occurs when the sense of biological, psychological, and social integrity is threatened due to unexpected events such as death, illness, divorce, loss of job, moving, unwanted pregnancy, or natural disaster. "Potential crisis areas occur during the periods of great social, physical, and psychological change experienced by all human beings in the normal growth process" (Auguilera and Messick, 1978, p. 132).

A maturational, normative, or developmental crisis occurs when the person is unable to make appropriate changes to new life situations, such as in marriage, beginning school, adolescence, or parenthood (Fig. 6-2). During periods of maturational crisis, the person learns to develop coping strategies for these new life situations.

Coping with Crises

Figure 6-3 describes the balancing factors that determine health. The paradigm illustrates how health, well-being, and integrity of self are dependent on the person's ability to cope with crisis, adapt to life stresses, and maintain a homeodynamic state. Likewise, the person unable to cope with crisis and adapt to stress suffers a breakdown in homeodynamic processes and resulting illness.

Figure 6-4 is a paradigm of the development of crisis, originated by Aguilera and Messick (1978, pp. 68–69). Figure 6-5 is an illustration of the paradigm using two students' responses to the same event (failing an examination). This example shows how a stressful event experienced by two individuals can lead to different outcomes, depending upon which coping mechanisms the person uses. Note that maladaptive coping hinders problem solving, and adaptive coping enhances it. The coping behaviors used may make the difference in whether a stressful situation becomes a crisis or not.

The positive outcome of crisis is that persons may function at a higher level than before. Therefore, the nurse focuses on the person's strengths and abilities to change and adapt and provides positive reinforcement by pointing out the person's past successes. Nurses often provide support during crisis periods. In a situational crisis such as acute illness, they identify persons' strengths and provide emotional or physical support (*e.g.,* being a sounding board or giving physical care). During developmental crises nurses provide guidance to give persons the necessary skills for helping themselves.

Figure 6-3

Balancing factors for health. *(From Aguilera DC, Messick JM: Crisis Intervention: Theory and Methodology, 3rd ed, pp 68–69. St. Louis, CV Mosby, 1978)*

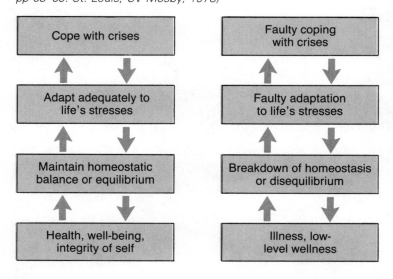

Using the Concept of Adaptation

Nursing's function is to assist persons in their adaptation to a variety of life experiences. Nurses need to consider the following factors when they help clients with their adaptations:

- The person and his strengths and needs
- The environment and its characteristics
- The interactions of the person with his environment

Individuals who do not cope successfully with stressors may experience crisis. Because so much of nursing practice deals with critical life events, nurses, as well as other health professionals, identify strongly with the concept of crisis.

Crisis Framework

Figure 6-6 presents a crisis framework for working with individuals. The columns in this figure identify four change phases: preparation for change, motivation to change, coping with change, and acceptance of change. Each identifies the way in which a person deals with change.

```
              ┌──────────────────────┐
              │    Human organism    │
              └──────────────────────┘
                         │
              ┌──────────────────────┐
              │ State of equilibrium │
              └──────────────────────┘
                         │
Stressful event →   ┌──────────────────────┐   ← Stressful event
              │ State of disequilibrium │
              └──────────────────────┘
                         │
              ┌──────────────────────┐
              │     Felt need to     │
              │ restore equilibrium  │
              └──────────────────────┘
```

A
Balancing factors present

B
One or more balancing factors absent

*Realistic perception of the event

Distorted perception of the event

plu...   and/or

*Adequ... situational ...   ...ate ...pport

plu...

*Adeq... coping me...   ...ng ...sms

resu...   ...n

Reso... of the ...   ...m ...ed

Equilibrium regained

Disequilibrium continues

No crisis

Crisis

*Balancing factors

Figure 6-4
Effect of balancing factors in a stressful event. *(Aguilera DC, Messick JM: Crisis Intervention: Theory and Methodology, 3rd ed., p 68. St. Louis, CV Mosby, 1978)*

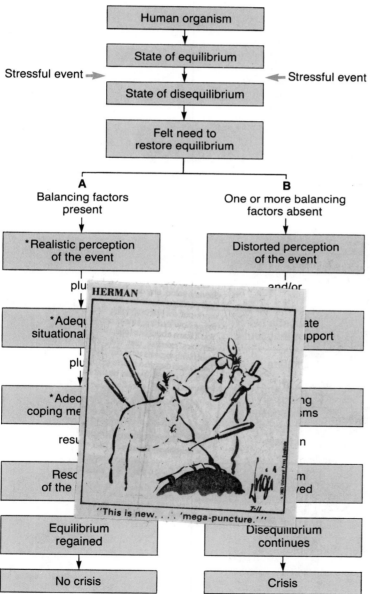

HERMAN

"This is new. . . . 'mega-puncture.'"

The nurse analyzes the person's behavior to recognize the level at which the person is coping. Once this is identified, the following goals can be established: crisis prevention, crisis precipitation, crisis intervention, and crisis resolution. These help the nurse determine what actions will best assist the person to adapt successfully to his situation. For each goal there are related nursing actions. The desired outcomes for each coping state are identified at the bottom of each column.

Change Phases in Crises

The following is a description of each of the four change phases identified in Figure 6-6:

1 *Preparation for change.* The client is unaware of an impending crisis such as the onset of menstruation (menarche).
   - The goal is prevention of crisis.
   - The nurse anticipates this crisis by preparing the client for change by **anticipatory guidance** (assisting the client to develop necessary knowledge, skills, or attitudes). For instance, the nurse might teach some basic anatomy and explain the process of menstruation.

2 *Motivation to change.* The client is partially aware of a problem but outwardly denies that it exists (e.g., an alcoholic who denies his excessive drinking to his family).

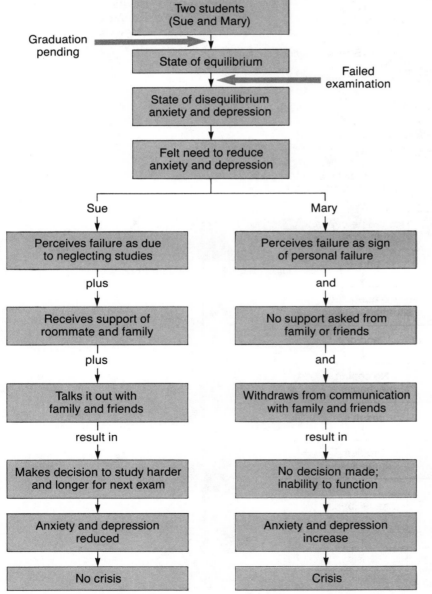

Figure 6-5
Illustration of effect of balancing factors in a stressful event. *(Aguilera DC, Messick JM: Crisis Intervention: Theory and Methodology, 3rd ed, p 69. St. Louis, CV Mosby, 1978)*

- The goal is crisis precipitation, which is accomplished by **confrontation** (helping the client to face the reality of the situation).
- When a crisis is precipitated, the nurse must be prepared to provide the support needed for the person to cope. Therefore, this is a highly sophisticated goal that should only be attempted by experienced nurses.

3 *Coping with change.* The client is aware that a crisis situation exists but is unable to cope on his own.
- The goal is crisis intervention.
- The nurse's action is **alteration** of the situation by providing support, working to reverse the stressors, or referring the individual to other support persons. For instance, the nurse might elevate the head of the bed and administer appropriate medications for a person experiencing an asthma attack.

4 *Acceptance of change.* The client is aware of a crisis situation and has begun to change in response to it.
- The goal is resolution of the crisis.

- Nursing actions are directed toward **rehabilitation.** The nurse reinforces the positive behavior the person exhibits and teaches, counsels, or provides adaptive devices. For instance, the nurse might teach safety techniques to an individual who has recently lost eyesight and reinforce use of his remaining sensory abilities, such as smell, touch, and hearing.

In some instances, persons move through each change phase or stage of adaptation in sequence. For example, the person who is prepared for impending change may be motivated to change, then copes with the change, and finally achieves a stage of growth or acceptance of the change.

Figure 6-7 summarizes the ways that the concepts of crisis, adaptation, and health relate to each other. There are four major nursing goals related to crisis:

- Crisis prevention
- Crisis precipitation
- Crisis intervention
- Crisis resolution

Figure 6-6
Change-phase table. Nursing actions that facilitate adaptation using a crisis framework. *(From Harms M, Del Vecchio A: Facilitating Adaptation Using a Crisis Framework. Unpublished manuscript, 1980)*

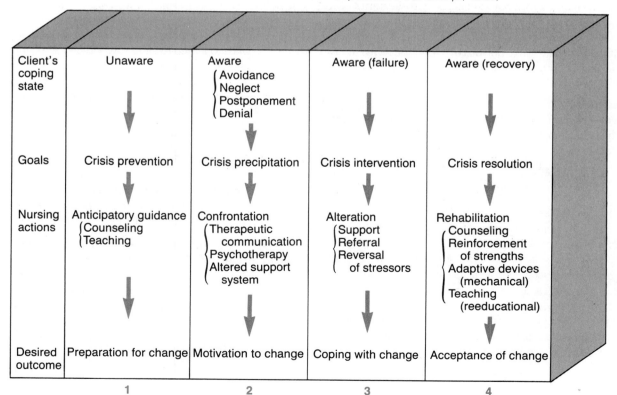

Client's coping state	Unaware	Aware { Avoidance Neglect Postponement Denial	Aware (failure)	Aware (recovery)
Goals	Crisis prevention	Crisis precipitation	Crisis intervention	Crisis resolution
Nursing actions	Anticipatory guidance { Counseling Teaching	Confrontation { Therapeutic communication Psychotherapy Altered support system	Alteration { Support Referral Reversal of stressors	Rehabilitation { Counseling Reinforcement of strengths Adaptive devices (mechanical) Teaching (reeducational)
Desired outcome	Preparation for change	Motivation to change	Coping with change	Acceptance of change
	1	2	3	4

Model I. The nurse   Model II. The patient/client

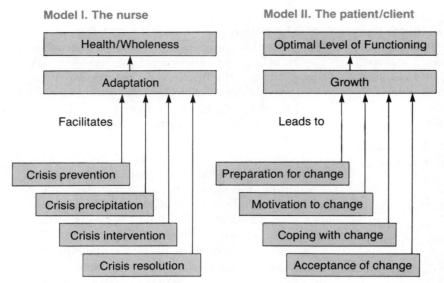

Figure 6-7

Facilitating adaptation using a crisis framework. *(From Harms M, Del Vecchio A: Facilitating Adaptation Using a Crisis Framework. Unpublished Manuscript, 1980)*

The desired outcome of each goal is adaptation, which leads to health and wholeness of the person (see Model I).

Model II illustrates the desired outcome for the client, resulting from the change process. Each of the change phases leads to individual growth. Notice that in both models the desired outcomes of the helping process are health, growth, and optimal functioning of the person.

The following is an example of a client who has experienced a situational crisis.* The elements of the adaptation process (stress, anxiety, coping, and crisis) are evident in this situation. The client has experienced a crisis and has begun to cope with it. Her task is acceptance of change (the fourth column of the change-phase table).

Example □ Jan is a 42-year-old female client who underwent a hysterectomy 1 month ago. After leaving the hospital she noticed that her surgical wound had reddened, was swollen, and had begun to drain pus. She was readmitted with a wound abscess. Jan also has been diabetic for 12 years and takes daily insulin injections. She is very knowledgeable about her disease and has developed a strict schedule for herself in order to control it.

Jan has a difficult family life. She states that her mother has a history of emotional problems and relies on her to make even the simplest decisions. Her father is experiencing memory loss due to aging and often forgets where he is. Jan expresses concern about caring for her parents. Jan is very close to her sister and a niece and has many friends in her church group. She also has a dog whom she describes as "almost human . . . we really understand each other." Jan is unmarried.

Jan weighs 242 pounds. She states she often feels lonely, depressed, or anxious and overeats to "feel better." She is trying to change by recognizing her habits and developing new eating behaviors.

In the hospital, Jan's infected wound is cleaned and bandaged three times daily. Jan will need to do this for herself after discharge. She experienced blurred vision soon after this hospital admission, for which no physical cause could be found. She states, "I realized that I was probably feeling overwhelmed at having to take care of my parents and their problems after I went home, on top of doing all those dressing changes and watching my diabetes. I guess my vision problem was a way to get out of all of the demands on me. As soon as I recognized this, my blurred vision went away."

Jan has established a strict routine in the hospital. When this routine is followed she feels comfortable in the hospital environment. However, if the nurses do not include her in planning her care, such as determining times for dressing changes, she becomes visibly anxious and angry.

Jan is open and expresses her feelings readily. She can identify her own weaknesses and strengths and is usually able to solve problems. She assumes responsibility for as much of her hospital care as possible, yet asks for assistance when she needs it.* □

Several elements of the adaptation process can be identified in this situation. Jan is currently experiencing several stressors. These include her parent's increasing dependence on her, her own health problems, and hospitalization. She is undergoing a situational crisis because her usual coping methods

* Data contributed by Charlotte Myers

are not effective in helping her deal with those stressors. Notice that when Jan felt totally unable to cope with stress she developed a physical symptom (blurred vision). This illustrates the relationship between health and adaptation. Jan had inadequate energy to cope with psychological stress; she drew energy from her biological subsystem, causing it to become less healthy also. Her usual coping mechanisms include overeating, controlling situations through strict schedules or routines, and problem solving. Note that when the nurses interfere with one of her most important coping mechanisms (control), Jan has no way to deal with anxiety, as evidenced by her reaction of anger.

Since Jan is recovering from her crisis, the desired outcome is acceptance of change. Nursing care focuses on crisis resolution. This requires knowledge of Jan's strengths, her current level of anxiety, her past methods of coping, and the current stressors in her life. Because Jan is in a moderate state of anxiety, her nurse can help to think of new ways of dealing with her situation. The nurse and Jan set goals together for crisis resolution. Because control is the coping mechanism that Jan is currently using, her nurse develops ways of returning a sense of control. This involves teaching her to care for her infected wound, following her schedule as closely

as possible, and encouraging her to make her own decisions about her hospital care. The nurse might also talk with Jan about how she can use her social supports to help her deal with her parents' health needs. Other resources, such as a community-health nurse or social worker might be called to give additional support after her discharge from the hospital.

Conclusion

This chapter has described the process by which persons adapt to changes in their environment. Adaptation is dynamic because movement or change from one condition to another is expected all of our lives. As stressors impinge on us, we respond accordingly. Although the number and type of stressors may vary, there is no escape from them. Therefore, each of us is involved continuously in the process of adaptation. Because adaptation is vital to the health and growth of persons, nursing's goal is to facilitate this process. Nurses have the knowledge and skills to deal with planned change of persons and their environment. In this way we assist persons to achieve their potential.

Study Questions

1. Describe several theories of adaptation. How can nurses use these ideas in their practice?

2. Describe the difference between the concepts of crisis, anxiety, stress, and coping.

3. Give three examples of life events that may lead (a) to situational crisis and (b) to maturational crisis.

4. How is the process of change related to adaptation?

5. List some ways in which the nurse may facilitate adaptation of persons.

Glossary

Adaptation: The process of changing throughout life by persons when faced with new, different, or threatening experiences without loss of health, sense of wholeness, or integrity of self.

Alteration: Therapeutic action consisting of support, referral, or reversal of stressors used to help persons cope with the biopsychosocial or environmental changes brought on by illness; nursing goal is crisis intervention.

Anticipatory guidance: Therapeutic action consisting of counseling or teaching used to prepare persons for impending biopsychosocial or environmental change; nursing goal is crisis prevention.

Anxiety: A diffuse, unpleasant, vague feeling of apprehension, nervousness, or dread expressed both somatically and psychically.

Behavior: An emitted response (action or reaction); it is overt, observable, and measurable.

Confrontation: Therapeutic action consisting of therapeutic communication, psychotherapy, or altered support system used to motivate an individual to change; nursing goal is crisis precipitation.

Coping behavior: Adaptive or maladaptive responses consisting of cognitive function, motor activity, affect, and psychological defenses. Consists of actions or reactions in response to stress.

Crisis: A turning point, a crucial period of increased vulnerability and heightened potential; may be biological, psychological, social; individual experiences disequilibrium when usual coping behaviors are not operating.

  Situational (accidental) crisis: Unexpected or hazardous events such as illness, catastrophic circumstances, natural disasters.

  Maturational (normative, developmental) crisis: Expected life changes such as birth, puberty, marriage, pregnancy, *etc.*

Culture shock: Profound disorientation suffered by the person who has plunged without adequate preparation into an alien culture (Toffler).

Distress: A state induced by unpleasant stimuli.

Environment: An open system composed of the social, natural, and man-made subsystems and their variables; the external system.

Eustress: A state induced by pleasant stimuli.

Health: A broad concept; refers to the biological, psychological, and sociocultural well-being of persons; the quality of life. (See Chap. 5 for definitions from a variety of perspectives.)

Health behavior: Actions by persons who believe they are well to avoid an encounter with illness.

Health–illness continuum: A bipolar model of health on a horizontal scale used to define health or illness.

High-level wellness: An integrated method of functioning that is oriented toward maximizing the potential of which the individual is capable within the environment in which he is functioning (Dunn).

Homeodynamics: A reciprocal interaction of living systems that maintains a balance within each system and a balance among them.

Illness behavior: The initial response of the person to psychological and somatic cues that are perceived as incapacitating, therefore, signs of illness.

Maladaptation: The process of using inadequate ways of dealing with stress in an attempt to maintain equilibrium.

Rehabilitation: Therapeutic action consisting of counseling, reinforcement of strengths, adaptive devices (mechanical), and teaching (reeducation) used to help individual to accept a new or modified life-style following a change; nursing goal is crisis resolution.

Stress: The nonspecific response of the body to any demand made upon it (Selye). Everyday wear and tear of living.

Stressor: Anything that induces stress; the stimulus that places demands on persons to prepare for change, *e.g.*, pain, cold, a test.

Bibliography

Aguilera DC, Messick JM: Crisis Intervention: Theory and Methodology, 3rd ed. St Louis, CV Mosby, 1978

Allport GW: Pattern and Growth in Personality. New York, Holt, Rinehart & Winston, 1965

Auger JR: Behavioral Systems and Nursing. Englewood Cliffs, NJ, Prentice-Hall, 1976

Bergerson BS: Adaptation as a unifying theory. In Murphy JF (ed): Theoretical Issues in Professional Nursing, pp 45–60. New York, Appleton-Century-Crofts, 1971

Bronowski J: The Ascent of Man. Boston, Little, Brown, 1973

Byre ML, Thompson LF: Key Concepts for the Study and Practice of Nursing. St Louis, CV Mosby, 1972

Cannon WB: The Wisdom of the Body. New York, WW Norton, 1939

Caplan G: Principles of Preventive Psychiatry. New York, Basic Books, 1964

Dabrowski K: Positive Disintegration. Boston, Little, Brown, 1964

Dubos R: Man Adapting. New Haven, Yale University Press, 1965

Erikson E: Childhood and Society, 2nd ed. New York WW Norton, 1963

Germann DR: Too Young To Die: The Case for Staying Healthy and Alive Through Preventive Medicine. Rockville Center, Farnsworth, 1974

Goosen GM, Bush HA: Adaptation: A feedback process. Adv Nurs Sci 1:51–65, July, 1979

Hartl DE: Stress management and the nurse. Adv Nurs Sci 1:91–100, July 1979

Henderson V, Nite G: Principles and Practice of Nursing, 6th ed. New York, Macmillan, 1978

Holmes TH, Rahe RH: The Social Readjustment Rating Scale. J Psychosom Res 11, No. 2:213–218, August, 1967

King I: Toward a Theory for Nursing. New York, John Wiley & Sons, 1971

Lamott K: Escape From Stress. New York, GP Putnam's Sons, 1975

Levine ME: Introduction to Clinical Nursing. Philadelphia, FA Davis, 1973

Mattsson A: Long-term physical illness in childhood: A challenge to psychosocial adaptation. In Garfield CA (ed): Stress and Survival: The Emotional Realities of Life-Threatening Illness, pp 253–263. St Louis, CV Mosby, 1979

Monat A, Lazarus KS (eds): Stress and Coping—An Anthology. New York, Columbia University Press, 1977

Nightingale F: Notes on Nursing. A facsimile of the first edition printed in London, 1859. Philadelphia, JB Lippincott, 1966

Rogers M: An Introduction to the Theoretical Basis of Nursing. Philadelphia, FA Davis, 1970

Roy SC: Introduction to Nursing: An Adaptation Model. Englewood Cliffs, NJ, Prentice-Hall, 1976

Selye H: The Stress of Life. New York, McGraw-Hill, 1956

Selye H: Stress Without Distress. New York, Signet, 1975

Sheehy G: Passages: Predictable Crises of Adult Life. New York, EP Dutton, 1974

Sigman P: Stress management and the nurse. Adv Nurs Sci 1:85–90, July, 1979

Sutterley DC, Donnelly GF: Perspectives in Human Development: Nursing Throughout the Life Cycle. Philadelphia, JB Lippincott, 1973

Toffler A: Future Shock. New York, Random House, 1970

Adaptation of the Elderly Person

Sharon Hein Jette

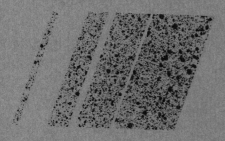

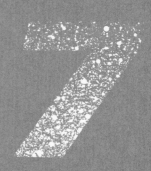

After completing this chapter, students will be able to:

● State five common myths about aging.

● Identify three theories of adaptation to aging.

● Recognize aging as a period of possible developmental crisis.

● Describe adaptation to functional changes of aging.

Have you ever heard the statements, "You're as old as you think you are" or "He's young at heart"? These are common ways of expressing the fact that each person adapts to aging in a unique manner (Fig. 7-1). Aging, as a growth process, begins at birth or even conception. Whereas peak physiological functioning may occur in the twenties, peak psychosocial maturation is more likely to occur in old age. Throughout life, various changes related to growth and the aging processes alter the person's ability to function in his environment.

This chapter will provide an introduction to the adaptations older persons use to meet their human needs. Functional changes of aging are presented as parallel to Maslow's hierarchy of needs. It is not the purpose of this chapter to describe in detail the biophysical and psychosocial alterations of aging. For that, the reader should refer to additional readings at the conclusion of this chapter for more detail.

The care of older people has evolved through centuries; the study of older people and how they adapt, that is, **gerontology,** has only occurred in the past 20 years. Since then, the field of **geriatrics**—professional care for elderly people who are sick—has become a specialty. Two other terms bear defining: **senescence,** denotes the normal, healthy process of growing older; in contrast, **senility** is an outdated, nonspecific term describing abnormal behavior in older persons. Unfortunately, the myth that "senility is inevitable" prevails in public thinking. A decade of research has shown that such difficult behaviors as confusion, incontinence, and aggression are often caused by specific physical abnormalities that are not inevitable but often treatable and preventable.

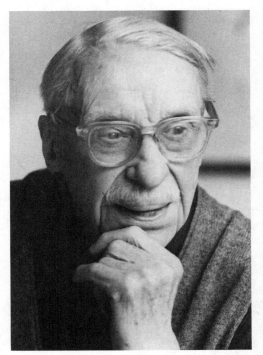

Figure 7-1
Each person adapts to aging in a unique way. *(Photo by Bob Kalmbach; University of Michigan Information Services)*

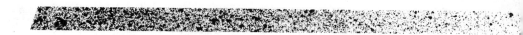

Myths and Attitudes About Aging

Myths about aging and old people arise partly from the fears of growing older, partly from generations of tales and jokes, and mostly from inexperience in living and dealing with elderly people. Listening carefully to older persons, withholding judgment, and caring for them as mature adults will dispel even the most persistent myths, such as those listed below.

Myth: Old Age Equals Sickness

Aging itself does not cause disease, but the probability of having chronic disease is higher in older people. However, even with two or three major chronic diseases, older people can adapt their life-styles and their environments.

Only about 5% of the 25 million Americans over age 60 are now living in institutions such as nursing homes, although many more eventually will spend some time in or die in such institutions (Butler and Lewis, 1977). Another 5% to 6% of elderly people are estimated to be sick, frail, and homebound. The remainder, almost 90% of all older persons, are adapting successfully in their homes and communities with the help of families and professionals as needed (Fig. 7-2). Because nurses typically care for the 10% who are sickest and most dependent, we often forget about the vast numbers of independent elders.

Myth: After 65 People Age Dramatically

The arbitrary age of 65 was chosen in the 1930s when the federal government needed to establish an age requirement for old-age assistance benefits. A person simply does not wake up "old" on his sixty-fifth birthday. Some bodily changes associated with aging occur typically in a person's forties, such as graying hair and decreased visual acuity. Other body functions vary enormously throughout old age depending on heredity, diet, occupation, environmental factors, life-style, and mental attitude. A person can be "old" at any age if he decides to exist without living fully, or he can be "young at heart" forever.

Figure 7-2
Most elders are successfully adapting in their homes and communities. *(Photo by Bob Kalmbach; University of Michigan Information Services)*

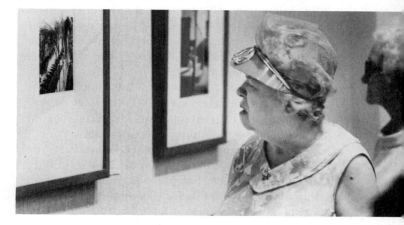

Myth: Older People Form a Homogeneous Group

Hardly! The arbitrary age of 65 begins what is often referred to as the first of two subgroups of elderly: that is, the "young–old" of 65 to 74 years, and the "old–old" of more than 75 years. Some authorities further designate the "extreme-old," over 85 years. The stage of life called "old-age" encompasses two and sometimes three distinct generations of people. In addition, today's elders include very diverse groups of successful retirees, indigent migrants, active politicians, isolated loners, educated professionals, first-generation immigrants, and proud ethnic peoples. There is no such single entity as "the elderly."

Myth: Older Years Are Tranquil, Golden Years of Pleasure

Sometimes called the "rocking-chair" myth, this one is neither true of nor desired by a majority of elders. Those who expect peaceful pastime are increasingly bitter at the inflation rate that steals their fixed pensions. Those who never contributed to pensions or security plans, such as domestic or migrant workers, cannot afford to retire to the rocking chair. Many elders find themselves raising their grandchildren while the parents work. For others, retirement is a waste of their talents; these people seek meaningful unpaid work or start second careers. (Colonel Sanders started Kentucky Fried Chicken after age 65.) And for those lonely, isolated elders confined to rocking chairs in urban ghettos and nursing homes, life is seldom golden. Lifelong living is a challenge of adaptation, and so is old age.

Myth: Older Persons Are Rigid, Fixed, Unable to Change

The "can't teach an old dog new tricks" myth results from experiences with cautious elders. Older persons require more time to integrate new knowledge, to respond, and to make decisions (Botwinick, 1973). But this is not rigidity. Oftentimes the tasks to be learned are meaningless, even childish, to older people; small wonder some older people appear uninterested and unmotivated. Other factors such as cultural style of learning, limited formal education, language barrier, enviromental distractions, drug effects, and sensory and memory alterations may change a person's ability to adapt to a new situation. One must consider that older people are learning some of the most difficult tasks of life: looking back, looking ahead, saying goodbye.

Theories of Adaptation to Aging

At this point in the brief history of gerontological research, no single unifying theory of aging exists. Instead, a set of controversial and often conflicting concepts of how people age has emerged.

Biological theories attribute aging to a combination of hereditary and environmental factors: these theories focus on the decline of ability and function as cells, organs, and systems age. This decline is variously attributed to a failure in deoxyribonucleic-acid (DNA) replication, an autoimmune malfunction, or virus invasion (Wallace, 1977).

Psychosocial theories of aging attempt to explain the causes of aging in terms of the interaction between self and others. The **disengagement theory** proposed by Cumming and Henry explained how older persons adapt successfully by withdrawing from social interaction and relinquishing social roles in order to prepare for death (1961). This controversial theory was challenged by the **activity theory,** which equates successful aging with the maintenance of social interactions and meaningful roles (Havighurst, 1963). Still another theory, the **continuity theory,** proposes that the older person adapts in order to maintain continuity of his personality (Neugarten, 1964). Essentially, this theory explains that personality remains constant throughout life; a hostile young man becomes a hostile old man and a creative young woman becomes a creative old woman.

Further theories show the links between biological and psychosocial theories, but all attempts to theorize on the process of aging show a complex combination of highly variable factors.

Developmental Tasks of Aging

As described in Chapter 3, Erikson's "eight stages of man" identify the task of maintaining integrity *versus* despair for the older adult (Erikson, 1968). Integrity involves the acceptance of one's life and one's self. If the person does not develop such a sense of acceptance, he may fall into despair of or disgust with his life.

R. C. Peck presents another perspective in his listing of psychological adjustment tasks for old age (1968). First, the task of ego differentiation *versus* work-role preoccupation challenges the retired person to define his ego in terms other than the work role. Next, the older person faces body transcendence *versus* body preoccupation and must adapt to bodily changes by overcoming physical limitations. Finally, the aged encounter ego transcendence *versus* ego preoccupation; the challenge here is to accept one's mortality and to extend oneself to future generations.

Spier identifies the life situations faced by older persons as follows: retiring from a work role; changing relationships with significant persons; maintaining income; meaningful productivity, and sexuality; and making adjustments to loss and death (1980). For most older people who have adapted well to earlier life, these adjustments are accomplished well; for others, these changes can become crises.

Adaptation to Functional Changes of Aging

All persons, regardless of age, share common human needs. Using Maslow's hierarchy of needs, this section will describe how older adults meet their needs and adapt to changes of aging.

Biophysical Needs

Aging alters several of the biophysical systems, with resulting changes in physical appearance, mobility, strength, and endurance. Alterations in the older person's mobility, for example, result from changes in his musculoskeletal and cardiovascular systems. All muscle becomes less elastic, less firm, and less strong with age, although much muscle function can be maintained by physical exercise. Older bones become more brittle, increasing the risk of fracture. The joints stiffen and affect movement, posture, and gait; arthritic pain is a common limitation of movement.

The respiratory and cardiovascular systems in older people produce less efficient circulation and ventilation. Breathing becomes more shallow as the ribcage expands less. The heart and lungs do not function as efficiently under stress when less oxygen is delivered to tissues (Campbell and LeFrak, 1977). At rest or under typical daily activity, the normal aged person is able to ventilate adequately, but under stress or exertion ventilation declines. Immobility may also cause decreased blood flow and pooling of blood in the legs. Reduced cardiac output and obstructed vessels combine to produce diminished circulation to extremities; this results in a characteristic feeling of chill and cold in many older persons.

The older person copes with these changes by slowing his speed of movement, by pacing his activities to avoid fatigue, and by changing his living environment to promote safety. Nurses assist elders to adapt by working at their speed, assessing their fatigue, and ensuring their safety. Although the older body reacts more slowly, older people can make accurate decisions and movements if given enough time (Welford, 1977).

Skin loses elasticity, moisture, and fatty tissue as it ages; this results in wrinkled, dry, fragile, and often tender skin that needs additional protection from heat, cold, and pressure. The nurse assists the older person to maintain skin integrity by careful assessment, teaching, and intervention.

Nutrition and elimination needs vary with activity level in older adults. Whereas the active elder may require the same caloric intake as a younger person, the immobile elder would require fewer calories to prevent an overweight state. Sometimes altered eating patterns and slower intestinal motility produce constipation. Older people learn to adapt by using natural-food laxatives, increasing exercise, adding bulk and fluid to the diet, and scheduling elimination times. Lessened bladder capacity may likewise produce frequency and urgency of urination, necessitating hurried trips to the bathroom.

Sensory changes commonly occur in older adults. With declining vision resulting from eye-muscle weakness and lens thickening, elders recognize their decreased ability to function in dim light and in glare. Changes in visual acuity usually demand corrective lenses. Accordingly, elders adapt by moving more slowly and cautiously to compensate for decreased accommodation, color perception, depth perception, and peripheral vision. Furthermore, nurses assist them to compensate by increasing the light received, eliminating glare, providing high-contrast colors, and giving navigational assistance as needed.

Hearing changes become more pronounced in the elderly. Many elders compensate for hearing loss so well that we do not recognize their impairment. Many others ae frustrated in their attempts to communicate because they cannot hear high-frequency sounds, especially high-pitched voices, and cannot distinguish speech sounds from background noise. Certain sounds, especially the consonants f, v, z, s, sh, t, th, and p become blurred, making it difficult to distinguish certain words, such as "thirst," from "first" or "verse" (Oyer and Oyer, 1976). Such changes can be misinterpreted as mental confusion in elderly. Nurses may assist by lessening background noise, writing notes and using touch, speaking slowly and distinctly, and lowering the pitch of the voice. Loss of sight and hearing together place an older person at risk of sensory deprivation due to inadequate reception of environmental stimuli. Sensory deprivation is discussed further in Chapter 17.

Safety and Security

Needs for safety and security cover a wide variety of issues. In the most basic sense, the elderly have the same needs as any other age group for safety from accidents, and they have special needs to avoid falls and burns. In another sense, the elderly need to feel safe from threats of violence. Elders in many urban neighborhoods commonly fear theft, assault, and rape. Indeed they become nighttime prisoners behind their own locked doors.

However, the most pervasive security need among the elderly derives from a common fear of neglect. To know that someone will respond to one's crisis is the most obvious form of security from neglect. In the field of child welfare, much has been accomplished to prevent and detect child abuse and neglect; so, too, have many laws recently been enacted to prevent "elder abuse" by families and caretakers.

Love and Belonging

The longer a person survives in this world, the greater the number of losses he will encounter in terms of family, friends, meaningful roles, and possessions. The general concept of loss as a lifelong readjustment process is presented in more detail in another chapter. For our purposes here, however, it is important to note that older persons especially must adapt to loss of loved ones and loss of belonging to meaningful groups, although new groups may be formed in place of previous ones.

People who survive into extreme old age in all likelihood have outlived one or more spouses and most of their siblings, as well as several groups of friends and neighbors, generations of pets, and perhaps some of their own children. Older workers are increasingly forced to retire and leave behind a lifetime of patterned productivity. Older homemakers find either the labor or the cost of home maintenance excessive and therefore are forced to leave their family homes. A fixed income may limit the ability of older people to indulge in the pleasures of retired leisure time. Living in a mobile society means they see children and grandchildren less and less often if the distance, cost, or effort of traveling is great. All of these changes make the elders' search for love and belonging more difficult.

Sensory changes common in aging also alter the ability to interact with loved ones and friends. Although some become socially isolated, most elderly learn to adapt.

Societal or subcultural norms may make it difficult for an older person to use sexuality as an expression of self. The lack of affectionate or sexual expression also threatens the need for love and belonging. Elders may also experience what Burnside calls **touch deprivation**—lack of touch stimuli that results in insecurity and anxiety (1973b). Elders, particularly disabled ones, are lifted, moved, turned, and walked, but seldom touched in a spontaneous caring way. To convey a sense of caring through touch, the nurse can offer purposeful nursing interventions in the form of relaxing massage, holding the hand, or gentle touching; these actions transmit caring, love, and belonging.

Self-Esteem

The older person gains his self-esteem by adapting successfully to the challenges of his life and environment. One challenge is to maintain memory. Although an older person may not retain less meaningful information from the recent past, he characteristicaly remembers meaningful information and events from the remote past. He may recall in vivid detail a trip to an exciting city years ago and yet be unable to recall yesterday's trip to the paperstand. Intermittent memory loss demands that the older person devise compensations such as reminder notes and daily routines. The essence of self-esteem may also be threatened, unless the individual sustains meaningful life roles or replaces those roles that have been lost. Should an older person lose decision-making control over his life, he is at risk of suffering lowered self-esteem, helplessness, hopelessness, and worthlessness. Such loss of control typically occurs in hospitalized or dependent elders.

Self-Actualization

Self-actualization demands that elders use all of their potential for further growth. It is therefore among the most difficult need for elderly persons to fulfill in this society. Despite the misunderstanding and fear of aging that pervade American society, most elders do find some expression for accumulated years of wisdom, knowledge, and experience. Some elders maintain active careers or second careers; others begin new projects, hobbies, or affiliations (Fig. 7-3). In addition to helping friends and family, older persons often reach out to help other elders through mutual-help programs. Volunteer programs

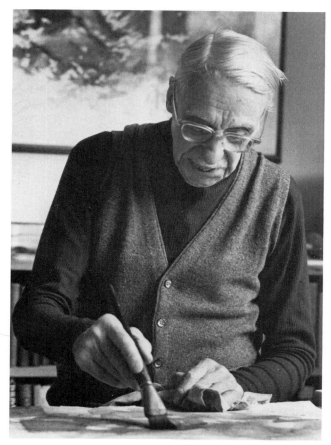

Figure 7-3
This older person has maintained his active career.
(Photo by Bob Kalmbach; University of Michigan Information Services)

to work with troubled children and families provide still other outlets for creativity.

Self-actualizing opportunities exist for the elderly person, and future generations of elders will demand more creative opportunity. There is also unlimited opportunity for creative adaptation to the challenges of relocation, of rehabilitation, and, ultimately, of dying. One prerequisite to self-actualization, however, is the satisfaction of basic and preceding needs; for this satisfaction, many elderly do depend upon nursing services to keep them healthy and to help them adjust to change.

Conclusion

For the most part, the foregoing life changes occur so gradually that the aged person learns how to adapt over a period of months or years. Sudden, unexpected losses provoke more difficulty in coping, but this is a characteristic of all life stages, not only of old age. The coping methods older people choose to employ can be effective if they are allowed adequate time and given support to solve their own stressful problems.

The elderly have much to learn and much to teach those who follow. If nurses can relinquish damaging myths and stereotypes about older persons, if we can see aging and dying as developmental processes of growth, and if we can understand the changes of aging, we can assist elders in a lifetime of adaptation.

In the eastern United States, a very old custom of personalized obituaries documents the older person's adaptation to life changes. The following is a typical tribute.

Example ☐ Mrs. Lydia (Turner) McRaddle died last Tuesday evening at the home of her only remaining son, Thomas McRaddle of 104 Cook Street. At age 87, she was Dorrville's second oldest citizen. Mr. Joseph McRaddle died 9 years ago, and their eldest son, Joseph Jr., died last summer in a traffic accident. An infant daughter survived only 3 weeks. Born the eldest of seven children of Johnson and Abigail Turner, Lydia McRaddle was a member of St. Stephan's Catholic Church, where a Mass for the Dead will be held on Wednesday, November 27th, at 9 A.M. The family invites all who remember her smiling face and clear soprano voice to join in the prayer on her behalf. Until she was 85, she sang in the parish choir by memorizing the hymns she could no longer read. But dim eyesight never prevented her from growing the finest herb garden in the Wells Valley. Her herb butters and vinegars consistently won top honors at the Wells fairground. Mrs. McRaddle would request that instead of flowers, donations be made in her name to the Lyons Club Fund for the Blind. Burial will be in St. Stephan's Cemetery next to her dear deceased husband. ☐

This tribute describes a lifetime of adaptation and learning to deal with the stress of life.

Study Questions

1. How might nurses assist elderly clients to alter their home environments to adapt to the biophysical needs of aging?

2. In what ways do health-care providers diminish the individuality of hospitalized elderly persons?

3. What effects do media (*e.g.,* televisions, newspapers, magazines) have on our images of elderly persons?

4. How can elderly persons remain healthy in spite of increasing age and diminishing physical abilities?

5. What does it mean to prepare for your old age while you are young?

Glossary

Activity theory: Psychosocial theory of aging that equates successful adaptation with the maintenance of social interactions and meaningful roles.

Continuity theory: Psychosocial theory of aging proposing that the older person adapts in a way that maintains continuity of personality.

Disengagement theory: Psychosocial theory of aging describing successful adaptation as withdrawing from social interaction and relinquishing social roles in order to prepare for death.

Geriatrics: Professional care for the sick older person.

Gerontology: The study of older people and how they adapt.

Senescence: The normal healthy process of growing older.

Senility: A general and outdated term used to describe abnormal behavior in older persons.

Touch deprivation: Lack of touch stimuli, resulting in insecurity and anxiety.

Bibliography

Botwinick J: Aging and Behavior. New York, Springer, 1973

Burnside I: Touching is Talking. Am J Nurs 73:2060–2063, December, 1973

Burnside I (ed): Nursing and the Aged, New York, McGraw-Hill, 1976

Burnside IM: Psychosocial Nursing Care of the Aged, New York, McGraw-Hill, 1973

Burnside IM, Ebersole P, Monea HE et al: Psychosocial Caring Throughout the Lifespan. New York, McGraw-Hill, 1979

Butler RN, Lewis M: Aging and Mental Health: Positive Psychosocial Approaches. St Louis, CV Mosby, 1977

Campbell EJ, LeFrak S: How aging affects the structure and function of the respiratory system. Geriatrics 32, No. 6:68–74, 1978

Cumming E, Henry WE: Growing Old. New York, Basic Books, 1961

Eliopoulos C: Gerontological Nursing. New York, Harper & Row, 1979

Erikson EH: Childhood and Society. New York, WW Norton, 1963

Havighurst RJ: Successful aging. In Williams RH, Tibbetts C, and Donahue W (eds): Processes of Aging, Vol 1. New York, Atherton Press, 1963

Lynn-Davies P: Influence of Age on the Respiratory System. Geriatrics 32:57–60, August, 1977

Murray R, Huelskoetter MM, O'Driscoll D: The Nursing Process in Later Maturity. Englewood Cliffs, NJ, Prentice-Hall, 1979

Murray R, Zentner J: Nursing Assessment Through the Lifespan. New Jersey, Prentice-Hall, 1979

Neugarten BL: Personality in Middle and Late Life. New York, Atherton Press, 1964

Oyer HJ, Oyer EJ: Aging and Communication. Baltimore, University Park Press, 1976

Peck RC, Berkowitz H: Psychological developments in the second half of life. In Neugarten BL (ed): Middle Age and Aging, pp 15–43. Chicago, University of Chicago Press, 1968

Rockstein M, Sussman M: Biology of Aging. Belmont, CA, Wadsworth Publishing, 1979

Schrock M: Holistic Assessment of the Healthy Aged. New York, John Wiley & Sons, 1980

Spier BE: Developmental tasks of the aged. In Yurick AG, Robb SS, Spier BE (eds): The Aged Person and the Nursing Process, pp 191–217. New York, Appleton-Century-Crofts, 1980

Wallace DJ: The Biology of Aging: 1976, An Overview. J Am Geriatr Soc 25:109–111, March, 1977

Yurick AG, Robb SS, Spier BE et al: The Aged Person and the Nursing Process. New York, Appleton-Century-Crofts, 1980

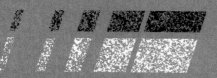

Health Care

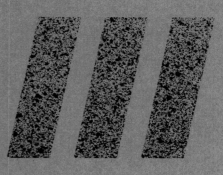

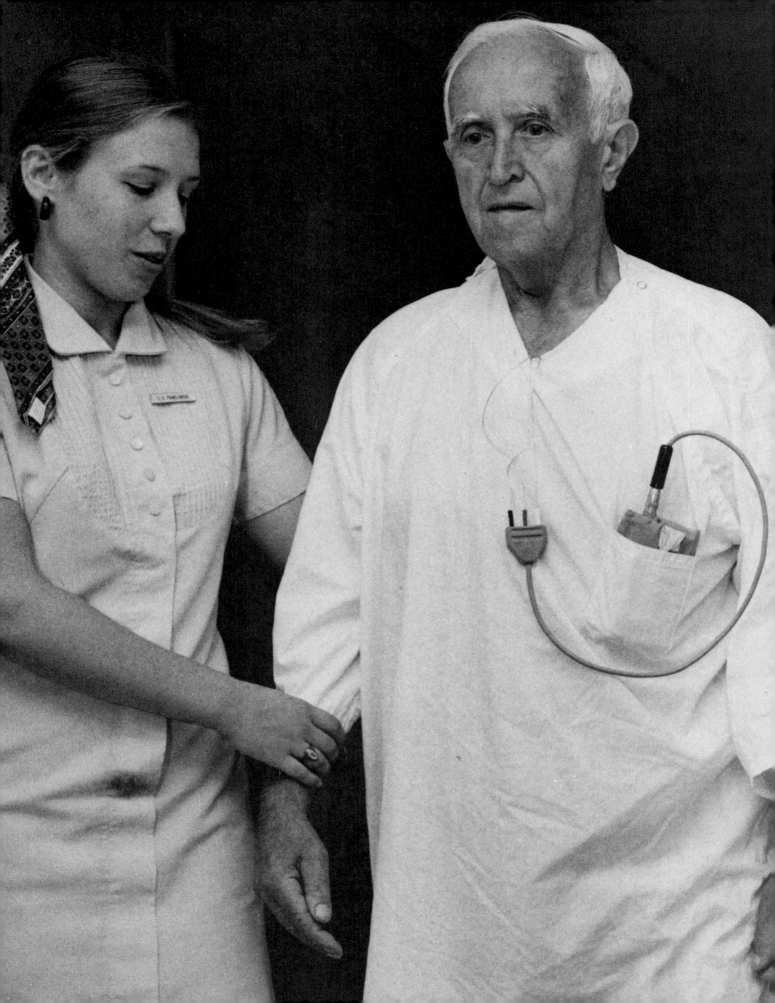

III

Health Care

Health care encompasses the services of many providers, of which nurses form the largest group. Although Americans are relatively healthy, billions of dollars are spent on health care each year. Health-care delivery is thus a major and costly national industry that has been shaped by historical influences and modern technology. It is both illness oriented and in a continuing state of crisis. As a result, individual persons may find health care to be both expensive and unsuited to their concerns. They may feel dehumanized by it or discouraged from seeking the care they need. The first chapter in this section presents many health problems of persons in the United States, as well as problems related to health-care delivery. Current means of managing health-care delivery are also discussed.

A person-centered approach to health-care delivery suggests that increasing attention be paid to persons as holistic individuals with greater emphasis on maintaining health. These ideas are developed in the chapter called comsumerism and preventive health care.

Health-Care Delivery

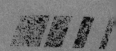

Mary L. Hunter

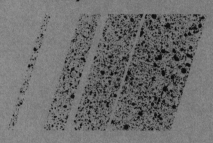

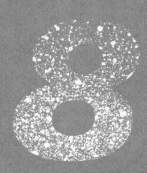

After completing this chapter, students will be able to:

● Differentiate between system and industry as these terms pertain to health-care delivery in the United States.

● Identify the major problems of health-care delivery.

● Discuss health manpower statistics and the contribution of nursing to health-care delivery.

● Discuss the historical influences on the delivery of health care.

● Identify health problems of each age group.

● Identify current and potential solutions for health problems.

● Discuss several ways in which government and the private sector have attempted to manage health-care delivery.

● Contrast the management of health-care delivery in traditional health-care systems and health maintenance organizations.

For at least 20 years, health-care delivery in the United States has been described as being in a state of crisis, possibly because we do not have the resources necessary to address all the needs that exist. Interestingly, however, most of the literature on crisis indicates that a crisis state cannot be maintained and sustained for more than about 6 weeks. Beyond that, stress to the system causes a complete breakdown and cessation of function. When crisis is the result of physical disease, such as cardiac failure, the person often must obtain relief within a few minutes for life to continue. How is it then, that we could have sustained the health-care crisis within this country for so many years!

Actually, some programs, agencies, and persons providing and seeking care *have* stopped functioning. However, health care continues to be given within the context of a crisis situation. The purpose of this chapter is to help the student examine health-care delivery as a concept and to consider strategies toward a more person-centered approach.

Health-Care Delivery as a System

A careful look at **health-care delivery** as we know it today may provide an understanding of why it is in crisis. Some of the literature on the methods and approach to health care in this country describe it as a "system." As indicated in Chapter 2, a system has been defined as an organized unit with a set of components that mutually react and function as a whole or total entity. Health-care delivery is composed of thousands upon thousands of smaller systems. The question is whether or not these smaller systems are subsystems of a greater system. In small towns for example, the doctors' offices, the pharmacies, the health department, and the community hospital may function as components of the town's larger system of health care. Other kinds of agencies, such as Heart or Diabetic Associations, the Visiting Nurse Association, and the United Way, may all work together with the other components of the system. When this is the case, health-care delivery in the area can be described as a system.

If, however, a person in that town is referred to a large medical center, he may find himself in a totally unfamiliar environment that appears very "unsystematic" in comparison to his previous experiences. Too often, persons entering large health-care facilities feel lost or overwhelmed by the "system." They encounter various specialists from several professions, many clinics, painful diagnostic procedures, and general difficulty in finding their way around. Moreover, conditions attached to the various payment plans are difficult to remember and fre-

quently result in unexpected heavy expense. This can be devastating financially and also very stressful.

We note too that procedures, policies, and payment plans vary among agencies and states. If one is buying a car, purchasing a house, or entering an educational institution, these variations can be tolerated. However, where health is concerned, the added stress of trying to enter and cope with a health-care system may increase the person's susceptibility to disease. The frustration described by persons who have attempted to obtain health-care services indicates that physiological changes can actually occur as a result of the stress experienced. To cite one example, a person who had asthma reported experiencing respiratory distress after a frustrating wait in a hospital clinic.

Walter Reuther, president of the United Auto Workers of America, made the following statement about his attempt to find comprehensive health-care plans for the auto workers, "Health care in the United States is in deep crisis—not because we lack the resources, not because the medical profession lacks the competence; we are in crisis because we lack a sound, modern, universal system for financing and providing comprehensive, high quality health care" (1969, pp. 14–15). Reuther's concern over the lack of an effective health-care system revolved about the difficulties of financing health care. Certainly the financial component is a major consideration. But what other factors are of concern?

Consider experiences which you, your family, or friends have encountered with health-care delivery. Perhaps you have known someone who needed several services in the course of one illness. Perhaps the person has seen a family doctor and then been sent to a surgeon who is part of a large hospital system. Here he has been referred to the social-service department for financial assistance; he has been given physical therapy; and he has received nutritional counseling from a dietitian. After leaving the hospital and returning home, he has been visited by a public-health nurse and has bought medicines and supplies from the nearest pharmacy. Consider this example and the following questions:

- Is there a common philosophy of health and health care among the agencies and care givers?
- Are the person's basic needs considered when care is planned?
- Is there effective transfer of records and appropriate data about the person among agencies, care givers, and the person seeking health care?
- Do nurses function as coordinators of care?

If you have answered "no" to these questions you have validated for yourselves that the word "system" does not apply to health care. Not only, as in Reuther's words, are we lacking a comprehensive system for financing health care, we also do not have an overall plan or philosophy from which the program flows. In order to solve these problems we do not necessarily need a single controlling body such as the federal government, although government agencies will be involved. Any solution requires that leaders from all health-care professions establish and put forth a philosophical framework on which the delivery of care can be based.

Problems in Health-Care Delivery

At the present time the most appropriate word to describe health-care delivery is that of "industry." Health care is a huge, unwieldy business that offers a multitude of products and services for sale, some of which emphasize illness rather than improved health. Some of the broad problems associated with our current structure of health care are listed below:

- Emphasis on crisis and illness rather than preventive health care and promotion of health
- Inadequate standards to ensure quality of care
- Minimal consumer participation
- Lack of coordination of services
- Poor communication among providers of services
- Extremely high costs

These problems will be evident throughout the discussion in the remainder of the chapter.

Health-Care Providers

Those who provide health care constitute a major component of the health-care delivery system. Table 8-1 lists the statistics for the approximate numbers of professional health-care workers in this country. These figures indicate that the nursing profession is twice the size of any other health profession. This fact clearly indicates that nursing ought to have a great effect on the health of this nation. Nurses in hospitals provide a tremendous amount of health and illness care that is difficult to quantify (Fig. 8-1). Significantly, nursing is the only group to provide regular, consistent, around-the-clock care. For real changes to occur in the health-care delivery industry, nursing leadership in collaboration with other professionals must be as evident as the numbers here indicate it should be.

Other health-care professionals and providers include nutritionists, dietitians, physical therapists, occupational therapists, optometrists, and audiologists. These persons also contribute many skills to health-care delivery. Other professionals closely associated with the health-care industry assist with rehabilitation (*i.e.*, social workers, psychologists, speech therapists, and vocational rehabilitation counselors).

Table 8-1
Approximate Numbers of Active Health Professionals

Projections for 1980

All active health professionals	1,885,370
Nurses (R.N.s)	1,099,600
Physicians (M.D.s, D.O.s)	466,800
Pharmacists	146,000
Dentists	126,000

Number of Health Professionals per 100,000 Population

All active health professionals	830.8
Nurses	484.5
Physicians	196.9
Pharmacists	64.4
Dentists	55.6

The Supply of Health Manpower, 1970 Profiles and Projections to 1990. DHEW Publications No. (HRA) 75–38, p. 15. Washington, DC, US Department of Health, Education and Welfare, December, 1974

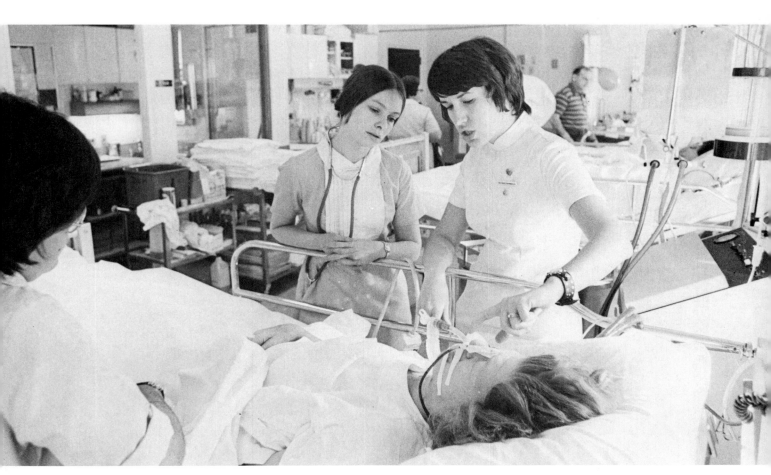

Figure 8-1
Nurses provide a significant amount of the health care delivered in hospitals. *(University of Michigan School of Nursing)*

Studies are frequently done by the health professions and the federal government to determine whether current manpower supplies are meeting society's needs. With the information obtained, plans may be made to raise or lower the numbers of professionals in a particular group. It is useful to note that changes in one group may have an impact on the functions of another. For example, if there are not enough physicians to meet medical care needs, nurses may discover that others consider them to be capable of performing tasks and procedures heretofore considered to be medical in nature. As the number of physicians increases, nurses may find that these very same people may no longer consider nurses to be competent for those duties.

The functions, as well as the supply, of health-care providers should also be considered. The team approach is often thought to be essential for effective care. Each professional has a set of skills that he

believes is necessary to provide the kind of care the person is seeking. He wishes to work with that client to provide a part of total person care. Unfortunately, we can overwhelm our clients when we ask them to relate to a team that may consist of nurse, doctor, pharmacist, dietitian, physical therapist, social worker, and chaplain, to name a few. Clients' needs will vary and they may indeed need direct care from these professionals. However, as nurses, you are encouraged to consider the many skills you have. As the person who has the most direct contact with the client, you act as a **coordinator of care.** You can help the client use other professional resources. You can relate to the team while your client relates to you as the care giver. You can assist the client in making more effective use of the physician. You may find that persons will seek out the nurse as a care provider at least as often as they seek the doctor, especially in the community.

Historical Influences in Health-Care Delivery

Table 8-2 indentifies the changes that have occurred in the United States since World War II. The advances in science and technology, with the accompanying movement from the country and farms to industrial areas and the cities, have resulted in changing needs for health care. We must realize, however, that some needs may have existed long before they were recognized. For example, a growth in the number of nonwhites was followed by an increased incidence in the health problems for this segment of the population. Yet this phenomenon may reflect the improvement in census activities rather than an increase in actual numbers.

Changes in family structure, civil rights dem-

Table 8-2
Historical Influences in Health-Care Delivery

Changes	*Influences*

Population dynamics since 1940	Increase in
	  General population
	  Nonwhite population
	  Life expectancy and birth rates among nonwhite persons
	  Proportion of foreign-born persons

Urbanization	Movement into suburbs
	
	Increase in
	  Marriage and divorce rates
	  Illegitimacy and teenage pregnancy
	  Pregnant women who do not receive prenatal care
	  Unemployment rate
	  Adult crime and juvenile deliquency
	  Numbers of persons living in substandard housing
	  Numbers of persons living at the poverty level
	  Older adult population
	  Automobile accidents, homicides, and suicides
	  Infant mortality rate and birth defects

Industrialization	Decrease in
	  Farming
	  Self-sufficiency once common among rural population

Literacy and education	Increases in
	  Knowledge about health care
	  Demand for more care of higher quality

Economic status	Wider range between high and low economic status Increase in government and private health-insurance programs
Advances in science and technology	Control of infectious diseases Development of drugs for control of many serious illnesses New and life-saving surgical techniques Life-maintenance techniques and equipment Hazardous industry Pollution resulting in increase in lung cancer and heart disease

onstrations, and the emergence of the consumer movement have affected our current method of health-care delivery. People who grow older in our society stay productive and are able to maintain their own homes for a longer period of time than was previously true. They often continue working at their careers or engage in more meaningful recreational, social, and charitable activities. Many older adults are more independent than their forerunners and, as a result, do not often live with their adult children. When these persons become less active due to disabilities or diseases, they often need nursing-home care. This need has added greatly to the costs of national health care.

Changes in nursing have also influenced health-care delivery. In the process of pursuing its professional development, nursing has become more autonomous and independent. Nurses are recognizing

Changes	*Influences*
Family structural changes	Breadwinner other than father
	New family structures, *i.e.,* communal living
	Single-parent families
	Working mothers
	Grandparents in own homes, far from adult children
Civil rights movements	Equality in health care as a right
	Equality regardless of race, creed, sex
	Women's liberation movement
Consumerism	Change in consumer concept of health and illness
	Self-help groups
	Increase in litigation
Nursing profession	Increased sense of accountability and responsibility
	Greater independence and autonomy
	More involvement in health policies and politics
Legislation	Hill–Burton Act (1946)
	Amendments to the Food, Drug and Cosmetic Act:
	Durham–Humphrey (1952)
	Kefauver–Harris (1962)
	Department of Health, Education and Welfare (1953)
	Regional Medical Program (1965)
	Comprehensive Health Planning Program (1966)
	Social Security Amendments:
	Title XVIII Medicare (1966)
	Title XIX Medicaid (1966)
	Comprehensive Drug Abuse Prevention and Control Act (1970)
	Health Maintenance Organization Act (1973)
	Professional Standards Review Organization Act (1973)
	National Health Planning and Resources Development Act (1974)
	Generic and Brand Names for Drugs Legislation (1977)
	Legislation prior to World War II:
	United States Public Health Service (1978)
	Pure Food and Drug Act (1906)
	Social Security Act (1935)
	Federal Food, Drug and Cosmetic Act (1938)

their unique contribution and finding more creative ways to distribute their services to society. They are beginning to affect health-care legislation and the politics of health-care delivery. The section on Professionalism will discuss these influences further.

Legislation represents another historical influence on health care. Over the years, health-care legislation has attempted to address a number of issues in health-care delivery. Legislation has provided monies for physical facilities, often hospitals, resulting in a prominence of tertiary care. **Tertiary care** can be defined as that care which takes place in highly specialized institutions that provide sophisticated diagnosis and treatment. Although persons may receive care in either the hospital or the ambulatory-care setting, it is generally considered to be long-term care.

Legislation has attempted to place controls on the accessibility, quality, and cost of health care. Specific legislation has been enacted to ensure the safety and efficacy of the drugs that are developed and distributed for general use in society. Several of these pieces of legislation will be discussed later in this section.

Health Problems of Persons in the United States

In spite of the many health problems discussed in this section, we should emphasize the fact that Americans are a very healthy people and have become progressively more so since 1900. Consider the following facts from the book Healthy People (DHEW, 1979, pp. 1–4):

- Diseases such as tuberculosis, gastroenteritis, diphtheria, and poliomyelitis—major causes of disability and death in the early years of this country—are nearly nonexistent today.

- With the advent of antibiotics, many of the bacteria-related diseases, which used to carry a high mortality rate, have become readily treatable.

- In 1900 the death rate per year was about 17 per 1000 persons; today it is 9 per 1000.

- Between 1950 and 1977 the mortality rate for children aged 1 through 14 years was cut in half.

- The life expectancy in 1900 was 47 years, whereas in 1977 it was 73 years.

Advances in our national health resulted from a variety of developments: improvement in sanitation, housing, and nutrition; the advent of antibiotics and

immunization programs, as well as the development of numerous drugs to control diabetes, hypertension, and other diseases; a growing awareness of the impact of certain life-styles and habits on our health; and the emergence of more self-help groups and self-help techniques.

When the health statistics of the United States are compared to other industrial nations, it is frequently observed that certain other Western nations have better national health programs than the United States does. The facts and figures may verify this view and reflect our faulty methods of health-care delivery. However, the United States has a population far greater and more diversified than countries such as Sweden and Japan. In addition, because of its complexity our society produces many more stressors that contribute heavily to health problems.

Since World War II, the United States has been a refuge for people fleeing political persecution and warlike conditions in Europe, Asia, and South America. That we may not provide proper care for these people is only one issue in a very complex problem.

In truth, we have made numerous advances. Consider the fact that it is now possible for women with diseases such as diabetes and heart problems to conceive and give birth. Consider the fact that many persons now survive serious illness and injury because of improved medical science, although they are often left with residual disabilities or compromised health. That we do have many preventable and treatable health problems must certainly be recognized. In this regard, we should be aware that statistics do not tell the whole story.

Health Problems Across the Life Span

Several examples of health problems that may occur across the life span have been listed in Table 8-3. As you can see from this table, the list is long and varied.

Solutions

Many solutions for these problems have been proposed and, indeed, policies, procedures, and community activities are already in place to deal with them. Some of the solutions are associated with preventive health care. Table 8-4 suggests some of the current programs available.

The aim of health-related programs is to increase society's awareness of existing needs. It is an attempt to help people realize their options and take better care of themselves, thereby retaining control over their lives.

(Text continues on page 120)

Table 8-3
Health Problems Across the Life Span

Age	Health Problems	Rank as a Cause of Death
Infants	Accidents	1
	Congenital anomalies	2
	Influenza and pneumonia	3
	Birth injuries	
	Low birth weight	
	Unfavorable resolution of trust *vs* mistrust	
Children 1–14 years	Accidents	1
	Malignant neoplasms	2
	Congenital anomalies	3
	Abuse and neglect	
	Dental caries	
	Inadequate school functioning	
	Lead poisoning among inner-city children	
	Learning disorders	
	Problems begun in childhood as precursors for adult problems	

	Unfavorable resolution of
	    Autonomy *vs* shame and doubt
	    Industry *vs* inferiority
	    Initiative *vs* guilt	

Adolescents and young adults 15–25 years	Accidents	1
	Homicide	2
	Suicide	3
	Alcohol and drug abuse	
	Injuries	
	Life-style and behavior pattern as precursors for chronic disease	
	Mental illness	
	Risk-taking behavior	
	Sexually transmissible disease	
	Smoking	

	Unfavorable resolution of
	    Identity *vs* role confusion
	    Intimacy *vs* isolation	

	Unwanted pregnancy	

(Continued)

Table 8-3
Health Problems Across the Life Span *(Continued)*

Age	Health Problems	Rank as a Cause of Death
Adults 26–44 years	Accidents	1
	Heart disease	2
	Malignant neoplasms	3
	Alcohol abuse	
	Cirrhosis	
	Diabetes	
	Feelings of stagnation and self-absorption	
	Homicide	
	Hypertension	
	Mental illness	
	Obesity	
	Peridontal disease	
	Unfavorable resolution of generativity *vs* stagnation	
Adults 45–64 years	Heart disease	1
	Malignant neoplasms	2
	Cerebrovascular disease	3
	Other problems similar to those in the age group 26–44 years	
Older adults 65 years and older	Heart disease	1
	Malignant neoplasm	2
	Cerebral vascular disease	3
	Arteriosclerosis	
	Decreased ability to care for self	
	Dependency	
	Depression	
	Diabetes	
	Fluid, electrolyte, and metabolic disturbances	
	Influenza and pneumonia	
	Injuries	
	Insufficient finances to meet basic needs	
	Neglect, loneliness	
	Nutritional deficiencies	
	Overmedication	
	Preventable and reversible mental deterioration and behavioral changes	
	Stress of loss and grief	
	Unfavorable resolution of Ego integrity *vs* despair Visual and hearing alterations	

Table 8-4
Possible Solutions for Health Problems

Solution	Examples
Community support systems	Abuse prevention Parent counseling Runaway centers Stress control Suicide prevention
Counseling programs	Family planning Genetic counseling Nutritional counseling
Educational programs	CPR classes Health education through the school year Nutritional education Physical-fitness activities and programs Information about signs of cancer Unemployment programs, teaching youth how to be employable
Health and safety protection	Automobiles designed for safety Changes in fabric (not inflammable) Childhood immunizations Control of firearms Control of disease, *i.e.,* veneral disease, hypertension Fluoridation of community water supply Lowering speed limits Occupational health and safety programs Poison control centers Proper reporting of diseases, regulations, and use of statistics Seat belts in moving vehicles Toxic-substance control Toy manufacturing safety regulations
Prevention programs	Dental hygiene Papanicolaou ("pap") smear Prenatal care and mental health Self breast examination
Screening programs	Screening and diagnosis for high-risk factors across age groups Screening programs for diseases such as diabetes and hypertension

Management of Health-Care Delivery

We have employed many strategies over the years to try and manage this unwieldy industry called health-care delivery. These strategies have involved the government, the private sector, and often a combination of both. The following discussion presents several key points in the history of health-care management. Perhaps consideration of these ideas will suggest new ideas for future solutions to the problems.

Government Structures

The Department of Health, Education and Welfare (HEW) was established in 1953. Its purpose was to organize the various health and welfare agencies of the government under one administrative unit for more coordination and efficiency. There were four major branches at that time: the Public Health Service, Social and Rehabilitation Services, the Social Security Administration, and the Office of Education. The department is now called the Department of Health and Human Services. Education now has its own organization. In the future the Department may be altered further to meet the needs of the time.

Of the above-mentioned branches, the Public Health Service is of major concern to nursing. It was established by a congressional act in 1798 and is the oldest of the organizations making up the department of HEW. It established a vehicle for health professionals and scientists to discover and apply knowledge in order to conquer disease and improve health.

Table 8-5 lists the six major agencies that comprise the Public Health Service, the combined purpose of which is to provide better health services for the American people. Activities of the service include:

- Review of health care—the quality and appropriateness of medical care provided to Medicare and Medicaid subscribers
- Provision of grants to study widespread health problems such as venereal disease and hypertension
- Assistance with plans to raise public awareness of serious health problems
- Operation of hospitals for national health problems such as narcotics addiction, tuberculosis, and mental illness
- Research on health problems
- Provision of training grants to educational institutions in the health sciences
- Publication of vital statistics pertinent to public-health programs

The Reagan administration's emphasis on decreased expenditures may alter the philosophy and functions of the Public Health Service.

Financing Health-Care Delivery

Health-care costs have mounted alarmingly since 1900. Many agencies can no longer be supported by fee for service alone and must rely on voluntary contributions or tax dollars. Many people cannot afford to pay for health care and find it necessary to join insurance programs or to receive help from the government.

Table 8-5
Agencies of the United States Public-Health Service

Agency	Mission
National Institute of Health	Research
Food and Drug Administration	Regulation related to consumer protection
Health Services Administration	Establishment of responsibility related to the delivery of health care and quality of care
Center for Disease Control	Responsibility for preventive medicine and public health
Health Resources Administration	Development of health-service resources and improvement of their use
Alcohol, Drug Abuse and Mental Health Administration	Development of strategies to deal with medical problems

Funding Health-Care Agencies

Agencies are funded from two basic sources: tax support and private support. Tax-supported agencies receive public aid through city, county, state or federal agencies and funds. Often several levels of government combine to provide assistance. These agencies are not necessarily free to those they serve and usually charge a fee for service in order to offset operating costs.

Most tax-supported agencies are nonprofit. Those that make a profit return monies to the agency for expansion of services and the purchase of new equipment. Examples of tax-supported agencies include health departments from all levels of government, many hospitals, Bethesda hospital complex, other army, navy and veterans' hospitals, state mental hospitals and neighborhood health clinics.

Non-tax-supported agencies include private, profit-oriented agencies such as pharmacies, some hospitals, nursing homes, and private practices that are run on a fee-for-service basis.

Private, nonprofit agencies are supported by fees for service and voluntary contributions. Examples of this kind of agency include certain hospitals, the Visiting Nurses' Association, and programs such as Motor Meals. Most voluntary agencies are also private and nonprofit oriented. They usually concern themselves with a single problem. The American Cancer Society, the American Heart Association, and the National Foundation (The March of Dimes) are examples of voluntary agencies. Figure 8-2 indicates the funding structure of health-care agencies.

Financing Personal Health Care

Private Insurance

Private insurance is one way of financing personal health care. Nonprofit, tax-exempt organizations such as Blue Cross–Blue Shield provide payment for the health-care needs of many Americans. Private, profit-oriented insurance companies also deal with the payment of health-care needs. To become insured, members must pay monthly premiums either by themselves or in combination with an employer. The best method of buying insurance is as a member of a contracting group through a union, an employer, or a club. This approach reduces the cost of insurance, because the pooled risks of all group members determine charges. These plans commonly pay about 80% of health-care costs, and the client must pay the remainder.

There are many other insurance plans available which offer varying coverage. Many do not cover preventive health-care costs or screening procedures such as routine chest x-rays. Some include benefits for psychiatric care and cancer follow-up care, but often coverage is limited for long-term disease. A certain amount of time must elapse between hos-

Figure 8-2
Funding of health care agencies.

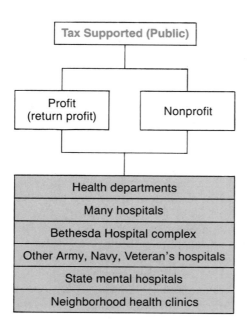

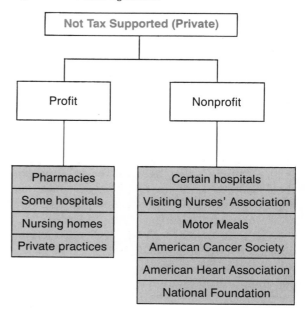

pitalizations for a given disease, before benefits resume.

It is not possible for nurses to know what each insurance program has to offer. We can be aware, however, that our clients need to understand the coverage they have as they make decisions about the health care they need. Even though one does not usually question the need for emergency or intensive-care treatment, there may be other treatment plans that can be considered and chosen. As nurses, we can help clients with that decision making.

Medicare

Medicare (Title XVIII of the Social Security Act), which has been in existence since 1966, is another prominent insurance program. It is administered by the federal government and is thereby uniform from state to state. Medicare serves persons age 65 or over regardless of financial resources. It also covers disabled persons under 65 who have been entitled to social-security benefits for 2 consecutive years and certain other persons with renal failure. These people are insured through a monthly premium deducted from their social-security benefits, with an additional amount being paid by the federal government. These monies are placed in trust funds that pay medical expenses for insured persons. Medical expenses covered include costs of physician services, home health care, and outpatient services such as rehabilitation therapy. Hospital insurance under Medicare is financed by workers' payroll deductions. Hospital expenses covered include semiprivate rooms, meals, the intensive-care unit, drugs, laboratory and x-ray tests, operating room use, dressing supplies, appliances such as wheelchairs, and rehabilitative services such as occupational and physical therapy. Psychiatric hospital care is covered for up to 190 days.

Services sometimes covered include certain hospital and home health-care agencies, independent laboratories and x-ray services, some ambulance firms, chiropractors, and a variety of independent practitioners. Agencies and independent practitioners can make the decision not to accept persons insured by Medicare. Because there is bookkeeping that must be done to qualify for reimbursement, certain agencies and individuals find this too time consuming and expensive.

Services not covered by Medicare include personal services in hospitals, such as television and telephones, private rooms or private-duty nurses, routine physical examinations and tests, routine foot care, eye and hearing examinations, eye glasses and hearing aids, and immunizations for infectious diseases. To be covered, care must be considered reasonable and necessary. Care that can be provided by unskilled care givers such as home health aids in not covered. Drugs or meals delivered to the home are also not covered.

Nurses who provide care for persons receiving Medicare should be aware of the following facts:

- Persons should always carry their Medicare cards and present them whenever seeking services.
- The person's claim number should appear on any bills or correspondence sent to the claims offices.
- The agencies and services the person is seeking should be checked beforehand to determine that they are approved for reimbursement by Medicare and that they accept Medicare.
- The services covered within a given agency should be clarified before the agency is used.
- Persons disagreeing with the coverage by Medicare in a specific instance have the right to appeal.
- All persons insured by Medicare should have a copy of *Your Medicare Handbook*, distributed by the U.S. Dept. of Hew (1979).

Nurses should be aware that Medicare does not address certain common needs of persons age 65 or older. Refer to Table 8-3 and note that preventive and promotional health-care coverage is inadequate.

Medicaid

Medicaid (Title XIX of the Social Security Act), a third way of financing personal health care, has also been in existence since 1966. It is administered by both federal and state governments in a partnership arrangement. The states develop their own programs within federal government guidelines. As a result, benefits vary from state to state. The program provides benefits for certain eligible needy and low-income persons who are under 65 years of age. In addition it pays for certain expenses for persons over 65 who are below a certain income level, including services that Medicare does not cover. Medicaid pays for medical expenses incurred by persons with complete visual loss and those classified as disabled, as well as by members of families with low income and dependent children. The program is funded by federal, state, and local taxes. Table 8-6 lists services covered by Medicaid.

As with Medicare, nurses can assist clients who are eligible for Medicaid by providing them with information concerning the program, making sure that they understand the necessity of always carrying

Table 8-6
Services Covered by Medicaid

Covered	Covered in Some States
Inpatient services	Dental care
Outpatient services	Prescribed drugs
Skilled nursing-home care	Eye glasses
Physician's services	Intermediate-care facilities' services:
Laboratory services	Diagnostic
X-ray procedures	Screening
Diagnosis and treatment of children under 21	Preventive Rehabilitative
Home health-care services	
Family planning services	
Rural health-clinic services	

their Medicaid card, and checking agencies to determine whether they accept Medicaid clients and which services are covered. Nurses will want to stay current with government reimbursement policies related to Medicare and Medicaid. As the administration of all levels of government changes, programs and their rules, regulations, and benefits change also.

Both programs expect high standards of care, and they support the development of needed services. They encourage innovations in medical-care delivery and require a review of the care provided. Both programs are also concerned about cost containment. An amendment to the Social Security Act, called the Professional Standards Review Organizations (PSRO), was enacted in 1972. This mandated that physicians develop a mechanism for monitoring care and assuring quality care to beneficiaries of Medicare and Medicaid. Physicians were the first target group of this law. However, nursing is now included and nurses are involved in peer review and quality assurance programs.

National Health Insurance

The major proposed solution for the financing of health-care delivery in the United States is **National Health Insurance.** This would provide guaranteed coverage so that health care could be obtained by everyone. The Advisory Committee on National Health Insurance, charged by President Jimmy Carter, was instructed to develop a plan that would provide the following (Mauksch, 1978, p. 1323):

* Fair and equitable treatment
* Redistribution of health-care resources
* Meeting manpower needs
* Training of health-care professionals
* Quality assurance systems
* Illness prevention means
* Planning and control of resources
* Origin and delivery of services
* Administrative simplicity
* Eligibility standards

This list indicates that the Carter administration wished to examine other major problems in addition to financing. Other administrations will have their own view of the issues. The Reagan administration, for example, halted most of the discussions on this proposal.

Overall, the proponents of a national health insurance program seek to reflect the generally agreed-upon notion that everyone is entitled to health care. A national health insurance program would attempt to deliver health care that is financially equitable, accessible, available, comprehensive, and uniform in quality of care.

Two nursing leaders, however, caution us to be alert to the limitations of national health insurance. Mauksch states, "The crucial issue here is that a national health insurance package that does not alter the manner in which care is administered or change the attitudes fostered by care givers simply will not meet the needs of the people." She goes on to explain, "The true success of national health insurance depends to a large extent upon the way providers and consumers deal with it. ... [They] will need to mount a national effort toward the improvement of health and illness care attitudes, so that the new system [national health insurance] may serve society well" (1978, p. 1327). In the same vein, McGee cautions, "It should be kept in mind that national health insurance deals only with cost coverage, not the health care system itself" (1980, p. 37).

It behooves us to be aware of these concerns. Federal legislators are asking nurses to testify during hearings on national health insurance. Proposed nursing solutions could make a difference in the overall effectiveness of health-care delivery. For example, Barbara Nichols, president of the American Nurses Association (1978–1982), testified before the Senator Edward Kennedy hearing in Denver on November 29, 1978 (Brewer, 1979).

Nichols pointed out that the United States provides a medical or acute-care system designed to treat people after they become ill or injured, rather than to emphasize preventive services. She indicated that the acute-care focus relies heavily on physicians and institutions, thus adding significantly to national health-care costs. Ms. Nichols pointed out that Senator Kennedy's plan for national health insurance does not consider nursing services as a covered benefit. She indicated that a separate identification of nursing service costs would more accurately describe the financial situation and she suggested a number of key ways in which nursing services could deal effectively with many of today's health problems. For example, health education programs and plans for care of chronically disabled and dying persons in the home could provide cost-effective care.

Just a year later, Sister Rosemary Donley indicated that the Kennedy proposal now delineated nursing service as a separate factor. She stated that the proposal opens the possibility of expanding the system of reimbursing nurse practitioners (1979, p. 4). This suggests that nursing can have an impact on the development of national health insurance policy.

Several plans for national health insurance have been proposed, each of which covers a variety of services. Some would provide payment for catastrophic illness only. Catastrophic illness is defined in terms of cost. Other proposals suggest additional coverage and improved benefits for the aged, pregnant women, and children. Some would require membership of our entire population, and others consider voluntary participation to some degree. Some programs would be supported by tax dollars, whereas others might involve private enterprise.

Although, as times change, specific persons such as Senator Kennedy may not be as vocal in health-care issues, others will take their place. It behooves nurses to be proactive in shaping legislation that would delineate appropriate nursing services. In this way we may be able to protect our clients from exorbitant expense and to ensure that preventive health care becomes a priority.

Donley states, "The ANA is on record in support of comprehensive national health insurance. While none of the bills [currently being proposed] meets ANA specifications, the catastrophic plans are least compatible with ANA statements and principles. ANA is on record in support of nursing service as a benefit

and the professional nurse as a provider" (p. 4). Sister Donley urges us to push and press this issue.

Nurses will want to consider the following questions concerning any form of national health insurance:

- How does the government plan to deal with overuse of the system?
- Can we expect a change from illness-oriented care to preventive health care and health promotion?
- Will national health insurance provide reimbursement of nursing services?
- Does the federal government understand the difference between medical insurance and health insurance?

Health Maintenance Organizations: A Possible Solution

Health maintenance organizations (HMOs) are group health practices whose major distinguishing feature is prepayment. Members pay a fixed fee on a yearly basis and receive health care whenever they need it either for a nominal additional charge or no charge, depending on the plan. The HMO provides comprehensive health-care services that include wellness care as well as illness care. The program is arranged so that a broad group of specialists participate in care and are available for referral. Most HMOs have participating hospitals as well.

The emphasis on preventive health services and wellness care encourages people to seek care early in a disease process, thereby avoiding hospitalization. The healthier the clients are, the more financially stable the HMO remains. The traditional approach to health care has been to pay doctors and hospitals to provide care to the sick, thus giving incentives for illness care. The HMO has sought to change that by providing incentives for health care.

One of the most successful HMOs is the Kaiser-Permanente prepaid care plan, which provides medical and hospital services to more than 3 million people. Agencies and physicians over a large portion of the western United States, as well as Ohio and Hawaii, participate in this program. Kaiser-Permanente has developed six basic principles from which it operates:

- Group practice
- Integration of facilities (combining both hospital and outpatient facilities)
- Prepayment

- Preventive health care (emphasis on keeping the person well in addition to treating the sick)
- Voluntary enrollment
- Physician responsibility (for patient care, financing, planning, and allocation of resources)

Central to their operation is the principle that the program must be self-sustaining. Equipment and facilities are paid for by client fees and long-term loans. Less than 1% of Kaiser-Permanente has been supported by either private or government sources.

A summary of the characteristics of HMOs and traditional health-care delivery suggests the following differences:

- *Traditional care*—Fee for service to physicians and cost reimbursement for hospitals provides incentives for delivering illness care; third-party insurance coverage relieves the person from much of the cost of his health care, thus providing him with little incentive for questioning that cost.
- *HMO care*—Prepayment of fixed fees to hospitals and physicians provides a strong incentive to keep costs reasonable and to provide wellness care. When the cost barrier is removed, people come in earlier for care and thus avoid long-term and expensive illness problems.

Using the Kaiser-Permanente plan as a model, the federal government enacted the Health Maintenance Organization Act in 1973. This was developed to study various methods of health-care delivery in the hope of generating a model for comprehensive health care. The act was to deal with such issues as the distribution and availability of quality health care, cost containment, and quality control. It provided for members of HEW to collaborate with the PSROs to ensure quality of care.

The future of HMOs is uncertain at this point. Much depends on what course the government takes with regard to national health insurance. A combination of the two concepts is a distinct possibility.

Person-Centered Health-Care Delivery

Students, in their learning years, can be observers of health-care delivery. For example, watching and listening while sitting in waiting rooms of health-care agencies provide opportunities for obtaining information about the "system." Be aware of how often the person becomes a number and how often the needs of the agency or the practitioner take priority. The following example comes from a nurse and mother of a 20-year-old man waiting to have an angiogram (x-ray film of the vascular system using a radioactive dye) for a possible subclavian artery aneurysm.

Example □ Tony was to have had the angiogram at 10 A.M. that morning. However, just before we left the house a fierce summer storm began. Upon finally arriving at the hospital we learned that the electrical system was not functioning and an emergency generator was being used to keep essential equipment and lights in operation. Appointments for many x-ray examinations were being canceled. Tony was asked to stay because of the more serious nature of his problem, with the hope that electrical power would be restored later in the day. This created a great deal of anxiety for him, because he had planned to have the procedure over quickly and to know the extent of his problem. The receptionist gave as much assistance as she could under the circumstances. However, no nurse came to console him or others in the same predicament. At one point his doctor entered an office along the hallway, and I thought surely he would stop in for a moment to commiserate. However, he did not. I knew that just seeing him would have helped Tony feel better.

Despite my anxiety over my son's condition, I found myself viewing the situation as a professional nurse and systems observer. I watched the frustration and anxiety people demonstrated when their x-ray tests were canceled. I noted that professional persons did not come to assist the receptionist or help the clients. One doctor who appeared spoke generally to the waiting room and said, "We're sorry this has happened and we'll try to reschedule you as best as we can." With that he turned on his heel and walked away. Some clients blamed the receptionist and were unreasonable and offensive in their remarks to her. She became defensive and rude telling them loudly that it wasn't *her* fault!

I kept thinking how much difference a nurse would have made. Nurses, for example, have been taught to use a Maslovian framework to understand the feelings of anxiety and insecurity that this kind of situation creates in the person. They understand the reasons why frustrated persons heap abuse irrationally on whomever is available. They can be objective and use therapeutic communication skills to help the person focus on reality and do problem solving. If three people out of ten can be scheduled with the return of electrical power, nurses know to choose those with greater physiological needs, because they have been taught how to establish priorities. Their presence would provide leadership for persons who do not have these skills. □

Conclusion

The current approach to health-care delivery is complex, unsystematic, and often described as in a state of crisis. Historical influences shaped the system, making it illness oriented, industrial in nature, and extremely costly. Financing health care involves funding both the agencies and the private and government insurance plans to pay for the health-care services people need. Americans are basically healthy people, and the leading health problems in various groups are well known. Americans recognize, however, that health-care delivery in the future may require both a different focus and different management strategies to maintain and increase the nation's health. These changes seem likely because of both cost factors and consumer complaints about a health-care delivery system that dehumanizes the individual person.

Study Questions

1. Consider a health-care agency with which you are familiar (*i.e.,* hospital unit, pharmacy, doctor's office, crisis center).
   a. Identify the professionals and nonprofessionals in the agency. Consider how geographically accessible it is to a broad spectrum of people.
   b. Identify the philosophy and standards of care in the agency.
   c. Identify the larger system of which it is a subsystem.

2. Describe how the following historical events have resulted in problems of health-care delivery:
   a. Legislation that provided hospital building funds
   b. Control of infectious disease
   c. Increase in the general population
   d. Urbanization
   e. Advances in science and technology

3. Discuss the limitations of Medicare in providing for the health needs of the older adult.

4. Accidents are a major health problem for people across the life span. Describe some possible solutions aside from those listed in Table 8-4.

5. Considering the problems of health and health-care delivery, suggest some ways nursing could advance health in the United States.

6. Examine the ideas behind national health insurance and health maintenance organizations. Describe how these two concepts might work together toward a health-care delivery system for all Americans.

Glossary

Coordinator of care: One of the roles of the nurse; the act of helping the client utilize appropriately all resources available to him.

Health-care delivery: The methods of and approaches to health care, sometimes described as a system or as an industry.

Health maintenance organizations (HMOs): Group health-care practices whose major distinguishing feature is prepayment.

Medicaid: Title XIX of the Social Security Act, which provides health-care insurance for certain needy and low income persons.

Medicare: Title XVIII of the Social Security Act, which provides health-care insurance for persons over 65 years and for certain other persons.

National health insurance: A proposed insurance program that would provide guaranteed coverage so that health care could be obtained by everyone.

Tertiary care: That care which takes place in highly specialized institutions that provide sophisticated diagnosis and treatment.

Bibliography

Aiken LH: Nursing priorities for the 1980's: Hospitals and nursing homes. Am J Nurs 81, No. 2: 324–330, 1981

Aiken LH: The practice setting: An overview of health policy issues. In Aiken LH (ed): Health Policy and Nursing Practice, pp. 3–16. New York, McGraw-Hill, 1981

Archbold PG, Hoeffer B: Reframing the issue: A debate on third-party reimbursement. Nurs Outlook 29, No. 7: 423–425, 1981

Archer SE: A national health service: Rationale and implementation. Nurs Outlook 29, No. 6: 364–368, 1981

Brewer K: Inclusion of nursing services vital to any national health insurance program. American Nurse 11:1, January 20, 1979

Chaisson GM: Correctional health care beyond the barriers. Am J Nurs 81, No. 4: 737–738, 1981

Department of Health, Education and Welfare (DHEW): Healthy People: The Surgeon General's Report on Health Promotion and Disease Prevention. Washington, DC, Office of the Assistant Secretary for Health, 1979

DHEW: The Supply of Health Manpower 1970. Profile and Projections to 1990. DHEW Publ #(HRA) 75-38. Washington, DC, Bureau of Health Resources Development, 1974

DHEW: Your Medicare Handbook. HEW publication # SSA 70-10050. Washington, DC, Department of Health, Education and Welfare, March 1979

Donabedian D: What students should know about the health and welfare system. Nurs Outlook 28, No. 2: 122–125, 1980

Donley R: Will we allow candidates to dodge the NHI issue? American Nurse 11:4, November 30, 1979

Fagin C: Nursing as an alternative to high-cost care. Am J Nurs 82, No. 1: 56–60, 1982

Faherbaugh S, Strauss A, Suczek B et al: The impact of technology on patients, providers and care patterns. Nurs Outlook 28, No. 11: 666–672, 1980

Farber SJ: The future role of the V.A. hospital system: A national health dilemma. N Engl J Med 298: 625–628, 1978

Grimaldi P et al: Medicaid reimbursement of long-term nursing care. Geriatric Nurs 2, No. 2: 133–138, 1981

Jennings CP: Nursing's case for third party reimbursement. Am J Nurs 79, No. 1: 110–114, 1979

Johnston M: Ambulatory health care in the 80's: Decade of dilemmas. Am J Nurs 80, No. 1: 76–80, 1980

King E: Health and nursing issues in the 80's. NLN Publ 16-1839: 1–9, 1980

Lancaster J: Macro-system interaction: Communication within the health care delivery system. Top Clin Nurs 1, No. 3: 89–100, 1979

Mancini M: Medicare: Health rights of the elderly. Am J Nurs 79, No. 10: 1810–1812, 1979

Mauksch IG: Advocacy or control: Which do we offer the elderly? Geriatric Nurs, Nov/Dec 1980, 278

Mauksch IG: On national health insurance. Am J Nurs 78, No. 8: 1323–1327, 1978

McGee E: The national health insurance maze. Imprint 27:36, 37–107, April 27, 1980

Moses E, Roth A: Nursepower. Am J Nurs 79, No.10: 1745–1756, 1979

Murray R, Zentner J: Nursing Concepts for Health Promotion. Englewood, New Jersey, Prentice-Hall, 1979

Nordberg T: Third party payments. Diabetes Educ 6, No. 1: 23, 1980

Reuther W: The health care crisis: Where do we go from here? Am J Public Health 59:12–20, January, 1969

Rittinger K, Lesparre M: Panel retains funds for nurses in manpower bill. Hospitals 28:32, May 16, 1980

Sasmor JL: Dollars and Sense. Am J Nurs 81, No. 3: 546–547, 1981

Shaheen PP: Nationalizing health care: A humanitarian approach. Nurs Outlook 29, No. 6, 358–363, 1981

Smith HL: Nurses' quality of working in an HMO. Nurs Res 30, No. 1: 54–58, Jan–Feb 1981

Templin HE: The system and the patient. Am J Nurs 82, No. 1: 108–111, 1982

US National Center for Health Statistics, Health Resources Statistics, (DHEW Publ No [PHS] 79-1509) Washington DC, US Government Printing Office, 1979

Wightman F: The health mobile. Health Visit 53, No. 10: 422–423, 1980

Consumerism and Preventive Health Care

Mary L. Hunter and Martha Keehner Engelke

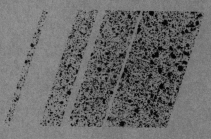

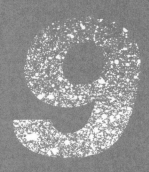

Consumers are people or groups of people who use a commodity or a service. As consumers, we use a continuous array of products every day. Even while we sleep, we consume. If the weather is cool, we use fuel to heat our houses. If it is warm, we use electricity to keep air conditioning or fans running. Many of us are consumers of educational services throughout a major portion of our lives, for either ourselves or our children.

All of us are consumers of health commodities and health services. Some of these services require the specialized knowledge and skills of health-care professionals. Many of the commodities, however, may be purchased by our own choice. Toothpaste, antidandruff shampoos, aspirin and bandages are just a few of the items we buy for health purposes. As we decide about these purchases, we become consumers of advertising and packaging. Often it is the sensory appeal of a color or the statement on the box that makes us choose a certain toothpaste or change from one type of aspirin to another.

The media, television, radio, newspapers, and magazines add to our knowledge of health products and health subjects. We read articles about our health and see messages from health organizations, such as the one issued by the American Cancer Society, providing a checklist of symptoms for certain diseases. We may also watch television programs that add to our information about ourselves and our health.

There are several problems associated with buying commodities and services. Although consumers want to spend money wisely and to receive something of value in return, they frequently settle for less than the best, possibly because of the expense, a lack of awareness, or a lack of time to find out about other available products. In times of illness, it is even more difficult to make effective decisions concerning health care. Anxiety about illness can frequently prevent us from making rational choices.

Unfortunately, consumers do not always shop for health-care services but rather accept those most readily available. When we buy products for our home or personal use, we read magazine articles about them and inquire as to their value per dollar. When we seek some kind of special service, we check with friends or the Better Business Bureau to learn more about the ratings of the suppliers who provide them. However, when it comes to purchasing health services, we are deplorably reluctant to check on the type of health care available.

Characteristics of the Consumer of Health Care

Consumers of health care, like all people, have certain characteristics that must be taken into account when health-care services are rendered. As such, these characteristics have important implications for nursing.

- **The consumer of health care has interrelated biological, psychological, and sociological concerns.**

    Consider the following example. A mother becomes ill with cholecystitis (inflammation of the gall bladder) and must be hospitalized. She is in severe pain and is scheduled to undergo surgery. As nurses, we are concerned about providing pain relief measures and giving her the best preoperative teaching possible. But unless we also consider her psychosocial needs, these actions may be ineffective. If this mother has a teenage daughter whose behavior has worried her seriously, being away from her now will increase her concerns. Because emotional stress is known to affect pain and learning, this woman's anxiety may make it difficult for her to learn at this particular time, thereby extending her postoperative course. This, in turn, could add to the stress of her family situation.

    Consider also a man who has experienced a serious heart attack and must be hospitalized for several weeks. When he is discharged, he is told to go home and rest; he is not to worry about anything except getting well. However, if this man has had financial concerns prior to the heart attack, being away from work for many weeks will more than likely

add to the burden. Relaxation will thus be difficult, if not impossible. The added stress may very well extend his convalescence and compound his financial burdens.

These examples have focused on physiological problems and suggest that psychosocial needs can increase the deleterious effects of physical illness. But these two examples can be viewed in another way, in that the preexisting psychosocial needs may have precipitated the physical problems. The interrelationship of these factors reinforces the need for nurses to consider the whole person when providing care.

- **The consumer of health care has a set of worries and concerns that may differ from those of the health-care providers.**

    Some people may not consider their long-term illnesses as health problems. If they have lived with a chronic disease for a long period of time, it may seem normal for them. One woman being interviewed in a clinic was asked, on the basis of a written questionnaire, if she knew what had made her "sick" (with diabetes).

    She answered, "Sick? I'm not sick. People with diabetes aren't sick. Even though I have to come into the hospital next week, it's just to get it straightened out; it's not because I'm sick. Now if they want to do something for me, I wish they'd do something about my heart. Ever since my heart attack 4 years ago, I haven't been able to get my housework done. Now that's a problem!"

    Martha Weinman Lear, in her book *Heartsounds*, described the last 3 years of her physician husband's life as he tried to cope with progressive heart disease. Although deeply concerned about his heart condition, he discovered to his horror that his mental abilities had declined following heart surgery. He had lost memory for recent events and he often could not grasp the meaning of printed monosyllabic words. Driving or shopping left him exhausted and confused. When he sought help for this problem from his cardiologists, he was told to be patient, to give his mind as well as his body time to recover. Some people reminded him that he was getting older, and that we all suffer from memory loss as we age. They did not understand why he was concerned about his memory when it was the heart disease which was life threatening.

- ● *The consumer of health care has a set of personal priorities.*

Public-health nurses who visit families in rural areas or inner cities may consider immunizations to be a top priority. A mother of such a family, trying to cope with chronic headaches and the need to keep food on the table for her children, is unlikely to take the time and energy required to go to an immunization clinic, even if the services are free, until she finds help for her other problems. The concern of the health-care professionals is not meaningful to her. The possibility of her children contracting a disease such as polio or smallpox seems too unlikely or irrelevant at this moment to represent a serious threat.

- ● *The consumer of health care has self-care abilities and a knowledge of personal needs.*

If we subscribe to the philosophy of self-care, we believe that persons have these abilities and this knowledge. However, persons cannot always communicate their knowledge or mobilize their strengths to meet their needs. That is why they become consumers of health care and why health-care professionals exist to serve them. As nurses, we provide services because we have been hired by consumers, not because we have the right to exert our authority over their choices.

Variables That Influence Health Behavior

Health behaviors develop from customs peculiar to one's social system, culture, and family; they are learned behaviors. A person will adopt a health behavior if he perceives it to have value, meaning, and relevance to his particular needs, and if it fits with his personal system of health practices and customs. Although care givers regard certain health behaviors as important, we sometimes discover that the person does not agree or, having agreed, does not proceed to practice those behaviors as expected. If we examine the variables that affect health behaviors, the cause of this variance between the ideal and reality becomes clear.

Biological Variables

The following physical symptoms are those that most commonly motivate a person to seek health care:

- ● Pain
- ● Respiratory distress
- ● Insomnia
- ● Visual and auditory alterations
- ● Dizziness
- ● The malfunction of a body part

The degree to which any symptom interferes with the person's functioning will also determine how quickly health care is sought. For example, the person who reads a great deal may want glasses as soon as his vision becomes impaired or altered. The person who experiences blurred vision but does not read very much may wait longer before deciding on glasses. Some persons neglect their dental health until they are affected by pain or have difficulty eating. Some people will seek health care as soon as they experience pain. Athletes, on the other hand, often function in their sport while suffering pain from former injuries and they continue to do so until the discomfort prevents them from performing effectively.

Psychological Variables

- ● *Timidity or hesitancy to consult a physician or to enter a health-care system.*

Consumers prefer to seek health care from professionals they know or have previously consulted. They wish to pay a price they can afford and avoid the confusion of a large health-care system. When their experience does not meet these expectations, they may become hesitant and put off seeking the care they need. Some persons have grown up in families that use home remedies rather than traditional care. These individuals may be suspicious of practices with which they are unfamiliar.

- **Anxiety that something is wrong: a fear of the worst.**

Some persons who are fearful that they might have a serious illness seek medical care immediately. Others minimize the symptoms, perhaps believing subconsciously that if the problem is ignored it will go away. Those who put off obtaining health care usually seek help once they accept the idea of coping with serious illness. This process often requires time.

- **Knowledge levels**

Our knowledge of health and disease frequently affects the way in which we seek health care. If we know a great deal, we can determine which symptoms are significant and can seek appropriate help. Knowledge of health services and health systems helps many of us to pursue health care with less difficulty than those who know little. Understanding where to go and how one is expected to function can decrease hesitancy to consult health-care professionals.

- **Self-esteem**

Our sense of worth affects when and how we seek health care and how we carry through with health practices. Frequently, feelings of self-esteem are not conscious; a person may not be clearly aware of how these feelings affect behavior. Persons with decreased self-esteem sometimes believe they will not receive attention and love unless they are ill. This may motivate them to seek health care repeatedly for the secondary gain it provides.

Sociocultural Variables

- **Availability or proximity of health-care services**

Persons generally desire health-care services that are near their homes. Healthy people prefer not to travel long distances for care. Those who are not feeling well may not be able to drive to distant facilities and may find public transportation difficult or unavailable.

- **Financial status**

For many years persons with limited financial resources had difficulty obtaining care. They may have refused or been denied health services because they were unable to pay. Today insurance programs cover a large percentage of health-care costs for those who can pay the program premiums. In recent years government programs have been developed that assist needy persons to obtain health care. These

have helped but they are not the whole answer. Some physicians and consumers overuse these systems, causing increased expense to the government and insurance companies. This results in increased consumer costs, either in taxes or insurance premiums. Moreover, the government has made decisions on how much it will pay for specific products or services. Some physicians and other health-care providers refuse services to persons using government-paid programs. They are reluctant to receive less remuneration than they feel is necessary to run their practices. They resent the paperwork and regulations involved in government programs. Nurses have recently been offering nonacute health care as a less expensive alternative to traditional care. Yet, persons who wish to use nursing services must pay for these themselves. To date, with few exceptions, neither the government nor private companies have agreed to reimburse nurses for the professional services they provide.

- **Alternative healing systems and specific religious philosophies**

Chapter 26 discusses folk medicine practices. Some individuals trust the medicine man or the curandero and practices such as yoga, acupuncture, or astrology more than they trust the Western cultural practice of calling the doctor. Some persons of the Judeo–Christian faith have been attracted by the laying on of hands and other faith-healing practices. Some of the alternative cultural practices are very effective. Remember, people have survived on this earth for centuries prior to the advent of modern medicine.

- **Media**

Television, radio, newspapers, and magazines have had a far-reaching effect on our lives, especially in the last 30 years. Through these sources we receive health-related information that is not always accurate and useful. Consumers need to be able to judge the quality of information from the media. As nurses, we can help our clients develop these decision-making skills.

In one instance, information from a television program helped an 11-year-old girl to save her brother's life. The boy accidentally electrocuted himself and would have died had the girl not performed cardiopulmonary resuscitation (CPR) and revived him. When asked later how she knew what to do, the girl replied that she had learned CPR from watching a television show about a hospital emergency unit.

The foregoing discussion suggests that all consumers of health care have their own definitions of health and illness. Decisions about whether and when to seek health care and to engage in health practices are based on many variables. Although often our health practices reflect our cultural and family customs, our uniqueness influences how we perceive health even more. Our total life experience and all the people who are meaningful to us are variables that influence our health-care decisions. If, as nurses, we believe persons are holistic, then we must consider the interaction between all variables that influence their perceptions of health.

Consumer Movement

Prior to World War II, people relied on intuition, prayer, some medicines, and a few surgical techniques to provide the health care they needed. Doctors made house calls and people kept their sick family members at home, often using the services of private-duty nurses to assist them. Families who could not afford special services were aided by friends and extended family members. Many women, especially those who lived in small towns or in rural areas, had their babies at home.

During this time, people were fearful of contracting dread diseases. Such illnesses as tuberculosis, nervous breakdown, pneumonia, strep throat, and polio evoked much anxiety. The summer months were stressful for parents who feared a polio outbreak and so kept their children away from crowded areas. A social stigma was attached to going to the sanitarium for tuberculosis. Nervous breakdowns often meant entering state hospitals from which people never returned.

Advances in medicine and science began to change this picture. In 1921 insulin was first used successfully in the treatment of diabetes mellitus. By 1940 to 1945, antibiotics were introduced to combat bacterial infections. These were miraculous drugs that turned formerly life-threatening diseases into short-term, treatable problems. Tranquilizers changed the whole concept of care for mentally ill persons. Steroids treated a range of inflammatory diseases such as arthritis and dermatology disorders. At the same time, surgical techniques and hemodialysis were developed and perfected, making a number of fatal diseases treatable or curable. In 1953 the polio vaccine arrived, solving one of our major national health problems.

Throughout the 20th century large numbers of new drugs became available, including medicines for hypertension and cancer and drugs for infertility and birth control. We were a nation of drug users long before the term came to mean something illegal and abusive. We believed there was a pill for everything. People often became resentful when told there was no remedy for their particular problem. Nor could they easily understand that antibiotics were effective against bacteria but not against viruses. Although penicillin cannot treat colds or flu, people frequently demanded it anyway and too often the physician would agree.

Eventually prescriptions, rather than the person's individual needs or self-care abilities, became the focus of treatment. Although drugs were often appropriate (as when antihypertensive drugs were prescribed for persons with high blood pressure), they were relied on completely without any thought given to other aspects of the person's life, such as are emphasized in the holistic view. It is conceivable that if people examined some of the factors precipitating hypertension, they might have learned other ways to control blood pressure. Professional nurses possessed skills to assist clients to do this. But the emphasis remained on the new miracle drugs and the easy solutions they seemed to provide for health problems.

For a while people were generally satisfied. However, as the age of science and technology moved along, consumers no longer remembered the effects of polio or strep throat. Discontent began to emerge. People noticed that health-care providers too often made statements like, "I know what's best for you; do as I say." Large hospitals and clinics usually did not provide the individualized care that might have been obtained in a setting in which the person was known. People began to wonder why they had so little voice in their health care. Specifically, they were concerned about the following:

- Drugs and other types of care which were supposed to help sometimes made them sicker.
- Advertising and packaging were often deceptive.
- Return visits to doctors were expensive and often seemed unnecessary or useless.
- The cost of health care was escalating beyond reasonable levels.
- Scandal was frequent: nursing-home administrators pocketed money provided from the state for patient care; physicians received percentages of prescription costs from pharmacists to whom they sent customers.

- Nurses, the ones who were supposed to care, were often perceived as unfeeling, uncaring, and not very available.

The consumer movement in health care originated from these concerns.

The consumer movement as we know it probably began with Ralph Nader's book, *Unsafe at Any Speed*, written in 1965. Nader berated car manufacturers for their failure to respond to the needs of the public and for their disregard for safety. Nader has continued his fight for consumer protection in a wide variety of products and services. Others have followed his lead, contributing to the growth of the movement.

As consumer pressure developed, consumer advocates were hired by hospitals and other health organizations. Hospital boards and committees were required to have consumer representation. Human subject protection committees developed in institutions where research was being done.

The consumer movement has produced many positive effects, especially in promoting protective and educational functions. Committees have been formed to set standards for many kinds of commodities and services. Organizations have created boards of review to ensure that these standards are followed. In the health-care industry the consumer movement has clearly established that persons have a right to receive information about their disease and treatment, to participate in the decision making, and to understand the charges for treatment. These rights have been outlined in the Patient's Bill of Rights, developed by the American Hospital Association (Table 9-1.) A variety of pamphlets and books have

---

Table 9-1
Patient's Bill of Rights

The American Hospital Association presents a Patient's Bill of Rights with the expectation that observance of these rights will contribute to more effective patient care and greater satisfaction for the patient, his physician, and the hospital organization. Further, the Association presents these rights in the expectation that they will be supported by the hospital on behalf of its patients, as an integral part of the healing process. It is recognized that a personal relationship between the physician and the patient is essential for the provision of proper medical care. The traditional physician–patient relationship takes on a new dimension when care is rendered within an organizational structure. Legal precedent has established that the institution itself also has a responsibility to the patient. It is in recognition of these factors that these rights are affirmed.

1 The patient has the right to considerate and respectful care.

2 The patient has the right to obtain from his physician complete current information concerning his diagnosis, treatment, and prognosis in terms the patient can be reasonably expected to understand. When it is not medically advisable to give such information to the patient, the information should be made available to an appropriate person in his behalf. He has the right to know, by name, the physician responsible for coordinating his care.

3 The patient has the right to receive from his physician information necessary to give informed consent prior to the start of any procedure and/or treatment. Except in emergencies, such information for informed consent should include but not necessarily be limited to the specific procedure and/or treatment, the medically significant risks involved, and the probable duration of incapacitation. Where medically significant alternatives for care or treatment exist, or when the patient requests information concerning medical alternatives, the patient has the right to such information. The patient also has the right to know the name of the person responsible for the procedures and/or treatment.

4 The patient has the right to refuse treatment to the extent permitted by law and to be informed of the medical consequences of his action.

5 The patient has the right to every consideration of his privacy concerning his own medical care program. Case discussion, consultation, examination, and treatment are confidential and should be conducted discreetly. Those not directly involved in his care must have the permission of the patient to be present.

(Continued)

Table 9-1
Patient's Bill of Rights (Continued)

6 The patient has the right to expect that all communications and records pertaining to his care should be treated as confidential.

7 The patient has the right to expect that within its capacity a hospital must make reasonable response to the request of a patient for services. The hospital must provide evaluation, service, or referral as indicated by the urgency of the case. When medically permissible, a patient may be transferred to another facility only after he has received complete information and explanation concerning the needs for and alternatives to such a transfer. The institution to which the patient is to be transferred must first have accepted the patient for transfer.

8 The patient has the right to obtain information as to any relationship of his hospital to other health care and educational institutions insofar as his care is concerned. The patient has the right to obtain information as to the existence of any professional relationships among individuals, by name, who are treating him.

9 The patient has the right to be advised if the hospital proposes to engage in or perform human experimentation affecting his care or treatment. The patient has the right to refuse to participate in such research projects.

10 The patient has the right to expect reasonable continuity of care. He has the right to know in advance what appointment times and physicians are available and where. The patient has the right to expect that the hospital will provide a mechanism whereby he is informed by his physician or a delegate of the physician of the patient's continuing health care requirements following discharge.

11 The patient has the right to examine and receive an explanation of his bill regardless of source of payment.

12 The patient has the right to know what hospital rules and regulations apply to his conduct as a patient.

No catalog of rights can guarantee for the patient the kind of treatment he has a right to expect. A hospital has many functions to perform, including the prevention and treatment of disease, the education of both health professionals and patients, and the conduct of clinical research. All these activities must be conducted with an overriding concern for the patient, and, above all, the recognition of his dignity as a human being. Success in achieving this recognition assures success in the defense of the rights of the patient.

Reprinted with the permission of the American Hospital Association, 840 North Lake Shore Drive, Chicago, Illinois 60611, copyright 1972.

been written to increase health consumers' knowledge and decision-making ability. These publications are available from government, private agencies, and individuals; the words "The Consumer's Guide" often appear in the title.

The consumer movement has helped to create **responsible consumerism.** Consumers control and provide input into those things that affect them as individuals. Responsible consumerism is an obligation. If people wish to receive value for their dollars, they have a responsibility to see that this happens.

A negative effect of the consumer movement is the proliferation of malpractice lawsuits. Consumers have recently discovered their rights and have taken to the courts. As a result, malpractice insurance premiums have become increasingly expensive.

Some persons who merit payment due to physician error would prefer to settle quickly without litigation. One such situation involved a women who was to have minor surgery for diagnosis of her infertility problem. Another woman was scheduled for a sterilization procedure on the same day. The physician confused the two women and tied the tubes of the one with the infertility problem. He stated, "As soon as I realized my mistake, I called a surgeon in another city who was well known for his ability to repair tubes and made arrangements for him to see this woman the next week. Then I called my attorney and told him we would have to make a settlement for my error. Attorneys for both parties were able to negotiate a reasonable settlement that included payment for future medical expenses as well as reimbursement for the emotional distress and pain incurred by this lady." Such reasonable settlement of problems might prevent malpractice insurance premiums from becoming prohibitive.

Still, many consumer complaints reach the courts. Some physicians may be reluctant to admit mistakes. Sometimes persons are looking for a reason to file suit in the hope of gaining special attention or a large sum of money. Some attorneys encourage this practice for their own financial gain. Whatever the reason for litigation, the result is increased malpractice insurance premiums, which are then passed on to the consumer through fees for professional service.

Although the increased incidence of malpractice suits is a real problem, it has had positive effects. The health-care professions have begun to review and evaluate their practices more carefully. Committees for standardizing diagnostic and therapeutic procedures are a part of most agencies that provide health care. Their purpose is to provide quality and safety in the care of the individual, as well as to protect the agency from litigation. These committees, concerned with both medical and nursing procedures, have attempted to set standards for the most common medical diagnostic tests and procedures and for most technical nursing procedures.

Nurses as Client Advocates

The dictionary defines an advocate as one who supports, upholds, defends, or intercedes on behalf of another. Nurses perform this function when they assist and support clients. The following list suggests several kinds of involvement nurses might practice in order to function as client advocates (Table 9-3):

- Uphold the Patient's Bill of Rights.
- Respond to the social and ethnic uniqueness of the person.
- Provide scientifically current nursing care.
- Establish continuity of care.
- Provide for client participation and decision making in all aspects of health care.
- Serve on a committee for standardizing agency procedures.
- Become involved in health care at the community level.

- Become involved in governmental programs that affect health care.
- Intervene on behalf of a person with any other health-care provider involved in that person's care.
- Coordinate all services used by the client in the attempt to restore, maintain, or promote health.

The following example describes a nurse who acted as a client advocate while she served on a standardizing committee at a large medical center.

Example □ The head nurse in a nursery intensive-care unit became concerned because of the large amount of blood that was being removed from the babies for the purpose of doing diagnostic tests. She pointed out that the amount of blood taken from the babies was often as much as that taken from adults for the same test. She stated that while 5 ml or 6 ml of blood was not a great deal for an adult to lose, it was too much for a baby. This was especially true when more than one test was to be conducted on a given day. On occasions when this subject was before the committee, laboratory personnel were consulted. Often they indicated that the amount of blood specified was necessary. On each of these occasions the nurse persisted in the following way: she remained composed, she came to the committee with data about her tiny clients, she elicited support from other members of the committee (often before the meeting), and she was willing to compromise. She stated, "I know this is difficult for the labs, but we must try to reach a better solution, because these little ones cannot tolerate the loss of so much blood." In this way she attained the respect of her colleagues and paved the way for protection of her clients. □

Nurses can become involved in the community in a variety of ways. They can serve on the board of directors for agencies whose activities are designed to meet consumers' needs. Because of their unique skills in understanding the biopsychosocial aspects of people, nurses can identify consumers' needs and how these can be met (Table 9-2). For example, one nurse sitting on a board of a community clinic, which served persons with special socioeconomic needs, was able to identify these needs for funding agencies. Using knowledge about perceptions of health and health behavior, the nurse could inform others more clearly of her clients' special needs.

Nurses can be advocates for individual consumers by assisting them in dealing with the process of entering a health-care agency, by helping them find information they need, and by encouraging them to solve problems and identify solutions for their health-care needs. Consumers often need someone who can consider their total needs; nurses, with

Table 9-2
Person-centered Health-care Goals

1 To receive care that subscribes to the philosophy of the whole integrated person with spiritual, psychological, physiological, and sociological components

2 To collaborate with health-care providers and direct the planning and implementation of one's own care

3 To receive information from health-care providers about his health concerns or disease to assist him in making appropriate decisions about his care.

4 To receive care that considers his unique needs when he has a diminished ability to participate

5 To communicate his knowledge about his unique needs and expect that health-care providers will incorporate these into the plan for his care.

6 To have his strengths assessed by health-care providers and mobilized toward supporting, maintaining, or promoting his health status

7 To have his unique characteristics (biopsychosocial–spiritual) assessed and care provided that is safe and relevant given those characteristics

8 To expect confidentiality concerning himself as a person and the care he is receiving

9 To be provided with the most modern and scientifically sound medical and nursing care available

10 To be advised of the rules, regulations, policies, and procedures of the agency or persons from whom he is seeking care

11 To receive continuity of care

12 To receive a full explanation of the expected costs of the health care for which he is contracting and the actual costs of it after completion

are in an ideal position to listen to their problems, identify their needs, and assist them in finding solutions. When the hospital nurse helps a client contact a dietitian for concerns about his low-sodium diet and when a community-health nurse helps a client identify an agency that provides needed financial assistance, both are acting as consumer advocates.

Journalist Fred Cook wrote about his wife's long battle against heart disease in *Julia's Story* (1977). The story is a tragic one, not so much because of the unhappy ending or even because of the constant stress Julia suffered at the hands of the various health-care delivery services she consulted. The real tragedy was that throughout their whole ordeal, she and her husband never really found anyone to whom they could turn. They needed someone who was willing to listen, to run interference for them, and to view them as whole persons. Nurses reading *Julia's Story* can hardly miss the need these people had for nursing care. Yet there are few nurses of any significance described in this story. The most helpful nurse they met arrived too late to be of real assistance.

Our challenge is clearly marked. As professional nurses, we have the knowledge, skills, and numbers necessary to make a difference to the health of individuals and groups of people. We can make ourselves seen and heard in a number of ways. We can insist on the consumer's right to have coordinated health care and, with other specialized professionals, help to provide this. We can assist the consumer to use his self-care abilities so that he will remain in control of the health care he receives.

Refer again to Table 9-1, which shows the Patient's Bill of Rights, and to Table 9-2, which presents another list of the rights of persons using health-care commodities and services. Perhaps the word "goal" would better convey the kind of care we want each person to receive. These goals reflect the philosophy of person-centered health care.

Preventive Health Care

The consumer movement that has produced increased participation in health care has also generated interest in maintaining personal health. People have begun to lose weight, to stop smoking, and to participate in sports in order to stay healthy. **Preventive health care** is a term to describe activities that promote health by reducing factors that contribute to illness and by reinforcing the person's strengths. As consumers have become interested in

their knowledge of biological, psychological, and sociocultural functioning, are well suited to this understanding. Since nurses spend more direct time with clients than other health-care providers, they

Table 9-3 **The Nurse as Client Advocate**
• Uphold the Patient's Bill of Rights
• Respond to the social and ethnic uniqueness of the person
• Provide scientifically current nursing care
• Establish continuity of care
• Provide for client participation and decision making in all aspects of health care
• Serve on a committee for standardizing agency procedures
• Become involved in health care at the community level
• Become involved in governmental programs that affect health care
• Intervene on behalf of a person with any other health-care provider involved in that person's care
• Coordinate all services used by the client in the attempt to restore, maintain, or promote health

preventive health care, the concept has received increasing attention from health-care providers. This section describes the concept of preventive health care and the nurse's role in health promotion.

Development of Preventive Health Care

Prevention is not a new concept in nursing. Consider the words of Florence Nightingale to the nurses of 1860, "There are five essential points in securing the health of houses: 1. Pure Air 2. Pure Water 3. Efficient Drainage 4. Cleanliness 5. Light. Without these, no house can be healthy. And it will be unhealthy just in proportion as they are deficit" (pp. 14–15).

Nightingale's principles demonstrate an awareness of preventive health care in an era in which communicable diseases presented the most serious threat to health. A person who lived in the 1860s was fortunate to survive beyond the age of 40 and to escape the dreaded diseases of tuberculosis, cholera, and rheumatic fever.

Today, the factors that affect a person's health are often related to their life-style, environment, and psychosocial response to stressors. The leading causes

of death have shifted from communicable diseases to conditions stemming from a complex interaction of heredity, environment, and personal health behavior. Death occurs for many people who might have lived longer had they altered those behavior patterns that compromised their health. In addition, many people are living restricted lives due to preventable conditions. The person with debilitating emphysema who continues to smoke, the child who develops polio because of a failure to be immunized, and the mother who delivers a low-birth-weight infant because of poor nutrition during pregnancy are examples of people whose quality of life has been impaired by failure to engage in preventive health care.

Society pays a price when preventive health care is not practiced. Increased technology, inappropriate utilization of hospitals, and the increasing complexity of health-care systems contribute to spiraling health-care costs. As the price of illness care climbs, interest in preventive health care increases. Nurses, physicians, and other health professionals are being challenged to collaborate with consumers in developing health promotion plans that focus on maximizing persons' strengths and modifying stressors before irreversible illness occurs.

Levels of Preventive Health Care

The concept of preventive health care can be applied at three levels: primary, secondary, and tertiary.

In **primary preventive health care,** the nurse intervenes with persons who have no symptoms at the time of the intervention but who are at risk for developing behaviors that could decrease their health. Exploring the implications of smoking with an adolescent who does not yet smoke, teaching the components of good nutrition to a 10-year-old child, and advocating the use of seat belts are examples of primary preventive health care.

In **secondary preventive health care,** the nurse identifies those risk factors in a person's life-style that affect physical or mental health. The nurse explores the significance of these factors with the person and assists him to minimize these risks through education, counseling, and treatment (Fig. 9-1). Assisting a new mother to adapt her life-style to the birth of her daughter, weighing and measuring a premature infant and comparing his growth to standards for his age group, and examining and protecting the bony prominences of a person confined to bed to avoid skin breakdown are examples of secondary preventive health care. In these in-

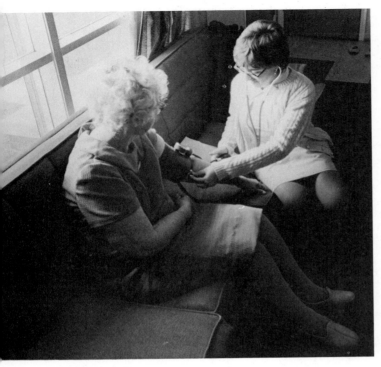

Figure 9-1
Secondary preventive health care involves evaluation and counseling related to health risks. *(University of Michigan School of Nursing)*

stances the conditions are ripe for the activation of stressors, but the nurse and client attempt to identify and eliminate those factors which contribute to the potential for physical or mental illness.

Tertiary preventive health care focuses on persons who have encountered significant stressors that have already compromised their health. Here the nurse's role is to facilitate an adaptive response to this stressor. Tertiary preventive health care emphasizes use of the person's coping mechanisms. This process is closely linked to rehabilitation. A nurse who facilitates the grieving process in a severely depressed widow or teaches range-of-motion exercises to the person who has experienced a stroke is providing tertiary preventive health care.

Consider the following example, which exemplifies how nurses can integrate all three types of health care into their practice:

Example □ Sharon Richards is a staff nurse in a hypertension clinic at a rural community hospital. She is often asked to speak to community groups about the causes and risk factors that contribute to hypertension. As she provides this service she is practicing primary preventive health care. She is interacting with a population that is assumed to be healthy and that hopes to maintain good health.

One day a month the clinic offers a hypertension screening program. During the screening clinic, Sharon Richards takes blood pressures, evaluates risk factors, counsels persons about their life-style, and refers persons with high blood pressure to the hypertension treatment clinic. At this time she is practicing secondary preventive health care.

In the hypertension treatment clinic, Sharon works with clients who have active disease. She teaches them about diet, medications, and exercise. She counsels and assists them in adapting their life-style to reduce factors that contribute to the progression of hypertension. Disease may have caused irreversible damage in these clients. However, Sharon supports them in developing health behaviors that will minimize the effects of disease and reverse or impede the illness process. □

As a nurse, your role may focus on one of the levels of preventive health care, but in all likelihood you will be involved in every level. You might work with a single client at all three levels. For example, you might teach a young woman how to do self breast examinations (primary) and help her to develop coping mechanisms to deal with the stress of impending motherhood (secondary). This client might also have a history of urinary-tract infections for which you have developed a plan of care together (tertiary).

Preventive Health Care Throughout the Life Span

The preceding discussion illustrates that consumers are entitled to an evaluation of their risk factors and preventive health-care practices. Table 8-3 in the previous chapter shows that there are specific developmental tasks and related stressors for specific age groups. Nurses can assist persons of all ages to identify the common stressors of their age group by using knowledge of growth and development. Many stressors are present throughout the entire life span because they affect basic needs such as good nutrition or a safe environment. Although a checklist approach to identifying stressors may be inadequate, knowledge of the individual's phase of development can assist nurses in planning preventive health-care appropriately.

Nursing Implications for Preventive Health Behavior

The variables that affect a person's ability and willingness to adopt preventive health behaviors are described earlier in this chapter. One important way that nurses can adovocate preventive health care is to help their clients explore their own health behavior. As clients become aware of their behavior they can be guided to modify those factors which they identify as stressors.

There are various ways to assist clients to develop preventive health behaviors. Exploring the client's health values and beliefs can help develop positive attitudes toward health. Health counseling enables clients to identify the existence of any risk factors for certain health problems and to develop strategies for maintaining health. Some individuals become so anxious and immobilized by fear of disease that they delay preventive health-care action. By exploring such fears, nurses can help these persons reduce their anxiety to a level that will enable them to seek health care. When persons believe that the positive value of seeking health care outweighs the barriers, they will be more likely to take action. Finally, teaching is an important nursing action that assists clients in developing programs for wellness (Fig. 9-2). Health education that actively involves the client has been shown to have a positive effect on willingness and ability to practice preventive health care.

It often provides an impetus for health action. For instance, telling a person to relax and avoid stress will have little meaning if his self-esteem is built around achievement at work. Specific information on how to incorporate techniques of relaxation into his life-style will be more useful in helping him to decrease stress. The processes of teaching and learning are described further in Chapter 28.

To develop strategies for preventive health care, nurses must synthesize knowledge and concepts from all areas of their education and experience. Interviewing and physical-examination skills increase nurses' ability to help clients examine their own risk factors. Knowledge of epidemiology and physiology serves as a basis for exploring strategies for health maintenance of clients. Knowledge of the principles of adaptation provides an insight for supporting clients to make changes in behavior that interferes with good health. The focus of preventive health behavior is assisting persons to identify and maximize their strengths. Building on strengths and facilitating preventive health behavior at primary, secondary, and tertiary levels are central to establishing a plan for health maintenance for consumers.

Figure 9-2
Teaching assists clients to develop programs for wellness. *(Photo by D. Atkinson)*

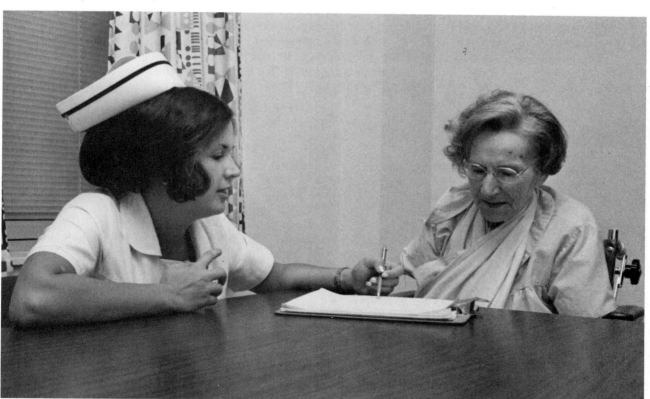

Conclusion

As nurses, you may work with persons who are having difficulty taking preventive health-care action. Specific points to keep in mind include the following:

- Extreme fear and a heightened sense of vulnerability may immobilize a person's ability to seek preventive health care.
- The person who does not believe that preventive health care is effective may be less likely to seek it.
- Perceived barriers may outweigh the perceived benefits of treatment and decrease preventive health behavior.
- A person who feels left out of the decision-making process might be less likely to initiate action.
- Lack of accurate, complete knowledge might inhibit a person's ability to seek preventive health care.
- The goal of secondary preventive health care is to initiate early diagnosis and intervention for a person known to be at risk.

Nurses will need to determine which of these factors may be relevant to a particular client. Exploring some of these ideas with the client can provide the information nurses need to plan care. Clients, as consumers of health care, with the help of their nurses, can learn to make appropriate decisions on how to take care of themselves.

Study Questions

1. Describe how the development of many new medications led to the consumer movement in health care.

2. Your client tells you she has discovered a lump in her breast. She begins to cry, saying she doesn't want the doctor to examine her. She tells you that her sister died a year ago from breast cancer. Discuss several factors that might be influencing this woman's health behavior.

3. You are a nurse in the outpatient clinic for diabetes care. After talking with Mrs. C., a 65-year-old client, you obtain the following information:
   a. She left home at 4 A.M., driving 200 miles to be seen in this clinic.
   b. The doctor she expected to see was out of town. Another doctor prescribed a new plan for her insulin dosage, but she was hesitant to tell him she didn't understand.
   c. The dietitian gave her a diet, which she said Mrs. C. must follow. However, it did not include her family's favorite foods.
   d. She forgot to bring her Medicare card with her.
   e. One of the clinic nurses scolded her because she used the bathroom but forgot to leave a urine specimen.
   Describe several ways you might function as a nurse advocate for Mrs. C.

4. Your client is an 11-year-old girl who is hospitalized with asthma. She is distressed because her parents are planning a divorce. Suggest some ways you might work with this girl, using the notions of primary, secondary, and tertiary preventive health care.

Glossary

Consumer: An individual, a group, or a community which uses a commodity or a service.

Preventive health care: Activities that promote health by reducing factors which contribute to illness and by reinforcing a person's strengths.

Primary preventive health care: Intervention with persons who have no symptoms but who are at risk for developing behaviors that could diminish their health.

Responsible consumerism: The act of controlling and providing input into those things which affect one as an individual; it is an obligation as well as a right.

Secondary preventive health care: Education, counseling, and treatment that assist a person to minimize factors which are a part of their life-style and which could affect their health.

Tertiary preventive health care: Care that focuses on persons who have encountered a specific stressor which has already compromised their health.

Bibliography

Becker MH (ed): The Health Belief Model and Personal Health Behavior. Thorofare, New Jersey, Charles B Slack, 1974

Benson R: The consumers' right to health care: How does the nursing profession respond? Nurs Forum 16, No. 2: 139–143, 1977

Bruhn JG, Cordova FD, Fuentes RG et al: The wellness process. J Community Health 2, No. 3: 209–221, 1977

Bullough B: Poverty, ethnic identity and preventive health care. J Health Soc Behav 13: 347–359, Dec 1972

Bullough B: The source of ambulatory health services as it relates to preventive care. Am J Public Health 64, No. 6: 582–590, 1974

Cook FJ: Julia's Story. New York, Kangaroo Book Publishers, 1977

Curtin LL: Is there a right to health care? Am J Nurs 80, No. 3: 462–465, 1980

Holder AR et al: Informed consent and the nurse. Nurs Law Ethics 2, No. 2: 1–2, 8, 1981

Kelly L: The patient's right to know. Nurs Outlook 24, No. 1: 26–32, 1976

Kohnke MF: The nurse's responsibility to the consumer. Am J Nurs 78, No. 3: 440–442, 1978

Lear MW: Heartsounds. New York, Simon & Schuster, 1980

Moffat S: Kaiser-Permanente—Prepaid care comes of age, pp. 125–137. Medical and Health Annual, Encyclopedia Britannica, 1978

Nader R: Unsafe at Any Speed. New York, Grossman Publishers, 1965

Nightingale F: Notes on Nursing. A facsimile of the first edition printed in London, 1859. Philadelphia, JB Lippincott, 1966

Quinn N, Somers AR: The patient's bill of rights. Nurs Outlook 22, No. 4: 240–244, 1974

Ricketts S: Can your citizens' advice bureau help you? Health Visit 53, No. 9: 386, 1980

Riley W: Citizen participation in community mental health center service delivery. Ment Health J 17, No. 1: 37–45, 1981

Zimmerman BM: Human questions vs. human hurry. Am J Nurs 80, No. 4: 719, 1980

Professionalism

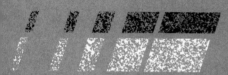

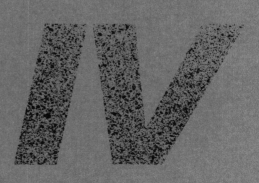

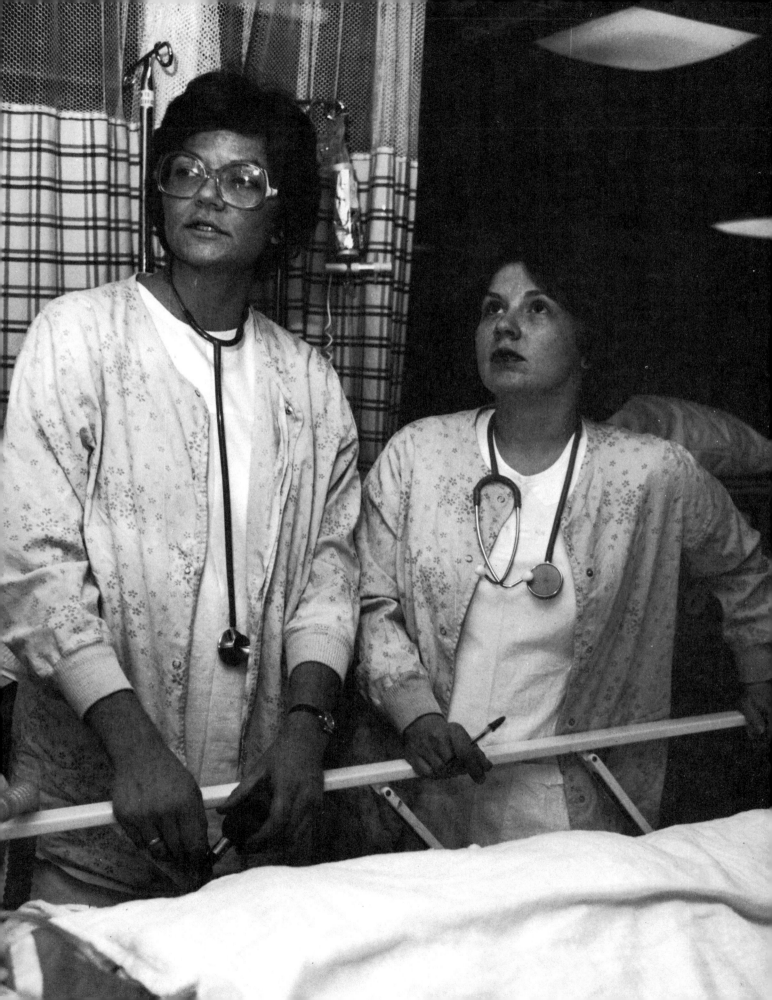

IV

Professionalism

The purpose of this section is to explore the concept of professionalism and its significance for both organized nursing and the individual nurse person.

To achieve professionalization, nursing must educate its practitioners about professional criteria and activities. Professional commitment and involvement begin appropriately with the introduction to professional nursing education. Today's issues are more easily understood if placed in an historical context. Legal and ethical considerations provide both opportunities for professionalization and constraints on practice. An understanding of professional issues, coupled with legal and ethical considerations, enables one to evaluate practice options rationally. Nurses need to know and use individual and group strategies to achieve personal self-actualization and to influence health-care policies.

Nursing, a Developing Profession

Janice B. Lindberg

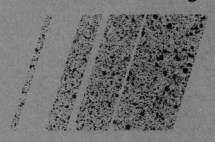

Objectives

Introduction

10

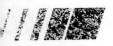

After completing this chapter, students will be able to:

• *Identify the characteristics of professions.*

• *Differentiate the casual and traditional use of the term "professional."*

• *Describe nursing's status in relation to each of the characteristics of professions.*

• *Describe the highlights of nursing history.*

Most of us use the terms "profession" and "professional" rather casually. In some instances, we intend to convey the impression that a person is an expert; in other instances, we use the term "professional" politely, as a title of distinction. Accordingly, we describe someone as a professional athlete, musician, or engineer. We may ask someone, "What is your profession?" when we mean, "What work do you do?"

Professionalism is defined as professional character, spirit, or methods. Professionalism also encompasses teaching and activities found in various occupational groups whose members aspire to be professional. **Professionalization** is a process of acquiring or changing characteristics in the direction of a profession.

The debate about whether nursing is a profession has stirred and divided nursing for decades. With attention focusing on educational preparation for entry into professional nursing practice, professionalism in nursing remains a current and pressing issue. Because the issues related to professionalism present implications and challenges for each and every nurse, the topic is one of importance to all of us.

The occupations traditionally accepted as **professions** are medicine, law, and the ministry. Many other occupational groups seek the status assigned to these professions. Whether society views these aspiring occupations as professions is another matter. You may or may not believe that nursing is a profession. Regardless, you are now being socialized to assume a nursing rather than a lay point of view about the matter. At the very least, you are probably being confronted with a view of nursing that is somewhat different from what you expected. Often beginning students imagine nursing primarily as the mastery of many technical procedures. Indeed, such technical mastery is important, but it is only a part of the larger scheme of professional nursing practice. Because nurses are conscientious and caring persons, beginning nursing students have much concern, conflict, and anxiety about whether they can perform all the technical procedures at the expected level. Sometimes students expect more of themselves than their teachers do.

As a student you may think, "It seems like there are a lot more important things to learn about than professionalism! I'm just a student after all." But a danger lurks behind this thought. The attitude of "just a student" today can lead to the attitude of "just a nurse"—any old kind of nurse—tomorrow. An introduction to professional attitude, behavior, and issues may increase your options about your potential development in nursing and about the kind of nurse you will become. The intent of this chapter is to increase your awareness of what professionalism means to nursing and to you personally.

Criteria for Professions

In general all professionals have the following characteristics (Schein, 1972, pp. 7–14):

- A body of knowledge on which skills and services are based
- An ability to deliver a unique service to other humans
- Education that is standardized and based in colleges and universities
- Control of standards for practice
- Responsibility and accountability of members for their own actions
- Career commitment by members
- Independent function

Let us consider each of these criteria for professions individually.

Body of Knowledge on Which Skills and Services Are Based

At one time in history, nursing skills and practice were based largely on intuitive knowledge. Today nursing, as a practice discipline, is called an applied science. If the person is the focus of nursing and man is a biopsychosocial being interacting with his environment, then nursing applies concepts from many different basic sciences. Some nursing leaders argue that nursing need not have a unique knowledge base. They believe nursing can be unique in its application of knowledge common to many disciplines. Other experts believe that nursing eventually will develop its own body of knowledge and its own theories. Some of the nursing theorists you may wish to explore include Rogers (1970), King (1971), Roy (1971), and Orem (1971).

Not until the 1970s did writings about nursing theory start to appear in the nursing literature. As late as 1970, it was rather unique for a doctoral dissertation by a nurse to focus directly on the outcome of specific nursing interventions. In 1973, the National Commission for the Study of Nursing and Nursing Education noted this lack of nursing theory. Most sciences have many theories about their particular disciplines rather than one grand theory. Regardless of whether nursing uses its own theories or those from other sciences, we can expect that many theories will influence nursing practice.

Ability to Deliver a Unique Service to Other Humans

According to Henderson, the unique function of the nurse is to assist the person in performing activities contributing to health and recovery, or a serene death, which the person would do for himself if he were able (1966). Further, the nurse does this in a way that encourages independence. The current emphasis on nurses' promoting self-care is consistent with Henderson's definition. In addition to a person-centered practice, the unique focus of nursing is often identified as health, not illness (as it is for medicine). Society validates its need for nursing by continuing to educate nurses.

The criticism that nurses are unable to agree on an explicit definition of nursing and also to document the effect of nursing actions is both justified and problematic. Nurses themselves often admit publicly their disagreements about what nursing is and how nurses should be prepared and should practice. Some nurses with a greater sense of independence seek an autonomy that clearly differentiates nursing from medicine as a separate health profession. If nurses themselves are unclear about the unique contribution of nursing, is it any wonder that society is confused about nursing service? Before nurses can demonstrate scientifically that their unique service makes a difference, they must state clearly what their unique service is. At the present time, it is foolish to argue that everyone called "nurse" provides the same unique service.

Standardized Education Based in Colleges and Universities

In the last decade, there has been a decrease in diploma nursing programs and an increase in all other nursing-education programs. In 1977, there were 1372 basic nursing programs. These included 349 baccalaureate programs with 101,430 students, 656 associate-degree (A.D.) programs with 91,102 students, and 367 diploma programs with 52,858 students (National League for Nursing, 1978, pp. 2, 35).

In 1974, the New York State Nurses' Association proposed that by 1985 the baccalaureate degree become the minimal educational preparation for entry into professional nursing practice. This proposal generated controversy among nurses, other health professionals, and hospital administrators. The suggestion of collegiate education, however, was far from new. As far back as 1860, Florence Nightingale advocated training schools that would be considered educational institutions supported by public funds. Although she thought the schools should be closely associated with hospitals, she also believed that they should be administered separately. In 1909, a Minnesota physician, Dr. Richard Beard, proposed and strongly defended university education for nurses.

A significant development regarding collegiate education for nurses occurred in the 1950s with the introduction of associate-degree programs to prepare nurse technicians (Montag, 1951). Montag intended such nurses to have a 2-year collegiate education. Their functions were to be narrower in scope than the baccalaureate-prepared R.N. but greater than the L.P.N. who received a year of preparation at most. The success of these programs, coupled with the general increase in numbers of community and junior colleges, resulted in a proliferation of such

A.D. programs. Unfortunately, there has never been a consensus about the differences between professional and technical nursing. However, baccalaureate education leading to the B.S.N. degree (bachelor of sciences in nursing) generally is acknowledged as preparation for professional nursing. Associate-degree education leading to the A.D.N. degree prepares one for technical nursing. The question of how nurses should be prepared is a major and unresolved issue to be explored later in greater detail (Fig. 10-1).

Control of Standards for Practice

A **standard** is an authoritative statement or criterion by which the quality of practice can be judged. In the late 1950s, the American Nurses' Association (A.N.A.), nursing's professional organization, expressed formal concern for control of practice at a level above the minimum required for R.N. licensure. The A.N.A. first published "Standards for Organized Nursing Services" in 1965. These standards emphasized both systematic nursing plans providing for client participation and nursing actions to maximize health capabilities. The nursing-practice standards assume individual responsibility and accountability for meeting the standards.

The American Nurses Association recognizes excellence in practice through a process called **certification.** Certification identifies persons who have obtained specialized knowledge and is a mark of professional achievement. Certification also carries with it the endorsement of professional colleagues.

Responsibility and Accountability of Members for Their Own Actions

General Discussion

The dictionary defines accountable as answerable. According to the Michigan Nurses' Association, **accountability** is responsibility for the services one provides or makes available (M.N.A., 1971). The concept of accountability is not new to nursing. In fact nurses are probably more concerned about accountability than many other professionals. Accountability has several dimensions, including legal, peer-group, employer, and consumer accountability. Licensing boards can revoke licenses to practice for incompetence or certain violations of the law. Nurses are accountable to health-care colleagues with whom they are professionally associated, as reflected in the increasing use of peer review within the clinical

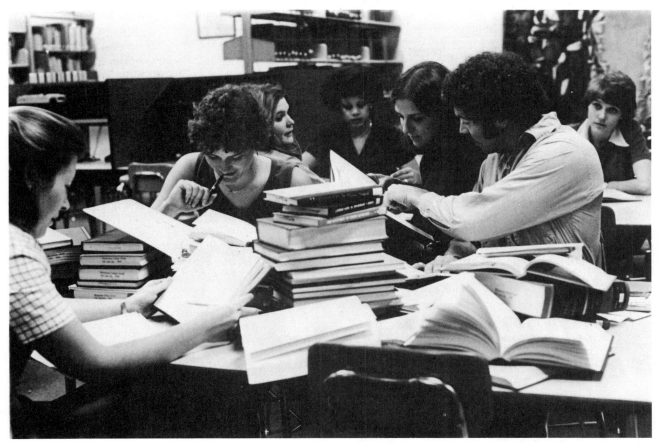

Figure 10-1
The question of how nurses should be educated is a major unresolved issue in the nursing profession. *(National Student Nurses' Association)*

setting. Such review may include evaluating the patient's health record in order to compare actual practice to the American Nurses' Association's nursing-practice standards. Because nurses are not generally independent practitioners, they are often also accountable to hospitals or other employing agencies. Increasingly, nurses describe themselves as directly accountable to their patients/clients.

During a study of baccalaureate nursing students in a large midwestern university, students responded to the following question about accountability: To whom are nurses primarily accountable for their practice? Eighty-five percent of the respondents answered that nurses are primarily accountable to individual patients; 15% of the students selected the remaining choices: hospital and other health-care institutions, doctors, the state, and patients' families (Lindberg, 1979).

The concept of accountability implies both that

one is responsible for the consequences of actions chosen and also that one accepts the consequences of choosing not to act in particular situations.

Primary care is a mechanism whereby health-care providers, including nurses, are accountable for the services rendered to specific clients. One usually thinks of acccountability in this more narrow sense of specific care situations. In the broader sense, one is accountable for moving the profession toward professional goals. The individual is also accountable to oneself for achieving maximum potential.

Code for Nurses

Another way professionals monitor conduct within their ranks is by formulating and enforcing a code of ethics. The Code for Professional Nurses was first outlined in the 1920s. It was finally adopted in 1950 and has been changed many times since (A.N.A.,

1968). This code not only guides members but serves as a proclamation to the public which nursing serves (Table 10-1).

Career Commitment by Members

A career is what you do as your major life work. It is sometimes described as the progress of a person through life. A career may be distinguished from a job, which is an individual piece of work done in the routine of one's trade or occupation. In earlier days, when women's life work was done primarily in the home, they had little opportunity for professional careers in the world of work outside the home. Today a majority of married women work outside the home. This fact reflects both economic necessity and a change in society's attitudes toward women's work. As women today consider employment, the choice between job and career is no longer made solely upon the length of time one expects to remain in the work force. Probably most nurses who work do so for more than a quarter of a century, or a third of their lifetime.

The characteristics of jobs and careers as listed in Table 10-2 may help distinguish between the two. The intent is not to imply that a career is inherently better than a job, nor is the contrast suggested as more than a guide.

According to Lysaught, one out of four registered nurses in America does not maintain a license to practice. An additional 25% retain the license but do not practice. Of the remaining 50%, 19% are employed part-time. This leaves 31% or approximately 650,000

Table 10-1
American Nurses' Association Code for Nurses

1 The nurse provides services with respect for the dignity of man, unrestricted by considerations of nationality, race, creed, color, or status.

2 The nurse safeguards the individual's right to privacy by judiciously protecting information of a confidential nature, sharing only that information relevant to his care.

3 The nurse maintains individual competence in nursing practice, recognizing and accepting responsibility for individual actions and judgments.

4 The nurse acts to safeguard the patient when his care and safety are affected by incompetent, unethical, or illegal conduct of any person.

5 The nurse uses individual competence as a criterion in accepting delegated responsibilities and assigning nursing activities to others.

6 The nurse participates in research activities when assured that the rights of individual subjects are protected.

7 The nurse participates in the efforts of the profession to define and upgrade standards of nursing practice and education.

8 The nurse, acting through the professional organization, participates in establishing and maintaining conditions of employment conducive to high-quality nursing care.

9 The nurse works with members of health professions and other citizens in promoting efforts to meet health needs of the public.

10 The nurse refuses to give or imply endorsement to advertising, promotion, or sales for commercial products, services, or enterprises.

**Table 10-2
Characteristics of a Job versus a Career**

Job	Career
A piece of work; may or may not be long-term employment	Life work; long-term commitment, long-term planning important, possibly involving a mentor
Variable initial training	Long training or education
Part time or full time	Usually full time
Intermittent retraining possible	Lifelong learning necessary
Job selects person	Person selects career
Administrator evaluation primarily	Peer evaluation primarily

full-time R.N.s. The impact of this number is deceptive, because the yearly turnover rate of R.N. staff nurses is actually greater than 70%, and probably fewer than 50% of the full-time R.N.s actually provide direct patient care. Some are administrators and educators.

Nursing continues to be predominantly a female occupation. The very name conveys a female connotation and, as such, implies that the situation is unlikely to change dramatically in the near future. It would seem, however, that the option for women to make a commitment to nursing as a career rather than as a job is more feasible than ever before.

Independent Function

During the first half of the 20th century, a view of nurse as handmaidens or assistants to the physician pervaded American thinking. The reason for this perception probably related more to deeply ingrained social values than to any inherent characteristics of nursing practice. State nursing-practice laws generally do not prohibit nurses from behaving in more independent ways consistent with their knowledge and skills. At the same time, nurses are clearly restricted in diagnosing illness and in prescribing independently for its treatment. These two functions are currently the prerogative of medical practice.

As currently practiced, nursing has acknowledged independent, dependent, and interdependent functions. Occasionally nurses hang out their shingles and practice independently. Society receives great benefit from nursing's independent practice in the form of voluntary service or charity. In fact, society often expects nurses to provide free advice and service in their neighborhoods and communities. It does not ask the same of law or medicine, in which most of the practitioners are men.

Additional Criteria

Two additional criteria of American professions identified by Lysaught are an active and cohesive professional organization and acknowledged social worth and contribution. In 1980, 180,000 R.N.s (approximately 1 out of 8) were represented by the American Nurses' Association, the official professional organization (Fig. 10-2). An additional 160,000 nurses belonged to other organizations, such as specialty groups or honor societies. The membership of these combined organizations accounted for less than one quarter of all registered nurses. Although lip service is given to the social worth of nursing, society has not provided comparable tangible reward of either status or economic compensation.

Historical Perspective

In the decade of the 1970s, nursing made enormous leaps in practice, education, and research. This opened the door to the 1980s as a "decade of decision," the theme of the 1980 biennial A.N.A.

convention. The decisions to be made in the 1980s are understood better from a brief historical perspective. For the same reason that other subcultures find their roots important, nursing is experiencing a surge of interest in its roots. Today a primary purpose of considering history is specifically to relate it both to the present and to the future. Some of the many references which do this very well include Kelly (1975), Ashley (1976), Chaska (1978), Kalisch and Kalisch (1978), and writings of the Bulloughs.

Time Line

Because Nightingale's era marks the advent of modern nursing, let us build a time line using it as a point of departure for discussing both the major issues of nursing and the role of the professional nurse today. The items in the nursing-history time line are listed in Table 10-3.

Lessons of the Past

Three lessons of the past worth learning would seem to be that

- Issues and problems facing nursing today are neither as new as we sometimes like to think nor as immobilizing as we pretend.

- In the past as now, individual persons make things happen as they work alone and together for common causes. Ideas and actions begin with one person. Although society shapes the nursing profession, persons within nursing have and will determine much of what happens to nursing. That group of persons includes us all.

- Just as yesterday's issues are today's history, today's issues are tomorrow's history.

Sometimes we forget that 100-plus years of history are not very long. It took over 50 years to enact women's suffrage after a national effort was mounted. As the 1980s began, the Equal Rights Amendment was still being debated as an addition to our Constitution. The Civil War, like other wars, had an impact in moving women from their place within the home to the wider world of work. "Modern nursing" originated during this Victorian age, which prescribed women's roles as secondary to those of men. Early training emphasized standard procedures, housekeeping tasks, and an ethic that supported medicine. At the turn of the century, both physicians and nurses treated patients primarily with concern and home remedies, because those were the treatments most available to health-care professionals and consumers.

Figure 10-2
Participation in organizational activities is one criterion of a professional. *(National Student Nurses' Association)*

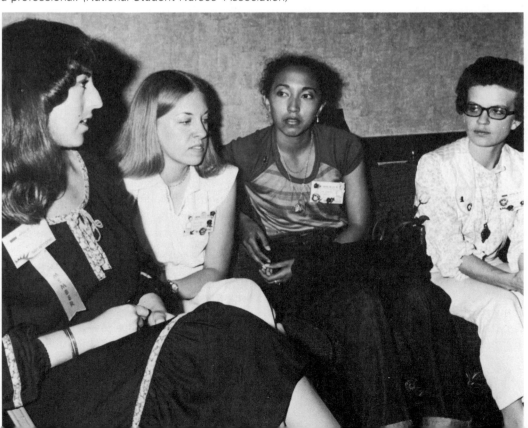

Table 10-3
Nursing History Time Line

1847	A.M.A. (American Medical Association)
1860	Florence Nightingale's London School
1869	National Women's Suffrage Movement began
1873	America's first trained nurse, Linda Richards, graduated
	Three "Nightingale" schools established in U.S.
	Bellevue Training School for Nurses, at Bellevue Hospital, New York City
	Connecticut Training School for Nurses at New Haven Hospital, New Haven, Connecticut
	Boston Training School for Nurses, at the Massachusetts General Hospital, Boston
1875	Practice options for nurses: ward nursing, superintendent of training school, private duty
1879	First "nursing" text published, *The New Haven Manual of Medicine*
1897	Nurses Associated Alumnae of the United States and Canada (renamed American Nurses' Association in 1911)
1900	First *American Journal of Nursing* published
1903	First Nursing Practice Act, North Carolina
1909	First University School of Nursing, Minnesota
1911	American Nurses' Association
1921	Passage of women's suffrage—19th Amendment
1922	Sigma Theta Tau, Nursing's professional honor society, established
1925	Frontier Nursing Service established, Kentucky
1930s	Students who gave most of care gradually replaced by R.N.s
	Junior colleges established
1950	Code of Ethics adopted by American Nurses' Association
1950s	Baccalaureate degrees for nursing faculty
1952	First associate-degree programs in nursing
1953	National Student Nurses' Association established
1957	Space Age began
1965	American Nurses' Association Position Paper on Baccalaureate Education issued
1971	Lysaught Report of the National Commission to Study Nursing and Nursing Education led to proliferation of expanded nursing roles.
1974	N-CAP (Nurses' Coalition for Action in Politics) established as political-action arm of A.N.A.
	Health Planning and Resources Development Act
1975	First nurses honored for certification by A.N.A.

Only after the turn of the century did medicine and nursing as practice disciplines become very divergent in the development of their applied sciences. A turning point for medicine might be identified in the second decade of the 20th century. In 1910, Abraham Flexner published a major study, *Medical Education in the United States and Canada.*

As a result of the Flexner report, medicine began to standardize its educational programs in colleges and universities. This was done in recognition of a need for a scientific base and support for research efforts. The Flexner report had specifically identified that society would be deprived of appropriate health care unless it was scientifically based and delivered. In addition to the attention it gave education, medicine began to give considerable attention to accreditation and licensing issues. The Flexner Report also made clear that society would need to pay for the necessary and improved education of physicians. Thus, the public expectation of payment for sophisticated preparation of medical practitioners was established, and an econometric model that recognized reimbursement consistent with long formal education and clinical experience was instituted.

Nursing, on the other hand, tended to remain charitable about the services it provided and unassertive about its economic welfare. In 1923 the Goldmark Report identified needs of nursing education and public-health nursing. This was the first of many studies by, about, and for nursing and its advancement. In spite of repeated studies, nursing proliferated a variety of programs without clearly or uniformly identifying the kind of practitioners it was preparing. It was not until the 1970s that two reports about the scope of nursing practice created a great deal of reaction, both within and outside nursing. These reports were "Extending the Scope of Nursing Practice," from the HEW Secretary's Committee (1971), and *An Abstract for Action*, from the National Commission for the Study of Nursing and Nursing Education, chaired by Jerome Lysaught (1970). The reports both validated the divergence of medicine and nursing and made it clear that nurses and nursing were not realizing their full potential. In 1980, at the biennial American Nurses' Association convention, Lysaught spoke about the contrasts in development of medicine and nursing. He described the transformation of American medicine between 1900 and 1980 as a miracle. Interestingly, he credits this fantastic change more to the efforts of basic and applied research than to the advancement of technology itself. A noticeable nursing-research effort aimed at improving nursing practice has just emerged since the 1970s.

Table 10-4 depicts a summary of the divergence between medical and nursing practice in the 20th century. Whether this divergence will continue is open to question, as indicated by the question marks at the bottom of the chart.

Conclusion

The criteria for professions and a brief historical perspective of nursing's development can help us understand modern nursing and its relation to other professions and the society at large. At this point we might conclude the following about nursing as a profession:

- Nursing has a briefer professional history than the traditional professions of law, medicine, and theology.
- Nursing has been and continues to be primarily a woman's occupation.
- Nursing's ranking on the criteria commonly used for professions is the subject of considerable debate.

Professionalization is a dynamic process. Some people describe nursing as a semiprofession or an emerging or marginal profession. Others call it an aspiring profession. Just as man is viewed as a being in the process of becoming, so might nursing be viewed. Thus the terms "developing profession" or "aspiring profession" are useful, because they convey a possibility of striving to achieve a potential. As man moves from basic needs through growth needs, so nursing must move from occupational to professional criteria before achieving full professional status. If the parallel drawn here holds true, nursing has perhaps reached early adulthood, not full maturity, as a profession.

Those who assess nursing as a profession tend to speak more of its health or illness than of its developmental phase. Sometimes they focus on nursing's many weaknesses or its ills. But health as a total concept includes both states of illness and of wellness. Health describes an idea that even in great wellness there are needs, while in great illness there are many strengths. A favorite book, *I Never Promised You a Rose Garden*, illustrates this point. The book deals with the growth of a young girl as she gains victory over a crippling mental illness. In one scene, the psychiatrist sits listening to a psychologist give a report from the battery of tests he has just administered to Deborah, the main character. He describes how the results of these tests diagnose Deborah as very ill with a serious form of schizophrenia. After listening to the report, the doctor leans back in her chair and says, "Someday, we must make a test to

Table 10-4
Divergence Between Medical and Nursing Practice

1900—Medical and Nursing Practice Similarities:

- Based on similar knowledge
- Characteristic of the individual
- Benevolent

1980—Medicine	*1980—Nursing*
Members educated largely in postgraduate university programs	Majority of members without baccalaureate education
Established scientific base	Developing scientific base
Established research effort	Developing research effort
Career commitment of members	Chronic instability of work force
Recognized professional autonomy and control of health care	Seeking professional autonomy and control of nursing
Strong professional organization	Struggling professional organization and some unionization of members
Fee for service collected privately and through third-party payers	Cost of services often not identified nor reimbursed through third-party payers
Dominated by men ?????	Dominated by women ???????

tell us where the health is, because in the end, it is our only ally." The doctor has described the need to find the uniqueness and strengths of the sickest patient in order to restore the state of wellness. This profound statement has great meaning for nursing in the way it views both its clients and itself.

The extent to which nursing achieves professionalism will depend in large measure upon finding where the health is in nursing and using it as our ally. The individual growth and activities of current nurses and those being socialized into nursing's professional ranks are very important. For this reason, the concluding chapter in the professionalism section will focus on the nurse person.

Study Questions

1. How do you feel about being a "professional" nurse?

2. How do you think nursing might have developed differently if
   a. The majority of practitioners were men?
   b. The majority of nurses were baccalaureate educated?
   c. All nurses accepted nursing as a career rather than as a job?

3. Using the criteria given, how do you rate nursing in comparison to other professions?

4. How has your awareness of professionalism changed?

Glossary

Accountability: Responsibility for services provided or made available.

Certification: A process by which a professional organization (in nursing, the American Nurses Association) recognizes excellence in practice; it identifies persons with specialized knowledge who have received endorsement of their peers.

Professionalism: Professional character, spirit, or methods; also activities found in various occupational groups whose members aspire to be professional.

Professionalization: The process of acquiring or changing characteristics in the direction of a profession.

Professions: Traditionally, the occupations of medicine, law, and the ministry.

Standard: An authoritative statement or criterion by which the quality of (nursing) practice can be judged.

Bibliography

American Nurses Association: Code for Nurses with Interpretive Statements. New York, The Association, 1968

American Nurses Association: Facts About Nursing '80–'81. New York, American Journal of Nursing Company, 1981

American Nurses Association: Standards for Organized Nursing Services. New York, The Association, 1965

American Nurses Association Convention: The '80's: Decade for decision. Am J Nurs 80:1317–1332, July, 1980

Ashley JA: Hospitals, Paternalism, and the Role of the Nurse. New York, Teachers College Press, 1976

Beard RO: The university education of the nurse. Teachers College Record 12:27–40, 1910

Chaska N (ed): The Nursing Profession: Views Through the Mist. New York, McGraw-Hill, 1978

Chrisman NJ: Nursing in the context of social and cultural systems. In Mitchell P, Lousteau A (eds): Concepts Basic to Nursing, 3rd ed, pp 37–52. New York, McGraw-Hill, 1981

Cohen HA: The Nurse's Quest for a Professional Identity. Menlo Park, CA, Addison-Wesley, 1981

Committee on Education: Position paper: Education for nursing. Am J Nurs 65:106–111, December, 1965

Flanagan L (compiler): One Strong Voice: The Story of the American Nurses' Association. Kansas City, MO, Lowell Press, 1976

Flexner A: Medical Education in the United States and Canada. New York, Carnegie Foundation for Advancement of Teaching, 1910

Goldmark J: Goldmark Report. New York, Macmillan, 1923

Greenberg J: I Never Promised You a Rose Garden. New York, Signet, 1964

Henderson V: The Nature of Nursing: A Definition and Its Implications for Practice, Research, and Education. New York, Macmillan, 1966

Jacox A: Address to the next generation. Am J Nurs 78:38–41, January, 1978

Kalisch P, Kalisch B: The Advance of American Nursing. Boston, Little, Brown, 1978

Kelly LY: Dimensions of Professional Nursing, 3rd ed. New York, Macmillan, 1975

King IM: Toward a Theory of Nursing. New York, John Wiley & Sons, 1971

Lindberg JB: Relationship Between Baccalaureate Nursing Students' Self-Esteem and Independent Behavior in Nursing. Ph.D. Dissertation, University of Michigan, 1979

Lysaught J: Action on Affirmation Toward an Unambiguous Profession of Nursing. Paper presented at American Nursing Association Biennial Convention, Houston, Texas, June 1980

Michigan Nurses Association: Position Paper on Nursing Practice. Lansing, MI, The Association, 1971

Montag M: The Education of Nursing Technicians. New York, GP Putnam's Sons, 1951

National Commission for the Study of Nursing and Nursing Education: An Abstract for Action. New York, McGraw-Hill, 1970

National League for Nursing: NLN Data Book, 1978, pp 2, 35. New York, National League for Nursing, 1978

Orem DE: Nursing: Concepts of Practice. New York, McGraw-Hill, 1971

Rogers ME: An Introduction to the Theoretical Basis of Nursing. Philadelphia, FA Davis, 1970

Roy SC: Adaptation: A conceptual framework for nursing. Nursing Outlook 18:42, 1970

Schein EH, Kommers DW: Professional Education, pp 7–14. New York, McGraw-Hill, 1972

Secretary's Committee to Study Extended Roles for Nurses: Extending the Scope of Nursing Practice. Am J Nurs 71:2346–2351, 1971

Simms LM, Lindberg JB: The Nurse Person: Developing Perspectives for Contemporary Practice. New York, Harper & Row, 1978

Steel JE: Putting joint practice into practice. Am J Nurs 81:964–967, May, 1981

Wandelt MA: Why nurses leave nursing and what can be done about it. Am J Nurs 81:72–77, January, 1981

Winsted-Fry P: The need to differentiate a nursing self. Am J Nurs 77:1454, September, 1977

Legal Aspects
and Ethical Issues

Janice B. Lindberg

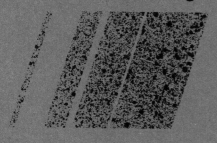

Objectives

Introduction

Legal Aspects
  Accountability
  Criminal and Civil Law
  Negligence and Malpractice
  Basic Human Rights
  Practice Acts
  Good-Samaritan Laws

Ethical Issues
  Person Focus for Bioethics
  Examples of Personal
  Bioethical Issues
  Theoretical Approaches to
  Bioethical Issues
  Moral Development
  Approach to Ethical Issues
  Larger Ethical Issues

Conclusion

Study Questions

Glossary

Bibliography

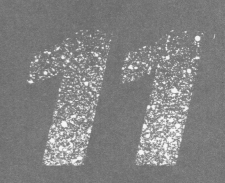

As a nurse you will confront many legal questions and ethical issues of health care. Both topics are subjects for comprehensive books. Obviously this discussion will be only a cursory introduction, presenting some of the more common ideas, terms, and concepts that are relevant for beginning students as practitioners. If you want specific legal advice, you should consult a lawyer or seek a primary source of legal information. Similarly, if you are concerned with a particular ethical issue, you will want to consult many primary references for varying viewpoints and detailed discussions. The field of bioethics is growing rapidly in both scope and prominence.

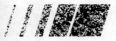

After completing this chapter, students will be able to:

● *Define accountability.*

● *Describe negligence and malpractice.*

● *Explain the need for personal liability insurance.*

● *Describe basic human rights.*

● *Identify practice acts as the state laws governing nursing practice and licensure.*

● *Describe a person focus for bioethics.*

● *Identify examples of personal bioethical issues.*

● *Contrast teleological and deontological approaches to bioethical issues.*

● *Describe Kohlberg's moral-development approach to ethical issues.*

● *Name three large ethical issues confronting nurses and other health professionals.*

Legal Aspects

Accountability

A major introductory legal concept is accountability. From your life experiences, you have internalized an everyday definition of accountability. Being answerable for professional conduct extends the concept to another dimension. This type of accountability was mentioned in the previous chapter in the context of peer, employer, and consumer relations.

In the introductory clinical nursing course of one baccalaureate program, faculty members have identified the following general behavioral objectives related to accountability and reliability.

The student will:

- Assume responsibility for own actions
- Demonstrate self-decipline in meeting commitments and obligations, *e.g.*, keeping appointments, submitting written assignments on time
- Prepare in advance for clinical experience
- Report unsafe patient/client practices
- Demonstrate awareness of patient/client rights
- Follow standard regulations and rules
- Apply safety measures to nursing interventions

The first objective, to assume responsibility, takes on new meaning for the professional nursing student. Although being a student gives the license to learn, certain prudent behavior nevertheless is expected, as indicated by the other objectives. The principle of reasonable care is considered in determining whether one has exercised such prudent behavior.

Hemelt and Mackert, in their book *Dynamics of Law in Nursing and Health Care*, define **reasonable care** as "that degree of skill and knowledge customarily used by a competent health practitioner of similar education and experience in treating and caring for the sick and injured in the community in which the individual is practicing or learning his profession" (1978, p. 11). Thus, just as a faculty member is expected to exercise appropriate judgment in making clinical assignments and supervising a student, so too is the student expected not to proceed without appropriate supervision if uninformed or unable to perform a certain skill (Fig. 11-1). Clients have a right to expect a student to perform at a safe level, even if not as skillfully as a licensed practitioner. Licensed practitioners them-

Figure 11-1
Student nurses practice accountability when they exercise reasonable care in their nursing activities. *(National Student Nurses' Association)*

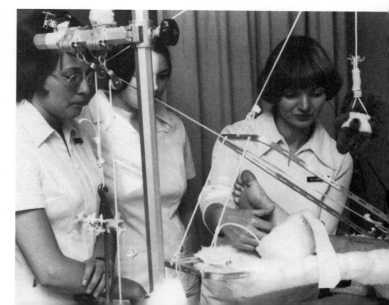

selves demonstrate accountability through consultation with informed peers.

Criminal and Civil Law

Laws are the civilized principles and processes by which people in society seek to resolve disputes and problems. **Criminal law** is concerned with behavior detrimental to society as a whole. **Civil law** deals with legal rights and duties of private persons. Criminal law is basically the State *versus* John Doe, whereas if Nurse Naylor were sued by Client Smith, the civil case would be Smith *versus* Naylor.

Generally health professionals are concerned with the category of law called torts. This concern is added to the legal rights and responsibilities the professionals retain as private citizens. **Torts** are civil wrongs that may be intentional or unintentional. The underlying concept of torts is the violation of reasonable behavior.

Negligence and Malpractice

Two commonly confused terms relating to torts and reasonable behavior are **negligence** and **malpractice.** Negligence is the more general concept. Although we often think of being negligent as being careless, the two are not necessarily synonymous. For example, Student Z, who injured Client Jones, would be negligent for attempting a procedure for which he had not received instruction even if he did it carefully. Malpractice involves negligence in carrying out professional services.

The term **liability** means responsibility because of position or particular circumstances. Thus, health professionals are liable or legally responsible for their professional behavior. Even though they proceed carefully, they could be found negligent. Their performance must be prudent in comparison with what similarly prepared health professionals would have done in the same circumstances.

Negligence related to nursing commonly includes such acts as failure to take appropriate precautions, to recognize dangers, or to report hazardous conditions. The nurse is responsible both for error in dependent nursing functions, such as administering physician-prescribed medications, and in professional judgment regarding more independent nursing functions, such as assessing client responses. The duty to take **affirmative action** when presented with a deteriorating situation (*e.g.,* unusual bleeding) refers to taking positive steps to bring such a situation under control.

Although opportunities for negligence abound, a formal charge is likely to be brought and a trial to occur only if harm results. Such a trial in court to settle issues is called **litigation.** Increasingly, patients or clients pursue litigation if they believe they have suffered mental or physical harm. Therefore, even careful students and registered nurses need the protection of liability insurance. Both the professional organization, the American Nurses Association, and the student organization, the National Student Nurses Association, provide such insurance service to their members at a reasonable cost.

Basic Human Rights

A **legal right** is a claim that is recognized and is enforceable by law. Persons who are hospitalized retain their constitutional rights, including those granted by amendments related to freedom of thought and speech, due process of law, and protection of minorities and the handicapped. Our society acknowledges basic human rights in other ways also. For example, health professions have codes of ethics governing behavior of profession members (see Chap. 10). Further, the Patients' Bill of Rights provides another acknowledgment of individual rights (see Chap. 9).

Complex health-care delivery systems such as hospitals are by their very nature confusing and intimidating to most persons. Although it may seem that individuals have little control over their personal situations in these systems, such is not the case. The nurse should be sensitive to the control and consent that each patient retains as his legal and moral right. **Consent** is a voluntary granting of permission. In many patient-care situations (*i.e.,* tests, operative procedures, and experimental treatments), consent must be explicitly obtained in writing. The consent must be accompanied by evidence of an appropriate explanation about risks and benefits. Patients even have such rights as refusal of injections. If that refusal is not heeded, patients have the right to bring assault-and-battery charges against health-care providers. Patients and clients also have other rights regarding intrusion, confidentiality of health-care records, and statements about their personal situation.

Practice Acts

The laws that govern nursing practice are state laws. The first nursing practice act was made state law in North Carolina in 1903. It was a **permissive** or voluntary law. Such laws permitted nurses to practice without a license if they did not claim licensure or use the R.N. initials. Currently, **mandatory** state

licensure for nurses requires all persons who nurse for compensation to be licensed. Many state practice laws have undergone recent revision. In 1972, New York's nursing practice act defined nursing's professional practice as "diagnosing and treating human responses." This or similar wording has been a model for many of the recently revised acts. This definition was also central to a recent social-policy statement by the professional organization (American Nurses Association, 1980).

Nursing practice acts define nursing practice and requirements for licensure in the particular state. They also create a board of examiners and specify their responsibilities. One of the requirements for licensure is passage of the State Board Test Pool Examination for Professional Nurses. Having the same examination for all states now facilitates state-to-state movement of R.N.s. Currently, the same examination is taken by graduates of associate-degree, diploma, and baccalaureate programs. This is partly because the purpose of licensure is to protect society by making sure that professionals demonstrate a minimal level of competence. Remember, according to the state, "R.N." designates the professional nurse in a legal sense, not according to the definition and criteria for a profession used earlier.

Many states are considering ways to test competency for R.N. relicensure, but it is proving particularly difficult to find a definition of professional nurse competency about which there is agreement. It is even more difficult and threatening to decide how competency should be measured. Nurses have a moral obligation, if not a legal one, to update their knowledge of nursing science and practice through some form of continuing education or learning.

Good-Samaritan Laws

Another kind of state law affecting nurses is a **good-Samaritan law.** Such a law is intended to encourage assistance of professionals in emergency situations. The coverage protecting nurses from liability varies from state to state. The legal, though perhaps not moral, choice exists for a nurse to pass by an emergency without fear of legal consequences. If care is offered a certain quality is expected, although the standard differs from a nonemergency situation. The standard would not be as high as that of reasonable prudent professional peers mentioned earlier, but it might be higher than for untrained lay persons. Good-Samaritan laws are meant to encourage participation but not to provide immunity if the "good Samaritan" is grossly negligent.

Ethical Issues

Person Focus for Bioethics

Ethics is a discipline involved with good and bad, moral duty, obligation, and values. It is concerned with social and political philosophy and also the philosophy of law. Only in the last decade has biomedical ethics been a well-recognized discipline. Since biomedical ethical issues have implications for other life and health sciences, we prefer the term **bioethics** to designate those health issues of an ethical nature that concern nurses. Although bioethical issues are of social and economic significance, the person is the focus for consideration of ethical issues and their implications for nurses.

The concept of client autonomy is a recurring theme of ethical issues. This means that the person is self-governing and independent regarding his decisions and activity. The autonomous person can be described as being rational and unconstrained. As Mappes and Zembaty state, the fully rational person has a number of abilities related to formulating and achieving personal goals (1981). Many persons who seek the services of health professionals may rightly or wrongly believe that their autonomy is threatened because of their dependency on others for care services. Ill and hospitalized persons are likely to believe themselves constrained even when they are aware and rational.

Two particular constraints that may be of concern are lack of ability and coercion. An example of the former constraint is the elderly person who lacks the strength to resist heroic lifesaving measures. Constraints on a person's autonomy can sometimes be justified to prevent public or private harm, to benefit the individual or others, to prevent offensive behavior in public, or to prevent self-harm (Mappes and Zembaty, 1981, p. 11). Fatherly interference with a person's autonomy is called **paternalism.** Although we usually think of paternalistic interference as compromising the rights of patients, it may not be intentionally limiting and often goes unrecognized.

Examples of Personal Bioethical Issues

Many of the life-and-death bioethical issues center on the underlying question, "When is a person not a person?" Names like Louise Brown (the first test-tube baby) and Karen Quinlan (a long-term comatose young adult) remind us of this underlying question about the nature of the person. An ad hoc committee of the Harvard Medical School proposed the substitution of irreversible coma for cessation of vital functions as the criterion for death. Their decision became timely when improved resuscitation and life-support measures maintained the lives of many who otherwise would have died. This action acknowledged the loss of personhood and incidentally made lifesaving transplant organs more readily available.

Anticipating the nature of ethical dilemmas may help you to understand moral values different from your own. To some professional nurses, the ideas of test-tube babies, termination of life-support systems, and abortion on demand are particularly distressing. Some other common but difficult ethical issues of a personal nature are highlighted in Table 11-1. Discoveries like manipulation of basic genetic material remind us that ethical issues will continue to pro-

liferate. The atrocities of World War II, with their terrible violations of human rights, led to formulation of the Nuremberg code to protect subjects of biomedical research.

Theoretical Approaches to Bioethical Issues

Most ethical theories belong to one of two opposing and mutually exclusive classifications. A **teleological** theory is one in which the ends justify the means. The outstanding example of a teleological approach is **utilitarianism.** The utilitarian approach is sometimes described as advocating the greatest good for the greatest number or choosing the least evil or least bad outcome. As you might guess, applied medical research supports this theory. The opposite

---

Table 11-1
Selected Bioethical Issues

Issues	Related Questions
Truth telling	Should a patient be told he is going to die if he seems unable to cope? if family members do not want him to be told?
Promise keeping	Should a spouse keep a promise not to remarry after the first mate dies?
Behavioral control or modification	Is patient welfare or staff convenience the intent of control? Are patient priorities considered?
Suicide	Under what circumstances, if ever, is suicide morally defensible? Does the nurse have the right to interfere?
Euthanasia	Is a severely defective newborn better off dead? Should a brain-dead person be considered a dead person? How can a living will preserve the dignity of a person?
Refusal of treatment	What if the nurse disagrees with the person's decision to refuse lifesaving treatment?
Irreversible coma	Is it morally right to hasten the death of a person kept alive by machines in order to transplant vital organs?
Opposing loyalties	Is the nurse obliged to keep hospital beds open if care for individual patients is compromised?

approach in its most extreme form is a **deontological** theory. For this theory, the moral right or wrong of an act is considered completely separately from the goodness or badness of consequences.

Teleological and deontological approaches can be illustrated with regard to abortion. Saving the mother's life justifies taking the unborn life in a teleological approach. In a deontological approach, on the other hand, any purposeful termination of life is morally bad, so the fetus would be spared.

A third approach, sometimes called a moderate deontological approach, is also called Natural Law and derives from the work of St. Thomas Aquinas.

Moral Developmental Approach to Ethical Issues

Moral development begins with the transition from instinctive thought to a higher form of thinking based on logic. The work of Kohlberg (1971) presents a hierarchical organization for understanding moral development (Fig. 11-2). This representation is somewhat similar to both Maslow's hierarchy of needs

(see Chap. 2) and Piaget's stages of cognitive development (see Chap. 3). Kohlberg's model helps one to refer individual moral growth to an accepted pattern of moral development for persons in contemporary American society.

Level-II development, according to Kohlberg, occurs at a time when children are moving from concrete operations to the formal operations of adult thought. This shift enables persons to envision various hypothetical alternatives relating to issues. Not only does the transition to formal thought occur at different ages for different individuals, but the cognitive shift precedes the moral development growth by several years for some persons.

Level-III development, the challenging of conventional morality, is an adolescent characteristic. For most nurses, the initial socialization to professional values occurs during late adolescence or early adulthood. At this point many persons may not have reached closure of the developmental process of stabilizing a moral prespective. Thus, adding professional responsibilities complicates coping with ethical issues. Growth beyond Kohlberg's stage of con-

Figure 11-2

Hierarchy of Moral Development. *(From Kohlberg, L: Recent Research in Moral Development. New York, Holt, Rinehart and Winston, 1971)*

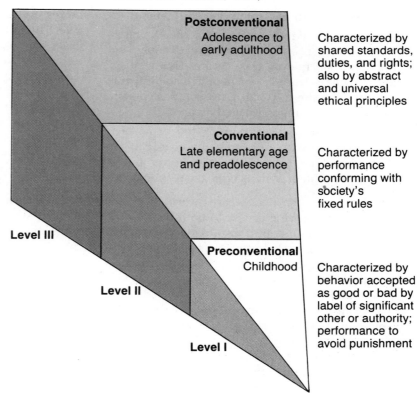

ventional morality makes one sensitive to universal ethical and moral principles and the value of unique persons and their differing views.

Larger Ethical Issues

When one reaches a stage of moral development characterized by awareness of universal ethical principles, a tangle of more abstract and larger ethical issues emerges. Although the same or similar questions may have arisen earlier, they assume greater significance when considered from an ethical perspective. Some of these questions are as follows:

- How do all citizens get access to health care?
- What should be the quality of health care?
- Who should control health-care decisions?

How do All Citizens Get Access to Health Care?

If access to health care is a right of all, inequality of access denies this right to some. Inequality of access then becomes an ethical issue. Some of the specific problems related to access are listed below:

- Access to health care is controlled largely by physicians who traditionally give illness care. If nurses are capable of certain health-care management, are they ethically responsible to try to have this management designated as part of the role of nursing? Nursing would then assume privileges of both control and accountability.
- Health-care services are geographically clustered. This distribution creates an advantage for the suburban middle class and a disadvantage for many elderly and poor people living in rural or inner-city areas. What is nursing's responsibility to serve underprivileged areas?
- Health-care costs are becoming too expensive. Even persons with moderate incomes can be devastated financially by a catastrophic illness or health problem. Who is ethically responsible?

Nurses and other health-care providers must work together to provide access to both health and illness care, better distribution of services, and affordable health care. The latter means that options other than the most expensive care must be appropriately available. Many persons have used an emergency room for nonemergent problems such as sore throats because it seemed the only service available. Screening in less expensive neighborhood clinics could reduce expensive visits to sophisticated specialty-care facilities. Nurses might assist clients to use health-care facilities appropriately or they might work to make such neighborhood clinics available.

What Should Be the Quality of Health Care?

Quality of health care becomes an ethical issue, because quality of health care is related to quality of life. The issues of access and quality are also, of necessity, related. If one does not have access to the system, the chances of receiving quality care are low. From a technological or medical perspective, the quality of health care may be high for those with access. However, if the quality of life is compromised by dehumanizing, depersonalized, and unwanted interventions, even those with access may perceive the quality of health care to be low. To provide quality health care and access to all persons would require major reordering of our national social and economic priorities. If we allot fewer health-care resources than are needed, how shall we decide who gets quality care?

Who Should Control Health-Care Decisions?

The concept of client autonomy is a recurring theme in ethical issues. A person-focused nursing perspective affirms the patient or client as the center of ethical decision making. High-level wellness is both relative and individual. Therefore, the client can be expected to make personal health-care decisions based on what the person, not the professional, defines as his concept of health. If the professional accepts this premise, then how the individual client views health care becomes more important than a case added to the research files or another notch on the surgeon's knife. The criteria for judging the success of clients' health-care decisions will change also. Effective coping and positive health-care decisions will be acknowledged by health-care professionals. Many trends, including the consumerism movement and home care for birth and death, suggest that persons are interested in controlling their own health-care decisions.

Tax dollars ought to support the health-care delivery that persons want and need. In spite of the billions of dollars poured into tertiary (*i.e.*, specialized) care, most persons will have only a minimal need for such services during their entire lifetime. It is possible that every state has more beds in nursing homes than in hospitals. Yet conditions in many nursing homes are such that one would not wish himself or a loved one cared for there. Nursing is the one health profession in a unique position to help persons use advances in scientific health care and reasonable self-care practices to increase their control over health-care decisions. The use of tax dollars to finance tertiary care is just one illustration that broader ethical issues related to health care are difficult to resolve. Resolution would require a profound social commitment and national priority for equality of human rights and valuing of individual persons.

Conclusion

This chapter introduces some legal aspects and ethical issues that are of concern to nurses. Nurses are professionally accountable for the services they provide, and they must practice within the restriction of criminal and civil law. Nurses must also demonstrate reasonably prudent behavior to avoid charges of negligence and malpractice. As autonomous practitioners, nurses have both their own practice acts and individual licensure. State practice laws define the legal practice of nursing further, while other state laws enable nurses to act as good Samaritans in emergencies.

A person focus and an awareness of contrasting theoretical approaches can guide the nurse's consideration of bioethical issues. Moral development is a personal developmental task of beginning practitioners who face ethical issues as professionals. Nurses and other health-care professionals must be concerned with both personal bioethical issues and larger ethical issues.

Study Questions

1. What are your personal feelings about assuming accountability for the professional nurse role?

2. What legal responsibilities do you have as a student? How can you influence the legal definition of nursing practice in the future?

3. Compare and contrast the role of the state and the profession itself in regulating the practice of nursing.

4. How do you feel about clients making ethical decisions with which you do not agree?

5. How do you feel about cloning to make biological carbon copies of plants, animals, and persons?

6. What ethical responsibilities do you have as a student?

7. What ethical responsibilities does nursing have as a profession?

Glossary

Affirmative action: Positive steps to bring a deteriorating situation under control, *e.g.,* intervening to control unusual bleeding.

Bioethics: A subspecialty of the discipline of ethics; issues of an ethical nature that concern health professionals.

Civil law: Law concerned with legal rights and duties of private persons.

Consent: Voluntary granting of permission, e.g., for treatment procedures or research.

Criminal law: Law concerned with behavior detrimental to society as a whole.

Deontological: A classification of ethical theory; belief that the moral right or wrong of an act is considered separately from the goodness or badness of consequences.

Ethics: A discipline concerned with social, political, and legal philosophy and principles of good and bad, moral duty, obligation, and values; rules of conduct.

Good-Samaritan law: A state law intended to encourage health professionals to offer assistance in emergency situations.

Legal right: A claim recognized and enforceable by law.

Liability: Responsibility or obligation because of position or particular circumstances; a legal responsibility for professional behavior.

Litigation: A trial in court to settle legal issues; a lawsuit.

Malpractice: Negligence in carrying out professional services; improper professional action.

Mandatory licensure: A kind of state law controlling nursing practice; requires all persons who nurse for compensation to be licensed.

Negligence: Failure to exercise that degree of care required by law for the protection of others.

Paternalism: Fatherly interference with a person's autonomy or independence.

Permissive licensure: A kind of state law controlling nursing practice; it permitted nurses to practice without a license if they did not claim licensure or use the R.N. initials.

Reasonable care: That degree of skill and knowledge customarily used by a competent health practitioner of similar education and experience in treating and caring for the sick and injured in the community in which the individual is practicing or learning his profession.

Teleological: A classification of ethical theory; belief that ends justify the means.

Torts: Civil wrongs that may be intentional or unintentional; violations of reasonable behavior.

Utilitarianism: An approach to ethics that advocates the greatest good for the greatest number.

Bibliography

American Nurses Association: A Social Policy Statement. Kansas City, MO, American Nurses Association, 1980

Aroskar MA: Anatomy of an ethical dilemma, the theory . . . the practice. Am J Nurs 80:658–663, April, 1980

Ashley JA: Hospitals, Paternalism, and the Role of the Nurse. New York, Teachers College Press, 1976

Beauchamp TL, Perlin S: Ethical Issues in Death and Dying. Englewood Cliffs, NJ, Prentice-Hall, 1978

Benoliel JQ, Berthold JS: Human Rights, Guidelines for Nurses in Clinical and Other Research. Kansas City, MO, American Nurses Association, 1975

Bullough B (ed): The Law and the Expanding Nursing Role. New York, Appleton-Century-Crofts, 1980

Cazalas MW: Nursing and the Law. Germantown, MD, Aspen Systems, 1978

Christman L: Moral dilemmas for practitioners in a changing society. Nurs Digest 6:47–49, Summer, 1978

Crisham P: Measuring moral judgment in nursing dilemmas. Nurs Res 30:104–110, March-April, 1981

Davis AJ, Aroskar MA: Ethical Dilemmas and Nursing Practice. New York, Appleton-Century-Crofts, 1978

Georgia's R.N.s defeat M.A.G. attempt to control nursing practice. Am J Nurs 80:576–577, 614–618, 1980

Hastings Center Report (Journal published by the Institute of Society, Ethics, and the Life Sciences, Hastings-on-Hudson, New York, 10706)

Hemelt MD, Mackert ME: Dynamics of Law in Nursing and Health Care. Reston, VA, Reston, 1978

Henderson G, Primeaux M: Transcultural Health Care. Menlo Park, CA, Addison-Wesley, 1981

International Council of Nurses: The Nurse's Dilemma: Ethical Conflicts in Nursing. New York, American Journal of Nursing, 1977

Kelly LY: Dimensions of Professional Nursing, 3rd ed. New York, Macmillan, 1975

Kohlberg L: Recent Research in Moral Development. New York, Holt, Rinehart & Winston, 1971

Kübler-Ross E (ed): Death, The Final Stage of Growth. Englewood Cliffs, NJ, Prentice-Hall, 1975

Levine ME: Nursing ethics and the ethical nurse. Am J Nurs 77:845–849, May, 1977

Mappes TA, Zembaty JS: Biomedical Ethics. New York, McGraw-Hill, 1981

Murchison I, Nichols TS, Hanson R: Legal Accountability in the Nursing Process. St Louis, CV Mosby, 1978

Piaget J: The Moral Judgment of the Child. New York, Free Press, 1965

Smith SJ, Davis AJ: Ethical dilemmas: Conflicts among rights, duties, and obligations. Am J Nurs 80:1462–1466, August, 1980

Steele SM, Hermon VM: Values Clarification in Nursing. New York, Appleton-Century-Crofts, 1979

Tate BL: The Nurse's Dilemma, Ethical Considerations in Nursing Practice. Geneva, International Council of Nurses, 1977

Thompson JB, Thompson HO: Ethics in Nursing. New York, Macmillan, 1981

Tishler CL: The psychological aspects of genetic counseling. Am J Nurs 81:733–734, April, 1981

Trials of War Criminals Before the Nuremberg Military Tribunals. Washington, DC, U.S. Government Printing Office, 1948

The Nurse Person: Issues, Practice Options, and Strategies

Janice B. Lindberg

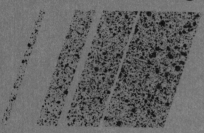

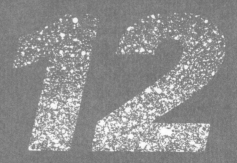

Who is the nurse person? The nurse person is every individual who was, is, or plans to be a nurse. To the nurse persons who have gone before, we and society owe a debt of gratitude. Down through the ages, nurses were the true health professionals. In the back woods, on the battlefield, and among the urban poor, nurses may have been the only health professionals. Nurse persons were there to comfort and encourage when needed. They greeted life and awaited death. Nurses helped people to learn about their bodies, manage their environments, and fulfill their potentials.

There are interesting stories about how nurses used herb teas and poultices to heal the sick. However, without fully realizing it, these nurses also had the tools to identify health. They learned to observe, to listen, and to focus on the uniqueness of each person they nursed. In doing so, they developed a person-centered dimension that made a difference in health care and gave a special purpose to nursing.

Today nursing is struggling to rediscover and understand more fully that sense of purpose and difference. Today nursing needs its nurse persons to focus some of their great skill, energy, and interest in wellness on the nursing profession and its contribution to society. The health of both nursing and society is at stake.

In this chapter we will consider a few of the many issues that affect nurse persons today and some of the practice options for nurses. The chapter concludes with some strategies the nurse person can use to achieve personal self-actualization and assist nursing to influence health-care policy.

Nursing's Self-Doubts

Historically, nurses were not always fully aware of their special contributions to health care. That is, they did not identify and articulate the essence of nursing. Sometimes nurses minimized their abilities to develop trust between themselves and those they nursed, to identify the healthy aspects of the person, and to help individuals mobilize their own health qualities to achieve their personal potential. Nurses recognized that although a person might have severe or even life-threatening physical problems, he was still a unique individual capable of growth. However, because nurses did not identify and articulate nursing's unique contribution completely, much of it was set aside as nursing entered an age of increased technology.

As technology flourished, much of nursing became "doing activities." Nurses and others measured their value by their skill in taking care of equipment. A unique nursing contribution was present in much of what nurses did, but it often seemed less important. It was not unusual for a patient to describe his appreciation of nursing care and for the nurse to think or say, "But I didn't do anything!" Perhaps the nurse listened with trust and therapeutic purpose and helped the patient to rediscover control of his life, to regain his sense of self-esteem, and to view his future with hope or a sense of well-being.

Many practicing nurses and students are not fully aware of this less tangible essence of nursing. They also may not comprehend fully the problems and issues before the profession. Yet, nurse persons who are the present and future nurse leaders will need to be the ones who provide, preserve, and develop today's nursing for tomorrow.

Problems Common to Nursing and Other Professions

If nurses are to control the service they provide to society, some current problems and issues will need to be addressed vigorously by nurses. In general, the problems faced by nurses and other professionals originate from the characteristics of professional occupations as discussed in Chapter 10. These include automony and independent decision making, career commitment, collegial relationships, and professional worth or rewards. Issues, in contrast to problems, are large questions about which there is no consensus on the right answer. Issues, therefore, are questions not easily answered with a simple yes or no.

Contemporary Issues

Control of Nursing Practice

One of the largest issues facing nursing is, who shall control nursing practice? Control is a primary issue underlying whether nursing will continue its professionalization toward independence and autonomy. Forces both within and outside nursing challenge the obvious answer that nursing should control its own practice. For example, medicine and hospital administration would gain much from controlling nursing, and some nurses are unwilling to assume this responsibility. If nurses do not assume control of nursing, then all issues related to future practice (*your practice*) will be decided by whatever group does control it.

Control of nursing practice has led to controversy about the so-called **extended** and **expanded roles** for nurses. A role is a pattern of behavior associated with a distinctive social position. An extended role is a role lengthened in a unilateral manner. For example, the role of the physician is extended through the use of another health worker. In this case, the authority base for extension is from the physician. Role expansion is a multidirectional spreading out. For example, an expanded role for the nurse may involve some extension into the physician's role, but this is a lesser part of the expansion. The authority base of expansion is primarily nursing knowledge and clinical expertise.

By 1970, various estimates had been made which suggested that perhaps there were 100,000 nurses who, with a modest additional training, could assist physicians in extending their medical services. If indeed medicine and nursing are different professions, the logic of extending medical services and calling this nursing practice is as questionable as expanding the scope of nursing practice and calling it medicine. What seems more reasonable is that the professions might work together to alter mutually the boundaries between them. Such an approach would require medicine to recognize that nursing is autonomous and should control nursing practice rather than serve medicine.

Relationship of "Control" to Other Issues

Other important issues are as follows:

* What services should nurses provide?
* How should nurses be educated?
* How should nurses receive payment for services?
* What should be the influence of organized nursing on American health-care policy?

If nursing demands its autonomy and retains control, then nurses, with their clients and society, will decide these issues together. Answers to the above questions, in turn, will influence the impact organized nursing has on even larger national health-policy issues. Many issues are more intertwined than they may appear on first inspection.

Lest you be discouraged about the problems facing nursing, remember that there is strength in numbers and that nursing is the largest group of health-care providers. To the extent that you are aware of the issues and choose to participate in their resolution, you may be able to influence the outcome.

You can expect that your views about various issues will change over time. In a study of baccalaureate nursing students, the majority of sophomores saw themselves as physicians' helpers in their professional roles. As seniors, the students saw themselves as more autonomous and began to perceive the nurse as a potential teacher and leader (Stein, 1978).

Stein thought that, as a result of their developing self-image, students experience a conflict between the ideal image portrayed by the school and the imperfect nursing found in hospitals and community agencies. Undoubtedly you have had or will experience a similar conflict. The mere fact that there are many issues facing nursing contributes to this conflict over what nursing is all about and what is the appropriate preparation for nursing. For students to ignore issues is tempting but shortsighted. The average baccalaureate nurse practices nursing as a student only one-seventh of the professional career. The issues you ignore today may seriously alter your career in years to come!

What Services Should Nurses Provide?

Those who contend that nursing is moving toward professionalization would argue the following principle: the profession, with help from the society it serves, should decide what services to offer. Other considerations are listed below:

* First, we must recognize that the health-care needs of society are changing because of changes in the nature of the population, technological advances, disease patterns, and life-styles. This reality affects or should affect the way health-care services are organized and delivered and also the scope of practice of various health-care professions, including nursing (A.N.A., 1979, p.8).

* Second, health care is an umbrella concept covering services of many professional and technical health-care providers. Health care is not solely medical care. Many health-care problems, especially chronic conditions, require other than medical management. The number of persons who require supportive nursing services to adapt to the lengthening life span will increase greatly.

* Third, nurses need to make known the nature of the service they are able to deliver. Both recipients of nursing care and other health-care professionals need this information. The authority for professional nursing practice legitimately comes from the skill and knowledge of the nurse provider.

The issue of what services nurses should provide is further complicated by the lack of unity within nursing itself. Nurses must unite to answer the issue of what services they should provide before they can address logically the issues of how nurses should be educated or paid for their services. Nursing must continue to strive for excellence in providing holistic person-centered care to the best of the capabilities of its practitioners at all levels.

How Should Nurses Be Educated?

Another issue for consideration is, how should nurses be prepared or educated? The answer is complex. Nursing knowledge is no longer simple and intuitive. Differences in education now undermine unity and development of the profession. Although the baccalaureate is advocated as the preferred professional preparation, associate-degree programs prepare approximately half the graduating registered nurses. Today some educators and employers see these programs as different in amount rather than kind of education. Therefore, they see associate-degree programs as a less expensive way to prepare registered nurses.

Two interesting points have been made about preparation for the inevitable increase in health-care technology. One is that as technology in health-care increases, more—not less—humanistic nursing is needed. The other point is that technological development may mandate that bioengineering technicians rather than nurses monitor equipment. Currently some people believe that baccalaureate programs do not place enough emphasis on technical skills. Others believe that B.S.N. programs (bachelor of science in nursing) continue to place too much emphasis on technical skills. Although many employers do not differentiate among R.N.s in the workplace, baccalaureate graduates should seek employment that will use their skills fully and compensate them for their additional preparation. Of course, the more expensive nurse to educate and employ should offer something obviously different and important.

Organized nursing's position on the kind of education its practitioners need is less confused than it may appear. The 1965 A.N.A. position paper stating the baccalaureate as the appropriate educational credential for entry to professional nursing practice was written when most current nursing students were starting elementary school! In reality, implementation of even the strongest pronouncements takes a long time when an issue is involved.

In 1979, the A.N.A. Commission on Nursing Education wrote (p. 10)

The new and emerging roles in nursing are an indication that today's professional nurse must acquire and utilize an expanded body of knowledge and a wide variety of skills. Today's professional nurse must be equipped with knowledge and skills that allow for flexibility and facilitate adaptability to particular situations. Today's professional nurse must have the ability to synthesize knowledge and translate it into reality-oriented action. Baccalaureate preparation in nursing equips an individual with a working knowledge of the biological, physical, social, and behavioral sciences. It provides educational opportunities that increase one's skills in critical thinking, clinical investigation, and decision making.

At the 1980 convention, the A.N.A. again reaffirmed the baccalaureate as the minimum educational preparation for professional practice. Although we need to avoid generalizations that devalue other educational programs, at the same time we need to demonstrate that differences in education do make differences in care. Additionally, we need to heed Toffler's predictions in *Future Shock* (1970). The fantastic knowledge explosion of our age will require all of us to be lifelong learners.

Although there is a shift in education to the graduate level for other health-care disciplines, only a small percentage of R.N.s are prepared with either masters degrees or doctorates. There is a need for masters-prepared nurses as clinicians, administrators, educators, and researchers. Doctorally prepared nurses are needed as leaders in all nursing areas. If one assumes that each facility in which nursing care is provided would benefit from having doctorally prepared nurses to stimulate research and practice, the shortage becomes very apparent. Imagine a hospital or other health-care agency with only one medical doctor! It will be increasingly difficult for nurses to be peers with other health professionals who are educated beyond them.

How Should Nurses Be Paid for Their Services?

This topic, like the others, is an issue because there is no consensus or easy answer about how payment should be made. This issue is closely related to control of nursing. Until nurses generate their own fees for service and bill directly, someone else will be holding the purse strings, controlling nursing monies, and deciding what services nurses should offer.

The majority of nurses are hospital employees. Even through many physicians may appear to be hospital employees also, the situation is not the same. Patients are billed for physician services separately, whereas nursing services are covered in a daily hospital rate or room charge. Often the nursing department does not exercise budget control. Physicians in hospitals may join medical service plans that operate on a share-of-revenue-generated basis. Obviously, the more patients seen and the more revenue generated, the greater the profit. Such plans may rent space and services, including nursing services, from a hospital. Physicians hiring nursing services expect to dictate what the nurses do. This control directly opposes the freedom professionals generally have, to determine both the nature and the cost of their unique services. When nurses are paid by hospitals or physicians, there is an incentive for both to pay as little as possible for the nursing services they require.

Increasingly, nurses employed by hospitals are entering into negotiated contracts with their hospital employers. The state professional organization, a branch of the American Nurses' Association, may serve as a local bargaining agent. Some nurses dislike having their professional organization participate in activities they believe characterize labor unions, not professional societies. Regardless of your personal viewpoint, it is a fact that the economic and general-welfare (**E. & G. W.**) activities of the American Nurses' Association require much of the professional organization's resources and efforts. Obviously, few members would disagree with the ends of economic security and fair compensation, but many members do not agree with the means deemed necessary to secure these ends.

Both the history of nursing service as a charity and the predominance of women in the occupation contribute to poor pay for members. Hospitals, physicians, and insurance companies resist efforts to introduce direct billing for nursing services. Health care is a major industry subject to the economic principles of big business; for this reason, hospitals oppose any additional private billing by their workers. Whatever the setting, increased use of nursing services may lead to decreased need for medical care; thus, physicians might resist direct billing that facilitates patient access to nurses, possibly in preference to themselves. Insurance companies are responsive to power politics and therefore inclined to support the side of organized medicine and hospitals. Nurses will achieve direct payment and financial security worthy of professionals when nurse persons individually and collectively are more assertive about the value of their services and take steps to muster a broad base of societal support.

What Will Be the Influence of Nursing on Health-Care Policy?

Unfortunately, nursing is attempting to influence health-care policy both locally and nationally at a time when organized nursing is fragmented and lacks a clear unity of purpose. Within local hospitals, the nursing department may not have an equal vote with medicine and hospital administration at the top level of decision making. Additionally, most nurses do not belong to the American Nurses' Association, the professional organization that could be the national voice of nurse power.

In spite of the many issues facing the profession and the lack of organized nurse power, nursing is beginning to value both the caring and scientific components of the profession equally. Nurses are recapturing the autonomy and independence which many of our nursing ancestors had. We are learning to put forth a nursing model of health care so that we will be viewed as colleagues of other health professionals rather than as extensions of them. We could learn much about influence from some of our nurse predecessors. Nightingale, Sanger, and Wald did not sidestep the issues of their day as they intervened to halt the miseries of the battlefield, unwanted pregnancies, and urban poverty, respectively. Neither did they always agree with nursing colleagues nor find support from them. They persevered because they believed they were right about the essence and nature and value of nursing service to society.

We need to remember that nursing is not the only profession with the problems of confusion about unique services, educational preparation, and payment for services. We should also remember that crises can be growth producing. Nursing is growing as a profession and its practitioners can grow as professional persons. From this perspective, many professional issues can be understood better as having maturational and situational aspects, as do other crises. The slow progress of nursing and the uphill struggle that is our fate, partly because most of us are women, is at times discouraging. Hopefully, we are taking the best of nursing art and melding it with scientific nursing to create a better health-care future.

Practice Options: Expanding Frontiers of Nursing Practice

Commonly Confused Labels Related to Practice Options

There are several commonly confused labels related to practice options. Some definitions that may be useful in understanding some common practice options are stated below.

Nurse practitioner is defined in some states as any nurse who renders service to a recipient. This term is also used to refer to an ambulatory-care nurse with advanced skills in assessment of the physical and psychosocial health—illness status of persons in a variety of settings, through health and development interviews and physical examination. The term may also be used to describe a nurse functioning in an expanded role, such as a pediatric nurse practitioner. Nurse Practitioner probably will be a general title describing the nurse of tomorrow, for whom the now-special practitioner skills will become commonplace.

A **clinical nurse specialist** is an expert in a particular practice such as psychiatric–mental health or medical–surgical nursing. This person gives direct and expert nursing care, models expert behavior for other nurses, and serves as a consultant or coordinator for persons needing nursing care in the area of specialty. This nurse usually has a masters degree and may have clinical nursing research skills, which are used directly or offered in consultation with other practicing nurses.

A **physician's assistant** (P.A.) is a dependent health worker who is selected by a physician and administratively reports to him. This is an example of what was earlier described as role extension. The P.A. is an extension of the physician and therefore does not have a nursing role. The authority for this role comes from the physician, which is why the P.A. is a dependent worker. This person is capable, under direction of an M.D., of performing functions now usually performed by physicians, such as physical and diagnositc examinations.

Many of the first P.A.s were corpsmen. It is not uncommon for physicians employing P.A.s to increase their practice size and income with relatively little cost to the physician.

The **nurse clinician** was first described by Reiter in 1966. This specialist was denoted primarily as a bedside or direct-care expert with an area of specialty and, possibly, advanced preparation. Today nurses designated as clinicians are usually baccalaureate prepared. In one large midwestern medical center, a clinical ladder of advancement provides a meaningful reward to expert nurses remaining in direct patient care. A nurse wishing to be identified as a clinician I or II presents a specific proposal or petition to be so designated and recognized. This is acted upon by a peer-review board.

Nurse midwifery, although recently more publicized as a practice role, has been in existence for much longer than other practitioner roles; the first midwifery school opened in 1931. "The American nurse–midwife always functions within the framework of a medically directed health service; she is never an independent practitioner." (Kelly, 1975, p. 509).

The **nurse anesthetist** usually functions under direct or indirect supervision of an anesthesiologist (medical specialist) whenever anesthesia is given. Preparation includes approximately 2 years in a school of anesthesia, which may or may not give credit toward an advanced degree.

Trends Related to Practice Options for Nurses

Several trends related to practice options for nurses are listed below:

- More practice options are available and possible than ever before.

- There is a trend toward more advanced preparation (*i.e.,* B.S.N. or M.S.N.)

- External barriers in relation to practice options are presently decreasing but have the potential to go either way.

- At least tentative attempts at collaboration between medicine and nursing are being made.

Practice options generally parallel the increased specialization that has occurred in medicine and other components of the health-care delivery system. There are nursing specialists for

- Age groups—pediatric, adult, and geriatric practitioners

- Illnesses—coronary disease, diabetes, cancer

- Abilities or disabilities—burns, rehabilitation, sexuality specialists, midwives

- Locales—ambulatory-care units, operating room, emergency room, home-care coordinator, and community-health nurses

Nurses can be care givers, teachers, and researchers in nursing. They can take on more independent functions and expand the frontiers of practice without leaving nursing. Within the broad categories of clinical practice, there are specific expanded roles yet to be defined. Clinician roles are only one example. Sometimes nurses are easily taken in by the name of a practice option rather than being sure they know what the option will actually offer them. Hopefully your talents will be used to best advantage for the benefit of yourself, nursing, and society. The expectation is that nurses will look beyond the labels of practice options to who controls, what preparation is necessary, and what the nurse will be doing.

Future of Practice Options

Nurses themselves must take the leadership role in deciding what part of health care is nursing and then follow through to control that nursing care. Given the size of the health-care industry, this leadership must come not just from nurses prepared in graduate programs, with masters and doctoral degrees, but from baccalaureate graduates as well. Never before have more practice options existed for beginning nurses prepared at the baccalaureate level. In other words, practice options can and will be defined by nurses like you.

Although some employers do not differentiate among associate-degree, diploma, and baccalaureate graduates, nurses need to find or generate job opportunities that allow them to practice as prepared and to grow to their full potential. Many students begin to explore practice options through part-time employment as a nurse assistant. The realities of the workplace look different from the student and the employee perspectives. During work experience, worrisome lack of practice with technical procedures, such as dressing, IVs, and injections, may be overcome. The opportunity to observe how a variety of nurses practice in different ways can be most instructive.

Nursing's Independent, Interdependent, and Dependent Functions

Nursing has independent, interdependent, and dependent functions. Remember that health care is medical and nursing care. Medicine and nursing are separate, although not always distinctly so. Traditionally nursing has assumed a subordinate position in health care and has performed functions auxiliary to medicine. The current image of the professional nurse, as advanced by nurse leaders, is that of a baccalaureate graduate who is a more independent career colleague of the physician.

Function is the kind of action or activity proper to a person. To describe someone's function we would note the person's behavior. Let us look at what characterizes independent, interdependent, and dependent behavior in nursing.

Independent nursing behavior is initiated as a result of the nurse's own knowledge and skills rather than as a result of delegated authority from the physician. Although some nurses may practice independently, this is not the norm for practice options. Even if most nurses do not believe that independent practice is currently feasible or something they want to do, they may be interested in independent behavior (Fig. 12-1). Mundinger prefers the term **autonomous** nursing practice to independent nursing practice (1980). She believes that although nursing may encompass some physician-directed activities, both nursing-theory components and unique nursing practice will be involved. Mundinger differentiates autonomous function from dependent function in the following way (1980, p. 4).

> Knowing why, when, and how to position clients and doing it skillfully makes the function an autonomous therapy. But, if physicians order it, how can it be autonomous? If physicians order an action nurses would not do in the absence of those orders, if they do not know why or when to do so, it is probably a dependent rather than autonomous function. But if the nurse has the knowledge and the skill to initiate and carry out the actions and answer for the results, then it is autonomous.

If nursing is a profession, most of the practice should consist of independent nursing functions!

Interdependent nursing behavior speaks both to the overlapping functions and to the desirability of collegial relationships in which each profession contributes according to its knowledge, skills, and focus. Gray overlapping areas may occur, especially in criticial-care units and primary-care centers. Often activities only seem more independent because they are more like physician behavior, such as monitoring complex equipment or ordering diagnostic tests. However, very strict regulations or prior agreements about steps to be taken in special circumstances may leave little room for autonomous decision making.

Dependent nursing behavior is performed under delegated medical authority or supervision or according to *a priori* routines. Routine administra-

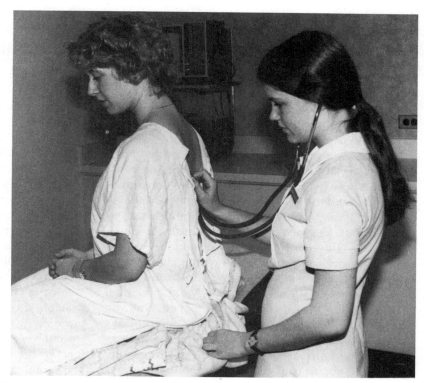

Figure 12-1
Using physical assessment skills to identify nursing problems is one example of independent nursing behavior
(Photo by Bob Kalmbach)

tion of prescription medications might be an example of a dependent nursing behavior. Much of traditional nursing activity has been giving care or doing treatments according to the dictates of the physicians' order book.

Independent Nursing Behavior Explored by Experts

Although one might expect that independent nursing functions would differ greatly form clinical specialty to clinical specialty and from practice option to practice option, such differences were not found in a recent study conducted by one of the authors (Lindberg, 1979). A group of nurse experts were unanimous about a number of independent nursing behaviors, including such activities as using physical appraisal skills to diagnose nursing problems, initiating teaching plans for patients, and asking the physician to change a medication based on nursing assessment of the client. Note that such behaviors are not confined to any one clinical area and that they may be practiced by nurses engaged in practice options with different names, such as staff nurse,

geriatric nurse, and so on. All forty experts valued independent behavior and shared similar spontaneous definitions of the term. They emphasized actions guided by one's own knowledge and skills rather than by an external person or source.

Baccalaureate Students' Views About Independent Behavior

In the same study described above, 317 baccalaureate nursing students identified most strongly with general independent behavior related to direct client care, such as using physical appraisal skills to diagnose nursing problems (Lindberg, 1979). They identified least strongly with independent behavior related to medical doctors or other non-nurse health professionals. Ninety-five percent of the students thought the opportunity for independent behavior in the ideal nursing job was important or very important. Students agreed that nurses who anticipate a long career favor independent behavior more than nurses who plan short-term employment. The students (97% of whom were female) did not believe independent behavior was a masculine characteristic. They did believe, however, that society *views* independent behavior as primarily a masculine characteristic. This discrepancy suggests that the behavior that nursing experts expect of students moving into contemporary practice options is in obvious conflict with students' perceptions of society's sexual stereotyping. This conflict, which is somewhat surprising given the recent women's movement, is an important issue to address openly.

Nursing as a profession has only recently begun to assert its autonomy. This means nursing must find ways to expand practice options to accommodate independent behavior of students now being prepared. Ways to function within the hospital setting without loss of professional identity and the desire for independent behavior should be researched more vigorously by the profession. At any time approximately 75% of nurses are hospital employed. Although students may not see the hospital as the ideal setting for nursing practice, they do expect to be employed there at least temporarily. Nurses generally do practice in acute-care settings upon graduation, partly because of the job availability and also to obtain valuable experience.

Strategies for Increasing Nurse Self-Actualization and Influence

Interrelatedness of Self-Image, Public Image, and Nursing Influence

A strategy is both a plan and action. It is the means to an end or goal. We are interested in the individual goal of self-actualization because we believe nurses themselves have inherent self-actualization tendencies just as their patients do. We are interested in the professional goal of influencing health-care policy because we believe nurses will move policy in the direction of helping other persons, namely clients of health-care delivery, to realize their inherent potential. According to Lysaught, 75% to 90% of the social worth of a profession is based on the profession's view of itself (1980). The profession's view of itself arises from the self-image of individual practitioners. Recent research suggests that nurses may have higher self-esteem and more positive attitudes toward independent behavior in their profession than has generally been assumed (Lindberg, 1979). Each nurse person needs to consider self-concept and its rela-

tionship to personal growth, the profession's image, and nursing's influence on health-care policy.

In the lay view, all nurses are the same. This view is largely one of the nurse as physicians' helper and nursing as a part of medicine with minimal independence and few intellectual aspects. This perspective may consider the nurse as a sweet young thing and not as a mature professional practitioner. The image of nurses and nursing is more of a reality issue and a challenge than most of us would like to believe. This issue is reflected in the public media (*i.e.*, magazines, television, and newspapers) and in the perception of nurses and nursing by fellow health professionals.

For nursing to influence health-care policy markedly is a big order. Nursing has been scorned by feminists and others as traditional women's work done by unassertive workers. In reality, nurses and feminists share some of the same concerns and are waging similar battles. Interestlingly, the women's movement has greatly influenced our society in recent years. Changes have been accomplished in part by increased self-awareness of women and also by mobilizing a sisterhood support system that nursing has virtually ignored. This suggests that the strategies nurses can use to achieve personal self-actualization and to influence health-care policy are both individual and group strategies.

Individual Strategies

Use of Information

Most professionals are well informed about their society and the world generally. They appreciate and understand society's development, its potentials, and its perils. They may have both a strong national consciousness and a humane view of world problems. Individual practitioners understand how their unique professional service to society relates to a larger scheme. Professionals recognize that knowledge is power, whether in science, economics, or politics. Some nurses have seen little need to be informed beyond their small sphere of practice. Yet nurses need to be informed about nursing specifically, health care generally, and the world beyond.

One of the ways the community of professionals maintains and advances its subculture is through an information network. The formal communication network consists of books, journals, organization newspapers, and so on. These provide for the scholarly expression of group goals and ideas. As a professional you will need to use the valuable information that passes through this network.

Learn to use the professional literature that is available to you through both service and educational institutions. Remember, the scholarly writing of today lays the groundwork for the nursing practice and research of tomorrow (Fig. 12-2). Using a variety of abstract periodicals will give you access to both the original basic-science research and other health-science literature.

Planning Ahead

Being well informed is necessary for the strategy of effective planning. All the strategies suggested here are intended to be points of departure for later professional growth and development. If you are tempted to explore such strategies more fully now, many books, like *Leadership for Change: A Guide for the Frustrated Nurse,* will be of interest (Brooten *et al,* 1978). Well-informed nurses need to learn much about leadership, change theories, economics, and politics to achieve individual and professional goals.

At this point in your career, it is probably difficult to imagine planning many years ahead. It is probably also true that few people in any field reach either their personal or professional goals unless they identify goals and plan appropriately. As Henning and Jardin suggest, taking a long-range look and deciding what you want can be the difference between surviving and winning (1978).

Know yourself. Unless you know what you want personally, it is unlikely you will get it. In order to control both your personal and professional lives, you must be active rather than reactive. Already you can ask yourself many questions. Do you anticipate working for most of your life? Most nurses who do work can expect a career of more than 30 years! Some economists suggest that within the next decade three-quarters of women will work for economic reasons alone. If you work, will you do this regardless of whatever else you do? What do you imagine yourself doing a decade from now? What must you do to reach that goal?

One reason for setting goals is to be able to identify obstacles in reaching them. With planning, it is possible to maintain a career focus even if you work part-time or anticipate time away from a career because of family or child-care responsibilities. Planning assists you to exercise freedom of choice and in that way to take control. An analogy may be made between the control we advocate for your career life and the control you encourage clients to assume for their health and self-actualization. Similarly, just as you plan short- and long-term goals for clients, it is appropriate to do the same for yourself.

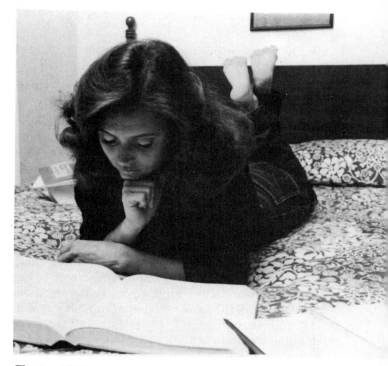

Figure 12-2
By keeping informed, nurses are able to positively influence health care. *(National Student Nurses' Association)*

Not all persons who make long-term career commitments may recognize potential conflict between being a high achiever and a successful woman. Matina Horner used the phrase "fear of success" to describe this phenomenon (1969). When external barriers to independent behavior are removed, such as when laws and policies are changed, internal barriers like fear of success and low self-esteem assume increased importance. Such unrecognized psychological barriers make some persons reluctant to plan and accept responsibility for their decisions. After all, hapless victims of circumstance are seldom held accountable for events beyond their control.

Do you share your planning and aspirations with your significant others to gain their understanding, support, and encouragement?

Participation

Being informed and planning ahead are dead-end strategies unless they are accompanied by active participation. Sometimes the person focus of nursing tempts us to judge participation by satisfaction in relationships rather than by achieved outcomes. Several questions to ask yourself about participating follow:

- Are you using your abilities and assets? to the fullest? to what end?
- Do you give positive feedback and unsolicited support to peers for accomplishment?
- Do you recognize the urgency of research participation by all nurses?

At the 1980 A.N.A. convention, Mauksch suggested that the research roles in nursing involve supporting research, being a participant or collecting data, initiating research, or being a consumer implementer. Further, she urged, any nurse [or student] can perform three of the four research functions. Research participation is needed to aid nursing's development and scientific credibility and, hence, its influence.

Experienced practitioners of nursing are always finding ways to participate as nurses beyond nursing. Increasingly, nurses are becoming appropriately visible in the media. One nurse gerontologist we know persisted until the local newspaper ran her column, "Ask Your Gerontologist." Others are taking the story of nursing's contribution to health care to radio, television, and popular magazines.

Participation involves risk-taking behavior. It implies conviction about goals and willingness to be identified with them. Sometimes participation leads to activities that fail to achieve their potential. Under these circumstances the participant accepts failure as a characteristic of the activity, not of the individual person involved. Participants come in many varieties. "Gray-shadow joiners" may be participants in name only, whereas "movers and shakers" seldom lack stimulation and a piece of whatever action happens. By definition and tradition, professionals are self-starters, initiators, and generally assertive persons.

> Living is the thing you do now or never ... which do you? (Hein, 1966)

Demonstration of Competence

Competence is both an individual strategy and a goal. The dictionary definition of **competence** is proper qualification or adequacy. Although the competence asked of you today is different than that expected of the licensed practitioner, the underlying concept is the same. Given your level of preparation and your professional intent, are your skills sufficient for the purpose? For example, how are your writing and speaking abilities? As an informed nurse person, you can begin to help others understand what nursing is trying to accomplish for health care. Nurses need to demonstrate competence in very public ways in order to change the media image of

nurses and nursing. Such change is critical to making nursing a potent force in shaping health-care policy. A major public-relations campaign is needed to advertise nursing's unique contribution to health care and also its independent functions.

Sometimes we use the term "competent" to mean taking responsibility for your own actions and making appropriate decisions. You need to feel a certain fundamental personal competence to be personally powerful and to control your own life. In this sense, personal competence is basic to the professional competence you will be learning. An extension of this competence is an ability to adapt to personal and professional stresses. Nurses need management skills to maintain the equilibrium necessary for their own adaptive living. Ideally, they also ought to be able to model the adaptive coping strategies they are advocating for their clients.

Recognition of women's competence may provoke a variety of responses. Nurse competence may challenge physician control explicitly and masculinity implicitly, since most physicians are male. Yet, it is in their everyday settings that individual nurses who have expertise and competence can anticipate making their initial and informal impact. Competent practitioners, managers, and leaders will be more effective change agents for improved health-care delivery.

Selected individual strategies for increasing self-actualization and nursing influence are summarized in Table 12-1.

Group Strategies

Informal Peer Groups

Informal peer groups are built from personal relationships. Since peer means equal, you will probably define your peer group initially to be your nursing classmates—perhaps friends in the same class studying for the same exam. As your own professional identity matures, you will come to identify other nurses and other health professionals as peers. Tomorrow your informal peer group may be an interdisciplinary team with common research interests. Hopefully such informal peer groups of practicing nurses and physicians can counteract some of the misunderstanding that occurs between health professionals under more formal circumstances.

Another type of informal peer group combines neophytes and experienced mentors. In corporations, politics, and academia such support groups are called, quite aptly, "old boy networks." They aid in climbing the corporate ladder or in moving from

---

Table 12-1
Selected Individual Strategies for Increasing
Self-Actualization and Nursing Influence

Use Information	**Plan Ahead**	**Participate**	**Be Competent**
Use person resources	Know yourself	Learn independently	Write and speak well
Gain access to professional literature through indexes and abstracts	Set goals	Interact with other health professionals	Project a professional image
	Share aspirations	Join health organizations	Assume accountability
Read widely		Mobilize support	Document practice
American Journal of Nursing		Provide curriculum input	Commit yourself to life-long learning
Nursing Outlook		Support research	Strive for excellence
Nursing 8–		Find a mentor	
Nursing Research Imprint		Fight sex discrimination	

---

junior to senior ranks. Some of the stressors that students and practitioners alike experience as "burnout" could be managed through peer support systems. Persons who understand the structure and function of informal peer groups and networks know that they are the glue that holds formal bureaucracies together. They are essential to successful functioning in hospitals and other large health-care organizations.

Formal Organizations

Formal organizations serve many important functions for professions, including providing social and moral support for individuals, setting standards, advancing and disseminating knowledge, and speaking for the profession (Merton, 1958).

Professional nursing organizations can form a significant power base. Until recently power was a foreign word to nurses. Now nurses are struggling to assert power within the health-care delivery system. Unfortunately, nursing's primary professional organization, the American Nurses' Association, has been losing rather than gaining members within recent years. At the start of the 1980s, one-fifth of professional nurses belonged to the A.N.A., whereas three-fifths of physicians belonged to the American Medical Association. At least two reasons for the drop in A.N.A. membership may not be readily apparent. First, beginning in 1968, nurses began to trade A.N.A. membership for membership in specialty-nursing organizations that were more closely associated with their clinical interests. Although these smaller groups may have met the needs of individual nurses for clinical interests, they did not meet the need of the profession for a strong central organizational voice for nursing. Second, many nurses find a conflict between the A.N.A.'s being both a collective bargaining agent and a professional organization.

Two professional organizations of special significance for students are Sigma Theta Tau, the nursing honor society, and the autonomous National Student Nurses' Association (Fig. 12-3). Another national organization that is concerned specifically with nursing is the National League for Nursing. Membership in this organization is not limited to nurses, although the organization aims to influence nursing education and practice.

Political Participation

"Nurses belong to one of the largest and most neglected groups in our voting population" (Kalisch and Kalisch, 1976, p. 29).

Most of us grew up believing in political action or decision making by majority vote. However, as children we also learned about decision making by authority. Even in the adult world, majority alone does not assure **power,** the ability to secure a particular outcome. Power among adults also comes from authority. **Authority** is recognized as an assumed right to control, whereas **influence** is the power of producing effects by less visible means.

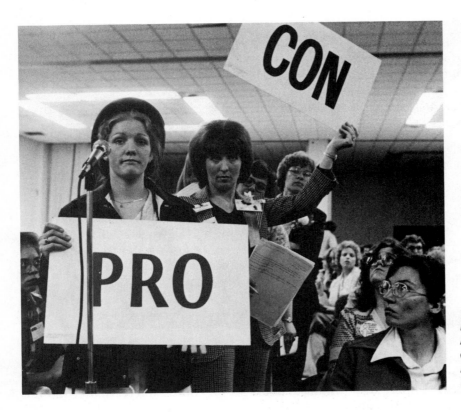

Figure 12-3
Active participation begins as a student: the National Student Nurses' Association Convention. *(National Student Nurses' Association)*

In its narrowest sense, political action means power in government. Increasingly, other kinds of political action or politics are advocated. For instance, *Sexual Politics* (Millett, 1970) and *Carl Rogers On Personal Power* are titles of recent popular books. In the latter volume, Carl Rogers describes **politics** as power and control and the extent to which persons, "desire, attempt to obtain, possess, share, or surrender power and control over others and/or for themselves" (1977, p. 4). According to the Kalisches, "Politics concerns the promotion of one's interest group and the use of whatever resources are available to protect and advance that interest" (1976, p. 30).

As a group, nurses have only recently become interested in political action. Nurses' Coalition for Action in Politics (N-CAP) is a nonprofit, nonpartisan program to improve health care through the political process. As the political-action arm of the American Nurses' Association since 1974, N-CAP has functioned to educate nurses politically, to encourage their participation in the political process, and to provide financial support and endorsements for political candidates who support issues of consequence to nursing and good health care. Nurses themselves are encouraged to run for elective office and to work for political campaigns. To date, few nurses are visible as legislators.

Many nurses have yet to learn the importance of political action as a strategy for advancing nursing and changing health-care policy. Obviously, nurses do not have to become legislators themselves to influence policy, but they must participate in local politics in some meaningful way. At the federal level, nurses have been noticeably absent from key decision-making positions related to health policy and allocation of health-care funds. Nurses' failure to participate in local and state politics has meant that federal monies shared locally seldom come to nursing. One congressman suggested that if 1000 nurses entered a national congressional office seeking support for a legislative issue, they would get results (Pursell, 1980, p. 107). His congressional district in Michigan has 4500 registered nurses. In 1979, the Carter administration attempted to nearly eliminate national funding for nursing education and research. Nurses, working with supportive congressional members, were successful in reversing this cutback attempt. One politically involved nurse's fascinating diary of this effort is presented in "It Could Happen Again" (Rinke, 1980).

Nurses do not have to wait for legislation to be introduced that relates to their issues. What nurses need to realize is that they can form bipartisan coalitions of their colleagues to draft legislation and then seek congressional sponsors. If nurses expect to influence health-care policy, they need to be informed, visible, and vocal in the local, state, and federal arenas. Political action should be seen as a group strategy that uses all the individual and group techniques presented. Hopefully, nurses are coming to a new awareness and involvement regarding political action. Nurses do not need to be the most neglected group of our voting populations.

In the keynote address to the Biennial American Nurse's Association Meeting in June, 1980, Rhetaugh Dumas proclaimed, "In a cost-conscious era, good intentions and unassuming, capable nursing work are essential, but no substitute for data, assertiveness, and political skill." Political nurse persons use power, control, and decision making. They trust themselves to say, "I think, I believe, and I accept the challenges." They are proactive persons whose mode of functioning is to create action rather than merely to react. They also recognize that there has been, within the last decade, a trend away from consumers who merely use resources to prosumers, who create resources. Just as the nurse encourages the client to assume control over his health by developing strengths, the nurse needs openly to assume control of nursing and its services. The political nurse person demonstrates by individual and group action that personal and professional power and freedom are created by nurses not given by others. As Mundinger reminds us, "Not to distinguish nursing's contribution is to lose it." (1980, p. 151).

Conclusion

This chapter focuses on the person who assumes the professional nursing role. Nursing shares common problems with other professions. These include the control of practice, educational preparation, and payment for services. In addition, these problems impinge on the issue of how nursing can influence American health-care policy. Never before have more practice options been available to professional nurses. Nurses are increasing their health assessment, illness management, and health-promotion skills. Practice is more likely to be based on knowledge rather than oriented to tasks. Increasing opportunities for independent nursing function are being identified and demonstrated. The so-called practitioner roles vary with community need and practice settings, legal constraints, and abilities of individual nurse persons. Nurses can use both individual and group strategies to increase nurse self-actualization and influence health-care policy.

Study Questions

1. Explain how the problems and issues identified in this chapter have the potential to stimulate the growth of nursing as a profession.

2. How might new practice options for nurses affect other health professionals and the health-care delivery system?

3. How does the independent functioning of nurses facilitate collegial relationships with other health professionals?

4. Describe what actions you as an individual nurse might take to improve nursing's public image.

5. Describe additional group strategies for increasing nursing's influence on health care.

Glossary

Authority: An assumed right to control someone or something.

Autonomous: Independent; self-governing.

Clinical nurse specialist: An expert in a particular practice area such as psychiatric–mental health or medical–surgical nursing.

Competence: Proper qualification; adequacy of performance.

Dependent nursing behavior: Those activities performed under delegated medical authority or supervision or according to *a priori* routines.

E. & G.W.: An abbreviation for economic and general-welfare activities of professional nursing organizations.

Expanded role: A multidimensional role change or alteration; authority for expanded nursing roles is primarily expanded nursing knowledge and clinical expertise.

Extended role: A role extended or lengthened in a unilateral manner; *e.g.*, the role of physician extended through another health worker, *i.e.*, P.A. (physicians' assistant), who is dependent on the authority of the physician.

Function: The kind of action or activity proper to a person in a certain role, *e.g.*, functions of a professional nurse.

Independent nursing behavior: Those activities initiated as a result of the nurse's own knowledge and skill rather than as a result of delegated authority from another, *e.g.*, a physician.

Influence: The power of producing effects by invisible or insensible means.

Interdependent nursing behavior: Those activities which overlap functions or activities of other health professionals; it recognizes the desirability of collegial relationships in which each profession contributes according to knowledge, skills, or focus.

Nurse anesthetist: A nurse who administers anesthetics, usually under direct or indirect supervision.

Nurse Clinician: An expert in bedside or direct care who usually has a specialized area of expertise and, possibly, advanced education.

Nurse Midwife: A registered nurse who specializes in assisting women and families to adapt to childbirth.

Nurse Practitioner: In some states, any nurse who renders service to a client; it is also used to describe nurses functioning in expanded roles, *e.g.*, pediatric nurse practitioner.

Physician's assistant (P.A.): A dependent health worker who functions as an extension of a physician and is accountable to the physician.

Politics: Power and control; promotion of an interest using whatever resources are available to protect and advance it.

Power: The ability to secure a particular outcome.

Bibliography

American Nurses Association, Commission on Nursing Education: A Case for Baccalaureate Preparation in Nursing. Kansas City, MO, American Nurses Association, 1979

American Nurses Association: Position paper. American Journal of Nursing 65, No. 12:106–111, December 1965

Bowman R: The nursing organization as a political pressure group. Nurs Forum 12, No. 1, 73–81, 1973

Brooten D, Hayman LL, Naylor MD: Leadership for Change: A Guide for the Frustrated Nurse. Philadelphia, JB Lippincott, 1978

Capuzzi C: Power and interest groups: A study of ANA and AMA. Nurs Outlook 28:478–482, August, 1980

Christy TE: Entry into practice: A recurring issue in nursing history. Am J Nurs 80:485–488, March, 1980

Diers D: A different kind of energy: Nurse-power. Am J Nurs 78:51–55, January 1978

Diers D: Research in Nursing Practice. Philadelphia, JB Lippincott, 1979

Hein P: Grooks 1. Garden City, Doubleday, 1966

Hennig M, Jardin A: The Managerial Woman. New York, Pocket Books, 1978

Horner MS: Fail: Bright women. Psychology Today 3:36, 1969

Kalisch BJ, Kalisch PA: A discourse on the politics of nursing. J Nurs Adm 6:29–34, March–April, 1976

Kelly LY: Dimensions of Professional Nursing, 3rd ed. New York, Macmillan, 1975

Kelly LY: Endpaper: Nurses of the third wave. Nurs Outlook 28:330, May, 1980

Lindberg JB: Relationship Between Baccalaureate Nursing Students' Self-Esteem and Independent Behavior in Nursing. Ph.D. Dissertation, University of Michigan, 1979

Lysaught J: Action in affirmation: Toward an unambiguous profession of nursing. Paper presented at American Nurses' Association Biennial Convention, Houston, Texas, June 1980

Masson V: On power and vision in nursing. Nurs Outlook 27:782–784, December, 1979

Mauksch I: Nursing Practice and Education for the 80's. Paper presented at American Nurses Association Biennial Convention, Houston, Texas, June, 1980

Merton R: The functions of the professional association. Am J Nurs 1:50–54, 1958

Millet K: Sexual Politics. Garden City, Doubleday, 1970

Mullane MK: Nursing care and the political arena. Nurs Outlook 23:699–701, November, 1975

Mundinger M: Autonomy in Nursing. Germantown, MD, Aspen Systems, 1980

Pursell C: Congressman urges greater nursing role in health policy formulation. Nursing and Health Care 2:107, 1980

Reiter F: The nurse clinician. Am J Nurs 2:274–280, 1966

Rinke LT: It could happen again. Nursing Outlook 7:449–451, 1980

Rogers CR: Carl Rogers on Personal Power. New York, Dell, 1977

Satir V: Making Contact. Millbrae, CA, Celestial Arts, 1976

Stein R: The emerging graduate. In Chaska N (ed): The Nursing Profession: Views Through the Mist, pp 21–34. New York, McGraw-Hill, 1978

Styles MM: Dialogue Across the Decades. Am J Nurs 78:28–32, January, 1978

Toffler A: Future Shock. New York, Random House, 1970

Communication

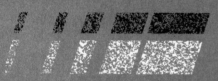

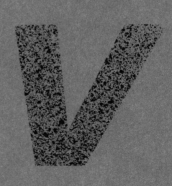

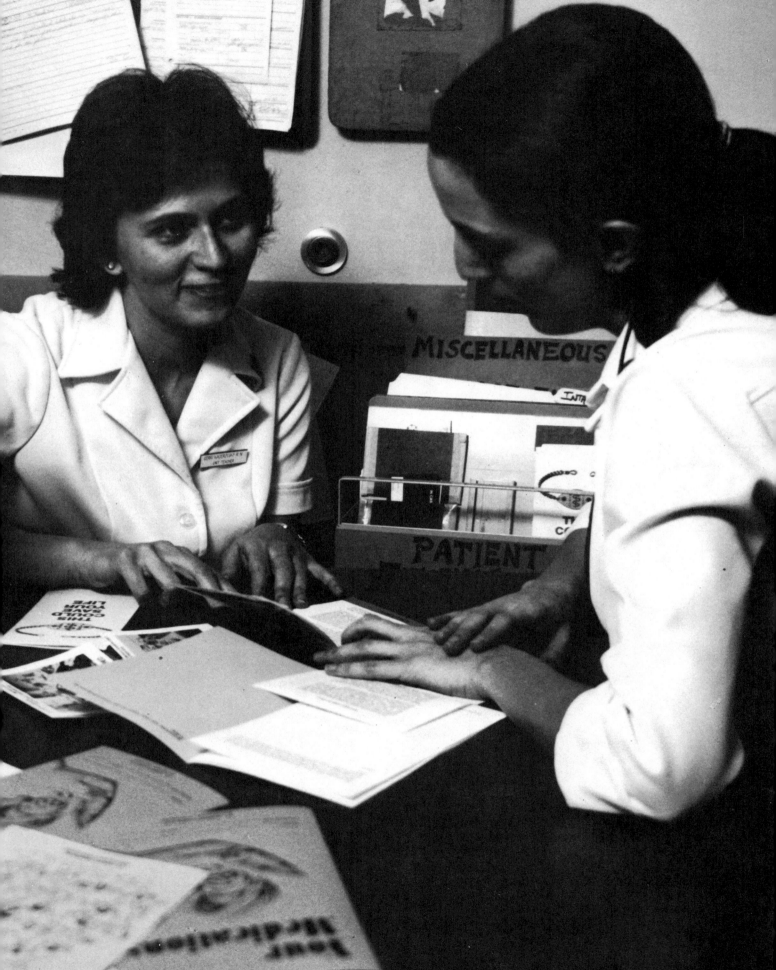

V

Communication

This section presents the concept of communication as an essential component of person-centered nursing practice. In previous sections we have discussed the person and his adaptations, health-care delivery, and professionalism. Communication is related to each of these concepts. Because nursing is an interpersonal process, effective communication is one of our most powerful tools for assisting persons to adapt to life changes. We use professional communication to share our knowledge with fellow nurses or other health-team members. And we use communication within the context of health-care delivery when we educate clients to be informed consumers or when we act as client advocates. This section presents communication in all of these contexts. Let us begin to explore this most important interpersonal skill: effective communication.

Interpersonal Communication in Nursing

Sharon Hein Jette

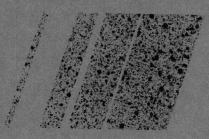

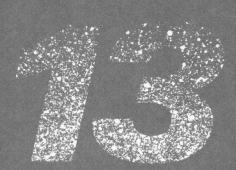

After completing this chapter, students will be able to:

●

Explain the importance of effective communications to good nursing care.

●

Contrast helping relationships with social relationships.

●

Explain the four roles of the nurse in a helping relationship.

●

Describe the phases of a helping relationship.

●

Describe the internal and external variables affecting communication.

●

Analyze verbal and nonverbal communication.

●

Describe the components of empathy.

●

Identify effective and ineffective communication techniques.

●

Distinguish assertive from passive and aggressive communication behaviors.

Locked in each person is a wealth of unique experiences and strengths, feelings and values. Effective communication is the master key that unlocks such human resources, enabling a nurse to understand, to care, and to help another person. The person, in turn, learns that the nurse does understand, does care, and will assist him. Such resonance between two persons, in this case between nurse and client, underlies a helping relationship and a most rewarding profession.

Human communication may appear to be the transfer of messages between persons; in reality, however, it is a complex process of the exchange of meanings between persons. When two persons exchange messages and derive a mutual understanding of their meaning effective communication occurs. One goal of any helping person, then, becomes rather straightforward—to exchange effective (mutually understood) communications. There is only one complication: humans cannot exchange meanings directly; instead, we must transmit messages in the form of behaviors—words or actions—and rely upon the human mind to decipher their meaning.

In nursing we must communicate effectively or risk the harm, the neglect, or even the life of clients whom we assist. But how does a nurse reach out and touch someone in distress, someone very different from herself, such as a frightened child recovering from surgery or a bereaved widow confined to a nursing home? Persons of all ages and backgrounds need nurses who can reach them, who can get through to them on a personal, individual level. Nursing demands creative, effective communication. Without it, we merely "go through the motions" of caring.

Fortunately, each nurse possessing a genuine desire to help can learn effective communication concepts applicable in nearly all situations. Communication skills and certain concepts of caring, of helping relationships, and of the communication process apply to all client interactions. By mastering such positive communication skills, the nurse demonstrates basic abilities to understand, to care, and to help.

Before continuing further in this chapter, reflect upon yourself as a communicator:

- Am I willing to admit that I must improve my communication skills to help others?

- Am I willing to unlearn old ways of dealing with people in order to learn more effective ways?

- Am I ready to try to understand another person's distress from his viewpoint?

- Am I able to support a distressed person and guide him toward health?

- Am I able to seek the support I need from others in order to help people?

If you answered yes to these questions, continue to read how to be an effective communicator, an effective helper, and an effective nurse.

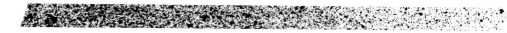

Nurse–Client Interactions as Helping Relationships

Most nurse–client interactions occur within the context of helping relationships, in which a nurse "has the intent of promoting the growth, development, maturity, improved functioning, improved coping with life" of the client (Rogers, 1961, pp. 39–40). In a traditional helping relationship, a client would identify a health problem or illness and seek help from a doctor; the doctor might then order nursing services to assist the client. Today, more clients are seeking nursing care directly in times of crisis. Nurses, too, are offering services more directly to prevent a problem or illness and to maintain the health of the client, the family, and the community. Thus helping relationships may be client-initiated or nurse-initiated. All helping relationships, however, have the same intent and share certain common characteristics (Table 13-1).

Characteristics of Helping Relationships

Carl Rogers's characteristics of a helping relationship were presented earlier in the text. Genuineness and acceptance of the other person are essential qualities for those who wish to help persons become healthier in mind and body. In exploring what it means to help another human being, counselor and behavioral-science researcher Laurence Brammer describes most distressed people as deprived, ignored, isolated, or deficient in knowledge or skill, rather than as diseased or ill (1979). This fact often surprises nurses who enter the field to work with "sick" people and subsequently learn the enormous needs of all deprived peoples for nursing services. Brammer outlines the characteristics of an effective helper as follows (p. 16).

- *Awareness of self and values*—The nurse needs to be able to answer Who am I? What do I believe? What is important to me? in order to help another person answer those questions. A certain level of insight precedes the use of a most important tool in nursing, the "use of self" as a caregiver.

- *Ability to analyze own feelings*—Nurses as helpers gradually learn to recognize and cope with their own feelings of joy and grief, power and anger, accomplishment and frustration.

- *Ability to serve as a model*—In order to show another person the route to health, a nurse necessarily maintains a certain level of health— in mind, body, spirit, and life-style.

Table 13-1
Characteristics of a Helping Relationship

- Awareness of self and values
- Ability to analyze own feelings
- Ability to serve as a model
- Altruism
- Strong sense of ethics
- Responsibility

- *Altruism*—Nurses characteristically convey a sense of altruism, that is, they receive self-satisfaction from helping people in a humanistic way.
- *Strong Sense of Ethics*—We strive to make the best possible judgments based on high principles of human welfare.
- *Responsibility*—Two dimensions of responsibility are inherent in nursing: taking responsibility for your own actions and sharing responsibility with others.

Professional versus Social Relationships

A successful helping relationship between nurse and client represents a different order of interaction than that which occurs in a friendship. This is not because of any superiority in the nurse but because of the mutual trust and the responsibilities for assisting others that characterize professional relationships. Although many elements of a professional relationship are warm, friendly, and social in nature, there is an underlying purpose in helping relationships that is beyond mutual enjoyment. Table 13-2 outlines the essential similarities and differences in the two types of interactions.

Many nurses are convinced that clients must like them and that a successful relationship is a friendly one. This attitude, while popular, is neither possible nor advisable in many helping relationships. Effken gives one example in which staff nurses were too affectionate to risk hurting or disappointing a client; it is equally ineffective to stereotype the client before knowing his unique values (1975).

Helping Roles

The nurse helps the client by acting in one or a combination of the following roles:

- Direct administration of physical care
- Advocacy on behalf of clients
- Psychosocial support
- Health education and counseling

Direct Administration of Physical Care. This is the traditional and time-honored role of the nurse. In the 1970s, this helping role evolved from one of performing service for others to one of assisting others to regain or retain the ability to care for themselves. The latter is the concept called self-care, which was described in Chapter 4.

Nurses provide direct assistance for those clients who are temporarily or permanently unable to care for themselves, but we encourage the majority of relatively healthy persons to retain responsibility for their own health care. Remember, helping means that control remains with the client; it does not mean taking over for the client to meet the nurse's need to feel needed. Contrast the following offers:

Nurse A: "Here, let me get that towel for you, Mr. N."

Nurse B: "I'll leave your towel within reach so you can get it when you need it, Mr. N."

Advocacy on Behalf of Client. The growing complexity of and rapid changes in the health-care delivery system make the client's search for satisfactory answers and solutions more difficult. Nurses perform an invaluable service by searching out the available solutions on behalf of the client as a consumer. In this way, the client can make informed decisions in meeting his own needs.

There are two levels of advocacy:

- The advocate seeks a solution on behalf of the client. "I found out about your medication for you. The pharmacist told me. . . ."
- The advocate relays to a client how to seek his own solutions. "I'll help you decide what to ask the pharmacist when you call him, Ms. S."

Psychosocial Support. The often-abused phrase "psychosocial support" includes a variety of methods by which the nurse sustains the emotions, the morale, the culture, and the spirituality of a client. Communication skills of empathy and assertiveness described later in this chapter are essential to this kind of support.

As nurses, most of us learn to react to the stress behavior of our clients; when someone shows signs of distress, we act to comfort and support them.

Nurse A: "Mrs. P. was so angry after her brother's visit, I had better go see if I can support her."

It is more effective, state Hein and Leavitt, to anticipate the need for support and equip the person to deal with it in advance (1977).

Nurse B: "Mrs. P. is likely to be very upset when she sees her brother. I had better help her prepare for his visit."

In such situations, skills of problem solving and anticipatory crisis intervention provide the client with basic psychosocial support. They prepare him by describing what to expect in a stressful situation

Table 13-2
A Comparison of Social Relationships and Professional Helping Relationships

	Social Relationships	Professional Helping Relationships
Impetus	Mutual need satisfaction and experiential sharing	Client need or concern
Goal orientation	Usually no definite goals	Always goal oriented and purposeful
Commitment	No stated responsibility to continue the relationship if problems occur	Responsibility to problem solve difficulties encountered
Acceptance	No expectations made of accepting the other person; acceptance qualified	Helper accepts the clients as he is; unqualified acceptance
Judgment	Value-based judgments are made to determine compatibility	Value-based judgments may occur, but mutual awareness and sharing of such perception is essential
Assistance	Voluntary assistance may be offered or refused	Obligation to provide assistance or resources for client to assist himself
Trust	Develops voluntarily, dependent on shared experiences and values	Helper obliged to build mutual trust
Confidentiality	No explicit obligation, although the degree of intimacy determines confidentiality	Helper operates under ethical duty of confidentiality to divulge knowledge only to responsible parties with client consent
Limits of interaction	Flexible to meet needs, interests, and convenience	Defined in advance, renegotiated to meet client needs or helper availability
Mutual understanding	Voluntarily sharing understanding	Obligation to use effective communication to understand client needs

Adapted and expanded from Gold HG: Therapeutic relationships—Social relationships. Unpublished manuscript, University of Michigan School of Nursing, 1973

and by providing sufficient information for him to make informed decisions and maintain self-esteem and self-control.

Health Education and Counseling. The effective nurse motivates a client to learn, grow, and change his health behavior as needed. The nurse's role as a health educator and counselor depends upon the ability to facilitate—not dictate—another person's growth. We teach our clients as if to say, "Here is the information you need. Make your own decision whether to use it or not. I will support you to cope with the consequences of your decision, positive or negative." This basic approach to teaching adults

can be altered somewhat when dealing with more dependent or unstable clients. The teaching–learning process is described later in the text as a specific example of the nurse's caregiving.

At any given time, a practicing nurse is likely to be enacting several of the above roles simultaneously. Teaching a new mother about infant care involves constant psychosocial support of her mothering abilities, as well as health education and counseling. Care of a dying person may include advocacy of death with dignity, along with physical care and psychosocial comfort to the dying person and his family. The four helping roles of the nurse overlap constantly in caring for, and caring about, people.

Developing Nurse–Client Relationships

Helping relationships as dynamic interpersonal processes do not automatically exist; they grow much the same way a garden grows. Careful preparation of growth conditions are a necessary first step. The progressive caring, feeding, and supportive direction given in a growth phase help any plant and any relationship to be self-sufficient and productive. Skillful nurses, like skillful gardeners, redirect disabled life back toward health, being ever careful not to neglect, oversupply, or destroy it in the process. Both gardeners and nurses eventually enjoy the satisfactions of a harvest, the closing of one growth cycle and the beginning of another. Throughout, there remains a mystical quality in the growth of a plant, the growth of a person, and the growth of a helping relationship.

Three Phases of Growth in Nurse–Client Relationships

In a growth process, helping relationships are divided into three phases:

- Opening (or initial)
- Working (or developmental)
- Closing (or terminating)

Introduction and preparation of the personal growth conditions take place in the opening phase. The working phase of a relationship fosters growth and change, problem solving, and decision making. The closing of a successful relationship can be considered a harvest of mutual satisfaction between nurse and client. These phases are not to be thought of as a rigid progression spaced equally throughout the interaction, as in Figure 13-1. Instead, imagine that these are flexible phases with overlap, each of variable length, as in Figure 13-2. When linked, the three phases form a chain of interactions, ending at a level higher than begun.

Trust

Growth in the interpersonal process is dependent on the development of mutual trust. Trust evolves when one person risks his own self-esteem, seeks supports from another, and finds it (Fig. 13-3). The helper fosters trust, not dependence, by making and keeping commitments, sharing responsibilities with the client, and ensuring confidentiality. "We cannot morally encourage disclosure about values, attitudes, and behavior unless we are certain that we can guarantee confidentiality" (Benjamin, 1976, p. 54).

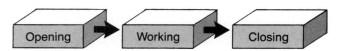

Figure 13-1

The phases of a helping relationship are not a rigid progression.

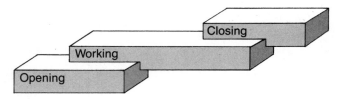

Figure 13-2

The phases of a helping relationship form a chain of interactions.

Few qualities of the helping professional are as essential as *confidentiality*. Imagine the damage to a growing trust relationship should a client discover that a nurse has inappropriately spread personal communications. Martin refers to the "duty of confidentiality" as a moral obligation binding the professional nurse (1978, p. 503). It is unlawful, unethical, and in many cases a breach of contract with the employment agency to break confidence. Sharing information that is vital to the health and safety of the client with other responsible caretakers is essential; however, the client has the right to be informed of a nurse's need to share vital information with others. Note-taking and other types of recording should never be the focus of an interaction, as in, "Hold it, I didn't get all that down." Secretive note-taking destroys trust. Ask the client's permission to take notes and share them with him. This acknowledges his control over the information.

Trust flows through a successful helping relationship. In the opening phase of the relationship, the underlying goal of both persons is to adapt to each other and establish trust. Throughout the working phase, both nurse and client strive to maintain trust during stressful decision-making and problem-solving encounters. The closing phase requires both to redirect trust, often by referral to another caregiver or by agreement that the client is self-sufficient again.

Guidelines for Successful Helping Relationships

Opening Phase

During the opening phase of a successful professional relationship, both nurse and client prepare to work together by establishing a contract, so to speak.

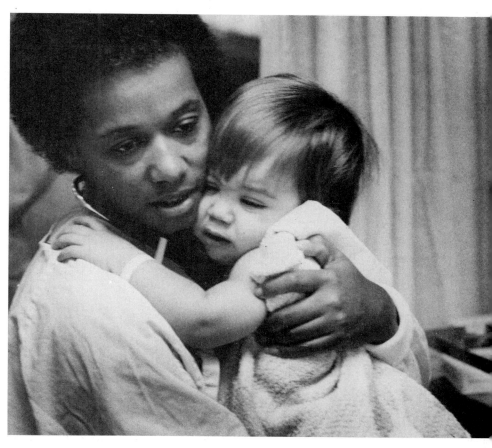

Figure 13-3
Trust evolves when one seeks support from another and finds it. *(Photo by Bob Kalmbach; University of Michigan Information Services)*

Whether formal or informal, this explicit agreement states the terms of the interaction, beginning with mutual introductions that clearly identify full name, preferred name (if different), and position.

Nurse: "Mrs. M., glad to see you again. I'm Susan J., the student nurse from Culler College. We met in the Diabetes Clinic last week. . . ." (pause for acknowledgement)

Client: "Oh yes, you wanted to visit me at home. . . ."

Sharing this information only in part or in haste leads to confusion at the very onset of the interaction. Giving a full and genuine introduction can prevent many misunderstandings and instill confidence between nurse and client.

The next step is mutual agreement on the purpose of the interaction. This step begins to make the interaction goal-oriented and purposeful, characteristic of the helping relationship.

Nurse: "I'm your primary nurse, the one who's responsible for helping you recover while you're here. I was hoping to spend about half an hour talking with you about your condition."

After stating the purpose, setting limits on the time and duration of interaction prevents later misunderstandings, such as this:

Client: "You won't be calling any more? But I thought you were going to be with me every Tuesday."

Setting time limits in advance allows the client to know when the nurse will, and will *not*, be available.

Nurse: "In an hour I'll be off for the day . . . is there any way I can assist you before I go?"

Early in a helping relationship, it is essential to make provisions for unexpected changes in the parameters of time and location.

Nurse: "If either of us wants to cancel or change a meeting, how shall we arrange it?"

In opening a helping relationship, the use of contracts, as suggested, will help the client (and nurse) adapt to a new relationship and to changes in the relationship.

One characteristic of the opening phase of many relationships is testing behavior, a common prelude to trust. Both persons establish a sense of security in the relationship by testing the limits set by the other; in its most extreme form, this behavior can be manipulative but usually is an adaptive behavior to see if the other person means what he says. The hospitalized client may express insecurity by calling the nurse repeatedly, thereby testing her patience and reliability. Clients of ethnic backgrounds that are different from the nurse's will test her willingness to understand them, sometimes with queries of, "How can you know what it's like?" The nurse who replies, "I know just how you feel," fails the test. Testing behavior is a direct indication of the amount of security and trust in a relationship; as interpersonal trust grows, testing behavior subsides. A clear indication of movement into the working phase of a relationship is the cessation of testing behavior.

Working Phase

At the point of completing a contract with the client, the nurse moves the interaction into the working phase by beginning the helping process. The working

Figure 13-4
During the working phase the nurse gives help that centers on the client's needs. *(Photo by Bob Kalmbach; University of Michigan Information Services)*

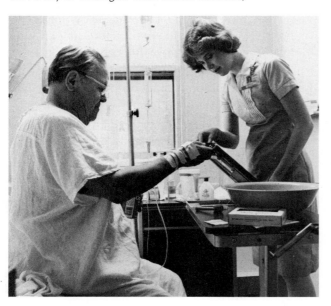

phase is the part of the relationship in which helping and growth occur, whether the nurse gives direct care, counseling and teaching, or psychosocial support. The care given centers on the client's needs and problems (Fig. 13-4). Therefore one of the most useful tools of the working phase is **problem solving,** the systematic process of identifying, clarifying, and resolving troublesome situations. Abdellah recognized the need for nures to use a basic structure of solving difficult clinical problems, regardless of the type of setting (1960). This process is rooted in the scientific method.

Problem solving, although widely adaptable to all nursing situations, must be enacted in the proper sequence of steps in order to be most effective (Johnson, 1970, p. 3)

*   Step 1—Recognize a troublesome situation and assess its characteristics.
*   Step 2—Identify the exact nature of the problem.
*   Step 3—Decide on a plan of action.
*   Step 4—Carry out the planned action.
*   Step 5—Evaluate the plan, the outcomes, and the new situation.

This process becomes circular when, upon reaching step 5, a new situation is uncovered, which demands that the problem solver return to step 1 to begin anew.

*   Step 1—Troublesome situation: after switching on a lamp, you remain in the dark.
*   Step 2—Identify the problem: the cord might be unplugged. Yes, it is.
*   Step 3—Plan of action: plug it in to see what happens.
*   Step 4—Act: plug it in.
*   Step 5—Evaluate: It is still dark. After another flip of the switch, it is still dark. . . . Now what? Is the bulb or the fuse blown? *Return to step 1.*

At times, identifying the exact nature of the problem can be difficult and time consuming, requiring that the problem solver turn the problem around to view it differently or emphasize another part of the complex problem. In working with a difficult family situation, for example, a nurse may begin to question whether the sick member of the family is really the source of the problem, or whether other members of the family, the community, or the environment are really the cause.

It is imperative, however, that the nurse not become so involved in problem hunting that she interrogates or otherwise forces clients, "Tell me your problem!" Many troubled persons do not recognize their concerns or problems, cannot verbalize them, or do not trust enough to share them (Geach, 1974).

As nurses adopt the concepts of self-care (*i.e.*, helping others to help themselves), we recognize that helping the client to solve his own problems, whenever possible, is preferable to problem solving for him. Therefore the following process of helping the client solve problems is recommended:

1 Explore what concerns he has about his past, present, or future health situation.

2 Use client-centered communication to identify the exact nature of the problem from his perspective.

3 Explore with the client what he has already tried to do to resolve the problem.

4 Explore what the client sees as possible alternative approaches to the problem now.

5 Explore what the client sees as positive and negative consequences of each alternative he proposes.

6 Explore what the client sees as barriers preventing him from taking action.

7 If the client is not able to suggest any approaches to his problems, the nurse now may suggest new approaches.

8 Explore the consequences and barriers he sees inherent in your suggested approaches.

9 If several approaches are suggested, help the client to decide which would be most appropriate for him to try first.

10 If the client indicates readiness to take action on his problems, provide him with the information, materials, and support he needs to begin. If he hesitates or shows unreadiness, return to step 6 to explore the barriers.

11 After the client tries a new approach, schedule contact with him to learn the outcome and to reinforce any progress. If new problems arise, begin again with step 1 to explore the concerns. If negative consequences occur, help him to deal with them as constructively as possible.*

This client-centered process of assisting the client to solve his own problems encourages self-esteem and independence in the client; this approach can be adapted to many nursing situations,

*Webb E: Helping the Client to Problem Solve. Unpublished Manuscript. Wayne State University College of Nursing, Detroit, 1976

even when the client is very ill or debilitated, allowing him to control decisions about his own health. At times, progress may be slow, especially in long-term relationships. Testing behavior may recur as a signal of frustration, unmet needs, or wavering trust.

☐ After a week's vacation, the nurse resumed visiting an older man in a retirement center, who pinched her and winked, "I needed you last week." She replied, holding his wandering hand, "I missed you, too." ☐

Closing Phase

Closing gestures are very likely to determine the client's perception of the entire interaction and, thus, his willingness to enter future helping relationships. Successful closing is planned in advance in order to allow time for adapting to the loss. It attaches value to the preceding interaction. The challenge is to focus on the client's achievement, rather than, "Look what I, the nurse, did for you!"

Nurse: "I've been working with you for 4 weeks now, and in that time you've gained enormous confidence in your ability to live alone. And you've taught me to slow down and listen to people like you who are hearing impaired. Thank you for that.

Interactions of longer duration often end in small celebrations or giftgiving. Gordy points out the necessity of examining the meaning of the gift when deciding to accept it (1978). Gifts may represent gratitude, guilt, or manipulation.

Mr. T. verbally expressed his thanks to the visiting nurse and offered her a new fountain pen, with his company inscription on it, saying, "You can never find a pen when you come. Here's one to remember me by."

S. K. offered the night nurse some of the candy at her bedside, saying "I don't need the calories. Besides, you've been so good to me ... I'd like to ask a favor. If you could visit me at my home, I'll fix a big dinner for us both. ..."

The nurse chose to accept Mr. T.'s gift; in contrast, she chose to decline the candy and to help S. K. find another solution to the underlying loneliness at home.

Testing behavior during closing is a common manifestation of separation anxiety, an insecure feeling of loss occurring at the end of meaningful relationships. Clients may withdraw as if to say, "I'll end this relationship before you leave me," as a protective, adaptive reaction to the loss. A realization

Table 13-3
Guidelines for Successful Helping Relationship

Opening Phase

- Establish understanding by stating the terms of the inter-action, beginning with mutual introductions.
- Agree on the purpose of the interaction.
- Set limits on time and duration of the interaction and make provisions for unexpected changes in the parame-ters of time and location.
- Establish a sense of security by meeting any limits set.

Working Phase

- Help identify, clarify, and resolve troublesome situations.
- Do not force client to "tell me your problem."
- Explore what concerns the client has about his past, pres-ent, or future health situation.
- Use client-centered communication to identify the exact nature of the problem from his perspective.
- Explore with the client what he has already tried to do to resolve the problem.
- Explore what the client sees as possible alternative ap-proaches to the problem now.
- Explore what the client sees as positive and negative consequences of each alternative he proposes.
- Explore what the client sees as barriers preventing him from taking action.
- If the client is not able to suggest any approaches to his problems, the nurse now may suggest new approaches.
- Explore the consequences and barriers he sees inherent in your suggested approaches.
- If several approaches are suggested, help the client to decide which would be most appropriate for him to try first.
- If the client indicates readiness to take action on his prob-lems, provide him with information, materials, and sup-port he needs to begin. If he hesitates or shows unreadi-ness, explore the barriers again.
- After the client tries a new approach, schedule contact with him to learn the outcome and to reinforce any prog-ress. If new problems arise, begin again to explore the concerns. If negative consequences occur, help him to deal with them as constructively as possible.

Closing Phase

- Plan for the closing in advance to allow time for adapting to any sense of loss that may result from the relation-ship's ending.
- Focus on the client's achievement.
- If client offers a gift, consider if it represents gratitude, guilt, or manipulation.
- Anticipate possible return of testing behavior or manifes-tation of grief or loss reaction due to the end of the relationship.

of waning interaction time often prompts clients (and helpers) to intensify the relationship near the end. Signs of grieving and loss reaction (outlined in Chap. 29) appear.

Just as the opening and each working step is planned, the closing is anticipated, planned, and enjoyed as the fruit of a successful relationship (Table 13-3).

Interpersonal Communication Process

Elements of a Human Communication Process

The interdisciplinary study of human communication combines the fields of biophysics, physiology, psychology, sociology, anthropology, and ecology. Indeed, these sciences form the basis of nursing study so that the educated nurse may use all of them to communicate effectively with clients as persons.

Communication has been described as a process, a continuous circular flow of energy. Most models of the communication process contain the following elements: source (also known as stimulus), message, transmitter, and receiver (also known as response). David Berlo described the human factors of sociocultural influence, environment, communication abilities, attitudes, and knowledge that modify the process (1960). Later communication scientists have added the element of **feedback** to complete a circular pathway of communication (Fig. 13-5). When a message proceeds in one direction from the source to the receiver, it is termed a **one-way communication.** A one-way communication neither expects nor encourages a response from the passive receiver. When the flow of a communication process includes a feedback loop, it is termed **two-way communication.** The receiver is expected and encouraged to participate actively in the exchange. A traditional lecture, for example, is one-way; the question–answer period afterwards is an attempt to establish a two-way dialogue. Effective nursing interactions are two-way communications involving both client and nurse as active participants.

Mass, Intrapersonal, and Interpersonal Communication

The field of human communication may be divided into three components: mass communication, intrapersonal communication, and interpersonal communication. Although each is a complex process, the three vary in scope.

Mass communication is the transmission of messages to a large audience of receivers. The modern media communicate information efficiently to the largest possible groups of receivers. For example, nursing literature attempts to reach the largest group of nurses possible. Because media messages are one-way communications on a large scale, they are rarely personal or confidential. This limitation of mass communication renders it less useful in helping relationships than intra- and interpersonal methods. One exception is the adaptation media for health education.

Intrapersonal communication, in contrast, occurs largely within the single individual when the mind or the body interprets messages for the person. The sensation of hunger, for example, is a physiological feedback mechanism that communicates needs to the person. The sight or smell of food percipitates the intrapersonal process of hunger sensation. Intrapersonal communication represents the unique interpretation of stimuli by each individual.

Interpersonal communication is the exchange of messages between two (or a small group of) persons. Effective interpersonal communication requires, in addition, the understanding of the meaning in such messages. The foundation of effective nursing lies in effective interpersonal communication.

Interpersonal communication is both a science and an art. As a science, it requires disciplined study of concepts and practice of technique to gain certain skill. As an art, it requires the fusion of the nurses's self with creativity, insight, and practice in order to achieve style. The distillation of art and science into a personal style of interaction is neither automatic nor innate. Study and practice are required to develop one's own skill and interpersonal style.

Figure 13-5
The Communication Process.

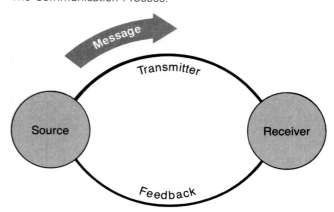

Interpersonal Process Applied to Nursing

In order to envision better the complexity of the interpersonal process, nursing-communication scientist Margaret Pluckhan has developed a concept of "intra–interpersonal" communication (1978). Since both source and receiver are biopsychosocial persons, not machines, each one's unique intrapersonal dynamics must be an integral part of any interpersonal model.

Each person processes a message stimulus by choosing whether to attend to it, by deciphering its meaning, and by choosing whether to respond. If a message fits the context of a person's experience, it is congruent and likely to provoke response. An incongruent message signals a misunderstanding.

When two persons interact, Pluckhan believes that the model of communication shown in Figure 13-6 depicts the process of exchange. This model is helpful in grasping the complex interaction within and between persons, as well as the range of internal and external variables that modify the nurse–client interaction.

Variables Affecting Communication

Internal Variables: Biophysical, Psychological, and Sociocultural

Within each individual, certain forces facilitate, while others disrupt, the ability to communicate effectively. The level of consciousness affects verbal expression; the unconscious person must communicate his needs by body language and depends upon a caregiver to interpret the needs correctly. Other biophysical variables hindering communication are sensory losses such as hearing and visual impairment, motor impairments, and any biochemical imbalance that causes confusion, especially drug intoxication. In contrast, a biophysical variable that aids communication is

Figure 13-6
Interpersonal communication model. *(Pluckhan ML: Human Communication, The Matrix of Nursing. New York, McGraw-Hill, 1978)*

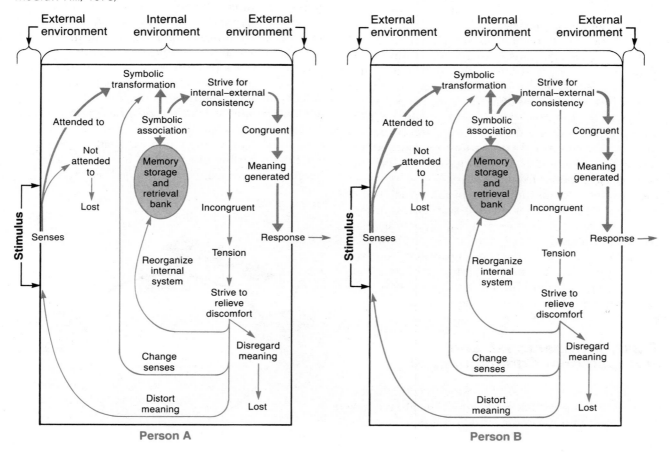

muscular coordination, which develops with the growing child into more and more effective speech and motor expression. Humans of all ages, however, can learn to overcome physical barriers to communication.

Selective inattention exemplifies a psychological variable affecting communication; with whatever conscious or unconscious motivation, a person simply chooses not to hear the message. Anxiety also affects the ability to communicate.

The entire realm of perception, the interpretation of stimuli, influences communication. Each human mind learns to perceive stimuli in certain patterns, influenced by personal values and attitudes. A typical example relates to age-perception; the adolescent calls anyone over 30 middle-aged and anyone over 50 old. The 60-year-old perceives himself as middle-aged, referring kindly to the old man of 80 down the street. Thus our perceptions are molded by our psychosocial experiences in life.

Sociocultural variables in communication present both obvious and hidden forces. Spoken communication obviously succeeds better if both persons speak in the same language; differing dialects and subcultural word connotations may prove to be hidden disruptors of understanding. Also hidden are individual values, which can block one's ability to understand the other's message. If a nurse values a stoic response to pain, for example, she may not even be able to listen to the whimpering complaints of a client after surgery or be aware of the reason for her feelings.

External Variables: Environment

All interpersonal communication occurs within the context of the surrounding environment. Anyone who has tried to concentrate on a lecture while sitting in an uncomfortable chair amidst construction noise knows how the environment can hinder communication.

Nurses can effectively structure the environment for optimal communication. This is another example of providing a supportive environment, as described earlier in the chapter. Rather than memorizing rules of environmental structure, such as furniture arrangement, the nurse develops a finer sense of assessment by using empathy in evaluating the physical environment:

> "If I were frightened or embarrassed in coming to this agency, how would I respond if interviewed in the waiting room? behind a curtain? in a private room?"

Application of Maslow's hierarchy of needs to interpersonal relations would suggest that the individual might not be ready to communicate highest-level concerns without some provision of environmental comfort and security. Before beginning interactions (especially lengthy ones) with a client, the nurse assesses his comfort level and security feeling. This can be done by using questions or observation. Physical comfort is augmented by such measures as body positioning, supplying drink or food, supplying pain medication, rearranging furniture, and controlling room temperature and ventilation.

Security, in this case a feeling of psychological comfort, results from specific relaxation techniques, respect for territoriality, and provision of privacy. The crucial element of confidentiality in interpersonal relations depends directly on the provision of as much privacy as possible. In addition, a private atmosphere lessens distractions to both nurse and client and diminishes interruptions that may connote disinterest.

What could you provide or adapt to increase comfort and security in the client's environment? Nurses have recently begun to address environmental alterations creatively, placing posters on ceilings above examination tables and replacing cubicle curtains with more solid and secure partitions. Minimizing distractions and securities can maximize chances of effective interactions.

Types of Communication Language

Humans communicate meaning to each other through the use of **language:** patterns of behavior designed to influence others. These patterns of behavior are learned responses and are culturally determined. Communication scientists have distinguished two types of communication behavior: verbal language, which conveys meanings through words, and nonverbal language, in which means other than words are used. For the purpose of study, we will first consider each of these languages separately, then, in order to view man as a holistic being, we will examine how persons combine verbal and nonverbal languages.

The nurse must first comprehend the verbal and nonverbal components of a client's message in order to analyze the combined meaning of both. Likewise, the client will seek to understand the nurse's meaning by examining verbal and nonverbal language.

Verbal Language

Consider the dollar bill. A rectangular piece of crinkled paper, it has very little significance until someone assigns meaning to it. In this case, the U.S. Treasury has assigned a value of 100 cents to it; other countries value the dollar differently in comparison to their own currency standards. A dollar bill is a symbol of some worth, a symbol exchanged to meet the needs of individuals.

In a similar way, a word possesses very little significance until assigned a meaning within a cultural or subcultural group. A word is a symbol of meaning that a person exchanges to meet his needs. Use of verbal language, then, is a symbolization process in which words are chosen as representative of an intended meaning. Commonly, the terms verbal and oral are used interchangeably (and inaccurately), because verbal language is the larger concept encompassing all use of words—oral (spoken) and written.

Oral communication serves as the most common vehicle of deliberate interchange among persons. As such, the spoken word is subject to many misunderstandings. Nurses should remember this in their oral communications with clients.

Written communications are of a higher order, being more formal and permanent than oral communications are. Although nurses orally transmit much information about client care, professional and legal responsibility for providing excellent care requires documentation in written form. The need for nurses to develop effective writing skills is crucial. Written care plans not only transmit important client information to other health-care team members, but they are also legal documents. Nursing publications convey creative and innovative nursing to even wider circles of practitioners and students.

Subcultural word differences may be subtle but significant. A person who believes he understands the language of another may discover that words, although identical in sound, differ in their meaning from one subculture to another. The word "bust" for example, is pronounced the same but quite likely interpreted differently by a sculptor, a fashion designer, and a drug addict. Words, then, are deciphered in context. Indeed, man searches for the meaning of words in the context of sentences or conversations; taking words or phrases out of context typically leads to misunderstanding.

The health professions, as a subculture, have created a language that changes the context of many common words. The use of such professional jargon increases the chance of misinterpretation between client and professionals. Consider this example, "You should void 2 hours post-op, and you're NPO after midnight." The nurse has knowledge of technical terms that may be unfamiliar to the client. The challenge is to establish a common language level by deciphering the technical words for the client and educating him about their meaning.

The meaning of words has two dimensions: **denotation** and **connotation.** Denotation, a standardized meaning, is derived from a cultural consensus on the usage of the term. In contrast, subcultural usage of a word determines its connotation or implies a judgment of its attributes. The noun "nurse," for example, denotes a person giving care to another in need; various connotations of the word include "handmaiden," "professional," and "manager."

Nonverbal Language

Symbols and actions other than words make up nonverbal language. Numerous studies have shown that nonverbal behavior expresses intended meaning, especially feelings, more accurately than does verbal behavior (Galloway, 1971). Yet we often ignore our clients' nonverbal expressions. Nonverbal language is culturally determined. To interpret the meaning of a body movement or gesture without consideration of cultural context equals stereotyping. A client may wish to call the nurse by pet names such as "honey" or "dear," for example, which represents long-standing cultural behavior. Labeling this behavior as rude and condescending is inaccurate.

In clinical practice, the nurse encounters many clients who are unable or unwilling to use verbal language—the infant and growing child not yet developed in speech, the comatose accident victim unable to speak, and the depressed person not yet ready to speak (Fig. 13-7). The practitioner must use astute observation skills in order to understand the needs of these clients.

Communication scientists Ruesch and Kees developed a classic system of describing nonverbal behavior as either sign language, action language, or object language (1956). Garland Lewis organized the realm of nonverbal language into sensory categories, and indeed this language involves perceptions of sight, sound, and touch (1973).

Sight

Behaviors in the nonverbal language that are observed by sight include those of facial expression, gestures, and body postures, as well as physical appearance. The finely coordinated muscles of the face often give the most subtle indication of mean-

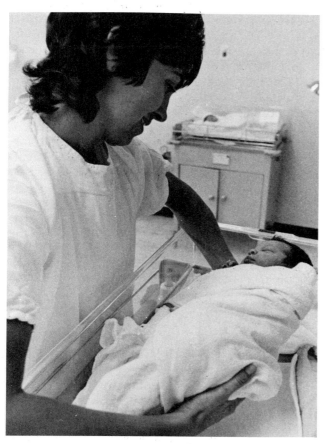

Figure 13-7
The nurse uses nonverbal language to communicate caring to the infant. *(University of Michigan School of Nursing)*

ings. One of the nurse's first observations is of the client's eye contact and eye movements. Eye contact conveys an open, sincere approach to another person; averted eyes may signal disinterest, diversion, or humility and often may raise tension in the interaction. In the extreme, however, a fixed and glaring gaze also serves to increase the anxiety of another, as if he were being scrutinized. Several barriers, such as surgical masks, hospital equipment, or telephone communication prevent open-eye contact in clinical situations. The nurse removes a barrier when she sits down to speak to children or to a person in a wheelchair or bed. Such a simple action establishes eye contact and avoids the authoritative position of towering over the client. Posture conveys meanings of interest and disinterest, of alertness, and of withdrawal. The client who curls into a fetal position communicates withdrawal just as surely as if he had said, "Leave me alone."

Other observations made by sight include that of muscle tension and rapid-breathing patterns that

are characteristic of anxiety. However, each individual manifests anxiety with his own pattern of nonverbal behavior, such as chain smoking, nail biting, pacing, and rocking. The nurse's ability to observe and validate such characteristic signs of anxiety increases the probability of understanding the client's meaning.

Appearance speaks of many traits. Let us examine the meaning of professional appearance. The student nurse in faded blue jeans typically does not match the client's perception of a professional nurse, thereby jeopardizing credibility and trust. A clean and neat appearance, uniformed or not, connotes such credibility immediately. Appearance can give the perception of sexual invitation, usually without the nurse's specific intention to do so. The lonely, insecure client will act upon such an invitation, usually startling the nurse. In this instance, recall that all such behavior is an expression of unmet needs, such as for affection or touch.

Color has language all its own. White hospital uniforms connote cleanliness; the recent popularity of colored and patterned uniforms seems to connote nontraditional values among younger nurses. Use of bright colored graphics provides stimulation to children's play rooms and hospital rooms that are otherwise stark and sterile.

Nonverbal Sounds

The skilled nurse trains the ear to observe speech sounds, because how something is said is as important as what is said. What is not said may be more important still. The skill of active listening involves listening for the nonverbal vocalizations such as sighs, cries, and voice inflections accompanying words. Contrast the following two consents:

> "Well, I guess I understand. ..." (deep sigh, chuckle)

> "OK with me ... when will it be?" (rising voice inflection)

Voice pitch, hesitations, and utterances, usually in combination with facial expressions, impart feelings of excitement, surprise, confusion, sarcasm, and mistrust. Such feelings can be heard by perceptive ears.

Silence as a nonverbal behavior holds a range of possible meanings, from boredom to contemplation, anger to introspection. Allowing the client to be silent during an interaction often causes anxiety in many nurses. The section on client-centered leads and responses explains the use and acceptance of silence.

Touch

Nursing is a touching profession; the intimate nature of many nursing tasks requires that caring be transmitted by touch. And yet, nurses have been cited as avoiding touch with seriously ill and aged clients. Touch is as essential for the elderly as for the newborn. The inability to reach out and touch a client may result from the nurse's own cultural definitions of what is an appropriate distance between persons. Although a nurse may prefer to know the person better before touching him or her, the nature of many short-term nursing interactions precludes lengthy introductions. In one study, hospital patients receiving spontaneous touch from nurses perceived that the nurses showed genuine interest in them within a very short time (McCorkle, 1974).

Space

Touch may intrude as well as soothe, and the observant nurse decides how and when to touch based on each client's response. Threatening touch represents intrusion into the personal space of another. Personal space can be envisioned as a bubble surrounding each individual and forming a part of his personal, portable territory.

Territoriality, or man's instinctive drive to protect his space from intrusion, provokes defensive behavior by the person suffering intrusion. A client may become angry should the hospital nurse touch articles on "his" bed. In turn, nurses can become defensive when clients or other professionals enter "their" workspace. Ardrey claims that possession of territory fulfills three of man's most basic needs: identity, security, and stimulation (1966). Nurses who threaten the territorial integrity of the client are threatening the fulfillment of these needs and hindering open communication.

Anthropologist Edward Hall created the term **proxemics** to mean the use of space in interpersonal relationships (1966). Space, or distance between communicators, is an extension of the concept of touch. Hall described four distances for interactions (pp. 109–120):

- Intimate distance (up to 18 inches) for privileged touching
- Personal distance (1½–4 feet) for interaction with well-known persons
- Social distance (4–12 feet) for impersonal business
- Public distance (over 12 feet) for formal speaking

Nurses are granted intimate distance with a majority of clients; we should maximize this privilege by deliberately maintaining this closeness. For example, the nurse who addresses a client from behind a desk sacrifices any chance for a closeness or privacy in the interaction. Many nurses fear touch will arouse sensuous feelings in clients. The mature and secure nurse learns to overcome this fear, learns how to increase the client's own self-esteem through touch, and promotes the use of therapeutic touch, such as massage, for relaxation, pain relief, and sound sleep.

Time

Closely related to special communication is the concept of temporal communication, the use of time and timing behavior to transmit meaning. American middle-class time orientation values the accomplishment and performance of tangible tasks. In nursing, sitting quietly with a client is often considered not doing anything. Other cultures, notably Navaho Indian and Japanese, value highly the vigil of sitting with a distressed person. Much of American culture stresses a "here-and-now," present orientation or an upward-bound, future orientation to time. This explains our insistence that very ill or disabled persons look ahead optimistically. But we cannot help the dying person to find satisfaction in his past if we ourselves cling to a future orientation.

Other considerations of time involve the length and timing of messages. The effective communicator will know and not exceed the attention span of listeners. Nurses working with children must modify treatments and activities to shorter, more frequent sessions to avoid restlessness. An interruption, another element of timing, prevents a complete message from being sent and usually leads to frustration and misinterpretation. Cultural variations in time perception need validation. For example, although some subcultures value punctuality, others do not; this could lead to misinterpretation when tardiness occurs.

Congruence: Matching Verbal and Nonverbal Behavior

In order to comprehend the holistic person, the nurse observes both verbal and nonverbal behavior and combines these to analyze the meaning. This analysis searches for congruence between verbal and nonverbal behavior:

Congruent: "I appreciate your help" (direct eye contact, soft smile)

Noncongruent: "I appreciate your help." (eyes averted, muscles tense)

Especially with distressed clients, the verbal behavior will often be incongruent with nonverbal behavior. Whereas congruence can be interpreted as an indication of open, trusting communication, incongruous messages signal the need for exploration of needs and feelings not expressed. The nurse mobilizes skills of empathy and validation to understand the client's conflicting messages and in this way maintains an open, trustful interaction.

Achieving Effective Communication

Use of Self

Even experienced nurses strive to improve three abilities in order to become more effective communicators (Pluckhan, 1978, p. 18):

- Knowledge—increased understanding of communication dynamics
- Insight—improved self-awareness of strengths and weaknesses
- Sensitivity—sharpened perception of other's needs

The term "use of self" represents the nurse's ability to integrate all three of the above abilities to produce successful interactions. Understanding the dynamics of the underlying communication process, its characteristics, and variables prevents communication problems. Nurses also learn how best to assist others when they become more aware of their own values and behaviors. Candidates for nursing often have a basic sensitivity to others; developing and expressing that sensitivity is a challenge throughout nursing practice. As nurses we bring ourselves, our past experiences, perceptions, and prejudices, to our helping relationships. The nurse who also brings a solid knowledge base, self-awareness, and sensitivity brings a valuable helper indeed to the helping relationship. Whereas knowledge is gained by disciplined study, sensitivity develops by mastering empathy.

Achieving Empathy

Empathy is the ability to enter into the life of another person in order to perceive his thoughts and feelings (Benjamin, 1976, p. 47). The nurse attempts to understand the client's life, his problems, values, feel-ings, and meanings, "to sense the client's private world *as if* it were your own but without ever losing the 'as if' quality" (Rogers, 1957, p. 99). Nurses who fail to separate the client's problems from their own risk emotional burnout; typically these nurses offer sympathy instead of empathy.

"I'm so sorry for you. I know just how awful it must be . . . it's too bad."

Few clients need this awkward compassion. Your empathic understanding, which consists of active listening, accurate observation, empathic response, and validation, is much more helpful.

Active Listening

Active listening is the cultivated skill of deriving meaning from the words or nonverbal expressions of another. While hearing refers to the passive reception of sound waves by the ear, listening encompasses active concentration and perception of another's message using all the senses. Because humans communicate their needs through verbal and nonverbal behavior, the nurse must employ sight, hearing, touch, and smell to listen actively. Hein advocates that the nurse listen for themes—patterns of communication behavior—in order to assess another's needs (1975). Common themes expressed by others include the following:

- Self-effacement (attempts to reduce one's significance)
- Poverty of resources needed to cope with a present stress
- Self-centeredness ("help me"), indicating insecurity
- Wellness or strength to deal with stress (often overlooked in our search for problems)
- Loneliness, creating despair
- Loss manifested in grieving behavior
- Humor, a coping mechanism of tension release

Accurate Observation

Accurate observation, the companion skill to active listening, involves not only looking at the client, but also identifying crucial facts about his nonverbal behavior. Knowing what to observe and recognizing how you observe are both essential.

How easy it is to jump to conclusions about what we observe and to offer solutions prematurely! Instead, we must be able to differentiate an observation from an inference or conclusion, in order to prevent misunderstandings. For an observed behavior, any one of several conclusions may be valid.

Observation

A woman wears a diamond ring on the third finger of her left hand.

Possible Inferences

The woman is married or engaged.

The woman likes diamonds.

The woman has inherited an heirloom ring that fits her third finger.

The nurse who jumps to conclusions ("I see you are married.") risks embarrassment and misunderstanding. Stating observations, not inferences ("I see you wear a diamond."), avoids communication breakdown.

Empathic Response

After careful listening and accurate observation, a nurse reacts to the client's message with a verbal, nonverbal, or combination response. Touch is a powerful and effective response to another person; it is often part of an empathic response. Nurses are privileged to hear intimate, painful, and moving accounts of the stress in others' lives. Successful empathic responses, or feedback, tell the client that the nurse is attempting to understand not only the client's situation but also his feelings and values.

There are three levels of empathic response that nurses use:

- *Level 1*—responding to situations (least effective)
- *Level 2*—responding to feelings ⎫
- *Level 3*—responding to values ⎭ (more effective)

At level 1, the helper responds to the situation, the facts and events stated by the client.

Client: "I was so upset and disappointed that I had to have another operation."

Nurse: "You had to have another operation?"

This response restates the client's situation only. Such a response is helpful to focus the interaction, but it is not considered an effective empathic response until it reflects feelings and values.

Level-2 responses can reflect feelings that are either stated openly or implied.

Client: "I was so upset and disappointed that I had to have another operation."

Nurse: "You became upset and disappointed when you heard you would need surgery again? Maybe frightened too?"

Such responses state the client's feelings, helping him to cope with these feelings by sharing them.

Level-3 responses reflect a deep awareness of another's values, of what is really important to him or her. Usually a helper is able to perceive a client's values after a trusting relationship has been established.

Client: Everything is so strange in a hospital. . . .

Nurse: It's important to you to be at home with your family . . . ?

Here, the helper perceives that this client's underlying value is being with the family; in questioning the client about this, a helper completes the empathic understanding by using validation.

Validation

It is necessary to gain some feedback from the client to know whether the empathic response is an accurate perception.

Nurse: "And is it important to you to be at home with your family?"

Client: (nods) "We really can't afford a babysitter for the entire 5 days I'll be gone. . . ."

The client affirmed her value of being with her children and raises her true concern of expense. At times our empathic responses are not accurate, and the client corrects our understanding.

Client: "Frightened? No, I've been through this before. I'm just angry that I got an infection the last time I was in this hospital!"

Validation completes a feedback loop, making empathy a two-way communication.

Learning the Empathic Response

Nurses who are just beginning to learn the empathic response will be frustrated to find that at first the response seems stiff, formal, and unnatural. The classic empathic responses to feelings, "You sound . . ." or "You look . . . ," are suggested as beginnings. The usual reflection of values ("So it's important to you that . . .") may help beginners to phrase emphathic responses. In communication study, as in any disciplined study, it is necessary to master the basic, the classic, before evolving a style of your own.

Eventually your empathic responses will flow naturally and spontaneously.

> "You know, Mrs. Y., your voice tells me that you're upset ... What is it?"

Some nurses become "turned-off" by the classic responses and never develop any empathy at all. This sad reflection is documented by numerous studies showing that nurses do not characteristically reflect high levels of empathy, warmth, or genuineness (Peitchinis, 1972).

Other Client-Centered Communication Techniques

The following techniques, some of which have been presented earlier, are useful in maintaining a client-centered interaction. The effective communicator chooses when and how to use these in relating to clients.

Silence

Murray and Zentner describe silence as a basic communication tool and outline four types of silence: blank, empty, or blocked silence; stubborn, resistive silence; fearful silence; and thoughtful silence (1979, pp. 75–76). Sensitive nurses encourage verbalization to replace empty silence if it will reduce anxiety of resistive and fearful silence.

> Seeing a client bite her lip and tense her facial muscles, the nurse waits a few seconds to ask, "What was it you almost said?"

Thoughtful silence, on the other hand, is a much-desired period of meditation or reflection that should be promoted in both nurse and client.

Stating an Observation

This skill allows the nurse to open a line of exchange and gather valuable information while avoiding the pitfall of stating an inference.

Nurse: "I see that you haven't eaten all your dinner."

Client: "It's not that I don't like it; my bowels are giving me problems."

Reflection

Reflection is the basic skill used to paraphrase or mirror the client's stated or implied feelings and values. In addition, it is an attempt to pinpoint the reason for his feelings.

Client: "I'm just not satisfied."

Nurse: "You're dissatisfied that the results of this test are negative?"

Client: "Yes. I'm not getting the truth."

Restatement and Summarization

Repeating the client's words almost verbatim is restatement.

Client: "There was nothing for me to say.

Nurse: "You had nothing to say."

At opportune times during a nurse–client interaction, a cumulative restatement called summarization can organize and focus the content.

Nurse: "Now so far you've described your relationship with your wife and two of your children. What about your son?"

Clarification

Pretending to understand a client can be very destructive to trust building. Many clients with speech difficulties have expressed a desire for listeners to stop and ask for clarification as often as needed rather than pretend to comprehend. If the helper does not hear or cannot comprehend the message, clarification is sought:

> "I couldn't hear you ... would you repeat that?"

> "I don't understand what you mean by incompetent?"

Explanation

Any client has the right to request and receive an explanation. Much anxiety can be prevented by giving explanations to clients before involving them in interviews and procedures.

> "Mrs. X., I will need to give you an enema this evening in order to help you empty your bowel for tomorrow's x-ray. Have you ever had an enema?"

Nurse-Centered Communication Techniques

In assertive behavior, the use of "I" statements is often very effective. However, most other "I" responses, or nurse-centered techniques, are harmful to the helping relationship because they do not allow the client to see his problems clearly.

False-reassurance responses sound impersonal and lead to mistrust.

Nurse: "I know just how you feel ... now, don't worry" (usually followed by a cliche, *e.g.,* "tomorrow you'll feel better").

Clients usually think, "You don't really know how I feel at all."

Advice giving is similar to false reassurance in that the helper generates easy solutions to a client's problems.

Nurse: "Now, I had the same problem; if I were you, I'd begin to volunteer to work with the disadvantaged. It worked for me."

Even well-intentioned suggestions, such as, "Why don't you try . . . ," are better generated by the client than the nurse.

Moralizing and preaching have no place in effective helping relations because they destroy the equal peer relationship of trust.

"You should (stop smoking, start exercising, stop worrying, *etc.*) if you want to help yourself."

Approval or disapproval messages place value judgments on the client and his behavior, making it nearly impossible for him to change his mind later.

Nurse: "That's good. I agree with your decision to keep your baby."

Client: "Well, actually, I haven't decided ... I may still want the abortion. . . ."

Criticism and its lighter version, ridicule, damage client self-esteem, making it difficult to reestablish trust.

Nurse: "Your plan was doomed to fail. I'm afraid it was too simple."

Denial and rejection are destructive because they undermine the seriousness of the client's problem.

Nurse: "No, you really don't have any problems with your children compared to some parents. . . ."

Threats or punishment are immature uses of authority to force the client's submission on one's advice or viewpoint.

Nurse: "You're going to fall unless you use that walker."

Most threats are desperate and lack any support on the part of the helper.

Nurses resort to defensive responses when they feel personally threatened or attacked by a client.

Client: "I never get any help with my bath."

Nurse: "We all try to give you some help, when we have time. . . . Anyway, you know you can do it yourself."

Had the nurse listened actively and avoided taking the complaint personally, she might have heard the real message and replied with empathy:

"You're feeling frustrated at having to bathe with that cast on your arm?"

Threatening responses are aggressive in nature and provoke only defensive client behavior.

Questioning

Questioning is the most commonly used and abused means of professional–client interaction, yet it need not be. The client-centered responses outlined earlier often communicate interest more accurately than questioning does. The choice of technique is often a matter of style and practice. Take a minute to emphathize with clients; would you be most responsive to nurses who listened to your problem or to those who asked only what interested them? The latter forms an unfortunate norm of nurse–client interactions in practice.

The challenge is to use, not abuse, the question when interacting. Overuse of the question–answer mode implies that the nurse knows best what is important to talk about. The pattern also implies that when we finish asking all the questions, we will come up with the solution! This is contrary to the problem-solving process of assisting the client to find his own solutions.

Questioning is abused when the nurse does any of the following:

* Threatens the client
* Interrupts the client or changes the subject
* Overloads the client with information or questions
* Asks meaningless questions
* Asks questions the helper cannot possible answer

Effective Use of Questions

When is it appropriate to use questions? Use questions when they will assist, not impede, the interaction:

- To ask for clarification, "Would you repeat that?"
- After an unavoidable interruption, "What were you saying?"
- As a restatement, "You did?"

The question and its effective variations are presented below.

Exploratory versus Closed Questions

Exploratory questions, also known as open-ended questions, exemplify the client-centered philosophy of Carl Rogers. They allow the client to explore and express his thinking. The client's response is unpredictable, open to his priorities and directions. The closed question, in contrast, usually limits the client to prescribed answers; only the very assertive client will venture to give more detail. Contrast the following:

"Is that medication working?" (closed)

"How well does that medication work for you?" (open)

Well-intentioned use of reflection is often transformed into an ineffective closed question by the addition of an unneeded query:

"You'd prefer that I leave, wouldn't you?"

Characteristically, the helper answers his own rhetorical question and proceeds without feedback from the client.

Exploratory questions present a range of open-ended options. The questions below are arranged so that each is succeedingly more open-ended:

- "What do you think is the next step in solving this crisis?"
- "What is your next move?"
- "Now what?"

Often the very cryptic, brief exploratory questions are the broadest in scope.

- "And?"
- "But what happened?"

Choose the exploratory question based on the client's concentration ability and level of abstract thinking. Asking, "And?" to a person who rambles off the topic produces mutual frustration; focusing him more firmly with "What's the next step you'll take?" will produce more concrete results. The toddler, with undeveloped abstract thinking, responds best to a closed choice:

"Jimmy, do you want orange or grape juice?"

The person who shows mental confusion or disorientation responds well to a closed question:

"Mrs. Jackson, it's Sunday morning, 9 A.M. Do you want to go to the chapel?"

Direct versus Indirect Questions

One way to avoid overuse of questions is to use the indirect question. This is actually a statement with the voice inflection of a question. Indirect questions soften the harsh effects of the straight or direct query.

"Are you worried about your mother?" (direct, closed)

"I wonder if you're worried about your mother?" (indirect)

Direct questions often catch the client off-guard and produce a startled, negative reaction:

Nurse: "What did you mean?"

Client: "Oh, nothing."

In contrast, indirect questioning makes it easier for the client to respond positively.

Nurse: "I'm not sure I understood what you meant."

Client: "Well, I was trying to say that. . . ."

Ineffective Questioning

Multiple questions overload and confuse the client. The client either stares in confusion, answers half the question, or gives a third answer not offered:

Nurse: "I wonder if you decided about the surgery, or whether you'll postpone it if your son comes home? He hasn't, has he?"

Client: "My son is a banker in Minneapolis."

A rapid-fire succession of questions, whether direct, indirect, closed, or open, forms an interrogation style best left to the police. The victim of such bombardment responds with confusion, frustration, even anger within a short time.

"When was your last visit?"

"April."

"This past April? What for?"

"Well, I had this pain in. . . ."

"Where?" (interrupts)

"In my groin."

"Put on this gown. Everything off underneath."

"But I came for glaucoma testing!" (angry)

Questioning may become threatening to a client not only by the manner in which questions are posed but by the very words that are chosen. The word, "Why?" is the most threatening word in the English language for gaining information.

"Why did you get out of bed by yourself?"

"I had to use the bathroom."

"I see that. Why didn't you call me?"

"I don't know." (defensively) "You never come!"

A less threatening approach is to state an observation.

Nurse: "I see you've gotten out of bed alone." (stating observation)

Client: "Yes. I felt strong enough to go to the bathroom by myself."

Nurse: "Then you are regaining your strength! But I'm concerned about your falling."

Client: "You don't want me to get up alone?"

Nurse: "Not yet. Let me show you how to get up slowly, so you won't get dizzy and fall." (offering self) "Tomorrow, you will be able to start walking again and I'd like you to do it safely."

Client: "So would I."

"Why" questions rarely produce the information sought. They usually provoke defensive "I don't know" answers or irrelevant excuses.

What power of authority does the nurse wield when asking, "Why didn't you keep last week's appointment?" To inhibit this aggressive approach, when you feel your lips pucker into a "why?", better whistle than threaten a client!

Client's Questions

In any interaction, the nurse encourages the client's questions. Just as the nurse uses questions at times to gain information, clients have the same need to ask questions. Some client questions seek clarifica-

tion or basic information, for instance, "What time is my clinic appointment?"

Factual answers are easily supplied, but how does the nurse react when the questions are more personal than factual? Indeed, we are often the ones to become quite defensive when a client's questions threaten us. Clients direct three types of questions to nurses: questions concerning others, questions concerning himself, and questions concerning ourselves (Benjamin, 1976, p. 74).

The majority of questions about others stem from curiosity and anxiety, such as, "What did my husband say to you?" The nurse has two options for answering such a query. First, a strict refusal on the grounds of professional confidentiality would be, "I'm not at liberty to discuss that," or, "You'll have to ask him." In contrast, responding to the client's underlying anxiety, the empathetic response might be, "He shared his concerns about the medications you take. You feel uncomfortable about his talking to me?" In such a way, the nurse betrays no confidence and refocuses on the client's anxiety.

When the client expresses questions about himself, listen carefully for an underlying concern. The strictly factual answer responds only to the presenting situation, whereas the empathy response acknowledges feelings:

Client: "When can I get out of this cast? It hurts."

Nurse A: "Two more days."

Nurse B: "Tell me what hurts about it."

Many nurses consider questions about themselves strictly off limits, and yet we reserve the right to explore intimate areas of clients' life-styles. Again, some personal questions reflect testing behavior; this will subside as trust is gained. In other instances, clients are sincerely attempting to be friendly. Very likely, however, personal questions represent an unmet need or underlying anxiety.

Client: "You ever been to the south side of this city?"

Nurse: "No, but I am trying to understand what it's like for you to live there, though."

Lengthy explanations focused on the helper often serve to raise the client's anxiety. Responding to the underlying need and refocusing on the client will meet his needs much more than lengthy explanations of your own personal life.

Client: "Say, have you ever used the Pill?"

Nurse: "No, I almost did, though, I have studied

about it. What questions do you have about your using the Pill?"

Graceful use of the refocusing technique requires practice to avoid harsh and abrupt subject changes.

Interviewing—Putting It All Together

Communication theory and skills have one purpose: producing an effective **interview** between nurse and client. Health interviews are either information-gathering interviews or helping interviews (or sometimes both):

- Information-gathering interviews are those in which the nurse seeks information from a client in order to plan or deliver nursing care.

- Helping interviews (also called therapeutic interviews) are those in which the nurse tries to help another to cope with stress. Chapter 14, Nursing Process, discusses how nurses identify health needs and plan, administer, and evaluate nursing care. Interviewing is essential to this process. A review of the interviewing techniques presented here will be useful when you begin giving nursing care to your own clients.

Unfortunately, the connotation of interview has evolved to mean cleverly forcing the other person to confess. Such tactics cannot promote trust in a helping interview. Nor is the monotonous, bureaucratic approach of "I just have a few (dozen) questions" acceptable. Successful interviewing uses a healthy balance of verbal and nonverbal behavior, empathy and assertive responses, and client-centered techniques, each chosen specifically to promote trust.

Kessler outlines the pitfalls of interviewing clients and recommends the following (1977):

- Do not create a negative first impression.
- Do not let personal biases interfere.
- Do not rush the interview.
- Do not accept inadequate answers.
- Do not follow a form or questionnaire too closely.

Assertive Communication

Learning to communicate effectively with other persons requires that several interpersonal skills be mastered. **Assertiveness,** a coping behavior, is a verbal communication skill that states one's own rights positively without infringing upon others' rights. Effective use of assertiveness prevents interpersonal misunderstanding and solves the inevitable conflicts that do arise.

Assertive communication reflects a certain level of self-confidence in nursing. A competent and confident nurse chooses to use assertive behavior rather than passive or aggressive behaviors in interpersonal conflicts. Many nurses who would not feel comfortable being totally passive or terribly aggressive have found that they can use assertive behavior to communicate their own needs (Simms and Lindberg, 1978). The assertive nurse takes responsibility, seeks workable compromises, speaks openly about his or her own feelings, and avoids projecting blame, needless apologies, angry or defensive outbursts, and silent smoldering. The following example contrasts passive, aggressive, and assertive responses.

Client: "Nurse, this soup tastes terrible and it's cold; I won't eat it."

Nurse A: (passive): "OK. Give it back to me." (silently thinking, "Why does everyone complain to me?")

Nurse B: (aggressive): "Well, it's not my fault. You'll have to speak to the dietitian. I can't help you."

Nurse C: (assertive): "That's disappointing. You can either have it warmed up or substitute something else. Which do you prefer?" (workable compromise)

Psychologist Manuel Smith described a Bill of Assertive Human Rights. Clinical nursing examples accompany each of these rights (1979, pp. 44–71).

Assertive Right I—You have the right to judge your own behavior, thoughts, and emotions, and to take the responsibility for their initiation and consequences upon yourself.

> **Nurse to supervisor:** "I, too, am disappointed that I couldn't finish my morning assignment; let me explain what I have done and we can work out a way to finish the rest."

Assertive Right II—You have the right to offer no reasons or excuses for justifying your behavior.

> **Nurse to colleague:** "I am not able to meet with you today at noon; can we reschedule?"

Assertive Right III—You have the right to judge if you are responsible for finding solutions to other people's problems.

Nurse to Client: "I can't tell you what is best for you, Mr. P. I am able to help you review your options and decide for yourself. I'll support your decision."

Assertive Right IV—You have the right to change your mind.

Nurse to aide: "I know that I said I didn't need your help, but I do. When can you help me lift this patient?"

Assertive Right V—You have the right to make mistakes and be responsible for them.

Nurse to client: "I was wrong, I checked and I am not able to drive you in my own car. We will need to work together to find you a ride."

Assertive Right VI—You have the right to say "I don't know."

Nursing instructor to student: "I don't remember the details of that procedure, but I can help you look it up."

Assertive Right VII—You have the right to be independent of the good will of others before coping with them.

Student nurse to instructor: "I understand you are trying to help me, and I don't mean to anger you, but I need you to tell me what I did wrong, not to lecture."

Assertive Right VIII—You have the right to be illogical in making decisions.

Nurse to administrator: "I can't explain why, but I need to change my assignment to a different unit. Can we work something out?"

Assertive Right IX—You have the right to say "I don't understand."

Nurse to physician: "I do not understand your reason for ordering this drug."

Assertive Right X—You have the right to say "I don't care."

Nurse to colleague: "I don't care to hear the details. I guess I prefer not to know all the client's gossip. . . ."

Assertive responses demand significant practice because many nurses must unlearn habitual passive or aggressive behavior before learning more effective behavior.

One of the most challenging nursing responsibilities is to teach assertive coping behavior to clients. Can you support the client who needs to express, "I don't understand what you say when you talk in those big words. Tell me in plain English"? Can you allow others—clients, colleagues, authorities—their assertive rights?

Conclusion

This chapter presents communication as both an art and a science essential to effective nursing. The nurse–client relationship represents a special helping relationship with inherent responsibilities and eventual rewards. Throughout the progress of helping relationships, nurses foster growth and trust by employing person-centered communication skills, especially empathy. Effective professional nurses choose assertive communication to express themselves with self-confidence. With continued insight and practice, nurses learn to conduct effective client-centered interviews and to generate conflict-free team interactions. Communication, and adaptive expression of man's needs, forms the foundation of humanistic nursing relationships.

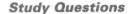

Study Questions

1. How do helping relationships differ from social relationships?

2. What are the three phases of helping relationships? How does the nurse maintain trust throughout these phases?

3. What biophysical, psychological, sociocultural, and environmental variables affect communication between nurses and clients?

4. What do the terms connotation and denotation mean in relation to verbal language?

5. List five components of nonverbal communication.

6. Why does the nurse need to observe both nonverbal and verbal behavior to communicate effectively with clients?

7. Describe several techniques that aid effective communication. Which techniques hinder communication?

8. What is the difference between empathy and sympathy?

9. How can the nurse use assertive communication effectively with clients? With peers?

Glossary

Active listening: The cultivated skill of deriving meaning from the words and nonverbal vocalization of another.

Assertiveness: A verbal communication skill that states one's own rights positively without infringing upon others' rights.

Connotation: A meaning of a word apart from its standard meaning; usually determined by its subcultural usage.

Denotation: The standard meaning of a word, which is derived from a cultural consensus on the usage of a term.

Empathy: Ability to participate in the life of another individual to perceive his thoughts and feelings.

Feedback: A return message from receiver to sender; part of the communication process.

Human Communication: The complex process of the exchange of meanings between persons.

Interpersonal communication: The exchange of messages between two persons or a small group of persons.

Interview: An interaction with a purpose.

Intrapersonal communication: Interaction that occurs within an individual when the mind or the body interprets messages for the person.

Language: Patterns of behavior designed to influence others.

Mass Communication: The transmission of messages to a large audience of receivers.

One-way Communication: An interaction in which a message proceeds in one direction from the source to the receiver.

Problem solving: The systematic process of identifying, clarifying, and resolving troublesome situations.

Proxemics: The use of space in interpersonal relationships.

Territoriality: The instinctive drive to protect one's space from intrusion.

Two-way Communication: An interaction in which a message proceeds from a source to the receiver and feedback occurs from the receiver to the sender.

Bibliography

Abdellah FG, Beland IL, Martin A et al: Patient-Centered Approaches to Nursing. New York, Macmillan, 1960

Ardry R: The Territorial Imperative. New York, Antheneum, 1966

Benjamin A: The Helping Interview. Boston, Houghton-Mifflin, 1976

Berlo DK: The Process of Communication: An Introduction to Theory and Practice. New York, Holt, Rinehart & Winston, 1966

Brammer LM: The Helping Relationship: Process and Skills. Englewood Cliffs, NJ, Prentice-Hall, 1979

Burnside I: Touching is talking. Am J Nurs 73:2060–2063, December, 1973

Effken J: Our affection for Mrs. Johns was hindering our nursing care. Nurs '75 5:14–16, June, 1975

Galloway CM: Non-verbal: The language of sensitivity. Theory Into Practice 9:227–230, October, 1971

Geach B: The problem solving technique as taught to psychiatric students. Perspect Psychiatr Care 12:9–12, January–March, 1974

Gordy HE: Gift giving in the nurse-patient relationship, Am J Nurs 78:1026–1028, June, 1978

Hall ET: The Hidden Dimension. New York, Doubleday, 1966

Hames C, Joseph D: Basic Concepts of Helping: Wholistic Approach. New York, Appleton-Century-Crofts, 1980

Hauser MJ, Feinberg D: Problem solving revisited. J Psychiatr Nurs 15:13–17, October, 1977

Hein E: Listening. Nurs '75 5:93–102, March, 1975

Hein E, Leavitt M: Providing emotional support to patients. Nurs '77 7:39–41, May, 1977

Johnson M, Davis ML, Bilitch MJ: Problem Solving in Nursing Practice. Dubuque, IA, WC Brown, 1970

Kalish B: What is empathy? Am J Nurs 73:1548–1553, September, 1973

Kessler AR: Pitfalls to avoid in interviewing patients. Nurs '77 7:70–73, September, 1977

Lewis G: Nurse-Patient Communication. Dubuque, IA, WC Brown, 1973

Martin AJ: Confidentiality—Its nature in law. Nurs Times 74:503–504, March 23, 1978

McCorkle R: Effects of touch on seriously ill patients. Nurs Res 23:125–132, March–April, 1974

Murray R, Zentner E: Nursing Concepts for Health Promotion. Englewood Cliffs, NJ, Prentice-Hall, 1979

Peitchinis JA: Therapeutic effectiveness of counselling by nursing personnel: Review of the literature. Nurs Res 21:138–148, March, 1972

Pluckhan ML: Human Communication: The Matrix of Nursing. New York, McGraw-Hill, 1978

Rogers C: On Becoming a Person. Boston, Houghton-Mifflin, 1961

Rogers C: The necessary and sufficient conditions of therapeutic personality change. J Consult Psychol 21:95–103, April, 1957

Ruesch J, Kees W: Non-Verbal Communication. Berkeley, University of California Press, 1956

Simms L, Lindberg J: The Nurse Person. New York, Harper & Row, 1978

Smith M: When I Say No I Feel Guilty: How to Cope Using the Skills of Systematic Assertive Therapy. New York, Dial Press, 1979

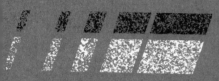

Nursing Process

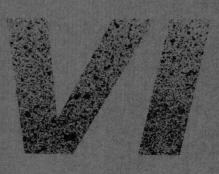

VI

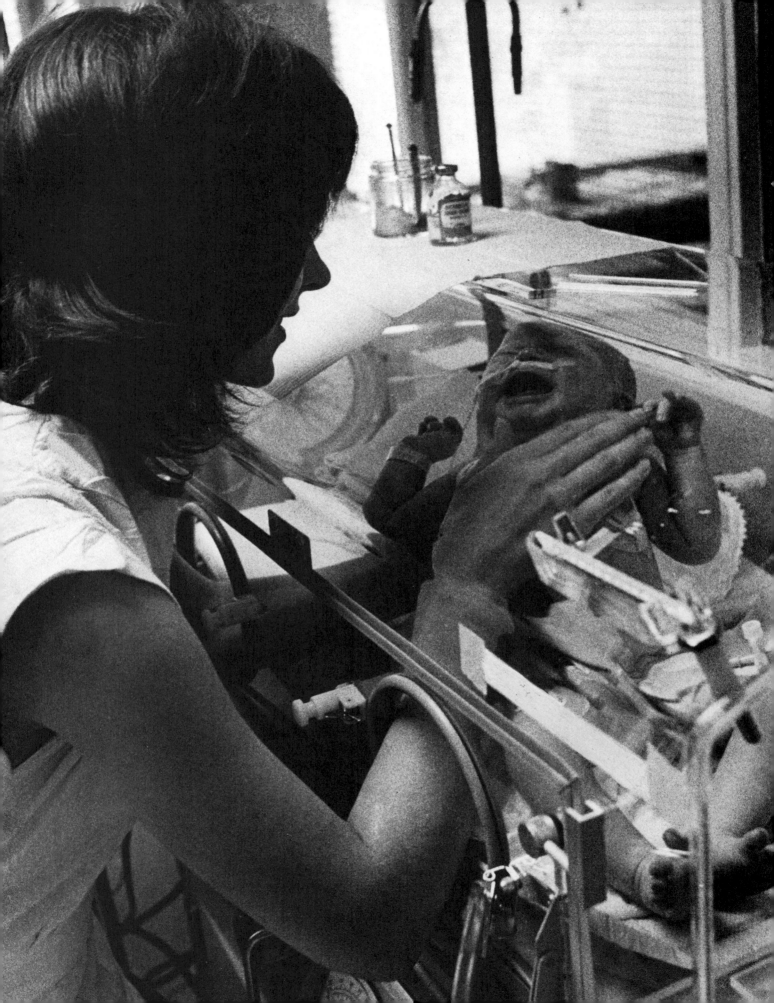

VI

Nursing Process

Nursing process is the framework through which nurses deliver their professional services. The term *process* can be defined as the act of moving forward toward completion of a goal or a continuous movement through a succession of developmental steps. Nursing process fits this definition because it involves a series of sequential steps and is goal directed. The steps involve assessing needs and strengths, planning and intervening, and evaluating results. The goal of nursing process is the optimal biological, psychological, and social function of persons who seek nursing care.

Nursing process, as the framework for the delivery of nursing care, integrates the concepts of person, health and adaptation, professionalism, health-care delivery, and communication, which were discussed in previous sections of this text. It incorporates the notion of persons as unique and holistic beings who strive to achieve their potential. Likewise, nursing process includes the concepts of professionalism and adaptation because this process is our professional method and the means by which we assist persons with their adaptations to attain health. Communication is essential to nursing process. Nurses use communication skills to establish trust with their clients, to identify clients' needs, and to assist them to adapt to stressors affecting their health. Nursing process is related to the concept of health-care delivery since it is implemented in a variety of settings and in collaboration with other health professionals within the health-care delivery system.

In Chapter 1, nursing process was described as a problem-solving process based on scientific method. Chapter 14 explores the relationship of nursing process to scientific problem solving and the implementation of nursing process in the delivery of person-centered care. The remaining chapters in this section describe applications of the nursing process to the care of persons with specific alterations in their functional abilities.

Nursing Process

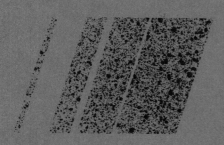

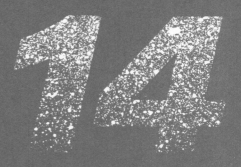

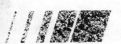

We must some day make a test to tell us where the health is ... in the end it is our only ally.

I Never Promised You a Rose Garden

The person who made this statement understood an important truth: all persons have strengths that can be used to cope with illness and promote greater health (Greenberg 1964, p. 19). This perception has profound meaning for nursing because, as a profession, nursing is concerned primarily with identifying that which is healthy and with helping people maintain, promote, and restore health. Through the development of the **nursing process,** nurses have, in essence, "made a test" as contemplated in the quote cited above. The challenge is to use this process well.

The nursing process is described as a series of scientific steps that assist the nurse in using theoretical knowledge to diagnose the nursing needs of persons and to implement therapeutic actions for the purpose of attaining, maintaining, and promoting optimal biopsychosocial functioning.

The nursing process proceeds logically from data collection to the provision of care. The literature describes the series of scientific steps taken, in various ways. Four major steps—assessment, planning, implementation, and evaluation—are always included as essential aspects of the process. We have chosen to describe these steps under three broad phases: assessment, which includes the assessment step mentioned above; therapeutic, which includes planning, implementation, and evaluation; and aggregation. Figure 14-1 depicts the sequence of steps in the nursing process.

After completing this chapter, students will be able to:

- *State the purpose of the nursing process.*

- *Discuss each phase of the nursing process.*

- *Describe how the concept of caring relates to the implementation of the nursing process.*

- *Discuss the relationship between self-care and the nursing process and how this relationship contributes to effective nursing care.*

Figure 14-1
The nursing process. Although this figure is developed as a linear model, note that each aspect may contribute to another in a more circular manner. For example, new nursing theory helps develop more effective interventions. If evaluation of your client's progress indicates a need to change the care plan, you will return to the assessment phase to collect new data before proceeding.

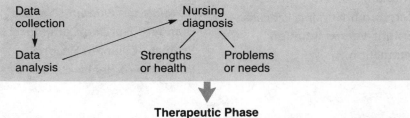

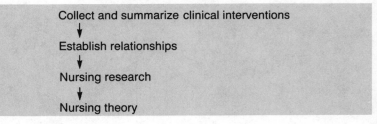

Overview

The Nursing Process as a Problem-Solving Process

The nursing process can be compared to the problem-solving approach and the scientific method, as shown in Table 14-1. These processes all follow a logical sequence of steps, beginning with the gathering of information and concluding with an evaluation of the outcome. Two particular components, interaction and goal direction, are part of problem-solving, which is more specifically suited to nursing process.

Let us first consider how we respond when confronted with a personal problem. Usually, we follow a series of steps to find a solution. We think about the problem carefully, discuss our ideas with others, and expect to achieve a certain goal by solving the problem. This process is directed toward a personal objective and, as such, concerns us directly. However, the problem-solving process from a professional nursing perspective changes our purpose from self-direction to person-direction, by putting us in the role of helping others to solve their problems.

Before the Nursing Process

Historically, nurses provided care that tended to focus on health problems or specific disease conditions rather than on the person for whom the care was provided. The nursing care provided was based

---

Table 14-1
Comparison of Nursing Process to Scientific Method and Problem-Solving Method

Scientific Method	Problem Solving Method	Nursing Process
Define the problem	Gather information in a situation	Assess the situation, collect data, analyze data, make a nursing diagnosis
Collect data from observation and experimentation	Analyze information and identify the problem	Set goals or expected outcomes
Devise and execute solution	Plan a course of action	Establish nursing interventions
Evaluate the solution	Carry out the plan	Implement interventions
	Evaluate the plan and its outcomes	Evaluate and revise the process

primarily on orders written by physicians, suggesting that nurses were extensions of physicians rather than health professionals providing a different service called nursing. As nursing expanded its knowledge base, this approach became unsatisfactory. Nurses began to think about planning care from a holistic viewpoint, a view that considers each person as a whole being with particular and unique needs. However, since nursing did not have its own process or professional theory base from which to operate, care plans often became lists and schedules of activities. The most important part of nursing, the process of caring, was rarely defined in these care plans. Thus, we began to look for a scientific base from which to practice our unique and caring profession.

Insight Versus *Intuition*

The nursing process was first articulated by McCain in her classic article, "Nursing by Assessment—Not Intuition." She stated (McCain, 1965, p. 82):

> This concept [*assessment*] incorporates the belief that the primary goal of nursing care is to assist a patient to attain and maintain a state of equilibrium as he reacts to internal and external stimuli ... The extent to which a patient does or does not achieve equilibrium is reflected in his physiological, psychological, and social behavior. Functional abilities then, become another way of expressing behavior ... In order to help him be a participant [in his care], the nurse must know his functional abilities as well as his disabilities.

McCain also wished to make the point that nurses to date had provided care that was often based on intuition and assumption rather than on a more systematic process. She therefore developed a nursing process that rendered nursing care more relevant and effective. Parts of the framework suggested in this chapter are developed from her original work.

To better understand McCain's thinking, let us consider the word **intuition.** The dictionary defines intuition as "the power or faculty of attaining direct knowledge" or "cognition without evident rational thought and inference"; or as "quick and ready insight." If nurses deliver care based on intuition, they risk acting without careful, systematic thought, relying perhaps on their own personal views or value systems. On the other hand, the word **insight,** which appears as part of the definition of intuition, is defined as "the act or power of seeing into a situation" and "the act or result of apprehending the inner nature of things." Such a perspective constitutes the basis of assessment, which has become an essential step in the nursing process and in the delivery of nursing care. For it is the ability of nurses to observe, listen, and involve themselves while applying their knowledge and skills that enables them to see beyond the obvious and into the very nature of things.

Historically we omitted assessment from our practice. Unfortunately, in our eagerness to establish a more systematic approach to nursing care, we embraced assessment as the vehicle for gaining insight; in the process we discarded intuition. However, we are beginning to recognize that both insight and intuition, when used together, represent a truer reflection of the very essence of nursing.

Interaction

As professional nurses, we have knowledge and skills that we can use in the helping role. The interactive component of the nursing process involves listening, observing, and responding for a purpose—providing meaningful nursing care. Our knowledge will help persons identify their needs, examine their goals, and make plans to attain those goals. Those who are more dependent and those who have complex needs may require more active involvement from the nurse. As each person gains independence and knowledge about his health, he can assume more control over his own care. It is sometimes difficult to achieve a balance between the decisions the nurse makes for the person and those he makes for himself. However, it is the goal of nursing to promote self-care abilities through appropriate use of the nursing process rather than to impose ideals.

Implementing the Nursing Process

The nursing process as presented here is somewhat of an ideal; that is, it represents the client as participating fully with the nurse in planning his care. Although there are many variations in both the individual nurse's approach and the individual person's response, we should strive for an ideal that envisions the person as an active participant in self-care and the nurse as a facilitator in attaining the goals of health promotion. We can remain alert to our ideal even though we will often modify the process to meet certain situations.

Assessment Phase

Data Collection

Data consist of facts, information, or findings gathered during assessment (Fig. 14-2). Depending on its source, data may be described as subjective or objective. **Subjective data** represent the person's verbal descriptions of his strengths, needs, perceptions, feelings, and experiences; **objective data** consist of information obtained from clinical observation, examination, and diagnostic studies. For example, if the client states, "I am very warm," then this statement represents subjective data. Objective data would be the temperature recording of 101 degrees.

Data collection is the process of gathering information or facts about a person, both to better understand his feelings, ideas, and values, and to identify his strengths and problems or needs. The data that are collected provide a basis for deciding what interventions can be used to cope with particular problems. The tools of data collection include the following:

- **Observation**—The act of seeing or sensing
- **Interview**—A conference held in a face-to-face meeting for the purpose of conferring on some point
- **Consultation**—The utilization of secondary resources to supplement data
- **Listening**—The act of purposefully paying attention in order to hear another person express his feelings, beliefs, strengths, and needs
- **Inspection**—A close and purposeful observation; the examination or testing of a phenomenon

Figure 14-2

Data collection is an information gathering process. *(Photo by Bob Kalmbach; University of Michigan School of Nursing)*

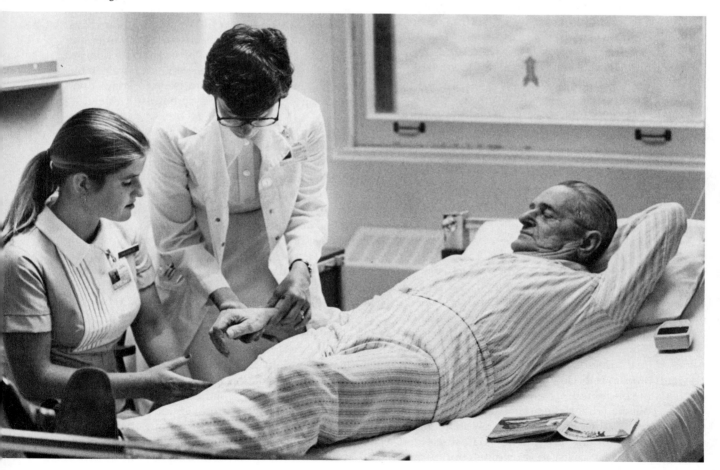

against established norms, such as the use of standard height-and-weight tables as a basis for comparison

- **Palpation**—Use of the hands or fingers to examine the external surface of the body to determine surface or underlying characteristics; for example, palpate to determine exact location of abdominal pain
- **Percussion**—Light but sharp tapping of an area of the body to determine position, size, and consistency of an underlying structure or the presence of fluid in a cavity
- **Auscultation**—The act of listening with a stethoscope for sounds in body cavities

Lamonica states, "Data collection is the continuous process of obtaining information needed in providing care" (1979, p. 2). In order to assist persons toward the goal of optimal health, we must first determine what their strengths and needs are. We are then in a position to plan nursing interventions that will provide meaningful care.

What must the nurse know about the patient? This is the central question in determining, in a professional responsible manner, the patient's requirements for nursing services. What must she understand of the intrinsic processes (physical, physiological, emotional), occurring within him? What must she know of the extrinsic factors (sociologic, economic) surrounding him, and the influence these exert upon him? How well does he manage himself in relation to the stresses he faces? What probable results can she expect from her nursing? When the nurse is able to answer these questions accurately, she is ready to provide appropriate comprehensive nursing. (Rothberg, 1967, p. 1041)

Approaches to Data Collection

There are numerous sources from which we can obtain information about our clients. The primary source is the person himself. Secondary sources include the person's written record, family members, friends, and other health professionals. Initial data from the client are collected and recorded by the nurse when the person enters the health-care system, at which time an interview and physical examination are usually conducted.

The collected data, when recorded, provide baseline nursing information about the person and serve as a basis for comparison when new data are added. Recorded data also assist in providing continuity of care because they offer one means by which health-care personnel can communicate with one another and share information about their clients.

The type of data collected relates to a variety of functional abilities, as indicated in the list of statuses and assessment guidelines found in Appendix A. This assessment guide presents a holistic view by combining information about all systems of the person's being.

Because the assessment guide in Appendix A is so inclusive and calls for information of a personal nature, students may wonder about the feasibility and suitability of trying to collect such extensive data. Actually, it is not necessary to obtain all this information about each client. Since there are many and varied approaches to data collection, each nurse will most likely develop an individual style for collecting information based on priorities related to the individual client.

Frequently these priorities become obvious in the first stages of the data-collection process. The initial consideration in the mind of the interviewer should be the person's current health status. For example, is he in pain or having difficulty breathing? Is he depressed or anxious? Is he unable to speak or communicate clearly? Is he confused or comatose? When problems such as these exist, the manner and type of data collected will differ from that collected when the person is feeling relaxed and comfortable. It becomes imperative, then, to learn to adapt one's interviewing skills to suit the demands of the situation.

If the person is unable to communicate his needs, it may be necessary to refer to secondary sources such as family members or the clinical record to obtain data related to his primary needs or concerns.

Although not all nurses are involved in the initial collection of data, there are numerous opportunities to gather additional information and augment the data base, because data collection is an ongoing process. Primarily, beginning students should develop skills of listening and observing as described in Chapter 13, while learning to record additional findings obtained from their interactions with their clients. A few appropriate and strategically placed questions will elicit much additional information that will be pertinent for planning care.

It is especially important to become proficient in collecting information that is of a personal nature. Although persons entering health-care agencies expect to be interviewed and examined, they may be reluctant to answer questions about their private concerns. A sensitive interviewer, while establishing an atmosphere conducive to the free expression of thought, will not try to force a confidence. As a trusting relationship develops over time, a client may feel more inclined to divulge information about himself.

Trust can be established by first developing a harmonious atmosphere and rapport with the person. Generally when the nurse demonstrates acceptance and empathy, the response will be one of trust. As the nurse continues with an honest, open, and respectful approach, a meaningful nurse–client relationship will occur. Table 14-2 suggests interventions that encourage the development of trust.

When collecting data, we need to remember that our purpose for doing so is to gather information that will assist in the planning of meaningful care to maintain and promote our clients' health. It is from this purposeful focus on others that we develop the intuition and insight that are, in essence, the means of carrying out person-centered care.

Data Analysis

Data analysis is a cognitive or thinking process whereby the nurse forms conclusions about the delivery of care. Referring to data analysis Thomas and Coombs state that "this thought process is influenced by scientific knowledge applicable to nursing, the definition of nursing, and past nursing experience" (1966, p. 55). Thus, in planning care, the nurse will compare facts gathered about the person with accepted norms in anatomy, physiology, psychology, and growth and development; at the same time, the nurse will draw upon accepted nursing knowledge and personal nursing experiences to recognize a pattern in or relationships among the data. Using this approach will lead to reasonable conclusions about the care that is needed. As in all aspects of nursing care, the person should participate as much as possible in this thinking process along with the nurse.

Consider the following situation. You are caring for a woman who has undergone abdominal surgery and is about to get out of bed for the first time following the operation. You note that her pulse rate prior to rising is 80, that her facial skin color is slightly pale, and that her lips are coral pink. She clearly states that she is determined to walk down the hall. After she begins to ambulate, her pulse rate rises to 92 and her face and lips become noticeably paler. However, she tells you that she is still determined to walk farther.

From your many experiences in delivering postoperative care, you know that the first attempts at ambulation should be limited to a few steps. From knowledge of physiology and nursing, you know that

a normal pulse range is 60 to 90 beats per minute and that skin color in light-pigmented caucasians should be pink. You are also aware, from your scientific understanding, that the changes you are observing could mean fatigue, hypotension, or even shock. You may decide to tell the person that her pulse rate has become somewhat elevated and that her color is slightly paler. You could also mention that the second ambulation will be easier and that she can walk farther at that time. By providing her with this information, you will undoubtedly help her to make the decision to return to bed.

In this situation you have pulled together quickly several unrecorded observations, drawn a conclusion based on experience and scientific knowledge, and shared it with your client. Together you have made a decision about how to proceed.

On other occasions you may be able to consider much more information, perhaps from a complete interview, in developing a total plan of care. An example in Appendix B demonstrates how one student used the nursing process to develop a comprehensive plan of care by thinking through and making relationships among a wide range of data collected on several different occasions.

The Nursing Diagnosis

Establishing the **nursing diagnosis** is the next step in the assessment phase of the nursing process and represents the conclusion drawn by the nurse and the person from the data collected and analyzed. Nursing diagnoses summarize the client's strengths and needs or problems within those specific functional areas for which nurses are qualified to provide support or care. Rothberg states, "Nursing diagnosis is the process which identifies the patient's resources and deficits, thus indicating his needs for nursing assistance . . ." (1967, p. 1041–1042).

Because the term diagnosis has long been associated with medicine, it is important to distinguish between nursing diagnosis and medical diagnosis. A nursing diagnosis arises from the nursing data obtained in assessing the unique functional abilities of the person, whereas a medical diagnosis identifies the disease entity that is present. In other words, the medical diagnosis generally describes the disease (i.e., diabetes mellitus, cancer of the lung, psoriasis), while the nursing diagnosis describes the strengths and problems or needs of the individual person.

The nursing diagnosis, then, contains two essential elements: strengths or inner resources and problems or needs. **Strengths** are biopsychosocial qualities that contribute to a person's character,

Table 14-2
Interventions to Develop Trust

Develop rapport:

- Demonstrate
  - Concern
  - Belief in the intrinsic value of the person
  - Unconditional acceptance of the person with his strengths and limitations
  - Empathy (see Chap. 13)
  - Compassion

Develop trust:

- Demonstrate
  - Consistency in behaviors exhibited toward the person
  - Willingness to clarify communications
  - Genuine interest
  - Truthfulness
- Remember that trust is not spontaneous but must be earned:
  - Spend time with the person.
  - Use a relaxed and unhurried manner.
  - Visit when there is nothing specific to do.
  - Address the person by name.
  - Do not invade privacy; hesitate at the door; ask the person if he feels like talking; ask if you may sit down.
  - Do not interrupt.
- Do not issue direct commands, such as "you should."
- Ask for clarification of statements you do not understand.
- Let the person know you remember what he has told you on another occasion. For example, ask how the situation is now; say, "I remember when you told me. . . ."
- Communicate that you wish to understand what the client is experiencing.
- Offer touch; assess the person's comfort level with touch, and start slowly and gently.
- Move your body toward the person as he speaks.
- Allow the person to tell his complete story, even when it is uncomfortable for you, or explain your discomfort honestly and find someone else to listen.
- Inform the person early of your time limitations.
- Be reliable. It is all right to forget or change your plans, but be honest about what you did and why.
- Be consistent in behavior.
- Facilitate the person to regain control over his care and his life.
- Help the person plan and carry out goals.

Kennison B: Personal communication, January, 1980

integrity, and uniqueness and that can be mobilized to cope with a problem and attain a goal. The person's strengths are the most important consideration when planning nursing care because they represent the person's inner health, which must be used to promote greater wellness. The following list suggests several examples of strengths.

- Has resolved developmental tasks favorably
- Meets own basic needs
- Values independence
- Relates warmly with spouse, children, and others
- Expresses strong religious faith
- Expresses a comfortable philosophy of life
- Verbalizes knowledge about health problems
- Displays a sense of humor
- Uses pain-control methods effectively
- Displays unique talents and interests (music, art, languages, cooking, woodworking, needlework, gardening, extensive reading, athletic endeavors, etc.)
- Demonstrates effective problem solving
- Accepts help from the nurse and others
- Expresses readiness to learn about health concerns
- Expresses readiness to start coping with health concerns
- Sleeps well
- Absorbs and digests food effectively
- Maintains a stable blood pressure

External resources, while not internal strengths, nonetheless need to be identified as sources of support in coping with health problems. Examples of external resources include the following:

- Supportive family
- Network of supportive friends and colleagues
- Financial stability
- Satisfying job
- Comfortable physical home environment
- Geographical proximity to shopping, recreational facilities, churches, health care facilities

The second element of the nursing diagnosis is the **problems** or needs that are identified. There are three possible classifications: actual problems, potential problems, or possible problems.

- **Actual problems** or needs are those which can be identified clearly from the data at hand. Some examples of actual problems or needs are as follows:

  Decreased endurance
  Respiratory distress with minimal exertion
  Anxiety related to forthcoming surgery
  Decreased mobility related to painful joints
  Chronic nausea
  Grief related to death of husband

- **Potential problems** or needs are those which the person is at high risk of developing given his particular situation. Some examples of potential problems or needs are as follows:

  Skin breakdown related to decreased mobility
  Maladaptive patterns of coping related to husband's death
  Abdominal distention associated with presence of nasogastric tube
  Diminished self-esteem related to alteration in usual functioning

- **Possible problems** or needs are those for which the nurse has obtained some data but not enough to identify an actual problem or need. An example of a possible problem or need would be possible financial problems. (This can be suggested by noting that a person who says he is not worried about his finances often wrings his hands and paces the floor when questions of money arise.)

Additional nursing diagnoses can be found throughout the nursing process chapters in this book.

A word should be said here about the National Conferences on Classification of Nursing Diagnosis. This group held its first meeting in 1973 and has met three times since then. These conferences are held in an effort to standardize and classify problems for which nurses provide care. The problems identified by these conferences focus on health status and alterations in health. Many of these nursing diagnoses are similar to ones identified in this text. For further reading on the National Conference and its work, refer to the books listed in the bibliography at the end of this chapter.

Considerations when Establishing the Nursing Diagnosis

Ideally, the nurse, together with the client, establishes the nursing diagnosis. However, there are times when the nurse will identify problems or needs that the person does not accept. Determining how to assist such a person is one of the challenges of nursing. Consider the following situation. On the basis of physiological principles and nursing knowledge, the nurse knows that ambulation following surgery is necessary to regain one's former level of functioning. The nurse may be able to identify a number of problems that might occur if a regular ambulation regimen is not followed. However, because of postoperative fatigue and pain, a patient may prefer to rest rather than ambulate. Standards of care developed through research indicate that we would be negligent if we did not intervene at this point. Providing the person with an opportunity to talk about the pain or any other concerns that may be troubling him and suggesting some coping mechanisms are usually effective means of gaining his participation. Establishing definite and agreed-upon rest periods will help relieve fatigue and facilitate ambulation as a necessary part of postoperative care. Nurses who can discuss potential problems with their clients and provide needed information are usually successful in gaining client participation. The person who is still unable to become involved in his own care may be expressing a deeper, unmet need, about which more data will need to be collected.

It is often difficult to respect a person's right to ignore or deny an obvious health problem, particularly if it has serious implications. However, if we learn to assess the meaning behind the behavior and to look at what the person perceives his real need to be, then perhaps we can help him to cope with the problem as he perceives it and to consider other problems as well. For example, a man who has hypertension may not take medications as prescribed. The nurse might identify the problem as inconsistent self-administration of medication. The person may brush the problem aside, saying that the pills are not very effective. The nurse who respects the person's right to make decisions about his health care can try to help with some other problem that the client has identified. Perhaps he is distressed because his family members do not communicate well. Working to solve this problem would be more relevant to him than trying to cope with the nurse's main concern. If the person is assisted in improving his family relationships, he may find it more worthwhile to take his medication as scheduled. Moreover, if he is happier in his family life, the hypertension may be less severe.

Therapeutic Phase

Goals or Expected Outcomes

Goals or **expected outcomes** are predictions of what the person hopes to attain given his strengths and needs. They are intended to maintain his identifiable strengths and to help him move toward solutions to his problems. Whenever possible, goals should be planned with the person and then recorded. It is helpful to remember that strengths can be mobilized to cope with the problems. If a person's strengths are not used, his needs may increase. In any situation, it may be necessary to adjust the goals periodically.

The criteria described below have been established for constructing goals.

• **Goals are written in behavioral terms and individualized to suit the person who expects to attain the result.**

It is the person's rather than the nurse's behavior that should be recorded. For example, a goal may be stated, "The person will maintain intact skin over pressure areas." It is more appropriate to state the goal in these terms than to say, "Maintain intact skin over pressure areas." The second example appears to suggest that maintaining skin integrity is the nurse's rather than the person's goal. The nurse's goal is to assist, but it is the person who will maintain intact skin. In essence, the person will attain this goal with the help of the nurse.

• **Goals are written in measurable terms.**

In the example above, the goal that the person will maintain intact skin over pressure areas is measurable, because the nurse will use her knowledge of what constitutes skin integrity to observe for any signs of skin breakdown. If a sign of poor circulation to the skin develops, nursing observations will identify this problem, and new plans for maintaining intact skin can be instituted. The person also can carry out his own observations, using knowledge the nurse has given him. The ability to participate in one's own care represents a strength that is mobilized to help attain the goal. Other examples of measurable goals include the following:

• The person will state that his pain has decreased following use of relaxation techniques.

• The person will state his diet from memory within 1 week after instruction begins.

• Before discharge, the person will demonstrate how to take a blood pressure reading.

• The person will smile three or four times a day.

• The person will verbalize feelings of increased safety and security.

- The person will ambulate in the hall 2 days after surgery.

There are some goals that cannot be structured within a time frame. For example, if the goal states that the person will verbalize feelings of increased safety and security, the word "verbalize" provides one means of measurement. However, the time frame is missing. The plan is to use interventions which will help the person feel more secure, so that eventually he will verbalize that sense of security. We need to remain aware of what is to be attained, no matter how long it takes.

• *Goals may be written as short-term and long-term goals.*

Not every strength or problem requires both short-term and long-term goals. Goals may be written to reflect plans for a relatively short period of time or for a more extended period. **Long-term goals** often refer to a broader accomplishment which, although realistic in the long run, can only be attained through a series of smaller steps. An example of a long-term goal might be that the person will lose 50 pounds over the next 12 months.

Short-term goals reflect smaller steps which can be pursued one at a time. They will be a means of demonstrating achievement, providing encouragement, and suggesting ways to attain the long-term goal. Consider the following examples of short-term goals established to meet the long-term goal of a 50-pound weight loss. The person will do the following:

- Identify his weight as a problem
- State his wish to lose weight
- Verbalize knowledge of good basic nutrition
- Plan with the nurse a realistic diet relevant to his needs
- Lose 1 pound per week for the next 6 weeks

As each of these goals is attained, additional goals reflecting continued loss of weight up to the 50-pound limit can be written and added to the plan.

We can summarize this discussion by saying that goals are planned with the client and reflect both his ability and his readiness to work toward attaining these objectives. Goals are written in measurable terms according to the behavior of the person who expects to attain the goal; they may be both long and short term; and they are revised as necessary.

Nursing Interventions

Nursing Interventions, nursing actions, or nursing measures are the steps taken to help the person attain the stated goals. They are directed toward promoting or maintaining health. They are planned with the person's strengths in mind and are used to develop those strengths to further his self-care capabilities (Fig. 14-3). Nursing interventions are derived from (1) scientific knowledge associated with the biophysical and behavioral sciences, (2) nursing theory based on research, and (3) past nursing experience.

Interventions can be categorized as diagnostic and therapeutic. Several examples of both classes of interventions are as follows.

Diagnostic Interventions

- Observe—Consider such items as nonverbal behavior, skin-color changes, progress in ambulation, and response to medication.
- Inspect—Examine a wound for signs of infection.
- Monitor—Check vital signs on a regular schedule, test urinary glucose and acetone four times a day, and weigh the person daily.
- Percuss—Determine changes in condition.
- Listen—Obtain data to detect changes in voice tones either for cues to respond in a specific way or for clues to a person's needs, concerns, or wishes; auscultate to determine changes in condition.

Therapeutic Interventions

- Listen—Provide opportunities for the person to verbalize; sit with and talk to the person; use touch, and acknowledge strengths.
- Problem solve—See Chapter 13 for strategies related to this intervention.
- Support physiological needs—Assist persons with activities of daily living as needed, irrigate wounds, and change dressings; encourage fluids to prevent dehydration; provide interventions for pain relief.
- Educate—Provide specific health information as needed and appropriate.
- Plan with—Plan a diet with the person, a stop-smoking regime, or a program of family discussions to improve relationships.
- Refer—Assist the person to find other profes-

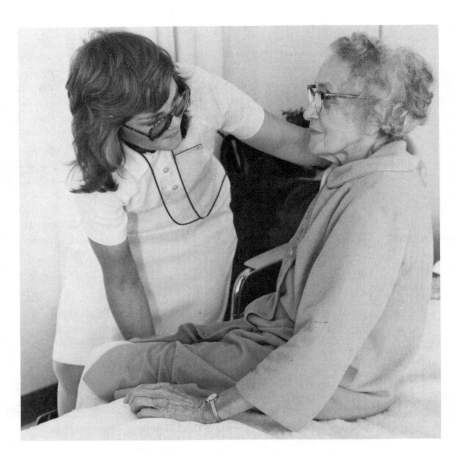

Figure 14-3
Therapeutic nursing interventions may involve care that meets a person's physical needs.

sionals, services, or facilities to help with his needs.

- Meet basic needs.
- Support developmental-task resolution.

Effective Interventions

Assessing and planning, although they represent formal steps within the structure of the nursing process, require approaches that are suited to the needs of the individual person. As mentioned in our discussion of holistic care in Chapter 2, all of a person's subsystems are interrelated, with the healthier parts contributing to any overall coping effort. However, if coping becomes ineffective, energy may be borrowed from stronger subsystems, causing them to become weaker. If too much energy is drained away, the result may be a feeling of hopelessness and helplessness in dealing with the stress of life, along with a sense of losing control over one's life and a diminished sense of self-esteem.

Interventions, to be effective, should be based on the concept of caring, as described in Table 14-3. Note that there are five basic areas to be considered when providing nursing care. The nurse begins first to develop a trusting relationship with the client and then gradually assists the person to maintain or recover control over his life. (Suggested interventions for achieving this goal are listed in Table 14-4.) As he perceives that he can control what happens to him, the nurse helps him establish goals, using a conscious effort to support and promote his strengths. This promotes a higher level of self-esteem. Gradually, as the person feels more positive about himself and his ability to cope, he can respond to the positive expectations that the nurse puts forth concerning his ability to take care of himself. A hopeful view of the future then develops and the cycle of trust, control, goal development, self-esteem, positive expectations, and hope repeats itself, resulting in greater control and less dependence on others.

Implementation

Implementation indicates that the nurse and the person together have put the plan into action. "Implementation is the actual giving of nursing care. It is nursing therapy or nursing treatments, each of

Table 14-3
The Concept of Caring

Interventions	Definitions
Develop a trusting relationship.	**Trust**—the assumption that another is responsible and honest and has integrity; the belief that we are safe with another; the ability to take risks concerning another person, a pet, or an inanimate object such as a car; the ability to act without fear of the outcome; a mode of positive expectation and hope
Assist the person to maintain or recover control over his life.	**Control**—the act of exercising restraint or direction over something or person
Assist the person to establish goals.	**Goal**—the aim or end toward which effort is directed
Assist the person to develop higher self-esteem.	**Self-esteem**—the individual's personal judgment of his own worth obtained by analyzing how well his behavior conforms to his self-ideal; the frequency with which his goals are achieved will directly result in feelings of increased self-esteem
Assist the person to develop a sense of positive expectations and hope.	**Hope**—expectation of something desired; confidence (trust) in another person, event, or outcome; promoting the promise of advantage or success
	Hopelessness—despondency, despair, abandonment of self to one's "fate"; inability to mobilize resources to cope; the sense that nothing can help, that the situation will never improve
	Despair—the state of believing that one has no further control over a situation, an event, or even of one's life
	Helplessness—weakness, dependence, ineffectiveness; inability to mobilize resources; being without hope
	Impoverishment—the state of feeling, in some measure, helpless–hopeless, sad, and fatigued, and often hostile and bitter; one's self-esteem is low and problem-solving skills are minimal.

Swain MA, Erickson H, Tomlin E, Steckel S, Hunter M, Boodley C, Kennison B, Kemp M: Personal communication concerning research project: Health promotion among diabetics: Comparing nursing systems. The Department of Health, Education and Welfare: The Division of Nursing, Grant No. NV00658-03, September 1978–September 1981

which is the giving of nursing care . . . Implementation of the nursing care plan contributes to comprehensive care because the plan considers the biopsychosocial aspects of the client" (Marriner, 1979, p. 127). Lamonica states, "Implementation . . . is the act of putting the nursing care plan (nursing interventions) into operation; it is taking action to meet objectives" (1979, p. 105).

Implementation is a complex undertaking. Certain activities, such as providing oral hygiene for a person with a dry mouth or teaching about the side-effects of a newly prescribed drug, are obvious interventions. However, other nursing action such as "providing support" are more difficult to discern because of differences in interpretation or insight. What does giving support mean? Interventions like those mentioned earlier (*i.e.*, encouraging verbalization, identifying strengths, and assisting with problem solving) are examples of how support may be given. However, the success of this goal will be influenced by other factors, including the communication skills of the nurse, the time available to provide support while attending to the needs of several persons, and the degree to which the nurse

> **Table 14-4**
> **Interventions to Assist the Client to Regain Control**
>
> - Help the person recognize and recall his strengths.
> - Respect the person's ability and right to make decisions about his care.
> - Support the decisions he makes and gear your interventions toward helping him carry out his plans.
> - Explain all nursing actions to the person and ask for his suggestions on how to proceed.
> - Use the person's ideas about his care and provide him with appropriate information so he can make safe decisions.
> - Acknowledge the person's accomplishments and express your respect. Remind him of other successful problem solving he has done.
> - Listen to the person's statements of how he feels. He knows better than anyone else what those feelings—both physical and psychological—mean.
> - Provide opportunities for the person to perform activities as he is capable.
> - Use a positive approach which indicates your expectation that he will become increasingly able to take care of himself.

is familiar with other support systems, such as the community resources that are available when needed.

In the initial stages of learning to implement a plan of action, students frequently turn to their instructors for guidance. Additional insights can be gained by concentrating on a limited number of nursing actions when caring for each client. Other ideas may be derived from textbooks, lectures, and one's own creativity. At the same time, however, it is important to be aware that interventions that sound logical, obvious, or sensible may require more definite thinking and preparation before being put into effect.

Evaluation and Revision

Evaluation and **revision** represent that part of the nursing process in which the person's strengths, needs, and goals, along with the planned interventions, are reconsidered and then revised as necessary throughout the period of need. "Evaluation is the process of assessing the patient's progress toward health goals" (Marriner, 1979, p. 217). In other words,

the stated goal or expected outcomes are used as a standard for evaluating the degree to which the person has improved his health status.

Evaluation begins with implementation of the nursing care plan. Throughout the delivery of care, it is important to consider the effectiveness of the plan in helping the client achieve his goals. Suppose, for example, that in implementing a nursing plan to teach an overweight man how to diet, you note that he still continues to gain weight despite his ability to learn the menu plan. It is clear that the plan is not working well. In fact, if the person is not ready to learn, teaching about diet at this point may represent a stressor rather than a therapeutic intervention. Therefore, you will want to reevaluate the plan and establish goals that identify smaller, more achievable steps. Perhaps you need to reassess the person's basic needs and deal with those concerns before continuing with the diet teaching. On the other hand, if you are caring for a client who has recently been diagnosed as having diabetes and who is truly ready to learn diet management, insulin administration, and a plan for exercise, then his immediate goal is to attain independence. You and the client together can decide to progress more quickly than the originally planned schedule.

The frequent revision of plans as a result of the evaluation of the client's progress may appear to be a backward step and thus may be discouraging. However, if the client has truly participated in the planning process, he himself is likely to arrive at the decision to revise the plan. Such participation will provide the control he needs and will help him recognize that he can make other revisions as his situation changes.

Although the purpose of this discussion of evaluation as a part of the nursing process has focused on the individual person and his attainment of health-directed goals, it is important to note that evaluation can be applied in a broader sense. It may be used to determine the quality of health care delivered in an agency or to judge the performance of the health-care personnel, either through self-evaluation or the peer-review process. Refer to the bibliography for additional readings on evaluation and quality assurance.

Aggregation Phase

Aggregation is the process of collecting and summarizing many nursing interventions and their outcomes and determining relationships among the outcomes. Predictions can then be made about the most effective interventions for a given age, sex, culture, health concern, life-style, and so forth. More importantly, however, aggregation is the process of synthesizing data collected from many persons and drawing conclusions by which nursing theory, nursing principles, and nursing knowledge are developed.

Providing care to many people in a variety of settings may reveal certain commonalities among their care situations. For example, it may become apparent that persons within a certain age or cultural group or those with a particular disease seem to respond in a similar manner to certain interventions. Identifying an apparent commonality may uncover a researchable problem that can be approached informally or formally. An informal approach may rely on careful observation and comparison to determine which interventions are most helpful. A more formal method may consist of conducting a research project to test a hypothesis. In either approach, if the data is analyzed carefully and recorded properly, the finding may be published and may thereby contribute to nursing theory.

However one decides to become involved in the aggregation phase, it is important to retain all data, care plans, journals, and written communications concerning client care and one's own experience (Fig. 14-4). At some point it may be possible to summarize and synthesize these items in order to contribute to the improvement of nursing and health care in general. Table 14-5 gives a succinct review of the steps involved in the nursing process.

Figure 14-4
Nurses may use each other's expertise when planning nursing interventions and comparing outcomes. *(Photo by Bob Kalmbach)*

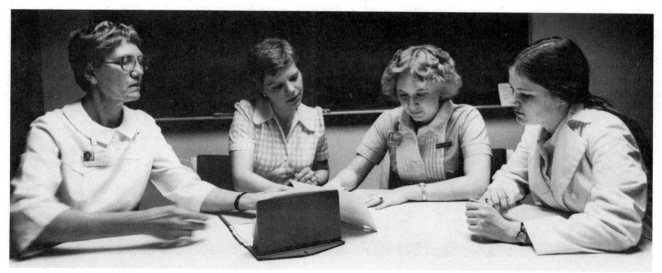

Table 14-5
Application of the Nursing Process

Phase	Step	Application
Assessment	Data	Subjective data Objective data
	Data collection	Tools of data collection: 　Observation 　Interview 　Consultation 　Listening 　Inspection 　Palpation 　Percussion 　Auscultation
	Data analysis	Cognitive process
	Nursing diagnosis	Strengths Problems or needs: 　Actual problem or need 　Potential problem or need 　Possible problem or need
Therapeutic	Goals or expected outcomes	Person behavioral Measurable Realistic or individualized Long- or short-term
	Nursing interventions	Diagnostic: 　Observe 　Inspect 　Monitor 　Percuss 　Listen Therapeutic: 　Listen 　Solve problems 　Support physical needs 　Educate 　Plan with 　Refer 　Meet basic needs 　Support developmental-task resolution
	Implementation	
	Evaluation and revision	
Aggregation	Collect and summarize nursing interventions	Develop nursing theory, principles, and knowledge
	Make predictions	

Recording the Nursing Process

The application of nursing process as described in several of the remaining chapters in this book will help identify specific problems and the kinds of outcomes and interventions that can be planned to meet these problems. How the care plan is recorded will depend to a great degree on the practices and policy of the agency in which the care is delivered.

An example of a recorded nursing process appears in Appendix B and was adapted from one written by a nursing student. Although only a representative sample of the statuses and care plan has been included, the data are descriptive, relevant, and clearly indicative of the fact that the student considered priorities when assessing the client.

Standard Nursing Care Plans

A standard is simply an approved model. A **standard nursing care plan** is one which has been developed to identify the problems, goals, and interventions that are considered typical for persons who have certain health problems or who are undergoing a specific diagnostic test or surgical procedure. Such plans may be identified as: "Nursing Care Plan for the Person with Hyperalimentation," or "Nursing Care Plan following Esophagoscopy."

Standard nursing care plans can be found in nursing textbooks and nursing care manuals. They are also developed by nurses on hospital units and in other health care-settings as a means of establishing standards of care for the clients of that agency. Specifically, these plans assist nurses to provide care for persons with needs unfamiliar to the nurse. They also address professional issues related to standards of nursing practice and quality control. In other words, they attempt to ensure that all clients of the agency receive care of high quality.

Although standard nursing care plans have several purposes, it is wise to remember that they are not individualized nor directed at the unique needs of the person receiving care. Of even greater concern is the fact that the individual's strengths are not considered in planning the goals or interventions. However, if we remember that these plans basically are models, we can use those parts that describe specific and necessary procedures for a given problem and then individualize the plan according to the strengths and needs of our individual clients.

Problem-Oriented Records

The **problem-oriented record,** often referred to as P.O.R. or P.O.M.R. (problem-oriented medical record), is a system for organizing the content of a person's health-care record within a given agency. The system was developed by Dr. Lawrence Weed around 1970 as a way to assist physicians in documenting their use of the problem-solving process. Dr. Weed was distressed at the incompleteness and disorganization of the usual medical record. He believed that physicians documented their activities but not the needs or problems of the client. P.O.R. has taken several forms, but the basic idea has enjoyed widespread use.

Since the problem-solving process is essentially the same for medicine as it is for nursing, the P.O.R. system is suitable in both specialties. The following objectives indicate the purposes of P.O.R.:

- To individualize care by focusing on the client and his needs

- To encourage health professionals to look for relationships among problems

- To promote communication among health-care members involved in direct care of the client

- To organize the health-care record so that all information from all health disciplines is recorded in the same way

The elements of P.O.R. are similar to parts of the nursing process and consist of the following items:

- Data base—the initial step, consisting of collected data about the client

- Problem list—conclusions based on the data and record of disturbances in functional abilities

- Initial plan—both expected outcomes and interventions for the problem. This should be completed in the first 24 hours after admission to the hospital, or on the first contact in an ambulatory care agency.

- Progress notes—the recorded results of nursing care and the person's progress. The recording is done using the acronym SOAP:

  S—subjective data or the person's description of his sensations or emotions

  O—objective data or the observations the nurse makes

  A—analysis or interpretations of what the data mean; the nursing diagnosis

  P—plan or immediate actions to be taken.

Consider this example. Data: A client who has

been on a 1000-calorie diet for 3 weeks is weighed. She weighs 144 pounds, (admission wt.—154 lb.). Client, smiling states, "My clothes even feel looser and I really feel better. I want to lose the rest of that weight." The entry on the progress note might look like this:

S—states feels better, clothes looser; "I want to lose rest of weight."

O—weight 144 lb. = 10-lb wt loss

A—clt losing weight; motivated to continue diet

P—continue 1000-cal diet; acknowledge successful efforts to lose wt

As new problems develop, they are added to the problem list and written in a "soap" note to document the progress. When a problem is resolved, it is marked as such on the problem list. Progress notes can be omitted as long as the problem remains solved.

- Flow sheets—three types: one for charting treatments and activities of daily living; a second for charting vital signs, intake and output, weights, and urine tests; and a third for documenting teaching provided for the client

- Discharge summary—a final progress note on each active problem at the time the person is discharged from the hospital or other health-care agency

The P.O.R. method has partially fulfilled some of its objectives. There has been improvement in the organization of health-care records, and both documentation of client progress and communication among health-care personnel have been facilitated. However, the philosophy and approaches put forth by the authors of this book place greater emphasis on a strength-oriented system. With this in mind, the sample "soap" note was written to underscore the maintenance and promotion of a strength. In this way we can adapt the process to reflect a more person-centered nursing philosophy.

Purposes of Health-Care Records

At this point it is appropriate to consider the general purposes of health-care records:

- Communication between health-care personnel

- Legal record—Because the record is a legal document and admissible as evidence in a court proceeding, all entries on a record should be clear and should include each of the following: the nurse's name, the date and time of entry,

any significant changes in the person's progress, and the nurse's observations and interventions.

- Evaluation—Report of client progress and the quality of health care. Groups of records may also be reviewed to evaluate the overall quality of nursing activities in helping clients achieve health-care goals.

- Education—Carefully kept records facilitate learning among health-care professionals as they analyze the thinking process and judgments of others.

- Research—Consideration of data present in a number of charts helps to identify researchable problems (*i.e.*, aggregation).

- Administration—Data from an agency's clients can be used to determine the needs of the agency so that it can better provide necessary services.

Conclusion

Nursing process is a scientific problem-solving method whose goal is the promotion of self-care abilities. Nursing process may be divided into three phases: assessment, therapeutic, and aggregation. The assessment phase involves collecting and analyzing data about a person's health status and identifying needs and strengths. The therapeutic phase includes planning goals and interventions, implementing nursing care, and evaluating results. Aggregation is the process of synthesizing the results of nursing interventions to make predictions about the most effective approach for a given situation.

Scientific assessment, planning, implementation, and evaluation enables nurses to give the most effective care possible. However, because nursing is a person-centered profession, nursing process must also be based on caring. Caring involves considering the person as a holistic being who has unique strengths and needs. A specific nursing approach using the concept of caring assists each person as well as groups of people, to become as healthy as possible.

Problem-oriented records and standardized nursing care plans are two methods of standardizing the implementation and documentation of nursing process activities. Both tools are useful, yet nurses must not overlook their clients' strengths and individuality when using such methods.

The use and continued reinforcement of nursing process stimulates the development of nursing research and theory and thus promotes nursing's growth as a profession.

Study Questions

1. Match the terms on the right with the correct choice on the left.
   a. Subjective data
   b. Objective data
   c. Nursing diagnosis (strength)
   d. Nursing diagnosis (actual problem)
   e. Nursing diagnosis (possible problem)
   f. Nursing diagnosis (potential problem)
   g. Expected outcome (goal)
   h. Nursing intervention
   i. Evaluation
   j. Aggregation

   _____ Data synthesis
   _____ Favorable resolution of intimacy *vs* isolation
   _____ Temperature 102°F
   _____ Decreased endurance
   _____ Person will ambulate t.i.d.
   _____ "I feel very tired."
   _____ A problem for which you need more data
   _____ Brainstorm problem-solving ideas
   _____ A problem for which the person is at high risk
   _____ Determining that health goals have been met

2. Suppose your friend, who is majoring in Business, asks you what nursing is all about. Using the ideas from this chapter about nursing process, development of trust, and the notion of caring, outline the main points you would use to answer this question.

3. Consider the following data—Mr. J., a 65-year-old widower, has been hospitalized for 2 weeks. His daughter Carol lives close by and has promised to visit several times. However, each time she has called to say she couldn't make it. You observe that Mr. J. has become sadder and no longer talks very much. He often sighs and occasionally states that he wishes Carol would come because there are things he'd like to discuss with her.
   a. Suggest additional data you would like to obtain as you proceed with care planning.
   b. What strengths can you identify in the data?
   c. Considering the concept of caring (Table 14-3), what problems do you see developing in Mr. J.?
   d. You plan to use a trusting relationship as a nursing intervention with Mr. J. Describe the steps you would take to develop a trusting relationship.
   e. Write a "soap" note for Mr. J.'s record.

4. Describe the differences between the standard and the individualized nursing care plan.

5. Identify a situation from your personal or professional experience in which use of the philosophy of self-care and the nursing process could have enhanced the person's recovery. Indicate how you would have applied these concepts to the situation.

Glossary

Aggregation: The process of collecting and summarizing numerous clinical interventions and their outcomes into classes of events and relationships among events, such that one can make predictions about the most effective intervention for a given sex, age, cultural background, health history, life-style, and so forth; the process by which nursing theory and principles are developed.

Assessment: The process of collecting information about the person to develop a base for delivering nursing care.

Auscultation: Listening with a stethoscope for sounds in body cavities.

Control: The act of exercising restraint or direction over; the act of making decisions that positively affect one's health.

Consultation: Utilizing resources to supplement data.

Data: Facts, information, or findings about a person.

Objective data: Information obtained from clinical observation, examination, and diagnostic studies.

Subjective data: The person's verbal description of his strengths, needs, perceptions, feelings, and experiences.

Despair: Despondence, a sense of hopelessness.

Evaluation: The process of assessing the person's progress toward health goals.

Expected outcome: A prediction of what the person would like to attain given his strengths and needs; the aim or end toward which effort is directed; a goal.

Goal: A prediction of what the person would like to attain given his strengths and needs; the aim or end toward which effort is directed; an expected outcome.

Long-term goal: A large accomplishment.

Short-term goals: Small accomplishments that can be pursued one at a time to attain a long-term goal.

Helplessness: Weakness, independence, ineffectiveness; inability to mobilize resources; feeling of being without hope.

Hope: Expectation of something desired; confidence in another person, event, or outcome; promoting the promise of advantage or success.

Hopelessness: Despondence, despair, abandonment of self to one's "fate"; inability to mobilize resources to cope; the sense that nothing can help, that the situation will never improve.

Implementation: Putting the nursing care plan into action; the actual delivery of nursing care.

Impoverishment: The state of feeling, in some measure, helpless-hopeless, sad and fatigued, hostile and bitter; having low self-esteem and minimal problem-solving skills.

Insight: The act or power of seeing into the situation; the act or result of apprehending the inner nature of things.

Inspection: A close, purposeful observation; the examination or testing of a phenomenon against an established norm.

Interview: A meeting of persons face to face for the purpose of a formal conference on some point.

Intuition: The power or faculty of obtaining direct knowledge or cognition without evident rational thought and inference: quick and ready insight.

Listening: Purposeful attention to hear feelings, beliefs, strengths, and needs.

Monitoring: Checking signs and symptoms on a regular schedule.

Nursing diagnosis: The conclusion drawn by the nurse or the nurse and the person from the data collected in the various functional areas; may represent a strength, a need, or a problem.

Nursing interventions: The steps the nurse takes to help the person attain his goal; nursing actions or nursing measures.

Nursing process: A series of scientific operations with three phases, which enables the nurse to utilize theoretical knowledge to diagnose the nursing needs of persons and to implement therapeutic actions that aim at attaining and maintaining the person's optimal biopsychosocial functioning.

Observation: The act of seeing or sensing.

Palpation: Use of the hands or fingers to examine the external surface of the body to determine surface or underlying characteristics.

Percussion: Light but sharp tapping of an area of the body to determine position, size, and consistency of an underlying structure or the presence of fluid in a cavity.

Problem: A situation that requires specific action to be taken.

   Actual problem: A problem that can be identified clearly from the data at hand.

   Potential problem: A problem the person is at high risk of developing, given his particular situation.

   Possible problem: A problem for which some data have been obtained but not enough to identify it as an actual problem.

Problem-oriented record (P.O.R.): A system for organizing the content of a person's health-care record within a given agency.

Self-Esteem: The individual's personal judgment of his own self-worth.

Standard nursing care plan: A plan that identifies problems, goals, and interventions considered typical for persons with certain health problems.

Strength: A factor that contributes to goal attainment; an ability; a unique characteristic; a healthy behavior.

Trust: The assumption that another is responsible, is honest, and has integrity; the belief that we are safe with another and can take risks; the ability to act without fear of the outcome; a mode of positive expectation and hope.

Bibliography

Atwood, J, Mitchell, P, Yarnall S: The POR: A system for communication. Nurs Clin North Am 9, No. 2: 215–228, June 1974

Bailey PA: Physical Assessment of the Elderly. Top Clin Nurs 3, No. 1: 15–19, Apr 1981

Berg HV: Nursing audit and outcome criteria. Nurs Clin North Am 9, No. 2: 331–335, June 1974

Blake BL: Quality assurance: An ethical responsibility. Superv Nurs 12, No. 2: 32–38, Feb 1980

Buchanan ME: Method of data collection. J Am Operating Room Nurses 33, No. 1: 137–149, Jan 1981

Calder, Landon A, Miller ML et al: How we won the health team's support for POMR. Nursing '81 11, No. 4: 137–143, Apr 1981

Campbell C: Nursing Diagnosis and Intervention in Nursing Practice. New York, John Wiley & Sons, 1978

Erickson HC, Tomlin EM, Swain MA: Modeling and Role Modeling: A Theory and Paradigm for Nursing. Englewood Cliffs, NJ: Prentice Hall, 1983

Fortin D, Rabinow J: Legal implications of nursing diagnosis. Nurs Clin North Am 14, No. 3: 553–561, Sept 1979

Gebbie KM (ed): Summary of the Second National Conference—Classification of Nursing Diagnosis, Clearing House for Nursing Diagnosis. St. Louis, University of St. Louis, 1976

Gebbie, KM (ed): Proceedings of the Third National Conference on the Classification of Nursing Diagnoses, Wakefield, Mass., Contemporary, 1979

Geden E: Nursing research: The basis of clinical decisions. Missouri Nurse 49, No. 6: 7, Dec 1980–Jan 1981

Gordon M: Nursing Diagnosis: Process and Application. New York, McGraw-Hill, 1982

Gordon M: The concept of nursing diagnosis. Nurs Clin North Am 14, No. 3, Sept 1979

Greenberg J: I Never Promised You a Rose Garden. New York, Signet, 1964

Hilger E: Developing nursing outcome criteria. Nurs Clin North Am 9, No. 2: 325–330, June 1974

Inger F, Aspinall MJ: Evaluating patient outcomes. Nurs Outlook 29, No. 3: 178–181, Mar 1981

Jacoby MK: Teaching assessment of client functioning. Nurs Outlook 29, No. 4: 248–250, Apr 1981

Kim MJ, Marity DA (eds): Classification of Nursing Diagnoses: Proceedings of the Third and Fourth National Conferences. New York, McGraw-Hill, 1982

King D, Barnard KE, Hoehn R et al: Disseminating the result of nursing research. Nurs Outlook 29, No. 3: 164–169, Mar 1981

Lamonica EL: The Nursing Process: A Humanistic Approach. Menlo Park, Addison Wesley Publishing, 1979

Lewis WR: Health behavior and quality assurance. Nurs Clin North Am, 9, No. 2: 359–366, June 1974

Marriner RR: The Nursing Process, 2nd ed. St. Louis, C V Mosby, 1979

McCain RF: Nursing by assessment—Not intuition. Am J Nurs 65, No. 4: 82–84, 1965

McKeehan K: Nursing diagnosis in a discharge planning program. Nurs Clin North Am 14, No. 3: 517–524, Sept 1979

Mundinger M, Jauron G: Developing a nursing diagnosis. Nurs Outlook 23: 94–98, Feb 1975

Niland MB, Beaty PM: A Problem-oriented approach to planning nursing care. Nurs Clin North Am 9, No. 2: 235–245, June 1974

Popkess SA: Diagnosing your patient's strengths, Nurs '81 11, No. 7: 34–37, July 1981

Reeves DM, Underly N et al: Nursing executive committee sets standard for clinical practice. Hospitals 55, No. 2: 71–72, July 1981

Rexilius B: Why not chart first? Superv Nurs 12, No. 2: 52–53, Feb 1980

Rothberg J: Why nursing diagnosis? Am J Nurs 67, No. 5: 1040–1042, 1967

Soares CA: Nursing and medical diagnosis: A variant of essential features. In Chaska N (ed): The Nursing Profession. New York, McGraw-Hill, 1978

Taylor J: Measuring outcomes of nursing care. Nurs Clin North Am 9, No. 2: 337–348, June 1974

Thomas MD, Coombs RP: Nursing diagnosis: Process and decision. Nurs Forum 5, No. 4: 57–64, 1966

Van Bree MS: Undergraduate research. Nurs Outlook, 29, No. 1: 39–41, Jan 1981

Watson AB, Mayers MG: Assessment and Documentation: Nursing Theories in Action. Thorafare NJ, Charles B Slack, 1981

Yarnall SR, Atwood J: Problem-oriented practice for nurses and physicians: General concepts. Nurs Clin North Am 9, No. 2: 215–228, June 1974

Yura H, Walsh MB: Nursing Process, 3rd Ed. New York, Appleton-Century-Crofts, 1978

Zimmer MJ: Quality assurance for outcomes of patient care. Nurs Clin North Am 9, No. 2: 305–315, June 1974

Zimmer, MJ: Guidelines for development of outcome criteria. Nurs Clin North Am 9, No. 2: 317–321, June 1974

Psychological Status

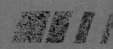

Janice B. Lindberg and Ann Z. Kruszewski

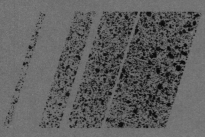

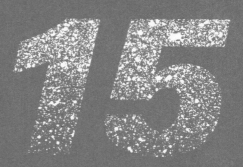

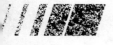

The psychological status of a person is a label applied to an important integrating function that encompasses cognition or thinking, emotions or feelings, and behavioral manifestations of both. We acknowledge this integrating status in all our references to man as a biopsychosocial being.

Psychological considerations have been addressed specifically and frequently throughout this text. Chapter 2 focused on the uniqueness of the individual person and on the human psychological needs each of us shares with other persons. In Chapter 3, psychological aspects of growth and development were discussed drawing upon the works of Maslow, Erikson, and Piaget. Chapter 28, Learning and Teaching, cites various psychological perspectives with specific reference to how persons are thought to learn. Additionally, attention to cultural status and sexuality highlights other important aspects of man as a biopsychosocial creature.

Appreciation for man as a holistic being has stimulated specific interest in the psychological aspects of health and illness and also in man's general adaptation to an ever-changing world. This chapter considers the nature of psychological functioning, factors that affect psychological functioning, general assessment of the psychological status, and nursing process applied to the common psychological problems of anxiety, altered body image, and low self-esteem.

The Elements of Psychological Function

"**Psychology** is the science that studies behavior and the unseen processes that shape behavior. Psychologists seek to explain, predict, and control behavior. Psychology is one of the behavioral sciences, but it is unique among that family of disciplines in that it emphasizes the individual" (Morris, 1973, p. 21). Today the study of psychology is divided into various specialties rather than into theories. Some of the adjectives used to describe the areas of specialization follow:

Physiological

Experimental

Developmental

Social

Educational

Industrial

Clinical

As scientists, psychologists use the methods of science to study behavior. However, because people are different from lower animals and because the real world is not a controlled laboratory, the study of man's behavior raises as many questions as it answers. Some of the deductive approaches to psychology underscore group norms of behavior, whereas some inductive approaches emphasize individual experience. Most approaches profess that both heredity and environment are major determinants of human behavior. Additionally, regardless of the theoretical perspective assumed toward psychology, some

of the large problems remain puzzling and virtually unanswered. For example:

- What are the real differences between man and animals?
- What is the relationship of the mind and body within the person?

Psychologists and nurses are concerned with three areas of psychological data or information. These are

- Cognition or thinking
- Operant behavior
- The affective domain or feelings

Cognition or Thinking

Cognition or thinking is a major concern of Chapter 16, The Mental Status. As you will remember from the study of evolution, the various parts of animal brains are developed according to special requirements of the species. Man, whose behavior is in large part learned as opposed to instinctive, has a larger brain which is capable of higher mental processes. The central nervous system is considered to be the focus of awareness, reason, memory, and emotions. Unfortunately much of the detail that would explain how these mental processes work is evasive because the human problem-solving process is adaptive. We know that man's ability to abstract information and to use the abstractions is virtually unlimited. We also know that there are limits to the human nervous system's capacity to process information in relation to serial numbers and short-term memory. Since man's most important tool is the mental process of thinking, it seems appropriate to devote a separate chapter to mental status.

Operant Behavior

Operant behavior is roughly equivalent to voluntary behavior. It is the kind of behavior that makes up most of the everyday activity of persons. Operant behavior is so named because " . . . the most important fact is that a person's own behavior brings consequences that change his action"(Carpenter, 1974, p. 10). Much of what we "know" about a person's general psychological functioning is inferred from observable behavior. Just as with data collection in other statuses, it is important for the nurse to report data objectively as observed, or subjectively as reported by the client. The inferences drawn from the data then become the nursing diagnoses or impressions. In this way, the nurse's conclusions or data analysis are open to validation by nursing peers and other health professionals.

Feelings or Affective Domain

Affect or **emotion** is the feeling tone of a person's reaction to other persons or situations. These two words are interchangeable in common usage. Feelings are complex, usually conscious experiences; however, they may be unconscious, especially during severe emotional conflicts. Common feelings include anxiety, fear, anger, grief, joy, and love.

Feelings involve overt behavior and also physiological changes, as we shall see when we discuss integrative mechanisms. These physiological changes may tell us something about the intensity of feelings but they do not explain causes. The overt behavior may involve facial expressions or gestures, body positions, distance between persons, and explicit acts of varying appropriateness. Occasionally, nurses will observe that the person's feelings do not seem to be appropriate to the situation. **Flatness of affect** is a phrase used to describe a dulled emotional tone. It is most frequently noted in severely disturbed emotional states. For example, a hospitalized person may show no emotional response when a significant other comes to visit.

Psychological Function as an Integrative Mechanism

We know that there are two major integrating systems of the biological person: the endocrine system and the nervous system. These two systems provide the coordinating mechanisms that send chemical and electrical messages to the cells and the larger structures of various parts of the body. Hormones create sexual and individual differences, affect metabolism, and influence emotional balance. The nervous system messages influence central and peripheral ner-

vous system function. The somatic portion of the peripheral system contains nerves that run from receptors to skeletal muscles. It primarily governs movement and reactions to external environmental changes. The autonomic nervous system, containing mostly motor nerves, serves inner muscles and glands.

True to the adaptive nature of man, the autonomic nervous system has two antagonistic mechanisms, which respond to sympathetic and parasympathetic stimulation. Sympathetic stimulation instructs the adrenals to produce epinephrine in preparation for "flight or fight." A review of a current physiology text will provide more details of these mechanisms, presented here in brief in Table 15-1.

The autonomic nervous system was once regarded as automatic. It is now considered to be more responsive to control by the person through his will than was previously believed. Conversely, we now also realize that chemical imbalances may affect psychological disorders and drug dependencies.

Man is both a thinking and a feeling creature. Each individual's **personality** is his unique way of feeling and responding to situations. As Morris says, "Personality is a person's own characteristic pattern of behavior, emotions, motives, thoughts, and attitudes" (Morris, 1973, p. 595). It is an intrinsic pattern of behavior that each person develops both consciously and unconsciously as a way of adapting to the environment.

Dynamics of personality are explained in terms of an energy system that has a limited amount of total energy. The energy which is leashed by unresolved conflicts of the past is unavailable for active problem solving. A strong ego, by monopolizing the energy store, has energy to invest in the development of higher psychological processes. In this way, the ego controls the cognitive functions. At times of stress and illness, usually healthy people may regress to less mature ego states. In such states, problem-solving abilities may be compromised. It is good to remember that mild anxiety can activate problem solving but severe anxiety can cause an irrational response and immobility. Nurses should recognize that implications for problem solving apply to themselves as well as to their clients.

Piaget reminds us "Any kind of behavior will always have an energetic or affective aspect to it as well as a structure or cognitive aspect" (Piaget, 1971, p. 231). Man's behavior is usually more obvious than either the cognitive or the affective aspects of the psychological status. Morris (1973) described the motives for man's behavior as physiological, stimulus, and learned (Table 15-2). What Morris calls psychological motives are what Maslow referred to as basic human needs. As described in Chapter 2, psycho-

Table 15-1
Effects of Sympathetic and Parasympathetic Stimulation

Sympathetic Stimulation (Thoracolumbar)	Parasympathetic Stimulation (Craniosacral)
Dilated pupils	Constricted pupils
Dry mouth	Slowing of heart rate
Increase in heart rate	Slowing of breath rate
Contraction of pilomotor muscles—"gooseflesh"	Increased digestion
Breath-rate increase	Blood-pressure decrease
Stopping of digestion	
Blood-sugar increase	
Perspiration increase	
Increased blood flow to skeletal muscle, heart, lung, and brain	
Blood-pressure increase	

Table 15-2
Motives for Man's Behavior

Physiological	Stimulus	Learned
Hunger	Senses	Fear
Thirst	Activity	Aggression
Sleep and dreaming	Exploration and curiosity	Social motives
Sex	Manipulation	Consistency
Maternal drive	Contact	
Aversive drives		

Morris CG: Psychology, An Introduction, p. 322–340. New York, Appleton-Century-Crofts, 1973

logical functioning integrates the holistic elements of each person.

Factors Affecting Psychological Function

The two major determinants of human behavior are heredity and environment. Both of these determinants contain several elements that affect psychological functioning, including general social consid-erations, interpersonal relationships, psychosocial development, and emotional adjustment. Some of these factors have been discussed elsewhere. Others will receive attention here as points to be considered during a general nursing assessment of psychological status.

General Social Factors

Nurses who recognize the potential impact of a variety of social factors on psychological status will be alert to intervention opportunities. By anticipating client needs they can teach their patients strategies that might limit disruption of psychological functioning. You will recall that in both situational and maturational crises, possibilities exist for growth-producing psychological change. People are usually less anxious when they know what to expect in unsettling circumstances. Their expectation gives them the necessary time to ready their personal strengths for the challenges they face.

A variety of social factors contribute to each person's psychological outlook and function. Included in these factors are social status, ethnicity, religion, occupation and economic resources, and residence.

Social Status

In an ever-changing society in which people move fairly easily from one social level to another, social status becomes increasingly more difficult to determine. This social mobility in turn results from many other social factors, including a transient and mobile work force, expanding educational opportunities, a credit-card economy, and instant worldwide communication. These factors make opportunities for social advancement more widely known and accessible to greater numbers of persons. A person often does not live his entire adult life in the same community. Even if he does, it may not be the community of his birth. Thus the continuity of social status that binds one generation to another may also be disrupted. Attempting to classify a person according to where he lives, how he dresses, or how he speaks may lead to biased and erroneous conclusions and offensive stereotyping—all of which contradict the very essence of person-centered care. Stereotyping tends to inhibit rather than to encourage open communication between nurse and client. On the other hand, how a person perceives and labels himself may offer significant clues to his unique strengths and needs.

Ethnicity

Part of a person's perception of himself frequently stems from ethnic background. In today's world people of particular ethnic origins wish to acknowledge their culture and be respected accordingly. The common and distinctive culture of an ethnic group such as Italians, Chinese, and Blacks may have an influence on beliefs, feelings, and behavior in relation to health care. Although ethnic identification should be respected for its possible contribution to beliefs, feelings, and behaviors, any cultural labeling or generalizing about individual persons runs counter to a person-centered approach and should be avoided by the nurse. (For further discussion see Chapter 26.)

Religion

Religious affiliation may also be a social factor influencing a person's psychological function and outlook. Religious values can hold special significance in times of illness. When physiological or psychological functioning is compromised, a person may become increasingly dependent on religious practices and beliefs, even if such beliefs have not played a major role previously. If religion has always been regarded as important, it may become an even more meaningful source of psychological comfort during times of illness. The nurse who recognizes the meaning of religion to the person will tap this source of comfort. If unable to provide religious support directly, the nurse may need to enlist the aid of other health professionals or clergy.

Occupational and Economic Resources

The manner in which a person earns a living and the amount of financial resources he has available play a part in shaping psychological outlook. A person's occupation may provide important information about sources of life satisfaction, self-esteem, and personal values. Since self-esteem is partially determined by life work and livelihood, considerable anxiety often occurs when health problems alter occupational status. Persons often consider appropriate health care a luxury beyond their means and they may experience considerable psychological distress related to anxiety and fear of catastrophic illness. They may also feel guilty if they are unable to provide adequately for loved ones.

Anxiety also occurs when a person's financial resources are limited or when difficult economic times occur, in general. At such times, young families and members of the middle class may find themselves caught in an economic squeeze along with the elderly, the unskilled, and disadvantaged minorities.

Residence

Where one lives and how independently one can function in that setting play a major role in psychological status. Persons who change residence often feel disrupted and in psychological disequilibrium until they adapt to new surroundings. This adaptation may require considerable energy, as evidenced by the struggles of college students away from home for the first time and of newlyweds and retired persons who move away from family and friends. These life events are among those implicated in causing high stress levels as identified by Holmes and Rahe (Chap. 6). The high stress level in turn often manifests itself in altered health status. This consideration of residence is especially pertinent to elderly people who may be forced to rely on other family members because of an alteration in health status. Frequently, they must face the need to leave their own homes. The psychological status of both the elderly person and the members of the family who feel responsible for his welfare will undoubtedly be affected by such circumstances.

Interpersonal Relationships

The number and types of interpersonal relationships available to a person will have a profound effect on how well he deals with alterations in his state of health. Included in this category are relationships with family, friends, and other significant people in his life—all of whom are frequently referred to as "significant others."

Family

Partly because of his higher mental capacities, man is extremely dependent on the nurturing family for both learning needs and socialization. Also, personality development is an interpersonal process (Fig. 15-1). For these reasons, when a person reaches adulthood, the family has deep personal meaning that can evoke intense feelings. Depending on the circumstances, families may impose a number of burdens, provide considerable emotional support, or offer a mixed blessing. In addition, the family as a unit conveys different meanings for different times, cultures, ages, and individuals. For example, in today's world more and more family units are composed of single parents or a combination of offspring from previous marriages.

Figure 15-1
Family relations affect how a person adapts to health alterations.

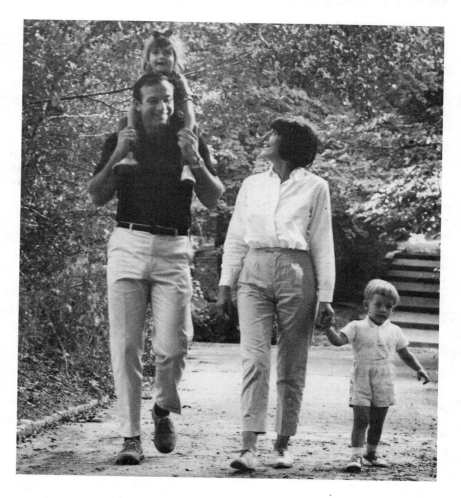

Peers

Although peer relationships are of prime importance during the formative years, it appears that families provide the most meaningful of human relationships throughout the life cycle. However, because relationships are an individual matter, it is important to identify which relationships provide the person with primary support and not to make assumptions about the meaning of any relationship.

Significant Others

Significant others may substitute for many family roles. In recent years many young adults have opted for meaningful personal relationships while postponing formal commitment to marriage and family. Other groups of people, such as senior citizens, mentally retarded adults, and emotionally disturbed persons, have found satisfying arrangements by living together informally as a family.

Psychosocial Development Level

Age, Sex, Sexuality

Even the basic personal characteristics of age, sex, and sexuality are significant factors in one's psychological functioning, as was previously indicated in Chapter 3 on growth and development and will be discussed in Chapter 27 on sexuality.

Human Need Fulfillment

Throughout this book, Maslow's hierarchy of needs has served as a major framework for delivering person-centered care. Because a person's needs are a factor affecting psychological functioning, one might attempt a general assessment of need fulfillment based on the Maslow hierarchy, try to determine the degree to which an individual has succeeded in resolving the developmental tasks identified by Erikson, and note the amount of personal self-esteem displayed.

Independence/Dependence

Relative dependence and independence and the manner of interrelating with others to meet one's needs is another facet of psychological status to be considered. Although in the past women and old people were considered to be dependent on husbands, sons, or other family members, these stereotypical roles have changed considerably in today's society. Even the traditional family roles have undergone considerable change as women have moved into the work force, and some fathers have opted to stay home to raise children.

Emotional Adjustment

Man has the capacity to adapt psychologically as well as biologically. Just as heredity and environment determine psychological functioning, they also help explain psychological malfunctioning. Because psychological functioning is an integrative mechanism, a disruption in the affective or feeling state is likely to be reflected in psychological dysfunctions of behavior or thinking abilities. For this reason, psychological adaptation is sometimes called emotional adjustment.

Adjustment and Coping Skills

Adjustment is the process and outcome of coping with life in society. **Coping skills,** as adaptive measures or means, enable a person to manage or overcome a psychological or social problem. This does not mean that life is easy or without struggle for people who cope well. Rather it means that the individual generally feels (affective element) and knows (cognitive element) that he is in control of his life situation. He perceives that he has adequate strengths or resources with which to manage life's problems. For the most part he will be functioning within society's legal and moral expectations. An exception might be the draft evader who follows his religious or moral convictions and violates society's law. In such instances, it is important to be aware that the person's thought, behavior, or feelings may reflect a developmental state, cultural norms, or views that are different from the nurse's.

Defense Mechanisms

Defense mechanisms are processes beyond a person's awareness that protect him against anxiety. Some common defense mechanisms are given in Table 15-3. All of us use defense mechanisms at some time in our lives. These mechanisms are inherently neither good nor bad. However, they are maladaptive when they are used to the exclusion of other coping strategies. The appropriateness of coping strategies also varies with different ages, cultural groups, and situations.

Common coping strategies include the following:

- Turning to a comforting person
- Displaying intense feeling

Table 15-3
Common Defense Mechanisms

Name	Definition	Example
Denial	Closing out painful or anxious situations or feelings	A high school senior who is failing all subjects sends in a deposit for college.
Displacement	Releasing bottled feelings on individuals less threatening than those who aroused the emotion	A teenager who dented the family car blows up at the younger brother who wants to borrow his bike.
Fantasy	Dreams satisfied symbolically through wishful thinking	A plain woman imagines herself to be a famous actress with many admirers.
Identification	Unconscious belief of likeness between one person and another	After treating his injured dog a boy decides to become a surgeon.
Intellectualization	Divorcing a feeling from an idea because the feeling is too painful to be admitted	A sterile woman devotes her life to teaching without allowing herself to experience grief.
Introjection	Taking another's values and ideas as one's own	A young woman from the country moves to Manhattan to work and share an apartment with her college roommate who is a native New Yorker.
Projection	Assigning one's own intolerable thoughts to others	A person who resents authority criticizes unruly juveniles.
Rationalization	Untruthful reporting of behavior, which is given a logical or socially acceptable explanation	A nursing student makes up a verbatim of a client interaction, saying it's legitimate because no one knows exactly what was said anyway.
Reaction formation	Masking of intolerable feelings by repressing the true feeling and reinforcing the opposite	A teenage girl who is jealous of her baby brother eagerly volunteers to take him everywhere and displays affection for him in public.
Repression, dissociation	Unconscious restraint from awareness of intolerable feelings	A woman is jealous of her sister's beauty but acts unaware of her feelings.
Suppression	Conscious restraint from awareness of intolerable feelings and thoughts	An athlete competing in an important meet has just received news of a friend's death but puts it out of mind to win the race.
Sublimation	Channeling of instinctual drives that are unacceptable to consciousness into socially acceptable activities	The aggressive young male becomes the football hero and team captain because of his take-charge attitude and successful tackles.

- Engaging in avoidance or withdrawal behavior
- Talking out the feelings
- Using symbolic substitutes (*e.g.,* prayer, an automobile)
- Relying on self-discipline
- Somatizing or expressing through body organs

The holistic or humanistic view assumes that man is inherently good and is striving to achieve his potential. To assist clients in their emotional adjustment, the nurse helps them to maximize their internal strengths and external resources.

Internal Strengths

Chapter 14 on the Nursing Process has stated that client strengths are important data to be gathered. Other chapters that apply nursing process also emphasize the importance of client strengths. The challenge to the nurse always is to plan interventions to enhance the strengths that have been identified. Remember also, it is the client who will make the emotional adjustment. How people feel about themselves, their general life situation, and their specific health problems will determine how the nurse is able to capitalize on their personal strengths to enhance biopsychosocial abilities.

One way to determine strengths is to begin with what you see as a problem and then ask, "What ability remains? What can the person do?" For example, what might be the strengths of a quadriplegic man who was paralyzed from the neck down in a driving accident? One such man who was unable to do his own care was eager and able to suggest what should be done—and also how and when. In this way, he was able to retain some control over his life situation. His planning skills were not affected by his physical disability.

Desire to assume control and responsibility for health situations is an important internal strength, as are both biological functioning and psychological ways of adapting to change. Physical strengths that might facilitate psychological functioning include such abilities as sleeping well or digesting and absorbing food. Other strengths might be the ability to assess situations realistically, the ability to accept assistance, eagerness and ability to learn new information, demonstrated past independence, and demonstrated past abilities. Perseverance, patience, and attention to detail are also valued strengths. Most persons have the cognitive abilities of thinking or of engaging in distraction strategies to control or minimize pain. An affective strength might be the ability to express feelings, whereas behavioral strengths might include strategies that have been useful in the past to deal with anxiety or crisis situations. Personal values and beliefs, related to religion, culture, helping others, and friendship, are strengths that might be called forth.

The nurse's ultimate goal is to assist the client to use strengths to be as independent, self-sufficient, and as self-actualized as possible given the circumstances. Although these strengths may be assessed on the basis of observation, it may be possible to obtain additional information by asking directly, "What do you see your personal strengths to be?"

External Resources

Most persons have a variety of external resources that can be used in times of need. Obvious ones may be money or insurance, which can buy services or provide the means to establish different environments. The factors that affect psychosocial function may also be considered appropriate external resources: family or neighbors, members of one's cultural or religious group, co-workers, formal organizations, and even pets. A general term for these particular resources is **social support systems.** Many resources that are available to the general public should also be considered (*e.g.*, crisis centers, social services agencies, or educational organizations).

Frequently the nurse, by bringing to the situation a sense of professional objectivity and an expert knowledge of resources available in the community, can put the client in contact with both his own internal strengths and appropriate external resources. If the nurse does not know the information firsthand, an appropriate inquiry can be made or the client can be referred to other health-care providers or even to a family member who can provide the assistance needed in a way acceptable to both resource and client.

Nursing Assessment of Psychological Status

General

Physical Assessment

Physical illness or disability is pertinent to a total assessment of a person's psychological function. Included in this category would be conditions that require emotional adjustment, such as threats to life and altered body image, or specific conditions, such as a history of seizures that might impose a different sort of alteration on psychological function. Similarly, the person's physical appearance, energy level, posture, and response to other people indicate something important about his perception of self.

Perception of Self

The nurse will want to know from direct report how the client perceives his personal world and translates events or circumstances concerning him.

- How does he see his health problem?
- How has this affected the significant people in his life and his relationship with them?
- How does he describe his life work or occupation?
- Is his income adequate to meet his needs?
- How does the health problem affect his life-style? Self-esteem? Body image?
- Does he report stresses?

Social Support Systems

Persons

- Who does the person turn to for support in his everyday concerns?
- Who does he turn to in times of difficulty?
- How do these persons or groups help the person?
- Are these usual support systems available to the person at this time?
- If not, what substitute support systems would he consider most helpful?

Ethnicity

- Is his race, culture, or ethnicity a major source of identity or belonging?

Religious or Spiritual Resources and Life Goals

- Does the person belong to an organized religion?
- How does he participate in religious activities?
- What does the person consider important in life?
- What are his plans for the future (even the next day)?
- What is his attitude toward his present life situation and toward the past?

Other

For some individuals, the support systems may be material objects such as their familiar home environment, their workplace, or perhaps financial holdings or family heirlooms.

Mental Status

A detailed mental assessment is also a part of the total psychological assessment. This will be discussed in Chapter 16.

Affective or Feeling States

- What kinds of situations cause anxiety or anger?
- How does the person feel in new situations or with strange people?
- How does he feel about accepting help for his health problem?
- How is his feeling tone reflected in his facial expression, body language, and behavior?
- Are anxiety or other emotions present or absent?

Behavior

Coping

- How does the person describe his adaptive behavior to stressful situations?
- What behaviors does he use to cope?
- How does he make decisions?
- Does he engage in health maintenance behavior? (See Person Assessment Guide, Appendix A.)

Life-Style

Sometimes we think of life-style in the context of activities of daily living, culture, or sexuality. A life-style is also a fairly consistent manner of functioning. It includes thinking, perceiving, and feeling and represents a way of responding to life in general rather than just to specific stresses. Healthy life-styles include satisfying social relationships, productive work, and behavior within societal norms (Fig. 15-2). Disruptive life-styles include impulsiveness, addiction, obsessive–compulsive behavior, and paranoid ideation (Wilson and Kneisel, 1979, pp. 316–377).

By now it should be obvious that it is not easy to isolate the various types of psychological function for assessment. Thoughts and feelings influence man's adaptive behavior. If nurses recognize that psychological functioning is an integrative mechanism, they will be alert to the constant interplay among thoughts, feelings, and behavior which occurs in the holistic person.

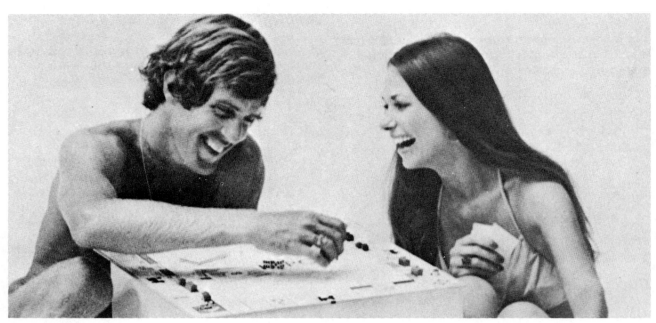

Figure 15-2
Healthy life-styles include satisfying social relationships,
productive work, and behavior within societal norms.

Nursing Process
Applied to Specific Psychological Problems

Anxiety

Assessment

Anxiety is a generalized feeling or emotion that occurs in response to an uncertain situation. It can be described as a state of tension and apprehension or as a sense of uneasiness that is felt when anticipating an unknown threat or danger. Because man is adaptive and his life situations are filled with uncertainty, anxiety is an inevitable result of living.

Anxiety can be contrasted with *fear*, which can be defined as an emotional state in which the object of the fear is an external threat of which the person is consciously aware. Both anxiety and fear are responses to some perceived interference in adapting to life situations. Both cause a physiological reaction. The energy of anxiety is not directly observed, but when adrenalin is released into the circulation, the flight-or-fight response occurs. As Brown suggests, muscle tension, the physical expression of anxiety, often braces the body without the person's being aware until after the anxiety-producing situation has passed (Brown, 1978).

Anxiety is often characterized according to behavioral responses. Some of the behavioral signs of the levels of anxiety are as follows:

- Mild—dry mouth, syncope, increased alertness to current happenings
- Moderate—perception narrowed
- Severe—discomfort increases, thoughts become scattered
- Panic—vomiting, loss of speech, withdrawal

Other behavioral signs of anxiety include nausea and vomiting, pallor and flushing, hives or red spots on the skin, increased motor activity such as wringing hands and pacing, incontinence, and inappropriate affect, usually laughing.

Nursing Interventions

Adapting to stressful situations may cause anxiety. Several strategies recommended by Brown (1978), among others, are listed below:

- Choosing to be less responsive to stressful situations
- Maintaining a less reactive physiologic state
- Intervening to ease physiologic responses
- Learning to recover more quickly

Although there are many situations that would produce anxiety in most persons, each person experiences anxiety in an individual way. Nurses can provide therapeutic assistance only to the extent that they understand this notion and do not make inappropriate assumptions.

On the other hand, it would be reasonable to expect that most persons find hospitals, unknown tests and therapies, and separation from familiar environment and support systems to be anxiety provoking. Therefore, reasonable explanations based on the person's age, level of understanding, and past experiences are appropriate interventions to reduce or minimize anxiety. Johnson (1974) found that anxiety and pain associated with tests or therapies could be decreased if nurses intervened by preparing persons for the sensations they were about to experience. When anxiety manifests itself in related physical symptoms, attention to these related "aches and pains" should be offered without value judgment. That is, the nurse should not make judgments about the pain someone else reports he is experiencing.

Another approach to reducing fear is to promote relaxation and distraction. It is thought that being in a state of physical relaxation is incompatible with anxiety. For this reason, biofeedback or simple relaxation techniques may prove useful. Knowles (1981) suggests the two exercises of round breathing and breath holding as activities that distract from anxious ideation.

Additionally, the nurse can capitalize on the fact that mild anxiety may motivate the person to learn new and necessary information and skills. An intervention appropriate to anxiety or other more specific feelings and emotions is to help the person identify, describe, express, and accept responsibility for feelings (Parsons and Sanford, 1979, p. 36).

Altered Body Image

Body image, or the way a person views his physical self, is based on his perceptions and knowledge about his appearance, boundaries, limits, and inner structure (Roberts, 1978, p. 267). This perception is developed throughout life by the way we interact with the environment and with those around us.

When body image is altered there is an accompanying period of grieving for the lost body part or function. With some health problems the loss will be visibly apparent, as in the case of an amputated limb. In other situations, such as the loss of reproductive organs following hysterectomy or mastectomy, the alteration in body image may not be as obvious to the casual observer.

Although the degree of physical disability is the most obvious factor affecting adaptation to altered body image, there are several other factors, including the reactions of others, cultural beliefs, and the person's own perception of the loss. Figure 15-3 illustrates the perception of loss by an 11-year-old girl with scoliosis. Note that a tree has become a metaphor for the body. Compare the twisted limbs of the preoperative tree drawing to the straighter trunk and limbs of the trees drawn after surgery. Nathan postulates, "This girl's ambivalence about surgery is indicated in the preoperative picture by the shining sun, that suggests optimism, while the tree itself has lost all of its leaves and appears to be weeping. The postoperative drawing of a tree, while straighter, is isolated and barren. The isolated, barren tree suggests apathy, depression and lack of interest in the environment, which is an accurate portrayal of most patients during the postoperative period. At one year follow-up the tree in her drawing is beginning to regain its leafy growth, and suggests the return of strength and vitality" (1977, p. 143).

Persons with the same disability do not necessarily grieve equally, although generally most experience the various stages of the grieving process: denial, anger, bargaining, depression, and eventual acceptance. Communication skills, particularly empathy skills, help the nurse to assess the amount of loss the person is feeling (see Chap. 13).

Assessment

Persons who are experiencing altered body image exhibit signs that the sensitive observer can interpret as manifestations of grieving. Unfortunately, not all health professionals interpret these signs correctly. A young student once commented that her client "sure was crabby today." This "crabbiness" was really anger; the client was mourning the impending amputation of his foot, a loss that would end his career as an automobile test driver.

This example illustrates the need to assess for signs of altered body image in any individual who experiences loss of a body part. These signs include verbal or nonverbal expressions of denial, anger, depression, or anxiety. Denial may be subtle, such

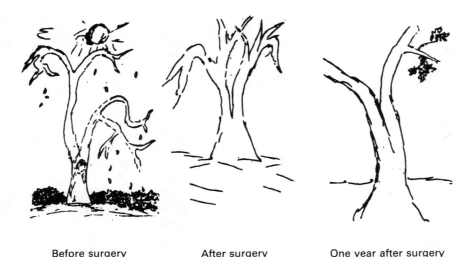

Before surgery   After surgery   One year after surgery

Figure 15-3
Tree drawings of an 11-year-old scoliosis patient: (A) before surgery, (B)
soon after surgery, (C) 1 year after
surgery. *(Nathan SW: Body image of
scoliotic female adolescents before
and after surgery. MCN J 6:139–149,
Fall, 1977)*

as refusing to talk about the loss or calling a paralyzed
body part by a name (*e.g.,* Homer), indicating that it
no longer is considered part of the self. Once altered
body image is identified, the nurse must use communication skills to help the person verbalize his
feelings about it.

Nursing Interventions

The nurse's role is to help the person adapt to the
loss and develop a positive body image. One of the
most important means of achieving this goal is to
display an accepting attitude. Nurses are often viewed
as "significant others" by their clients. As such, they
serve as mirrors through which clients gauge the
attitudes of others toward their altered bodies. If the
nurse conveys a sense of caring and acceptance, the
client will also be more inclined to accept his
limitations. Touching the person, spending time with
him, and being available to talk about his condition
are different ways of demonstrating acceptance.

Another approach is to encourage the individual
to acknowledge the loss by talking about it and even
looking at it. Nurses might gently encourage the man
with a recent leg amputation to view himself in a
mirror or assist the woman who has had a stroke to
talk about her paralyzed arm. Such interventions
help these people form a realistic picture of their
losses and incorporate these changes into a new
body image. To offer this guidance effectively, nurses
must feel comfortable with their own feelings about
these disabilities so that they can discuss them in
an objective manner.

The nurse can also help family members develop
acceptance toward the loss by helping them to look
at, touch, or talk about the changes that have taken
place. This is an important intervention because the

positive attitude of significant others will help the
person adapt more easily to his altered body image.
Table 15-4 shows a sample care plan for a person
experiencing altered body image due to an amputation of the left leg. Other nursing interventions for
the person experiencing loss are described in Chapter 29 (Grief and Loss).

Low Self-Esteem

Self-esteem is the part of self-concept that deals
with self-regard. A person's view of self is thought to
control both his behavior and his relationships with
others. Rogers suggested (1951, p. 507), "Most of the
ways of behaving which are adopted by the organism
are those which are consistent with the concept of
self." In the hierarchy of basic human needs, Maslow
(1970) places self-esteem between love and belonging,
and self-actualization. Branden (1969) emphasized
that an individual's self-evaluation is the single most
significant key to his behavior, because self-evaluation or regard affects thinking, emotions, desires,
values, and goals. Any threat to a person's functional
ability is also a threat to the person's self-esteem.

Assessment

The person with low self-esteem regards or evaluates
himself poorly in comparison with others and with
what he thinks his ideal self should be. There are
many formal tools that psychologists use to measure
self-esteem. Most are beyond the intent of nursing
assessment. However, one such instrument (Bills,
1975) provides us with positive and negative adjectives that persons might be asked to use to describe

---

Table 15-4
Sample Nursing Care Plan for Persons
with Altered Body Image Due to Mobility Problems

Problem	Goals	Interventions
Altered body image related to left leg amputation	Client will verbalize feelings about altered body image.	Convey warm, accepting attitude. Help person to view altered body part.
Depression and anxiety secondary to grief response	Depression and anxiety will decrease; client will verbalize the change	Provide opportunities for client to talk about altered motor function. Assist family to discuss impact of mobility problem. Assist client with physical appearance. Teach client new ways of performing motor function.

---

themselves (Table 15-5). A client may use some of the negative adjectives or may describe himself as the opposite of some of the positive words (*i.e.,* incompetent, without purpose, unworthy). Bills (1975) thought that the discrepancy between a person's self-esteem rating and his concept of his ideal self influenced both self-satisfaction and personal adjustment.

Other attitudes may be noted when assessing self-esteem. Does the client say that bad things always happen to him? Is this his expectation? Does he accept himself as he is? Do his words or actions suggest that he believes himself unworthy of help, close relationships, or professional concern?

This last point is especially pertinent because health professionals often expect clients to act on their own behalf and care for themselves. However, low self-esteem may be the cause of poor health practices such as overeating or failure to take prescribed medications. The relationship of such practices to low self-esteem may be overlooked if health providers expect clients always to care well for themselves. At the same time, we should remember that, just as anxiety can be motivating, temporary low self-esteem actually may precede a change toward heightened self-esteem.

Nursing Interventions

Rogers (1951) suggested that if persons are treated with unconditional positive regard by others, the likelihood of their viewing themselves with positive regard or esteem will be increased. This is perhaps the first principle underlying nursing intervention. A nurse operating on this principle behaves as follows:

* Does not express value judgments about the person's feelings, beliefs, or behaviors
* Considers the client's uniqueness in all care
* Handles the client's body and all interactions with respect and dignity
* Recognizes and encourages his strengths and adaptive coping behavior

---

Table 15-5
Adjectives to Assess Self-Esteem

Positive	Negative
Competent	Annoying
Dependable	Cruel
Mature	Fearful
Purposeful	Nervous
Stable	Reckless
Successful	Sarcastic
Useful	Stubborn
Worthy	Fault-finding

From Bills RE: A System for Assessing Affectivity. University: The University of Alabama Press, 1975

Through appropriate assessment, goals, and interventions, the nurse enables the client to achieve the small successes necessary to promote self-worth (Fig. 15-4). An essential aspect of this goal is to maintain physical appearance. Helping the male client to shave or the female person to apply makeup or perfume may be the first step toward rebuilding self-esteem.

It should not be surprising that problems of altered body image and low self-esteem frequently occur together. Teaching the person to deal with disabilities by acquiring new abilities is one way to foster a sense of independence. For example, a woman with a paralyzed arm will need to learn new ways of grooming, bathing, eating, cooking, and doing other activities. As she learns how to carry out these activities, the woman incorporates an understanding of her abilities and her limitations into a new body image. As she learns that she can perform many of her old activities by using new techniques, she will come to reestablish a sense of self-esteem.

In fostering new abilities, it is important that the nurse establish realistic expectations and teach skills that the person can successfully perform. Establishing unattainable goals only sets the stage for failure, intensifies frustration, and results in lowered self-esteem. Therefore, whatever intervention the nurse chooses to institute must be aimed at enhancing self-esteem in order to promote healthful behavior.

Figure 15-4
Small successes help in promoting self-worth. *(Photo by D. Atkinson)*

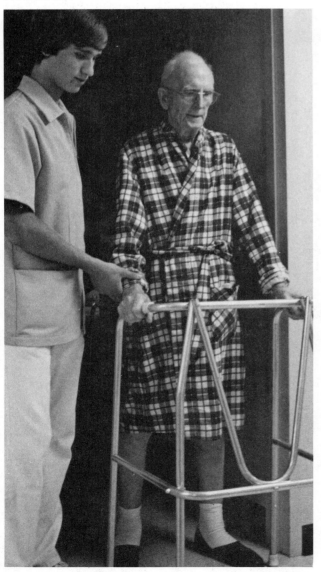

Emotional Support

To provide **emotional support** means to offer encouragement or to sustain someone with empathy. It involves acknowledging the need that all people have for interpersonal warmth. This need, which exists from birth, fosters growth and development and remains with us until death. Turning to a comforting person is a common and healthy coping strategy. Because nurses are perceived as sources of comfort and because they are the most available health professionals in most health-care settings, they are frequently called upon to offer emotional support in a variety of situations. In our personal lives, we are selective about the emotional support we offer. However, in a health-care setting, professional nurses are expected to attend to the psychosocial needs of the clients on demand. This expectation may be threatening to students and experienced practitioners alike. However, most of the strategies that your client would probably find most helpful are quite appropriate for beginning students to initiate.

Suggested strategies for providing emotional support include the following:

- Engaging in active listening and maintaining appropriate silence
- Assuming a friendly manner by introducing oneself when appropriate
- Smiling
- Supplying needed information and answering questions or finding someone else to do so
- Providing unhurried activity with the person

- Allowing and encouraging the client to maintain independence
- Anticipating the need for support and equipping the person to deal with a difficult situation in advance, either by direct personal action or by referral
- Being spontaneous and natural

On this last point, we should note that a spontaneous reaction on the part of the nurse may very well provide more comfort and support than a formal response. Thus, a comforting touch or hug, which initially may seem inappropriate, will nonetheless convey a sense of caring and concern and provide the emotional support that is needed. This is indeed an opportunity for therapeutic use of self. Additional insight into empathic responses can be obtained by reviewing the chapter on Communication.

Obviously, most of the strategies listed above are suitable for initial meetings or brief encounters. In life-threatening or long-term situations, other strategies might be more appropriate. Whatever the circumstances, the client needs to feel that the environment is psychologically safe. A major priority in this regard is to build a trusting relationship. Interventions for developing trust are listed in Table 14-3. In essence, then, providing emotional support is a widely applicable nursing intervention that enhances person-centered care.

Conclusion

Areas of psychological function of most concern to nurses are cognition or thinking, operant behavior, and the affective domain of feelings or emotions. The psychological status has been shown to be significant because the integrative function it serves enables the person to behave as a holistic thinking and feeling individual who is adapting to a complex world. Several factors affecting psychosocial functioning are: general social factors; family, peer, and significant other relationships; psychosocial developmental status; and emotional adjustment. The many social factors that contribute to each person's psychological outlook have special implications for nurses. Because man is a social being, both his strengths and his needs are enmeshed in his relationships with others. Psychological functioning has also been presented as a synthesis of basic personal characteristics and psychosocial development. Emotional adjustment is both the process and the outcome of meeting basic human needs and resolving developmental tasks.

Developing internal strengths and mobilizing external resources are important strategies in planning nursing care. Identifying these strengths constitutes an important part of the nursing assessment of psychological status.

Common psychological problems include anxiety, altered body image, and low self-esteem. Because anxiety is an inevitable and universal occurrence, the nurse will often be faced with the need to assist clients to adapt to stressful situations that cause anxiety. Altered body image may present as either an obvious or a subtle problem. Since it represents loss which is unique to the individual, this problem is especially challenging to the nurse who strives to give person-centered care. Self-esteem is a motivating factor of particular importance because it affects thinking, feeling, and behavior. Low self-esteem becomes a health concern particularly as it affects thoughts and feelings related to health behavior. Providing emotional support for persons facing all these problems represents a major nursing intervention in promoting healthy adaptation.

Study Questions

1. Anxiety is an unseen psychological phenomenon. What implications does this fact have for the nurse's communication and observation skills?

2. Defense mechanisms may be adaptive or maladaptive. Explain.

3. John S., age 14, is experiencing the turbulence of adolescence. He often releases his frustration by hitting out physically at other persons. What more satisfactory coping strategies might you suggest for John's use?

4. Karen T., 16 years old, is awaiting corrective orthopedic surgery. This is her first hospitalization. How will you determine what she is feeling?

5. Mrs. R. is awaiting a radical mastectomy for cancer. How do you think this surgery will affect her body image and self-esteem?

6. Mr. W. requires complete morning care, including a full bed bath. Explain how the nurse might use this time to provide emotional support to Mr. W.

Glossary

Adjustment: The process and outcome of a person's coping with life in society.

Affect: The feeling tone of a person's reaction to other persons or situations. Interchangeable with "emotion" in common usage.

Anxiety: A diffuse, unpleasant, vague feeling of apprehension, nervousness, or dread expressed both somatically and psychically.

Cognition: Thinking.

Coping skills: Adaptive response consisting of cognitive function, motor activity, affect, and psychological defenses.

Defense mechanisms: Processes beyond a person's awareness that protect the person against anxiety (see Table 15-3).

Emotion: The feeling tone of a person's reaction to other persons or situations. Interchangeable with "affect" in common usage.

Emotional support: Encouragement provided with feeling.

Flatness of affect: Dulled emotional tone; most frequently noted in severely disturbed emotional states.

Operant behavior: Roughly equivalent to voluntary behavior. The kind of behavior that makes up most of the everyday activity of persons. Called operant because a person's own behavior brings consequences that change his action.

Personality: An individual's unique way of feeling and responding to situations. A person's own characteristic pattern of behavior, emotions, motives, thoughts, and attitudes.

Psychology: The science that studies behavior and the unseen processes that shape behavior.

Self-esteem: The self-regard dimension of self-concept. It is thought to control both behavior and relationship with others.

Social support systems: External resources such as family, neighbors, co-workers, peer group members, and even pets.

Bibliography

Anxiety: Recognition and intervention programmed instruction. Reprint from Am J Nurs 65:129–152, 1965

Bills RE: A System for Assessing Affectivity. University, AL, University of Alabama Press, 1975

Branden N: The Psychology of Self Esteem. Los Angeles, Nash, 1969

Brown BB: Stress and the Art of Biofeedback. New York, Bantam Books, 1978

Carpenter F: The Skinner Primer. New York, Free Press, 1974

Cohn L: Coping with anxiety: A step-by-step guide. Nurs '79 9:34–37, December, 1979

Engel G: Psychological Development in Health and Disease. Philadelphia, WB Saunders, 1962

Francis G: The therapeutic use of pets. Nurs Outlook 29:369–370, June, 1981

Freud A: The Ego and the Mechanisms of Defense, rev ed. New York, International Universities Press, 1966

Hall CS, Lindzey G: Theories of Personality, 2nd ed. New York, John Wiley & Sons, 1970

Hazzard ME, Thorndal ML et al: Patient anxiety: Teaching students to intervene. Journal of Nurs Educ 4:19–21, January/February, 1979

Johnson JE, Rice VH: Sensory and distress components of pain. Nurs Res 23:203–209, 1974

Kalisch B: What is empathy? Am J Nurs 73:1548–1552, September, 1973

Knowles RD: Dealing with feelings: Managing anxiety. Am J Nurs 81:110–111, January, 1981

Maslow A: Motivation and Personality, 2nd ed. New York, Harper & Row, 1970

Morris CG: Psychology, An Introduction. New York, Appleton-Century-Crofts, 1973

Nathan SW: Body image of scoliotic female adolescents before and after surgery. Matern Child Nurs J 6:139–149, Fall, 1977

Parsons V, Sanford N: Interpersonal Interaction in Nursing. Menlo Park, CA, Addison-Wesley, 1979

Peterson MH: Understanding defense mechanisms: Programmed instruction. Am J. Nurs 72:1651–1674, September, 1972

Piaget J: Biology and Knowledge: An Essay on the Relationship Between Organic Regulation and Cognition Processes. Chicago, University of Chicago Press, 1971

Roberts S: Behavioral Concepts and Nursing Throughout the Lifespan. Englewood Cliffs, NJ, Prentice-Hall, 1978

Rogers CR: Client Centered Therapy. Boston, Houghton-Mifflin, 1951

Wilson HS, Kneisel CR: Psychiatric Nursing. Menlo Park, CA, Addison-Wesley, 1979

Mental Status

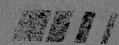

Sue Fink

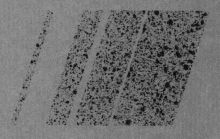

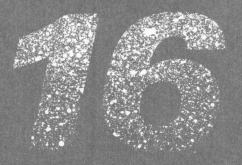

After completing this chapter, students will be able to:

- Identify factors affecting mental status.

- Describe the assessment of a person's mental status.

- Recognize alterations of mental status and their implications for the person's independent functioning.

- Explain appropriate nursing interventions for persons with altered mental status.

This chapter focuses on the assessment of a person's mental status and the implications that alterations in mental status have for nursing care. A person's ability to adapt to his environment is dependent on his mental functioning. When a client is alert and responds to our questions or asks questions of his own in a clear organized manner, we often assess this function without too much conscious thought. However, other situations may call for a more complete assessment to enable us to identify interventions that can be instituted to promote and maintain well being.

The nurse is often the health-care provider who is in a position to identify alterations in a client's mental status, regardless of the setting. For example, the nurse in a community setting may be the first to notice clues of deteriorating mental functioning such as changes in grooming or housekeeping. The nursing staff in an acute-care setting, through continuous assessment, can identify early changes in mental status that often accompany illness and hospitalization. Through complete assessment of the client, early interventions needed to promote health can be identified.

Alterations in a client's mental status affect all aspects of the nursing process. Initially, the assessment phase may need to be adjusted to fit the circumstances. For example, if the client has a problem with attention, it may be necessary to conduct the interview in several short sessions. If the client is unable to understand or use language to speak, secondary sources such as charts and family members will need to be used to obtain historical information. If the client responds slowly and requires frequent redirection, more time will be needed for the interview. It is often best in these instances to decide which parts of the interview are most essential for planning nursing care. Regardless of the degree of impairment, it should be remembered that the client himself is the only source of information about his perceptions and anxieties. When a client's thought or communication processes are diminished, the nurse must make increased efforts to understand the person, rather than to discount what he says. For example, a statement such as "the bugs are biting" may actually be the patient's perception of the discomfort caused by lying on a small object. Or the client's insistence of the need to "get those shoes out of here and burn them up" should not be dismissed without closer assessment to determine possible reasons.

The planning and intervention phases of the nursing process are affected in several ways by the client's mental status, including the degree to which he is able to participate in planning objectives and carrying out interventions. The comatose person may be totally dependent on the nurse, whereas persons with less profound alterations will have a greater ability to participate in their own care. Thus, the client's mental status must be considered when deciding what objectives are achievable. The mentally impaired person may be able to learn the concrete steps of self-care but unable to learn the abstract reasons for these steps.

Factors Affecting Mental Status

Alterations in mental status occur across all age groups and with many different health deviations. The school nurse will need to assess the child who falls and hits his head. The community health nurse will want to assess the person who is unable to follow the conversation or express himself as clearly as in past visits. Nurses in acute-care settings will monitor patients of all ages for any changes in mental status that may accompany the physiological and psychological stressors of acute illness.

While the focus of this chapter will be on assessment and intervention with the adult client, many of the same techniques can be used with children. When assessing children, the nurse should use the normal developmental patterns for the child's age to analyze the data. Interested students may wish to refer to the norms provided by Burns and Johnson (1980) for assessing children's mental status. The Denver Developmental Screening Tool is a helpful tool in evaluating the mental development of preschool children.

Man's response to his environment and his cognitive ability are dependent on intact brain function and therefore can be altered by any of the physiological processes that affect brain cell metabolism, as well as by direct injury to brain tissues. Also, emotional, social, and environmental factors can influence mental status, as indicated in Table 16-1. The older adult is particularly susceptible to impaired mental function because physiological changes brought on by age tend to lower reserve capacity and decrease the body's ability to adapt to stressors. Loss of social and emotional support often contributes to the elderly person's vulnerability.

Nursing Assessment of Mental Status

Level of Consciousness

Consciousness means awareness of self and the environment. Although such awareness cannot be measured directly, it is inferred from objective data about the person's behavior and response to stimuli. Clinically, **level of consciousness** generally refers to the degree to which a person is responsive to the environment—or state of arousal. The subjective component of consciousness—awareness of self—will be discussed in the section on orientation.

Recording Level of Consciousness

Many classifications and grading systems have been used to describe levels of consciousness. Terms such as "stupor," "semiconscious," and "comatose" are not clearly defined and should be avoided. Research has demonstrated that there is little agreement among observers when these terms are used for assessment (Teasdale, Knill-Jones, and Van Der Sande, 1978).

Figure 16-1 shows the Glasgow Coma Scale, which describes eye opening, verbal response, and motor response on a numbered scale. It has been used in a number of settings to improve observer reliability (Jones, 1979a and 1979b, Teasdale and Jennett, 1974). Settings in which a large number of unconscious or seriously ill persons are cared for

Table 16-1
Factors Causing Altered Mental Status

Central Nervous System Factors

- Trauma to brain tissues
- Space-occupying tumors or lesions
- Infectious processes such as encephalitis and meningitis
- Cerebral vascular problems such as stroke, thrombi, emboli
- Mental retardation and learning disabilities
- Degenerative brain disease

Systemic Factors

- Cerebral hypoxia due to respiratory or circulatory insufficiency
- Disturbances in fluid, electrolyte, and acid–base balance
- Metabolic disorders such as diabetes and pernicious anemia or hepatic, renal, or thyroid diseases
- Alcohol or drug intoxication and withdrawal
- Hyperthermia or hypothermia

Other Factors

- Sensory deprivation or overload due to social and environmental factors or sensory impairments
- Psychological reactions such as anxiety, stress, and depression
- Malnutrition

"Can be roused by vigorous shaking while calling his name."

"Moans and opens eyes, but forms no intelligible words."

"Moves all extremities spontaneously, but does not move to command."

"Unresponsive to verbal stimuli or touch. Withdraws from painful stimuli, but does not open eyes."

Stimuli

Impaired consciousness occurs along a continuum. As the level of consciousness deteriorates, the person responds more slowly and requires stronger stimuli to evoke a response. When the person responds to

Table 16-2
Assessment of Level of Consciousness

Observe eye movements, verbal response, and motor responses in each category:

1. Spontaneous activity
   - Verbal or nonverbal communication
   - Position changes and movement of body parts
   - Restlessness, frequency of movement
   - Eye opening
2. Response to environmental stimuli
   - Light
   - Noise
3. Response to verbal stimuli
   - Reaction when name is called
   - Ability to respond to questions
   - Ability to follow simple command (lift arm)
   - Ability to follow complex command (hand me the glass)
   - Ability to grip examiner's hands (compare right and left to test neuromotor response as well as ability to respond to command)
4. Response to tactile stimuli
   - Light touch
   - Vigorous movements
5. Response to pain
   - Treatments
   - Applied stimuli

are likely to have some standard format for assessing level of consciousness.

When no standard format is used, the nurse will need to describe the patient's behavior and the stimulus that was used to elicit that behavior. Vision and hearing acuity must be taken into account in evaluating responses to environmental and verbal stimuli. Table 16-2 lists some observations and stimuli used in assessing level of consciousness. Observations are generally made in the order listed, but tactile stimuli may be needed to arouse the person fully before other responses are evaluated. The following are examples of the nurse's written assessment:

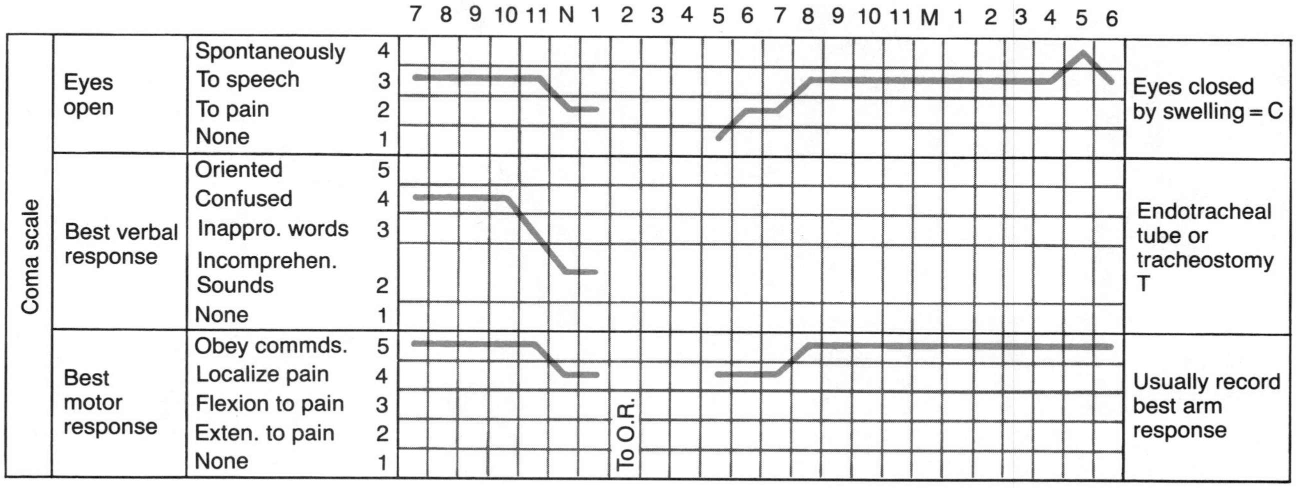

7 8 9 10 11 N 1 2 3 4 5 6 7 8 9 10 11 M 1 2 3 4 5 6

Coma scale	Eyes open	Spontaneously	4		Eyes closed by swelling = C
		To speech	3		
		To pain	2		
		None	1		
	Best verbal response	Oriented	5		Endotracheal tube or tracheostomy T
		Confused	4		
		Inappro. words	3		
		Incomprehen. Sounds	2		
		None	1		
	Best motor response	Obey commds.	5		Usually record best arm response
		Localize pain	4		
		Flexion to pain	3	To O.R.	
		Exten. to pain	2		
		None	1		

Figure 16-1

The Glasgow Coma Scale (GCS) includes three parts—assessment of eye opening, verbal response, and motor response. Each can be assessed hourly, given a numerical value, and plotted graphically. A patient's neurological status—unchanged, deteriorating, or improving—can then be monitored. In the GCS above, the patient remained stable until 10 A.M., deteriorated rapidly between 10 A.M., and 1 P.M., at which time he went to the operating room. Postoperatively, his GCS improved. *(Jones C: The Glasgow coma scale. Copyright 1979, American Journal of Nursing Company. Reproduced with permission from the American Journal of Nursing, Sept., Vol. 79, No. 9.)*

tactile stimuli, his response to pain does not need to be tested. If a painful stimulus is needed to elicit a response, applying pressure at the base of the fingernail has proven most reliable (Teasdale *et al.*, 1978). Other common methods of administering painful stimuli include applying pressure on the supraorbital notch or Achilles tendon and rubbing the sternum with the examiner's knuckles.

Pupillary Reaction

Pupils are always assessed along with consciousness. The sympathetic and parasympathetic pathways that control pupillary reactions are anatomically adjacent to brain-stem areas controlling consciousness. Therefore, assessment of the size, shape, equality, and light reactions of the pupils provides guidelines to the presence and location of brain lesions and edema. Since the pupillary pathways are quite resistant to metabolic changes, the presence or absence of the light reflex is an important sign distinguishing metabolic coma from brain injury (Plum, 1972).

The first step in examining the pupils is to observe them for size, shape, and equality. Remember that room light and various drugs affect pupil size. The pupillary response to light is then assessed by stimulating the pupil with a small bright light di-

rected from the side (Fig. 16-2). **Direct light reaction** is observed by watching the response of the stimulated pupil. **Consensual light reaction** is observed by watching the response of the unstimulated pupil.

Orientation

Assessment of Perception

Orientation refers to one's perception of time, place, and person. A person must be fully aroused before orientation can be accurately assessed. The client's behavior and responses, as well as the stimuli present, should be described. In other words, specific data rather than conclusions or labels are reported. Because terms such as "confused," "disoriented," and "senile" are used differently by different observers, these words should be avoided when observations are recorded. The term "senile" is particularly unfortunate because it implies that the altered status is due to age alone. As a result of this connotation, treatable causes of the altered mental state may not be sought.

Data to assess orientation are often obtained by observing spontaneous statements made by the client during conversation. At other times a more direct form of questioning may be necessary. If such as-

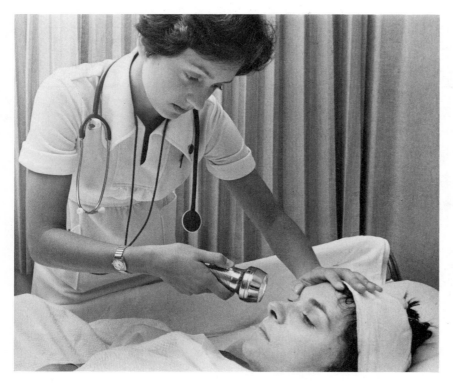

Figure 16-2
The nurse assesses pupillary reaction to light.

sessment must be carried out frequently, an explanation of why you are asking these questions is in order. For an accurate assessment, questions must be varied from time to time and should be phrased so that yes/no answers will not be given unless the person is unable to respond verbally. Examples of possible questions include the following:

- What is the name of this place?
- Where is it located?
- What day is today?
- What year is this?

Orientation to person is used to describe the client's perception of who he is and whether or not he recognizes others. The written assessment must clarify which of these aspects is being addressed. Orientation to self is broader than just the ability to give one's name. Of equal importance is the manner in which the client speaks of himself and whether or not he disregards some portion of his body. It is also important to note whether the client recognizes visitors and is able to describe accurately his relationship to them. Institutionalized persons are frequently confused about names and roles of various staff members. This seems quite understandable in

view of the fact that patients come in contact with a large number of staff who may wear similar clothing and perform the same tasks. However, when the person has had an ongoing relationship with the same care givers and has been able to recognize them, then confusion about names and roles is a significant sign of disorientation.

Assessment of the Sensory Environment

Man's ability to maintain orientation to his surroundings is dependent on the stimuli in the environment as well as on his ability to perceive and organize that stimuli. The nurse needs to be aware of the environmental stimuli to which persons are exposed in order to evaluate their responses. Frequently, the questions hospitalized persons ask indicate the strengths of their mental functioning rather than disorientation. For example, when an accident victim who entered the hospital in an unconscious state regains consciousness and asks what hospital this is, he indicates by his question that he has been able to use environmental clues to determine that he is in a hospital. Similarly, the person who was transferred to a different unit after surgery indicates by his questions about what floor he is on that he recognizes that he is in a different environment. However, when evaluting a person's orientation to time, it is important to remember that people cannot be expected to know the exact time or date when clocks and calendars are not visible or available.

Sensory Deprivation and Overload

Numerous studies have demonstrated that disorientation, disturbed feeling states, inability to think and reason, and phenomena such as **delusions** and **hallucinations** can result from altered sensory environments. The terms **sensory deprivation** and **sensory restriction** are used to refer to a reduction in the amount of meaningful sensory stimuli. **Sensory overload** refers to a marked increase in the amount or intensity of stimuli with a lack of meaningful patterns.

An accurate assessment of possible sensory deprivation or overload will depend on an understanding of the sensory stimulation levels to which a person is usually exposed. The amount of sensory stimulation that is "normal" is a highly individual matter. The gregarious, active person who seldom spends time alone might suffer sensory restriction in an environment which provides adequate stimulation for a person whose usual level of stimuli is less intense. Similarly, the person who lives alone and prefers a quiet environment may suffer sensory overload in an environment that is not overly stimulating to others.

The reticular activating system plays an important role in the processing of stimuli and behavior. It is thought that the reticular activating system adapts to certain levels of sensory stimulation. In healthy states, people behave in ways that either decrease or increase the sensory input to levels which maintain optimal states of arousal (Bolin, 1974; Linsley, 1961).

Any circumstance that alters the person's ability to control sensory input makes that person susceptible to subsequent mental alterations. The individual with sensory impairment or immobility may have difficulty maintaining his usual sensory input. The hospitalized patient may be bombarded by constant unpatterned stimuli that have little meaning for him, or he may be exposed to very little sensory stimuli. The person who is confined to bed in a single room with nothing to see but bare walls and ceiling has a restricted sensory input. At the same time, the continuous unfamiliar noises of hospital equipment and personnel and unrelieved pain may greatly increase his sensory stimuli. The elderly client who lives alone may have adapted well to impaired vision and hearing but may show signs of sensory restriction when there is a sudden decrease in mobility.

Perceptual Distortions

The term "disorientation" is sometimes used to refer to persons who experience **perceptual distortions.** These distortions range from mild images and spots before the eyes to **delusions** and **hallucinations** accompanied by high levels of anxiety and agitation. The milder forms may be assessed by asking the person if he has experienced dreams or has seen things he knew were not there. It is important to determine the presence of these perceptual distortions, because people are often worried about these experiences but do not mention them. A common statement from such persons is, "I'm glad to know those experiences are common. I thought I was losing my mind." Perceptual distortions can occur with or without disorientation to time, place, and person.

Memory

Short-Term and Long-Term Memory

Humans possess an elaborate memory system which enables them to retrieve information and incorporate new information. (Fig. 16-3). Information from our environment enters through the sense organs and goes to separate **sensory stores** that correspond to each sensory modality. The sensory stores receive a vast amount of information in the form of sensory patterns which have not been analyzed for meaning, but this information is held only briefly before it is either lost or transferred to **short-term memory.** The transfer of information to short-term memory involves pattern recognition. Since short-term memory has a limited capacity, **attention** determines which information enters short-term memory and which information is lost or decays. For example, when you are paying attention to something else, the classroom discussion does not enter your memory even though you hear the sounds.

Short-term memory has a limited capacity so information which is not rehearsed or transferred to long-term memory decays within seconds. Information may be maintained in short-term memory through **rehearsal.** Repeating a phone number to yourself as you cross the room to dial the phone is an example of rehearsal. There are individual differences in short-term memory, but these differences are probably due to the use of processing techniques

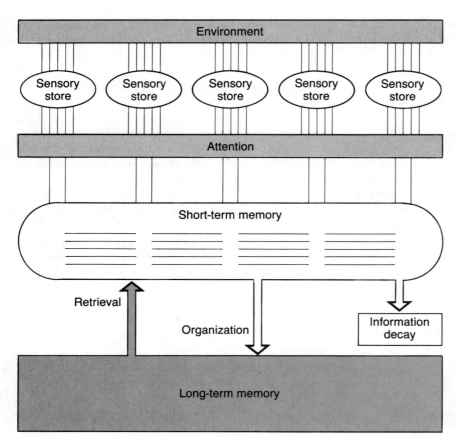

Figure 16-3
The human memory.

such as coding, rehearsal, and associations or grouping. Studies show that most people are able to hold about seven pieces of information in short-term memory at a time.

Information is transferred to **long-term memory** through rehearsal and various organizing techniques, which help us to fit the information into a new or preexisting framework that joins information into meaningful units. Long-term memory has a virtually unlimited capacity to store units of information. When information is used for problem solving, it must be retrieved from long-term memory and reentered in short-term memory. The process of forgetting may be due to interference or retrieval failure (Loftus & Loftus, 1976; Wolf, 1971).

Memory Impairment

Since short- and long-term memory rely on different processes, impairment can occur in one or both types of memory. The person who has undergone severe physical or emotional trauma may be unable to recall information from long-term memory al-though short-term memory is intact. Elderly persons may have difficulty with short-term memory while long-term memory is unaffected. This may explain why an elderly person relates events of the past accurately but cannot recall recent happenings. It also explains why the individual who elaborates thoroughly on a subject learned in the past may have more difficulty learning new material than might be anticipated. Laboratory memory tests indicate that age-related differences are due to slower learning by elderly people rather than to differences in recall (Craik, 1977).

Assessment of Memory

Clinically, a person's memory is usually assessed by his ability to recall recent or remote events. Both these areas need to be assessed on the basis of what is already known about that client. Persons with severe memory loss often give very believable but inaccurate answers to questions. This is called **con-fabulation.** Recent memory can be assessed by noting the person's recall of events over the past several hours. Although the inability to recall recent events is often interpreted as a deficit in short-term memory, actually it is a deficit in the ability to retrieve information from long-term memory. A more direct measure of short-term memory is the digit repetition test. In this test a person is given a series of nonrepeating numbers such as 519237 and is then asked to repeat them. Adults can normally repeat seven digits forward and four digits in reverse order.

Long-term memory can be assessed during the history taking process and by asking questions based on information that the client has previously learned. Asking the client to name the last three presidents or give his birthdate is a technique commonly used to assess long-term memory. Simple mathematics calculations, days of the week, and the alphabet are other types of questions that can be used.

The nurse should be cautioned, however, that clients may fail to respond to these questions because they see them as irrelevant or as an attempt to make them look foolish. The most successful assessment will be one in which the information needed is gathered during a meaningful interaction that is not viewed by the client as interrogation.

Persons with severe cognitive impairment often share with the nurse reminiscences about their personal histories, although they are unable to answer simple questions. These recollections would need to be validated by a family member if possible. Sometimes these "stories" can be verified, indicating an area of intact functioning; at other times they turn out to be stories that enabled the person to have a pleasant social interaction.

The nurse should ask clients whether they have noted any problems with or changes in their memory. Persons often need assistance in coping with relatively minor changes that would not be detected in the usual assessment. Elderly persons often voice concern about their memory. Studies have shown that persons who complain of poor memory often perform better on objective memory tests than those who report good memory. This discrepancy between objective measures of memory and subjective reports appears to be related to stereotypes of aging and depression (Zarit, 1979). When a young person misplaces his keys or misses an appointment, it is inconvenient or irritating, but it will not be viewed by him or others as a sign of beginning mental deterioration.

Even when it is clear from assessment that a memory loss exists, asking about it directly may help reveal how the client feels about it and adapts to it in his everyday life. Whenever any kind of impairment is identified, the nurse will want to assess how this affects the client's life so that assistance with adaptation can be offered when needed. Sensitivity to the effects of attention is also necessary. We all remember best the things that have meaning for us. The client whose wife always puts his pills on the table for him may refer to her when asked what pills he is taking even though he demonstrates in other ways that his memory is intact.

Mental Capacity

Knowledge of the client's education and type of employment provides clues about intellectual functions, although it must be remembered that such data are only clues. Past performance at times bears little relationship to current functioning. Therefore, formal education and socioeconomic status do not always accurately reflect mental capacity. One of the first things to note is the client's attention span.

- How long (in minutes) does the client concentrate on one topic?
- Does he change the subject or stop attending to what is being said?
- Does he show any nonverbal signs of inattention such as body movement and wandering eye movements?

The client's ability to understand ideas can be determined by asking him to state in his own words the ideas you have been discussing with him. Often this will happen spontaneously in the course of an interview or teaching session. The degree of understanding the client shows in discussing his current problems and situation may provide data about his grasp of both concrete and abstract ideas.

Clinically, several methods are used to assess the person's understanding of abstract ideas. The client may be asked to explain a proverb such as:

"Don't cry over spilled milk."

"Don't put all your eggs in one basket."

"A rolling stone gathers no moss."

The person who cannot deal with abstractions will interpret these sayings very literally. For example he might say, "If milk is spilled mop it up instead of crying."

Another objective measure of abstract thinking is to ask the person how a series of words is related to each other. For example:

- Car, train, airplane (used for transportation, require fuel)

- Apple, pear, orange (fruits, edible, grow on trees)
- Goldfish, dog, cat (pets)

Although these methods of assessment can be useful, remember that what the nurse really needs to know is whether the client is able to understand ideas without concrete examples. This has a bearing on health teaching. For example, because the inner workings of the body may appear to be very abstract to many persons, effective teaching about physiological functions and pathophysiology often requires concrete examples, analogies, models, or drawings.

The nurse's primary interest in assessing the client's intellect and judgment is to determine his ability to learn and perform self-care. A great deal of information about mental capacity is gained when the ability to understand ideas is assessed.

- How does the client express himself?
- Are thoughts presented in a logical organized manner?
- What kind of vocabulary and sentence structure does the client use?

Often the nurse will want to evaluate problem-solving ability in very specific instances. For example, how does the person plan to get to his appointment next week? or how would a person who lives alone get help in the event of an accident? Again, the nurse will want to assess how the client's mental functioning affects the way he adapts to his usual environment and to added stressors.

Communication

General Assessment

While interacting with the client the nurse will be assessing the person's capacity to communicate.

- Is the client able to hear you?
- Does he indicate by his verbal or behavioral responses that he understands what is being said?
- How does he respond?

Speech Patterns

Speech patterns and vocabulary are closely related to mental functioning. Normally, speech is easy and free flowing and thoughts are expressed in a fairly organized manner. The person whose thought processes are impaired will speak slowly in short simple sentences with few descriptive terms and a quite limited vocabulary.

Affect

Much of the emotional content of communication is conveyed through **affect.** Affect is the person's tone of voice, speed of delivery, and facial expression. When a person says, "I'm going away this weekend," his affect often tells us whether he anticipates or dreads the trip. However, it is important to remember that these clues can easily be misread. Therefore, verbal clarification is needed. Whether the person's affect matches the content of what he is saying should also be noted. For example, when a person says he is happy about something or angry about something, does his affect match what he says? Does his affect change according to the content or is it the same throughout the interview?

Body Language

Hand movements, gestures, posture, and general appearance are forms of **body language** that should be assessed. Body language is less consciously controlled than speech and is often a more accurate reflection of how a person feels. Body language may either reinforce or contradict the spoken message. If the nurse says, "I'd like to talk with you," and then sits back in a relaxed posture, the nonverbal communication reinforces her words. If the same verbal message is given while the nurse sits on the edge of her chair and glances at her watch, contradictory messages are sent. The body-language message, "I'm too busy now," is usually the one received. Similarly, the person who says he is not at all anxious but continuously crosses and uncrosses his legs and twists the buttons on his jacket is sending contradictory messages.

Language Disorders

Communication is a complex process which requires the ability to receive messages, interpret their meaning, and form a response. Disruptions may occur in any of these areas without emotional disturbance or cognitive impairment. For example, the person who has undergone laryngectomy or has vocal cord paralysis will have communication problems that relate to sound production. Some neurological deficits affect only the ability to control the musculature needed for clear articulation of speech. This is called **dysarthria.**

Aphasia

Aphasia, on the other hand, is the general term used to describe disruptions in the ability to interpret and respond to verbal and written language. Aphasia is most commonly caused by a cerebral vascular accident (CVA or stroke).

The left hemisphere of the brain is the dominant area for communication in most people. The message that a person hears is carried along neural pathways to the left temporal lobe. There it is received and interpreted. The message then goes from the temporal lobe to the frontal lobe where the motor patterns for speech are formed and sent to the speech muscles. Disruptions in any part of this circuit will cause aphasia (Norman and Baratz, 1979).

There are several types of asphasia. Depending on the area of brain damage, aphasic persons may have difficulty with comprehension, response, or both. People with primary impairment in comprehension are able to speak in an articulate and effortless manner with normal rhythm, intonation, and rate of speech. However, expression errors such as word and sound substitutions are common, because the person is unable to comprehend what he is saying. Errors in writing will be similar to those made in speech. Reading comprehension will parallel auditory comprehension. When the client's primary problem is in response, speech will be labored and he may only articulate a few words. Reading comprehension is usually intact, but writing will be impaired to the same degree as speech (Norman and Baratz, 1979; Piotrowski, 1978).

There are several levels of language: automatic, imitative, and symbolic. The lowest level, automatic speech, is the last to be affected by aphasia. Social gesture speech (*e.g.*, Hello, How are you, Fine), songs, prayers, and swearing are examples of automatic speech. Aphasic persons often produce automatic speech without conscious awareness. At the imitative level the person is able to repeat what is said to him but unable to form phrases on his own. Symbolic language is the ability to express thought fluently in words of one's own choosing (Piotrowski, 1978). It is helpful to be aware of these levels of language because the impairment of clients with only automatic or imitative speech may be misunderstood unless carefully assessed.

Mixed Impairments. Clinically, language impairments are rarely limited to either comprehension or response. There are usually multiple impairments and strengths in varying degrees. Many language deficits will be apparent in spontaneous conversation. Some additional techniques that are sometimes used for assessment include object identification, ability to follow directions, reading, and writing tasks. Table 16-3 summarizes some characteristic strengths and deficits of persons with aphasia. The reader is reminded that many aphasic persons demonstrate varying levels of both comprehension and response impairment.

There are several problems in assessing the aphasic person with mixed impairments. It is especially difficult to assess the comprehension of a

---

Table 16-3
Characteristics of Impairments in Language Comprehension and Response

	Comprehension Impairment	Response Impairment
Speech	Articulates effortlessly	Labored speech
	Rhythm, rate, and intonation normal	May articulate only sounds, a few words, or nothing
	Word and sound substitutions common	Automatic or imitative speech may be present
Writing	Word and sound substitutions similar to speech errors	Impaired to the same degree as speech
Reading	Impaired to the same degree as auditory comprehension	Usually intact (similar to previous reading level)
Motor Response to Verbal Directions	Impaired	Intact if required response is within person's motor capability
	May rely heavily on situational clues, gestures, and facial expressions	

person with expression impairment. Often the individual's ability to understand language is overestimated because he is able to respond appropriately by interpreting gestures, facial expressions, and situational clues. His reliance on these clues should be determined so that care can be planned accordingly. Variability in the person's comprehension often can be explained by the presence or absence of nonverbal clues. On the other hand, the person's inability to respond verbally may lead one to underestimate his comprehension unless other modes of assessment are utilized. Similarly, the effortless speech of the person with comprehension impairments may lead

to overestimation of his comprehension unless there is careful assessment.

It is essential for the nurse to identify the ways in which a client is able to communicate (*i.e.,* strengths) as well as the ways in which his communication functions are impaired. Does he use gestures that can be identified to signify certain needs? Can he use a word or picture pointer board to identify his needs? Is he able to write? Careful assessment of the person's capabilities and strengths, as well as his impairments, enables the nurse to plan individualized care that fosters the highest level of functioning possible.

Nursing Process
Applied to Common Mental Status Alterations

Altered Levels of Consciousness

Assessment

The goal of the nurse in monitoring all persons with altered consciousness is the early recognition and prevention of complications. Increased intracranial pressure (ICP) is a complication commonly associated with factors causing altered states of consciousness. Because the cranial cavity allows no room for expansion, any process that increases intracranial pressure causes brain cell anoxia and possible brainstem herniation. These processes lead to permanent brain damage or death.

Research has shown that the earliest signs of increasing intracranial pressure are subtle changes in the level of consciousness, restlessness, decreased mental clarity, and disorganized behavior. Changes in vital signs such as widening pulse pressure, slowing of the pulse rate, and respiratory irregularities are later signs of increased intracranial pressure (Mitchell and Mauss, 1976 and 1978). Assessment of pupil responses and sensorimotor responses are also important and were included earlier in this chapter's discussion of the assessment of the level of consciousness. These assessments are sometimes referred to clinically as a neurological assessment or "neuro check" (Table 16-4).

Altered states of consciousness result in reduced awareness of the environment and decreased ability to adapt to it. The unconscious person may be totally dependent on others for basic life-sustaining needs.

Maslow's hierarchy of needs provides a framework for determining priority of assessment and caregiving activities. Assessing respiratory status and providing an open airway and adequate ventilation always are first priority. Despite the priority of this physiological need, higher-level needs are present simultaneously and must be attended to.

Table 16-5 lists the problems identified after assessment of a person with altered consciousness. The nurse must carefully assess factors related to immobility and dependency, as well as neurological deficits, in order to plan nursing care that maintains and restores function.

Nursing Interventions

Maintaining Adequate Ventilation

Maintaining adequate ventilation is always the first priority of nursing care. The person with an altered

---

Table 16-4
The Neuro Check

- Level of consciousness
- Pupil check
- Blood pressure
- Pulse
- Respirations
- Movement of extremities
- Muscle strength

Table 16-5
Common Problems and Interventions for the Unconscious Person

Data: J.L. is a 24-year-old male construction worker. He was hospitalized 2 days ago after sustaining a closed head injury in an auto accident on his way to work. He does not open his eyes or make any verbal response to stimuli and is unable to respond to verbal commands. He has spontaneous movements of all extremities and his eyes are opened spontaneously at times. He withdraws purposefully from painful stimuli. Pupils are equal and react briskly to light. Temperature is 100°F rectally. BP is 110/60. Pulse rate is 62, strong and regular. Respirations are 18, regular, and unlabored. Lungs are clear to auscultation, and chest expansion is full. Oral secretions are copious and lips dry. A Foley catheter is in place and he has had no bowel movements since admission. He is being hydrated with intravenous therapy at present with plans to institute nasogastric tube feedings. Mr. L.'s wife has stayed at the hospital since his admission. She states that she sleeps "a little" in the family waiting room but appears very tired.

Problem	Expected Outcome	Nursing Intervention
Potential airway obstruction due to altered consciousness	Adequate respirations maintained	• Maintain in side-lying position with head elevated 30 degrees. • Keep suction equipment on hand and use for removal of oral secretions as needed. • Turn side to side every 2 hr. • Assess respiratory status every 2 hr.
Potential increased intracranial pressure due to closed head injury	Complication not experienced	• Monitor level of consciousness including pupil and motor responses every hour. • Monitor vital signs every hour. Report changes promptly after full assessment. • Maintain adequate ventilation and avoid elevated temperature. • Position carefully with head of bed. Avoid neck flexion, extreme hip flexion (>90°), and prone position. • Minimize stress (see interventions with next problem).
Potential emotional distress due to trauma and loss of control	Minimal stress experienced	• Talk to Mr. L. while providing care. Explain what you are going to do and provide orienting information. Determine preferred name from wife and call him by name. • Avoid bedside conversations with others about Mr. L. • Handle Mr. L. with respect and gentleness while providing care.
Potential skin breakdown due to immobility and altered awareness	Skin intact and without redness	• Inspect skin when turning. • Turn side to side every 2 hr. • Massage bony prominences when turning and use padding between knees. • Keep skin clean and dry. • Provide lubrication as needed.

(Continued)

Table 16-5
Common Problems and Interventions for the Unconscious Person *(Continued)*

Problem	Expected Outcome	Nursing Intervention
Potential contractures due to immobility	Full range of joint motion maintained	• Perform passive range of motion (ROM) exercises 3–4 times daily. • Position in functional body alignment. • Use footboard and hand rolls to maintain functional position.
Potential injury due to altered consciousness and spontaneous movement	Free from further injury	• Siderails up at all times unless care giver is at that side of the bed with full attention on patient. • Siderails padded to prevent injury from unexpected movements or convulsive activity that may accompany head injury. • Restraints avoided if possible because patient's resisting efforts may increase ICP and tissue injury. • Remove mitts or other protective devices for skin care and inspection.
Dependent for hygiene needs due to altered consciousness	Hygiene maintained	• Keep skin clean and dry. • Give mouth care t.i.d. or as needed. If patient is a mouth breather, give care every 2 hr to prevent drying of oral mucosa. • Apply cold cream or chap stick to lips. • Examine eyes for signs of dryness or irritation and instill lubricating drops as needed.
Dependent for nutritional needs due to altered consciousness	Adequate nutrition maintained: body weight, intake and output	• Administer intravenous fluids or nasogastric feedings as ordered. (See chapters for nursing interventions specific to these treatments.) • Monitor intake and output, hydration, electrolytes.
Altered urinary and bowel elimination due to altered consciousness	Free of urinary tract infection (UTI); free of fecal impaction	• Provide catheter care b.i.d. and monitor for signs of UTI. • Monitor bowel elimination and administer ordered stool softener, cathartics, suppository, or enema as needed. • Maintain usual bowel elimination patterns to aid in future retraining.

Problem	Expected Outcome	Nursing Intervention
Patient's wife anxious and becoming overtired	Mrs. L. will be able to cope with current crisis and maintain own health; will verbalize feelings about current situation; will identify and attend to own health needs	• Talk with Mrs. L. away from bedside. Make opportunities to answer her questions and focus on her feelings. • Plan mechanisms for giving Mrs. L. regular reports on husband's progress that are acceptable to her (*e.g.,* conference with nurse b.i.d., phone calls to or from nurse). • Foster realistic hope by pointing out Mr. L.'s strengths (*e.g.,* breathes well on his own, vital signs stable and normal, moves spontaneously, withdraws from painful treatments, excellent health prior to accident). • Promote normalcy during her visits by encouraging her to talk to husband and touch him. Role model this behavior and share with her the benefits of it. • Explore with Mrs. L. ways she might wish to be involved in husband's care (*e.g.,* holding him while nurse gives skin care, bathing). • Arrange referral to social services if further assessment of Mrs. L.'s needs and concerns is indicated.

level of consciousness should be placed in a side-lying position with the head of the bed elevated 30 degrees. This position prevents the tongue from obstructing the airway and facilitates handling of oral secretions. The person must be turned from side to side frequently to further aid drainage of secretions. In addition to the potential for atelectasis and pneumonia associated with the immobility of the unconscious person, inadequate ventilation may lead to elevated intracranial pressure in susceptible persons. The hypoxia and hypercapnia resulting from inadequate ventilation lead to vasodilatation, which further increases intracranial pressure.

Avoiding Increased Intracranial Pressure

Studies of patients whose intracranial pressure was monitored continuously show that various other nursing activities may cause this pressure to rise (Mitchell and Mauss, 1976 and 1978). The person should be positioned carefully to avoid neck flexion, extreme hip flexion (more than 90 degrees), and prone positions. All of these positions have been associated with increased intracranial pressure. Individuals who can move themselves in bed should be taught to exhale as they move to avoid Valsalva maneuvers, which are also associated with rising pressures. Hyperthermia is another factor to be considered since it can lead to increased intracranial pressure due to vasodilatation. It is the nurse's responsibility to monitor the person's temperature and institute measures for temperature control, such as administering ordered antipyretics, giving cooling baths, or using a cooling mattress.

Attending to Psychosocial Needs

The person with altered consciousness continues to have social and emotional needs. Even when people are nonresponsive they may be able to perceive stimuli. Hearing is thought to be the last sensation to diminish. In one case study a patient, on regaining consciousness, reported that the only way he had of knowing he was alive was the nurse's talking to him (Wisser, 1978).

Studies that monitored varied physiological responses suggest that the content of conversations to which the patient is exposed is important. Whereas talking *to* the nonresponsive person is helpful to him, conversations *about* him are stressful (Lynch, 1978; Mitchell and Mauss, 1978). Lynch reports one case in which heart rate increased as much while several staff members conferred about the patient at his bedside as it did when he was taken off the respirator and suctioned. Independent observers in several intensive care units found that the most disturbing stimuli were communications among staff members and that staff rarely talked to the patients while providing care (Noble, 1979).

Besides responding to sound, comatose persons are also responsive to touch. In one study, heart rate was significantly reduced when the nurse held the hand of unconscious patients or quietly took their pulse (Lynch, 1978). There findings suggest that the nurse's verbal and nonverbal communications remain vital to the person's well-being even when consciousness is altered.

Family Considerations

The needs of the unconscious person's family are also an important consideration for the nurse. Family members of seriously ill persons are often highly stressed and require nursing assistance to mobilize their resources and adapt to the crisis situation. The family experiences loss when the unconscious person is unable to respond. Usual roles and support systems are disrupted. Members of the family may feel angry or guilty about events leading to the person's condition. These feelings may lead to expressions of hostility and anger directed toward staff members. When the patient's prognosis is poor, anticipatory grieving often occurs.

Nursing research (Breu and Dracup, 1978; Dracup and Breu, 1978; Hampe, 1975) has identified the following needs of the spouses of seriously ill patients:

- Need for relief of initial anxiety through explanation of what is happening to the patient
- Need for information about the patient's progress
- Need to be with the patient
- Need to be helpful to the patient

- Need for support and opportunity to ventilate feelings

Common nursing problems and interventions for the unconscious person are illustrated in Table 16-2. The reader is referred to appropriate chapters of this text for further discussion of problems related to immobility, nutrition, and elimination.

Altered Orientation and Mental Functioning

Assessment

Disorientation in time and place is most often accompanied by some impairment in thought processes. The term **confusion** is often used to describe the person who is disoriented, has decreased memory function, and shows a limited attention span. A careful assessment of mental status, describing specific behaviors of the individual and the environment, is essential. Including the context in which behaviors occur is necessary to avoid subjective labeling. It is often presumed that the term "confusion" has a precise meaning. In fact, it is used to describe a wide variety of behaviors which are judged by nurses and others to be inappropriate to the present circumstances. One study showed that patients who were socially undesirable or presented problems that made the nurse's job more difficult were most often called confused, whereas the same behaviors in socially desirable patients were not labeled as confusion (Williams *et al*, 1979).

Physiological Causes

Any systemic compromise to cerebral support, such as hypoxia, fluid and electrolyte imbalance, and metabolic imbalances, can result in confused states in persons of any age. However, elderly people who are ill are especially vulnerable. Physiological changes due to age reduce the older person's reserve capacity and decrease his ability to adapt to stressors. Thus, a wide variety of medical problems such as heart attack, pneumonia, and influenza may cause disorientation and impaired intellectual function in elderly persons. It is important that these abrupt alterations in mental status be distinguished from the gradual deterioration in intellectual function, memory, and judgment that is associated with degenerative brain disease in the elderly.

Nursing actions to support, protect, and reorient the person will be similar regardless of the cause of his disorientation. However, nurses will need to determine the factors causing the confusion if they are to provide care that prevents or modifies this symptom.

Interrelated Causes

Disorientation and impaired thinking are most frequently due to a combination of physiological, psychological, and environmental factors. Therefore, the nurse will need to assess the total person and his environment. The confusion of the person with a pulmonary disorder is likely to be related to inadequate ventilation. In this instance, the nurse would monitor respiratory status closely and work with other members of the health-care team to ensure adequate oxygenation. At the same time, it is important to be aware of this individual's anxiety and the potential for sensory overload. Similarly, the mental functioning of the person with degenerative brain disease may be affected by depression and social isolation as well as by the disease process.

Early Detection

In community settings the nurse is often in a position to identify abrupt changes in mental functioning that require prompt medical evaluation. The teaching functions of the nurse are important in working with individuals and community groups; medical evaluation is frequently not sought because the importance of symptoms is not understood. When the person is elderly, it may be assumed that the mental changes are irreversible. But even when the person's disorientation and declining mental capacity are due to chronic degenerative disease, the symptoms and course are varied. Careful assessment of the person's strengths and impairments, his environment, and the available personal and community support systems assures interventions that meet both the person's need to function as fully as possible and his need for safety.

Nursing Interventions

Because of the multiple factors involved in disorientation and disordered thought processes, it is not possible to devise a plan of care that is appropriate for all such persons. Interventions need to be individualized and based on the nurse's assessment of the total person and his environment. Expected outcomes need to be evaluated carefully to determine the success of the interventions or the need for a different approach. General nursing approaches aimed at modifying or preventing confusion are summarized in Table 16-6.

Empathic Communications

Most nursing research about approaches to confused persons has focused on group work with elderly institutionalized persons with degenerative brain disease. A variety of different types of groups have been used. Reality orientation groups focus on reorienting the person to his current surroundings using a very structured format. Other groups focus on providing social stimulation through sensory experiences or reminiscence. Although being involved in a group has generally not significantly altered patient scores on orientation and cognitive functioning there have been other positive effects, such as improved ability to perform activities of daily living and increased socialization with others (Hogstel, 1979; Letcher, Peterson, and Scarbough, 1974; Shaw, 1979; Voelkel, 1978). Groups that produce these positive outcomes appear to have in common the fact that they provide a safe empathic environment that stimulates the person's remaining capabilities. These elements can be utilized in one-to-one relationships with confused persons as well as in group work.

Table 16-6
Nursing Strategies to Prevent or Modify Confusion

- Communicate clearly.
- Maintain oxygenation, hydration, and nutrition.
- Avoid extremes of sensory input.
- Provide an orienting physical and social environment.
- Provide physical and psychological safety.
- Avoid the use of restraints, both physical and chemical.
- Stimulate the person's capabilities.
- Focus on positive progress and achievements.
- Enhance body image and self-esteem.
- Maintain consistent staff and continuity in care.

Nursing interventions for patients in acute-care settings who experience episodes of disorientation and impaired thought processes have not been studied. Descriptive studies of these patients suggest, however, that an empathic trusting relationship with the nurse can help people to cope with this experience (Ellis, 1972; Jackson and Ellis, 1971; Williams *et al.*, 1979). It is often helpful if the nurse focuses her attention on the person's emotional reactions to his disorientation.

Recall our basic needs discussion in Chapter 2. Providing an environment in which the confused person is physically safe and feels safe assumes a higher priority than orientation to time and place. The anxious or frightened person requires a calm reassuring approach. Nonverbal means of communication, such as touch and gestures, are often more helpful than verbal assurances or directions.

Family Considerations

The nurse will often need to deal with the anxiety of family members as well as of clients. Reassurance that this alteration in mental functioning is related to the person's illness and is not permanent should be given when this is the case. Families should be told about the person's confusion and ways in which they can be helpful, rather than being left to find out for themselves.

When their own needs for reassurance and support have been met, family members can become a great resource to the confused individual. The visitors need to know that it is helpful to the disoriented person if they talk to him about concrete things in the environment and correct his misperceptions without argument. Both visitors and nursing staff need to talk with the confused person about topics that are meaningful to him and that focus on his capabilities and progress. For example, a conversation with a retired farmer might begin by pointing out the rain outside his window and mentioning the season. This might evolve into a conversation about the tasks farmers do in the spring.

Although it is important to assess the person's orientation at varying intervals, it is equally important to ensure that nurses' interactions with disoriented people stimulate their capabilities rather than focusing solely on their impairments.

Setting Realistic Goals

It is important for both the nurse and the client that realistic objectives be set when nursing care is planned for the confused person. If unachievable goals are set, the nurse is likely to feel that attempts to assist the person are futile and to withdraw from further interactions with him. When your objective is for the person to be oriented to time and place, you may not notice that he is less agitated even though he is still disoriented. It can be both challenging and frustrating to work with the confused person. When you are able to see positive results from individualized care, it is very rewarding. Often, though, the responses are small and the person's behavior is unpredictable and varied. Nurses must be in tune with their own feelings and seek the support and assistance of colleagues when needed.

The following vignette provides an example of individualized nursing care which helped a person and his family cope with an episode of disorientation. In this example, a consistent nursing approach was used to provide a safe and orienting environment. The nurses recognized the person's strengths and helped him maintain as much control over his circumstances as he could. They responded to the person's disorientation by increasing their efforts to communicate with him and personalize his care.

Example □ Mr. P., an 80-year-old retired barber, was admitted to the hospital after breaking his hip in a fall. Mr. P. was mentally alert and oriented prior to surgery. He voiced concerns about his wife being alone because she had had a stroke several years ago and depended on him for assistance. He was reassured when he learned that his son would stay with her. He also asked his son to call someone from his bowling league to let them know that he could not be there the next day. He told the nurse that there was nothing he hated more than inactivity, and that he hoped this accident wasn't going to keep him down for long.

The night after Mr. P.'s surgery he became disoriented and agitated. He insisted that he had to help his wife and was struggling to get out of bed. Since he could be moved safely to a reclining chair, the staff moved him rather than resisting his efforts to get up. The lights were turned on and his glasses found for him. While these activities were being carried out, the nurse spoke calmly and quietly to Mr. P. reminding him that he had fallen and was in the hospital. Once in the chair, Mr. P. recognized his surroundings but continued to express concern about his wife. Because the nursing assessment had included information about his family, the nurse was able to remind Mr. P. that his son was with his wife and would see to her needs. The nurse got Mr. P.'s watch and put it on for him. He was surprised to learn that it was 4 A.M. and was more than willing to go back to bed. Mr. P. did not want the room lights on but was willing to have the bathroom light left on. He stated that at home he always left the hall light on at night. The nurse raised the side rails on the bed and left the bed in the low position. She told Mr. P. that the rails would remind him that he needed help if he wanted to get up again, and she showed him how to work the call light, which was secured within his reach. Mr. P. slept through the rest of the night, but the staff continued to check him frequently.

The next day Mr. P. continued to be disoriented at times but responded to the nurse's orienting comments. In addition to providing orienting information, the nurse engaged Mr. P. in conversations about topics she thought would be meaningful to him such as bowling, his former work as a barber, and his family. The nurse acknowledged the many accomplishments Mr. P. mentioned in response to her questions. She encouraged him to share his knowledge of the city where she was a newcomer and he was a longtime resident. Mr. P.'s children visited and were told about their father's confusion and the ways in which they could help him regain orientation. They communicated with him in a manner that helped him to focus on reality. The family was asked to bring small personal items such as a picture of his wife and his own bathrobe.

During the next few days, the nurse encouraged Mr. P. to do as much of his own care as possible, and despite his recurring disorientation she continued to involve him in planning a daily routine. Once a routine had been found that met Mr. P.'s needs, it was communicated in his care plan to provide continuity. His intake and output was monitored, and because of his confusion he was offered fluids and the use of the urinal at regular intervals to prevent dehydration or incontinence. Efforts were made to have the same staff assigned to Mr. P. each day. Although it was several days before Mr. P. was consistently oriented and functioning with the mental clarity noted on admission, there were no further episodes of agitation. □

Altered Language Function

Assessment

Impairments in language function affect the whole person. His ability to identify his needs to others is limited, as is his ability to express his feelings. These problems often lead to frustration, anxiety, depression, and lowered self-esteem. The nurse's assessment should focus on identifying the person's remaining strengths and capabilities so that interventions can be planned which assist the person to use the strengths he has. The reader may wish to review the assessment process discussed earlier in this chapter.

Nursing Interventions

The goal of nursing care is to help the person function at his highest possible level. Talking to the person and encouraging him to use whatever capabilities he has stimulates language functioning. Topics should be ones that are meaningful to the client. Nurses will need to alter their speech to match the person's ability to understand. Short phrases accompanied by gestures are often useful. Encouraging the person to use those language functions that remain requires a calm unhurried approach. Environmental noise should be controlled, and situations in which the person's attention must be divided among several people should be avoided. Adequate time must be allowed for the person to respond.

Frustration interferes with the person's ability to communicate and may be indicated by the person's body language. Even though the use of remaining skills should be encouraged, the person should not be pushed. At times when frustration is high, it is often best to offer some gentle guidance such as filling in a word or phrase that the person is groping for or clarifying his statement. Gestures, pointing, or writing may be helpful to some. If the need is not an urgent one, taking a break and trying later may be the best strategy. Individuals react in varied ways to these approaches. What decreases frustration for some people increases it for others. Thus, it is essential that the individual's response be evaluated and successful approaches communicated.

Family Considerations

Families are often as frustrated in their attempts to communicate with the client as he is. Providing time away from the bedside to talk with family members gives them a chance to explore their feelings. Nurses can assist family members by sharing their knowledge of successful communication methods. Role modeling this behavior by talking to the client in the family's presence is a helpful nursing intervention.

Self-Care and Self-Esteem

The loss of communication skills can be devastating to one's self-esteem. To help overcome this problem, the person should be encouraged to take an active role in his care and rehabilitation. He needs information about what has happened, what is happening, and what is going to happen. He should be involved in planning his care and encouraged to participate in self-care activities within his physical limits. Personal possessions, cards, and family pictures can serve as useful reminders of his personal history and can foster a sense of security and belonging. Careful attention to personal grooming needs can support feelings of self-worth. Signs of progress and current strengths should be pointed out to the client. The care plan in Table 16-7 represents the type of problems nurses frequently encounter with aphasic persons or persons whose language functioning has been impaired.

Conclusion

Alterations in mental status occur across all age groups and are associated with many different health deviations. Physiological processes; emotional, social, and environmental factors; and a person's developmental level are important determinants of mental status. Nurses adapt their assessment of mental function to the unique characteristics of the individual. Mental status assessment includes level of consciousness, orientation, memory, cognitive ability, mental capacity, and communication.

Table 16-7
Common Problems and Interventions for the Aphasic Person

Data: Mrs. G. is a 58-year-old housewife who had a left CVA 2 weeks ago. She speaks in short phrases with long pauses between words. She pronounces words with difficulty and often uses the wrong sound or word. At times she is able to follow directions, but at other times she is not. Her posture is rigid and her face flushed when she tries to express herself verbally. She is often tearful and says she's not good for anything. Her husband visits daily but makes few attempts to talk to his wife.

Problems	Expected Outcomes	Interventions
Difficulty expressing needs and feelings due to aphasia	Ability to use current communication skills to express needs and feelings; increased ability to express self verbally	• Anticipate needs and ask about them. Keep grooming supplies and personal possessions available. • Encourage Mrs. G. to use gestures with speech by modeling and positively reinforcing this behavior. • Provide ample time for Mrs. G. to respond. • Talk to Mrs. G. while providing care. Describe activities as they are done by nurse or client. • When Mrs. G. is unable to find the word she needs, determine whether she can use alternate word, gestures, or writing. • Monitor Mrs. G.'s body language for signs of frustration, and attempt to supply missing word or expand what she says when this occurs. • Use clarifying statements (*e.g.,* Do you mean _____?) • Maintain a calm, relaxed environment.

Mental status alterations affect the person's ability to adapt to his environment and function independently. One such problem is altered level of consciousness. The goals of nursing care for persons with altered consciousness are early recognition of changes in mental status and prevention of related complications. A person-centered approach to care means that the nurse gives verbal support and explanations and communicates with touch even when the person is unconscious. The nurse is attentive to physical needs, as well as social and emotional needs.

A second problem of mental status is altered orientation and mental capacity. Persons experiencing this difficulty need nursing support which promotes feelings of safety in their environment. Nursing intervention begins with establishing trust with the confused individual. Reality orientation and touch or other nonverbal communication diminish the person's anxiety and increase his sense of security.

Altered language function is a third problem that may occur with impaired mental status. The nurse assists individuals with this need by stimulating their language capability, acknowledging their feelings, and assisting significant others to use helpful communication techniques. The goal of nursing care is

Problems	Expected Outcomes	Interventions
Difficulty understanding verbal expressions of others	Increased ability to understand	• Limit environmental distractions. • Slow your rate of speaking and use short sentences or phrases. • Avoid long series of instructions and interactions with more than one person at a time. • Accompany verbal message with gestures and situational clues.
Decreased self-esteem related to communication problems	Indication of feelings of self-worth	• Provide opportunities for Mrs. G. to discuss her feelings. • Explain past, current, and future events related to her CVA. • Call attention to strengths (*e.g.,* some ability to express self and understand others, identifying and sharing frustration), and signs of progress. • Involve Mrs. G. in planning her care, and encourage self-care activities within her abilities.
Lack of communication between husband and wife	Ability of couple to communicate in manner which is satisfying to them.	• Talk with Mr. G. privately and encourage him to express his feelings. • Assess couple's usual patterns of communication. • Assist Mr. G. in identifying and using successful communication techniques.

not only to promote the client's ability to communicate but also to enhance self-esteem.

Nursing interventions for mental status alterations are based on the unique needs of individual persons. Likewise, the nurse is attentive to the needs of the client's family members or significant others and includes them in the plan of care.

Study Questions

1. Persons with impaired mental status are often dependent on the nurse to meet safety needs. Remembering that safety needs include perceived as well as actual threats or dangers, what steps would you take to ensure the safety of the following persons?
   a.   The confused person.
   b.   The unconscious person.

2. According to Mr. L.'s care plan you are to observe for signs of increased intracranial pressure and do a neuro check every hour. Describe the assessment you will carry out.

3. During your assessment interview you note that Mr. S. speaks in short, single sentences and frequently changes the subject. Although he is alert and indicates that he hears without difficulty, he does not seem to understand the explanations that have been given to him about the reason for his hospitalization.
   a.   How will these facts affect your nursing interventions while Mr. S. is undergoing tests to confirm a possible diagnosis of diabetes?
   b.   What else will you want to know about Mr. S.? Describe your further assessment.
   c.   If diabetes is confirmed, how will these facts affect your plans to teach Mr. S. to care for himself?

4. Describe nursing interventions that assist the aphasic person in using his remaining communication skills.

Glossary

Affect: The feeling tone of a person's reaction to other persons or situations; interchangeable with "emotion" in common usage; also a person's tone of voice, speed of delivery, and facial expression.

Aphasia: A general term used to describe disruptions in the ability to interpret and respond to verbal and written language.

Attention: Concentrating one's awareness on only one internal or external stimulus.

Body language: Nonverbal communication, which includes facial expressions, gestures, and posture; the way individuals position their bodies in relation to each other when interacting.

Confabulation: Giving believable but inaccurate answers; making up answers to fill gaps in the memory.

Confusion: A general term often used to describe disorientation, decreased memory function, and limited attention span.

Consciousness: Awareness of self and the environment.

Consensual light reaction: The response of the unstimulated pupil to stimulation of the other eye with a small bright light.

Delusions: A false notion created without appropriate external stimulus or relation to one's own knowledge and experience. Unlike hallucinations, it does not involve false excitation of the senses.

Direct light reaction: The response of the stimulated pupil to a small bright light.

Dysarthria: The inability to control musculature needed for clear articulation of speech.

Hallucinations: A faulty perception bearing no relation to reality or external stimuli; may be visual, auditory, or olfactory.

Level of consciousness: The state of awareness varying from fully alert to coma.

Long-term memory: That stage in the memory process which accounts for remembering material long after it was learned.

Orientation: A person's perception of time, place, and person; involves the ability to comprehend and adapt.

Perceptual distortions: Experiencing of stimuli that is inconsistent with reality; distortions range from mild images and spots before the eyes to delusions and hallucinations. May be accompanied by anxiety and agitation.

Rehearsal: The process of repeating in the short-term memory, which leads to material being transferred into long-term memory.

Sensory deprivation: A severe deficit or restriction of a person's usual sensory input; may involve one or more senses; may involve altered function or environment.

Sensory overload: High, intense sensory stimulation that may lack meaningful patterns.

Sensory restriction: See sensory deprivation.

Sensory stores: The first stage in the memory process based on sensory information from the environment; separate sensory stores correspond to each sensory modality.

Short-term memory: The temporary conscious memory storage; uses the active process of repetition or rehearsal to retain the small number of items held in it.

Bibliography

Adams N: Prolonged coma: Your care makes all the difference. Nurs '77 7:21–25, 1977

Bartol M: Nonverbal communication in patients with Alzheimer disease. J Gerontological Nurs 5:21–31, 1979

Bolin R: Sensory deprivation: An overview. Nurs Forum 13:241–258, 1974

Breu C, Dracup K: Helping the spouses of critically ill patients. Am J Nurs 78:50–53, 1978

Burns K, Johnson P: Health Assessment in Clinical Practice. Englewood Cliffs, NJ, Prentice-Hall, 1980

Burnside I: Clocks and calendars. Am J Nurs 70:117–119, 1970

Burnside I: Touching is talking. Am J Nurs 73:2060–2063, 1973

Burnside I: Working with the Elderly: Group Process and Techniques. North Scituate, MA, Duxbury Press, 1978

Burnside I: Nursing and the Aged. New York, McGraw-Hill, 1981

Burnside I, Mochrlin B: Health care of the confused elderly at home. Nurs Clin North Am 15:389–402, 1980

Chodil J: The concept of sensory deprivation. Nurs Clin North Am 5:453–465, 1980

Conway B: Neurological and Neurosurgical Nursing. St Louis, CV Mosby, 1978

Craik F: Age differences in human memory. In Birren J, Schaie K (eds): Handbook of the Psychology of Aging, pp 384–420. New York, D Van Nostrand Reinhold, 1977

Dracup K, Breu C: Using nursing research to meet the needs of grieving spouses. Nurs Res 27:212–216, 1978

Ebersole, P: Reminiscing. Am J Nurs 76:1304–1305, 1976

Ellis R: Unusual sensory and thought disturbances after cardiac surgery. Am J Nurs 72:2021–2025, 1972

Fox M: Patients with receptive aphasia: They really don't understand. Am J Nurs 76:1596–1598, 1976

Gardner D, Stewart N: Staff involvement with families of patients in critical care units. Heart Lung 7:105–110, 1978

Gerdes L: The confused or delirious patient. Am J Nurs 68:1228–1233, 1968

Guyton A: Physiology of the Human Body. Philadelphia, WB Saunders, 1979

Hahn K: Using 24-hour reality orientation. J Gerontological Nurs 6:130–135, 1980

Hampe S: Needs of the grieving spouse in a hospital setting. Nurs Res 24:113–120, 1975

Hirchfield M: The cognitively impaired older adult. Am J Nurs 76:1981–1984, 1976

Hogstel M: Use of reality orientation with aging confused patients. Nurs Res 28:161–165, 1979

Jackson C, Ellis R: Sensory deprivation as a field of study. Nurs Res 20:46–53, 1971

Jones C: Glasgow Coma Scale, Am J Nurs 79:1551–1553, 1979a

Jones C: Monitoring recovery after head injury: Translating research into practice. J Neurosurg Nurs 11:192–198, 1979b

Kroner K: Dealing with the confused patient. Nurs '79 9:71–78, 1979

Letcher P, Peterson L, Scarbough D: Reality orientation: A historical study of patient progress. Hosp Community Psychiatry 25:801–803, 1974

Lindsley D: Common factors in sensory deprivation, sensory distortion, and sensory overload. In Soloman P (ed): Sensory Deprivation, pp 174–194. Cambridge, Harvard University Press, 1961

Loen M, Snyder M: Psycho-social aspects of care of the long term comatose patient. J. Neurosurg Nurs 11:235–237, 1979

Loftus C, Loftus E: Human Memory: The Processing of Information. New York, John Wiley & Sons, 1976

Lynch J: The simple act of touching. Nurs '78 8, No. 6:32–36, 1978

Mahoney E: Alterations in cognitive functioning in the brain damaged patient. Nurs Clin North Am 15:283–292, 1980

McCorkle R: Effects of touch on seriously ill patients. Nurs Res 23:125–132, 1974

Miller L: Neurological assessment: A practical approach for the critical care nurse. J Neurosurg Nurs 11:2–5, 1979

Mitchell P, Mauss N: Intracranial pressure: Fact and fancy. Nurs '76 6, No. 6:53–57, 1976

Mitchell P, Mauss N: Relationship of nurse activity to intracranial pressure variations. Nurs Res 27–4–10, 1978

Noble M: Communication in the ICU: Therapeutic or disturbing? Nurs Outlook 27:195–198, 1979

Norman S: The brain damaged patient: Approaches to assessment, care, and rehabilitation. Am J Nurs 79:2126–2130, 1979

Norman S, Baratz R: Understanding aphasia. Am J Nurs 79:2135–2138, 1979

Nowakoski L: Disorientation: Signal or diagnosis? J Gerontological Nurs 6:197–202, 1980

Piotrowski M: Aphasia: Improving nursing care. Nurs Clin North Am 13:543–553, 1978

Plum F: The Diagnosis of Stupor and Coma. Philadelphia, FA Davis, 1972

Shaw J: A literature review of treatment options for mentally disabled old people. J Gerontological Nurs 5:36–42, 1979

Skelly N: Aphasic patients talk back. Am J Nurs 75:1140–1142, 1975

Teasdale G, Jennett B: Assessment of coma and impaired consciousness: A practical scale. Lancet 2:81–84, 1974

Teasdale G, Knill-Jones R, Van Der Sande J: Observer variability in assessing impaired consciousness and coma. J Neurol Neurosurg Psychiatry 41:603–610, 1978

Trockman C: Caring for the confused or delirious patient. Am J Nurs 78:1495–1499, 1978

Voelkel D: A study of reality orientation and resocialization groups with confused elderly. J Gerontological Nurs 4:13–18, 1978

Wallenhagen M: The split brain: Implications for care and rehabilitation. Am J Nurs 79:2118–2125, 1979

Wilkinson O: Out of touch with reality. Am J Nurs 78:1492–1494, 1978

Williams M, Holloway J, Winn M et al: Nursing activities and acute confusional states. Nurs Res 28:25–35, 1979

Wisser S: When the walls listened. Am J Nurs 78:1016–1017, 1978

Wolanin M: Physiologic aspects of confusion. J Gerontological Nurs 7:236–242, 1981

Wolanin M, Phillips L: Who's confused here? Geriatric Nurs 1:122–126, 1980

Wolanin M, Phillips L: Confusion: Prevention and Care. St Louis, CV Mosby, 1981

Wolf V: Some implications of short-term, long-term memory theory. Nurs Forum 10:150–165, 1971

Worrell J: Nursing implications in the care of the patient experiencing sensory deprivation. In Kintzel K (ed): Advanced Concepts in Clinical Nursing, pp 130–143. Philadelphia, JB Lippincott, 1977

Young S: Understanding the signs of intracranial pressure. Nurs '81 11, No. 2:59–62, 1981

Zarit S: Helping an aging patient to cope with memory problems. Geriatrics 34 No. 4:82–90, 1979

Special Senses and the Environment

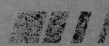

Janice B. Lindberg and Ann Z. Kruszewski

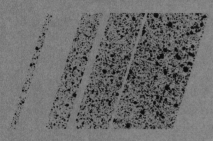

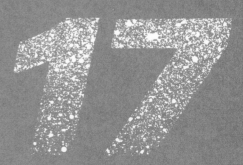

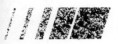

The special senses mediate between the stimuli in the environment and the sensations experienced by the person. The purpose of this chapter is to consider the concepts both of special senses and of environment as they relate to nursing care of the person. The senses to be highlighted are: sight, hearing, taste, smell, and touch. Basic nursing assessment and interventions will be presented for each sense. Selected problems related to alterations in vision, hearing, and touch will receive special emphasis. The environment will be discussed in relation to general safety and specific adaptations needed for altered abilities.

Man's special senses function within normal ranges that are determined by general human characteristics and age. Alterations of these senses in the individual occur as a result of heredity and environmental factors. For the nurse interested in person-centered care, the loss of any function related to the special senses requires special consideration. This consideration will recognize the way the person perceives the alteration as well as his unique strengths in coping with it.

Although the nurse does not diagnose the sensory deficit, determine its cause, or prescribe medical treatment, the effect of the alteration on the person's activities of daily living is an important nursing concern. The environment is a nursing consideration both because it contributes to perception of sensory stimuli and because altered sensory function affects adaptation to the environment. A knowledge of human anatomy and physiology enables the nurse to recognize and interpret certain alterations and also to alert clients to seek medical attention when indicated.

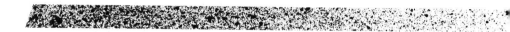

Factors Affecting Function of Special Senses

Man's sensory organs are some of his most vital aids to adaptation, operating on stimuli present in both his internal and external environments. A **sensation** is an awareness of internal and external conditions resulting from the stimulation of sensory receptors. Sensations may be categorized as cutaneous, visceral, olfactory (smell), gustatory (taste), visual, auditory, and positional. The cutaneous sensations relate to touch, heat, cold, and superficial pain. The visceral sensations include hunger, thirst, nausea, distention of the bladder and bowel, and deep pain.

For each of the five special senses we will consider (sight, hearing, taste, smell, and touch), there is a unit of sensory function that includes the sense organ or receptor, an afferent pathway to the brain, and a sensory area in the cerebral cortex. A general state of arousal is necessary before the person can even tend to the stimuli in conscious awareness.

Age

The arousal for sensation occurs in the reticular activating system (RAS). In the infant this response is undifferentiated and may be checked by purposefully startling the infant by striking the surface on which he rests. The normal baby will respond with a defensive reflex that consists of drawing its arms across its chest in an embracing manner. With maturation a more selective response will be made.

Once a sensation reaches the cortex, a complex analysis and interpretation occurs which organizes the sensations into perceptions. A **perception** then is an elaboration of the sensory impressions. It is the mental mechanism by which the nature and meaning of sensory stimuli are recognized and interpreted by comparing them with stimuli associated with past experiences. Obviously, the ability to interpret the sensations of the environment increases with age, experience, and the maturing mental abilities or thought processes. However, even *in utero* the fetus responds to the sound or sensation of the mother's heartbeat. This realization has led to the manufacture of crib toys that play a recorded maternal heart sound, simulating the comfort of the womb. The rhythmic "whoosh" is intended to soothe a restless infant.

Although the child is equipped with all the special senses at birth, some alterations in function occur during the growth process. Two examples are the normal ability of the eyes to focus and the visual defects of refraction that may occur in later childhood. Other alterations may be the result of injury or disease processes. Some hereditary and congenital disruption (*e.g.*, deafness) may become apparent with a lag in developmental abilities such as language. Many of the alterations in vision that occur in later life are a result of the normal aging process. Other alterations, such as certain hearing deficits, result from environmental factors.

Heredity

To many people, the term "hereditary" connotes a condition that is present at birth and is hence inherited. However, an abnormality may be present at birth (**congenital**) and not be genetically determined (**inherited**). Congenital conditions may be the result of drug exposure or an infectious process such as rubella, which can affect the special senses and result in cataracts, blindness, and deafness.

Actual hereditary or genetically determined abnormalities may cause sensory defects, including deafness and inborn errors of metabolism such as Tay-Sachs disease. Tay-Sachs, a disorder found in children of Mideastern extraction, is due to a missing hormone. It causes lipid accumulation within brain neurons, retinal degeneration, blindness, and possibly early death, usually before school age.

Other eye conditions that may be inherited include **strabismus** (cross-eye), color blindness, and retinoblastoma. Retinoblastoma, a malignant tumor of the retina, is a dominantly inherited condition. Even though the condition is treatable, it results in loss of eyesight in the affected eye. Nearly 50% of the children born to a person who has had retinoblastoma will inherit the disease. Color blindness is an example of a less serious, sex-linked genetic disorder, occurring primarily in males.

Environment

Environment affects sensory function as it affects so many of man's other abilities. In fact, sensory stimulus has been identified as an important motivating factor in man's behavior (Morris, 1973). The idea of man's functioning in dynamic equilibrium suggests that there are ranges of sensory stimulation within which a person can function effectively and comfortably. For example, there is a narrow range of temperature changes that man can tolerate without resorting to artificial adaptations.

Being aware of heat and cold through cutaneous sensations serves as a basic protective device. The environment provides many cutaneous stimulations. We adapt to most of these automatically as we handle the elements of our environment and go about the activities of daily living. However, illness can modify seriously our range of tolerance to sensory stimulations. If you have ever had the "flu" you can remember how even the weight of the bed covers was an unwelcome and painful sensation. Imagine an illness which is so confining that you are unable to shift position to alleviate the pressure caused by prolonged immobility!

To maintain his adaptive powers, man relies on an extensive amount of visual and auditory stimulation from his environment. Sense organs such as eyes and ears are specialized for their particular stimulus, such as light and sound. Although these organs are very sensitive, sufficient light is necessary to see, and adequate sound is required for hearing.

To the average young person with intact senses, this may seem to be an insignificant point. Yet, for the elderly person who has diminished sight and hearing and is in a strange environment, adequate sight and hearing may require that certain adjustments be made in the surroundings. The same is true when taste is diminished. The stimulus of inviting, colorful and attractive food with a pleasant aroma may help compensate for this deficit.

Learning about the environment through the senses is facilitated by stimulation of more than one sense. For example, seeing and touching a new object at the same time that it is being described helps us to learn and remember.

One can, however, get too much or too little input or sensory stimulation. In other words, we can suffer from sensory deficit or sensory overload that carries psychological and sociological implications, along with other problems. For example, as most of us know, too much light can be an environmental hazard for unprotected eyes. That is why workers in blast furnaces and artists tending potter's kilns know to protect their vision with appropriate shielding.

Most of us are aware of the danger of retinal burn that can result from viewing a solar eclipse or nuclear explosion. However, the hazards of deafness due to prolonged exposure to environmental noise are either not as well understood or are discounted as untrue. Too frequently, fans of rock and disco music and workers exposed to industrial noise pay the price of deafness from sensory overload.

Sensory Deficit or Deprivation

Normal sensory function depends on getting the appropriate amount of stimuli from the environment and being able to organize information and make some sense of the stimuli we receive. In this way, we orient ourselves to our environment.

If a person does not get enough stimulation or gets too much or if he is bombarded with stimuli that have no meaning for him, psychological disturbances can occur. This type of problem may arise for persons in health-care institutions who have little control over the amount and kind of sensory stimulation they receive.

The reticular activating system (RAS), identified as the arousal center for sensation, is thought to adapt to certain levels of stimulation. When stimuli are increased or decreased or distorted, the usual balance of the RAS is disturbed and a compensatory adjustment comes into play. However, with continued disturbance, the adjustments may fail and cause disorientation to time, place, and person, as mentioned in Chapter 16. The integrative mechanisms of psychological function are thus threatened. Cognitive thinking abilities are compromised, feeling states are altered, and extreme perceptual events like hallucinations and delusions may be experienced. Behavior also becomes disorganized. Some of what we know about sensory deficit comes from reports of victims of brainwashing or from persons who were inadvertently isolated when lost in the wilderness or at sea. Their strange experiences have been reported in fact and fiction for years.

Although research on sensory deprivation abounds, it has produced divergent and often inconclusive results. In addition, laboratory experiments involve more extreme conditions than those encountered in clinical situations. However, some helpful clinical implications may be suggested from the research.

Persons hospitalized in either acute-care situations or in nursing homes may experience **sensory deprivation.** First, hospitals impose unfamiliar surroundings and other restrictions. Isolating patients or clients because they have a serious infection or illness or because they are dying imposes further deprivation. Nursing homes or average hospital rooms may be monotonous environments if confinement is prolonged. There may be less to see, hear, and touch than in more familiar surroundings. Both perceptual deprivation due to restriction of external stimuli and kinesthetic deprivation due to immobility are often imposed. Immobility, decreased sensory input, and anxiety lead easily to sensory deprivation (Fig. 17-1).

Manifestations

Persons experiencing sensory deprivation report daydreaming, increasing anxiety, bodily aches and pains, and floating sensations. The reactions may be mild or extreme depending on the circumstances. As West wrote, "I woke—or dreamed I woke—in absolute darkness and absolute silence. I was—or dreamed I was—floating in an undetermined space in a timeless continuum" (West, 1973, p. 293). Such was the perception described by the main character of *The Salamander* as he talked about his feelings during an earlier period of solitary confinement, a world of complete darkness without any sensory stimulation.

Disturbances in RAS balancing function result in increased sensitivity to stimuli as attempts are made to restore the balance. This explains why hallucinations may occur. When dealing with someone who is experiencing hallucinations, it is important to realize that this person needs an explanation of what

is happening. He needs to be reoriented to the reality of the situation and assured that he is not losing his mind. Without this explanation, a change in affect, including an increase in anxiety, is virtually assured. At times the situation can be so frightening that such changes occur even when an explanation is offered. The result can be anxiety elevated to the level of panic.

If the void in sensory deprivation is not filled constructively or by hallucinations, boredom may result. Boredom and continued inactivity may lead to sleeping the day away. This, in turn, can interfere with nighttime sleep, as will be discussed later. Boredom and sleep patterns may therefore be early cues to sensory deficit. Other symptoms of sensory deprivation such as labile emotions, poor concentration, incoherent thinking, and regression of behavior may also be observed by an astute nurse who spends time with the person. These symptoms may influence relationships with family and staff and also

Figure 17-1

Visual restrictions can lead to sensory deprivation. *(Photo by Bob Kalmbach)*

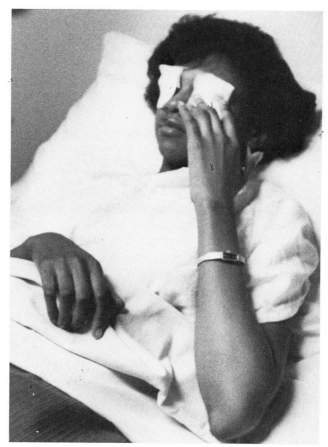

the ability to learn self-care or other information and skills. Table 17-1 summarizes factors that contribute to sensory deprivation.

Nursing Interventions

Although perception may be decreased for a variety of reasons—including alterations in the environment, problems with the sensory organs themselves, or drugs and pain that narrow perception—nursing interventions are required. Even the simplest interventions of assuring adequate light or providing eyeglasses or a hearing aid should not be overlooked. Other possible interventions follow:

- Supply activities that allow exploration of the environment (Fig. 17-2).
- Give the person meaningful objects that stimulate exploration and manipulation.
- Encourage goal-directed conversation to focus thinking on meaningful topics.
- Provide reality orientation.
- Encourage self-care.
- Give the person goals such as, "The tube will come out in 3 more days and then you can eat."
- Provide "reference points" of clocks and calendars and help the person to use these.
- Increase environmental stimuli like radio, television, and social contacts.
- Meet needs for closeness, security, and self-esteem.

Because sensory deprivation can lead to long-term depression, especially in the elderly, it is im-

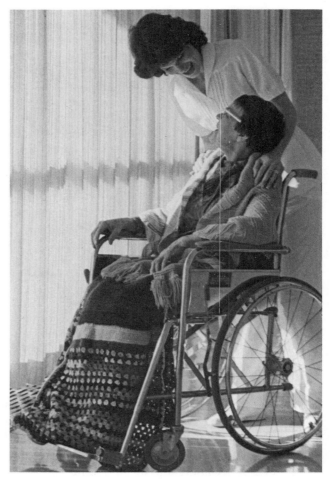

Figure 17-2
Exploration of the environment helps avoid sensory deficit. *(Photo by Edward J. Bonner)*

portant to keep personal belongings and mementos in view as a source of familiar stimulation in an unfamiliar environment. M. Kennedy, an Iranian hostage in 1980, described the importance of maintaining a personal environment amid hostility; he and fellow hostages arranged their meager belongings to create a make-believe "house." At the same time, we need to remember that even familiar environments must change to keep being stimulating. However, the patterns of change must be meaningful to the person involved.

Sensory Overload

Sensory overload can be equally if not more distressing than sensory deprivation. **Sensory overload** may be defined as high, intense stimulation that may lack meaningful patterns. Actually, symptoms for both

---

Table 17-1
Some Factors that Contribute to Sensory Deprivation

- Decreased vision, hearing, or touch
- Immobility
- Social isolation
- Isolation for disease control
- Fewer stimuli in the environment (*e.g.,* bare walls, no television)
- Medications (*e.g.,* narcotics, hypnotics)
- Lack of "reference points" (*i.e.,* clocks, calendars, routines)
- Anxiety

sensory deficit and sensory overload may be the same. This is not too surprising, considering that both conditions involve a disruption in the normal adaptation to the environment (Fig. 17-3). Symptoms for both deficit and overload include changes in the following:

- Affect—anxiety, fear, depression, panic
- Perception—hallucinations, paranoia
- Cognition—decreased ability to think coherently and problem solve, decreased ability to concentrate, disorientation

As we noted in our discussion of anxiety in Chapter 15, the hospital environment can be overwhelming to those who are unfamiliar with it. One factor contributing to overload is the degree of hustle and bustle with which hospitals operate, irrespective of the time of day or night. This alone can be disorienting. If pain and anxiety are added components, the stimulation in this highly active environment may be even more intensified. To some people, even the clothes worn by hospital personnel may provide sensory overload, because they do not provide easy identification of workers with their roles. Strange or casual uniforms in place of the traditional whites may be overstimulating to others.

Many of the factors that contribute to sensory overload are summarized in Table 17-2. Several of these factors are prominent in an intensive-care unit

Table 17-2
Some Factors that Contribute to Sensory Overload

- Hospital equipment that is not meaningful to the person
- Increased noise, especially nonpatterned noise such as the constant hum of machinery, but also loud conversation of staff
- Increased light, especially nonpatterned light that does not distinguish day from night
- Number of activities surrounding the person including frequent examinations, procedures, and large number of attending personnel
- Pain

(ICU) and in the environment of the actutely ill person. An additional source of sensory overload, especially for those who are very ill or restrained by life-sustaining equipment, is verbal communication among staff members. In a study by Noble, "Eleven independent observers agreed that the most dis-

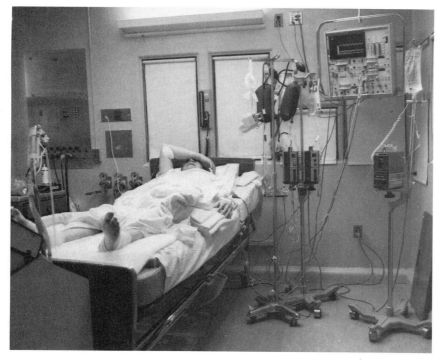

Figure 17-3
The intensive-care unit environment may lead to sensory overload.

turbing stimuli in the ICU were staff communications—not machine noises, constant artificial light, or the proximity of patients to each other as suggested by the literature. Aside from endogenous pain, the nurses themselves and other staff, communicating with patients and one another, appeared to be the single greatest source of exogenous disturbance for patients'' (Noble, 1979, p. 196).

Nursing Interventions

The nurse who recognizes that a person is suffering from sensory overload can institute appropriate interventions. Even though it may be impossible to change the general hospital environment, it is possible to modify environment of the unit. One of the first steps that can be taken is to reduce stimuli coming from personnel and equipment and to organize essential interruptions for minimal confusion. Explaining the purpose of the interruption may also be helpful because some of the overload comes from the person's failure to organize existing stimuli meaningfully (Fig. 17-4). It may also be possible to supply other more meaningful stimuli, such as the presence of a significant person.

Although we often think of sensory overload as visual or auditory, other input, such as cutaneous stimuli related to pain and itching, may contribute to the total sense of overload. Some appropriate interventions for sensory overload are summarized in Table 17-3.

Because nurses take the hospital environment for granted, they must purposefully assess for sensory deficit and overload and then initiate interventions suited to the individual circumstances. Sometimes just letting the person rest undisturbed with lights out and the door closed will enable him to establish equilibrium.

Table 17-3
Some Appropriate Interventions for Sensory Overload

- Decrease noise, equipment, personnel (decrease meaningless stimuli).
- Allow rest periods between activities.
- Supply meaningful stimuli (familiar objects, clocks, calendars, social visits).
- Decrease pain, itching, or other sensory stimuli.
- Provide reality orientation.

Nursing Assessment of Special Senses and Environment

The purpose of this discussion is not to teach the student to do a complete physical examination of each sense in order to establish a diagnosis. Several excellent assessment guides, including volumes by Bates (1979) and Malasanos and co-workers (1981), serve this purpose. Rather, our intent is to enable even the beginning student to assess special senses in order to determine the effect that an alteration will have on adaptation to the environment and on activities of daily living. Further, such assessment will enable the nurse to make appropriate referrals of clients for medical treatment. Also, appropriate teaching can be instituted to help the person prevent deterioration or further damage to these precious special senses.

Figure 17-4
Nurses' explanations help to reduce sensory overload in the intensive-care-unit.

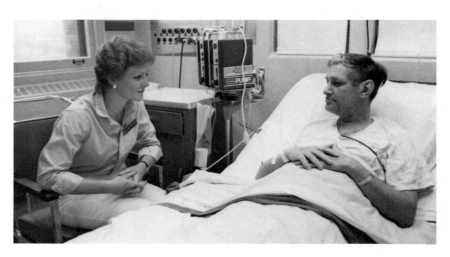

Sight

By knowing the persons at risk, the nurse can assess carefully for potential sight problems. Table 17-4 gives examples of some persons at risk and their related visual problems.

Structural Defects of the Eye

A review of anatomy will remind the reader of common structural defects of the human eye.

Myopia or nearsightedness occurs when the eye focuses images in front of the retina. The refractive power of the eye may be too great or the eyeball too elongated. This condition decreases distant vision and requires a negative or concave lens for correction.

In **hyperopia** or farsightedness, the refractive power of the eye may be too weak or the eyeball may be shortened, causing images to focus behind the retina. This condition decreases near vision unless a positive or convex corrective lens is used. Myopia is more common than hyperopia.

Other defects include astigmatism and presbyopia. **Astigmatism** is an irregularity of the cornea which causes blurred vision. Perpendicular or horizontal lines appear distorted without corrective lenses. **Presbyopia** is a condition of aging in which decreased elasticity of the lens hinders accommodation to close vision. The person may state that he can no longer see to do close work or he may be observed reading the newpaper at arm's length if the condition is uncorrected. Presbyopia is usually the reason persons in the 45-year range begin to wear bifocals. However, presbyopia affects eyes differently depending on whether they are myopic, hyperopic, or normal. For example, the nearsighted person with reduced accommodation may actually see better as a result of presbyopia.

Legal blindness means a functional ability of less than 20/200 vision with eyeglasses.

With growth, the refractive power of the healthy eye may change. The teenager who has myopia may notice that stronger lenses are needed with each change in eyeglasses, indicating that his vision is "getting worse." Such a person may fear blindness, not realizing that vision will stabilize after the growth spurt. The sensitive nurse can anticipate this fear and provide anticipatory guidance.

Assessment

Symptoms

Although the Person Assessment Guide (Appendix A) does not include a history component for special senses, there are several points that need to be assessed in determining whether a client is at risk for a visual problem. The following list of symptoms suggests those conditions which should be evaluated.

• Pain	Inflammation, foreign body, corneal abrasion, increased intraocular pressure leading to blindness
• Halos around lights	Glaucoma
• Diplopia or double vision	Muscle disturbance or inflammation

---

Table 17-4
Some Persons at Risk for Vision Problems

Persons at Risk	Related Visual Problem
Infant	Congenital blindness from mother's rubella or venereal disease
Preschooler	Strabismus or amblyopia
School-aged child	Refractive errors, *i.e.*, myopia, hyperopia, strabismus
Middle-aged to elderly adult	Presbyopia, glaucoma, cataracts
Post-stroke persons	Blindness, decreased visual fields
Diabetic persons	Retinopathy, blindness, cataracts, glaucoma

- Floaters or spots — Infrequent: benign, and, with aging; frequent: retinal detachment

- Photophobia or light intolerance — Conjunctivitis or cataract

- Frequent head-aches — Refractive error, eyestrain

- *Known defects*
  Does the person have any of the following?

- Myopia or hyperopia
- Diminished night vision
- Presbyopia
- Astigmatism
- Color blindness
- Legal blindness
- Visual field defect

- *Corrective devices*

- Does the person wear eyeglasses, contact lenses, or a prosthesis?
- If glasses or contact lenses are worn, what can the person see without them?

- *Physical assessment*

- Can the person read such things as mail, the newspaper, or a menu? These observations assess near vision.
- Can the person see objects at a distance?
- If vision is severely decreased, does the person perceive light from dark?

- *Field of vision*
  Depending on the circumstances, this may or may not be part of your assessment. The only equipment needed for a cursory assessment is an object like a pencil or a penlight.

- Have the person close one eye and look straight ahead at the object.
- Bring the object in toward a center line from the ears and also from above and below the eye.
- Ask the person to tell you when the object becomes visible.
- Normally, peripheral vision allows the person to see
    60 degrees nasally
    90 degrees temporally
    50 degrees up
    70 degrees down

- *Extraocular movements*
  The extraocular movements (EOMs) can be examined similarly without elaborate equipment.

- Hold your finger or penlight approximately 4 inches from the person.
- Check the person's ability to follow the movement with his eyes.

- *Other considerations*
  The eye provides a window to view the condition of blood vessels. This direct visualization may give important data about persons with diabetes, hypertension, or arteriosclerosis. Additionally, abnormalities of the eye may indicate other disease processes. Therefore, jaundiced sclera, pupillary reflexes, and ptosis or drooping lids are important findings. Bilateral edema, protruding eye (exophthalmos), and sunken eyes reflect other general disease problems.

Hearing

Some persons at risk for hearing loss include those listed below:

- Infants whose mothers have had rubella or mumps in pregnancy
- Those exposed to environmental noise or ototoxic drugs including aspirin or the "mycin" antibiotics
- Those who have had a stroke or have a family history of hearing loss
- Elderly persons

There are two basic types of hearing loss: conductive loss and sensorineural loss. **Conductive hearing loss** is due to a problem with the external or middle ear. It may be related to infection, the presence of a foreign body, or otosclerosis. **Sensorineural hearing losses** are caused by inner ear or central nervous system problems. This type of loss is not totally correctable with a hearing aid. Sometimes the loss may be of a mixed nature.

Assessment

Again some knowledge of the person's health history will be helpful.

- Were there frequent upper respiratory infections as a child?
- Was there exposure to environmental noise?

Presbycusis is hearing loss due to aging. With it comes a decreased ability to distinguish higher frequencies and perhaps some difficulty in hearing female voices.

Are there signs of decreased hearing, such as

- Asking frequently that statements be repeated
- Inability to hear at a distance
- Need to see the person who is talking
- Leaning forward or turning an ear toward the speaker
- Answering inappropriately
- Talking too loudly
- Inability to carry on a phone conversation
- Strained facial expression

Hearing problems may also cause behavior changes, which will be more noticeable to family members than to the examiner.

- Do significant others or co-workers notice inattentive, suspicious, withdrawn, or hostile behavior? Remember that the person who has a hearing loss that has not been properly assessed may be seen as confused, retarded, senile, and so on.
- If there are defects, does the person lip read or use a supportive device?
- Does the person experience unusual sensations in either or both ears, including roaring sounds, ringing, or buzzing noises known as **tinnitus?**

Physical Assessment. Hearing may be tested by determining how well the client can hear a whisper. The whisper test is especially appropriate for determining the effects of hearing losses on activities of daily living. If the person is unable to hear an audible whisper spoken within a few inches of his ear, he should be referred to a medical specialist for further examination. The person who fails to hear a barely audible whisper has inadequate hearing, whereas one who hears only loud whispers has a moderate hearing loss, meaning that his hearing level for conversational purposes is borderline (Boles, 1971).

Taste

The taste buds, located primarily on the tongue in the papillae, serve as the sensory receptors for the sense of taste, which is mediated by the facial (VII) and glossopharyngeal (IX) cranial nerves. Therefore, persons who suffer injuries to the tongue, the afferent nerves, or the related sensory area of the central nervous system lose this sense.

The basic tastes sensed by the tongue are sweet, sour, bitter, and salty. The tongue is also sensitive to touch and temperature, which in turn influence taste. **Appetite** is the pleasurable desire for food that generally occurs when we think about food, smell it, or see it. Taste remembrance also contributes to appetite, whereas interference with smell decreases appetite. This is partly why we lose our appetites when we have a cold that interferes with our sense of smell. In some illnesses and other circumstances, altered taste, because of its relation to appetite, may contribute to nutritional deficits.

Taste may also lead to overindulgence in favorite foods. Additionally, persons with altered taste sensations may use a high intake of salt and sugar to compensate. The use of these products has been related to higher incidences of such diseases as diabetes, heart disease, hypertension, and obesity (Ahrens, 1974; Finnerty and Linde, 1975).

It has been assumed that taste itself decreases with age. However, research evidence raises a question about this assumption and suggests that there are other aspects of our knowledge about taste function that remain ambiguous (Beidler and Smallman, 1965; Grzegorczyk *et al.*, 1979; Murphy, 1979). Taste complaints in the elderly generally relate to the food's being bitter or sour. Schiffman (1979) suggests that food may be made more palatable by enhancing its odor with artificial flavors. However, artificial sweeteners and other additives themselves often leave a bitter aftertaste. From a holistic viewpoint, it is important to remember that elderly persons frequently have a variety of chronic health problems and diminished functional abilities that may contribute to altered taste sensations.

Assessment

Two measures for assessing taste include having the person differentiate between two different flavors and asking him to respond to direct questions about taste changes if appropriate. It is especially important to note whether the person wears dentures or has a long history of smoking. Both of these conditions are known to decrease taste sensation. Asking about mouth care habits is also part of assessment. Good oral hygiene is thought to be a major contributing factor in maintaining optimal taste function.

Smell

Smell may diminish with aging, sinus infections, skull injuries, and such procedures as tracheostomy.

Assessment

As with taste, a brief assessment involves actually having the person differentiate between two dissimilar odors and also questioning him directly regarding any change in the sense of smell.

Nursing Interventions

Because smell contributes to taste and appetite, interventions similar to those used for decreased taste are appropriate here as well. Additionally, smell serves a safety function, especially for gas leaks and smoke.

Because unpleasant odors may occur with certain diseases or be present in the hospital environment, deodorizers should be used when possible. It is important to remember that the best deodorizer for unpleasant odors is fresh air, which dilutes the odorous particles that stimulate smell. Failing this, one must resort to commercial deodorizers as an adjunct to the usual cleaning procedures. However, some deodorizers are as offensive as the odors they attempt to mask. A person-centered approach, based on a trusting relationship, suggests that the person be consulted for his preferences in this regard if he is able to provide them.

Touch

Touch is one of the cutaneous sensations, along with the senses of heat, cold, and superficial pain. Touch also serves as an important safety function in preventing tissue damage. However, some diseases may result in a diminished sense of touch. For example, one woman with diminished sensation in the legs associated with diabetes told of finding open blisters on her feet after a day of shopping. "I had no idea I had hurt myself until I saw that injury," she stated.

To assess the touch sensation, the nurse gains information by asking the person about the presence of any unusual sensations or by testing for pain, temperature, vibration, and pressure. Light touch is often tested by brushing the person's skin with a ball of cotton or by pricking the skin with a pin. Deep pressure may be tested by squeezing the calf muscle, Achilles tendon, or arm muscles.

A few terms related to alteration in touch include the following:

- **Paresthesia**—a feeling of tingling or numbness, which may be related to a central nervous system disorder, hyperglycemia in diabetes, peripheral nerve damage, or electrolyte imbalance.

- **Anesthesia**—the loss of sensation that may occur in disease conditions such as diabetes and substance abuse such as alcoholism. Persons who have had a cerebral vascular accident (CVA or stroke) or spinal cord injury will experience anesthesia in the affected parts. In the case of a stroke, the anesthesia may affect one entire side of the body. In spinal cord injury, the anesthesia will extend downward from the site of injury.

- **Hyperesthesia**—an exaggerated feeling or pain that may follow peripheral nerve injury or an inflammatory process such as shingles.

General Safety in the Environment

Environment, as a major factor affecting man's general adaptation, was discussed in Chapter 3. The discussion here will focus on nursing assessment of the environment in relation to general safety. Specific adaptations needed for altered sensory functions will be considered briefly under nursing process applications.

We need to be cognizant of the fact that merely removing a person from familiar surroundings and placing him in a strange environment—whether a hospital, nursing home, or professional office—will trigger some need for adaptation, because change of this type has an impact on all senses. Thus, the person will need the nurse's assistance in adapting to environmental change in accordance with his state of dependence or independence. At the same time, we are also concerned with increasing a client's awareness of the hazards present in his environment and with the opportunities for achievement that are available in one's surroundings regardless of the setting.

Assessment for Dependent Persons

When caring for a dependent person, the nurse will need to monitor the environment to assure that his basic physiological needs are met. To the extent that he is immobilized, debilitated, or otherwise incapacitated, he will be unable to get from the environment even that which is necessary to sustain life. For dependent persons and those with severe deficits, it is especially important that their surroundings be structured to allow them to function at their maximum ability.

- Is the environment equipped with an adequate means for summoning assistance?

- Is the call-light cord readily accessible and within sight even for persons who normally wear eyeglasses but may not do so because of illness?

- If the person's hearing is severely compromised, is there an alternative means of answering the call light other than the intercom?

- Is there a clear path from bed to toilet? Are cords and equipment safely out of the way?

- Is the bed in the lowest position and securely locked?

- If the person is elderly with diminished sight and hearing, are the side rails used at night as a reminder that assistance is needed when moving about in this strange environment?

Environmental hazards related to oxygen and fire, for example, may be greater for dependent persons with multiple sensory deficits.

Because the dependent person is particularly prone to the hazards of sensory deprivation or overload, the nurse will be concerned about the intensity, pattern, variety, and appropriateness of sensory stimuli. Thus, it is especially important to note patterns of activity, light, noise, and color.

The nurse should also be aware of certain limits created by special circumstances. For example, isolation for infection control physically limits the person and may contribute to sensory deprivation, especially if a hearing problem already exists. Personnel attending such a person frequently stand at the door of the room and ask hurried questions which often cannot be heard clearly. Or they wear protective clothing including a face mask that muffles their voices and prohibits lip reading, thereby compounding the person's hearing problem. In the same way, the operating room or intensive-care unit can be especially frustrating when persons who normally rely on supportive aids for sensory deficits—corrective lenses or hearing aids—are not able to wear their devices in these settings.

Whether the dependent person remains in a hospital environment or is transferred to an extended care facility such as a nursing home, the environmental concerns related to sensory problems will remain the same.

Assessment for Independent Persons

Hospitalized persons who are more independent will need less intervention for environmental adaptation than severely dependent persons. A person who has a visual or hearing deficit and yet functions very independently in familiar surroundings may need some orientation to a strange environment. Even persons without sensory deficits will need some environmental orientation, including cautions about potential safety hazards.

As for the home environment, some information about living space is essential to help the person adapt to a sensory alteration. In this regard, the nurse will want to know about the following:

- Type of dwelling (*e.g.*, apartment, house)
- Architectural barriers
- Privacy, warmth, lighting.
- State of repair
- Space for work and play
- Usual environmental stimuli
- Length of residence

Additional information concerning the neighborhood is also pertinent:

- Nature of the neighborhood (*i.e.*, rural, urban, residential, commercial)
- Presence of any pollution
- Transportation facilities and access to services

Refer to the Guide to Person Assessment (Appendix A) for specific questions that may be appropriate.

Although information about home health and safety features and hazards are a consideration for all clients, such information is especially important for those who have some kind of special sense impairment or motor ability problem. Specifically, the nurse is concerned about hazards that could contribute to accidents or disasters.

- Are there obstacles, slippery surfaces, or poorly lit areas like stairs?
- Are there emergency phone numbers, smoke detectors, and disaster plans that increase security? Older persons, especially, who are recognized as blind or deaf, may fear assault and robbery.
- Are there locks, lights, and other security systems?

Nurses need objective and subjective data to make nursing diagnoses and plan appropriate interventions. The client needs to understand that the nurse does not make value judgments about the person's environment, as Lentz and Meyer (1979) so vividly point out in "The Dirty House."

Nursing Process
Applied to Specific Special-Sense Problems

Vision Problems

Decreased Vision or Blindness

Visual impairment may be temporary, permanent, partial, or complete and may affect one eye or both. In partial blindness, the person may perceive shadows, light and dark, or he may have a central or peripheral defect. Consistent with a person-centered approach to care, the nurse will want to assess the person's adaptive mechanisms before assuming that a problem exists. A blind softball pitcher told a T.V. news reporter that he wished people would find out what his abilities were rather than making assumptions about his blindness and its limitations.

Several possible problems may occur in the presence of decreased vision or blindness: anxiety and depression, decreased sensory stimuli, potential injury, and difficulty in carrying out activities of daily living. Possible nursing interventions for such problems are presented in Table 17-5.

Most blindness is preventable. This fact suggests that the nurse's most important intervention is health teaching for vision maintenance. The following list offers some suggestions for teaching clients about ways to maintain vision:

- Avoid rubbing eyes.
- Avoid eyestrain.
- Avoid damage from ultraviolet rays.
- Protect eyes from foreign bodies.
  - If foreign bodies are not easily removed by pulling the upper lid forward and down, professional treatment should be sought.
  - If large foreign bodies have penetrated the eyeball, do not attempt to remove. Rather, place a clean cloth over the eyes to decrease movement and seek immediate medical attention.
- Keep eyeglasses clean, protected, adjusted.
- Avoid nonprescription eyedrops and seek attention for symptom.
- Avoid cleaning eyes or contact lenses with soiled articles.
- Use caution with aerosol sprays.
- Use caution with ammonia, lye, and so on.

- Flooding the eye with water is the immediate and most important step that can be taken after an irritant has been splashed in the eye.
- Visit physician frequently if you are prone to eye problems.
  - **Ophthalmologists** and **oculists** are medical doctors who specialize in eye conditions.
  - **Optometrists** have college level training and can fit eye glasses, but they are not medical doctors.
  - **Opticians** are technically competent to grind and mount lenses, that is, to tend a lens dispensary. They work from the prescription of an ophthalmologist or optometrist.
  - Initial assessment of a refractive error is most appropriately performed by a physician who would recognize a pathological condition that needs medical treatment. Because contact lenses are not suitable for all persons, these also should be prescribed by an opthalmologist.
  - The type of eye care specialist to whom a person is referred will depend on the person's health problem and need.
- Know danger signals that indicate serious eye problems:
  - Persistent eye redness
  - Pain or discomfort especially after injury. Severe pain indicates an emergency condition which should be treated immediately. Sudden increased intraocular pressure due to acute glaucoma, for example, can lead to optic nerve damage within a day if left untreated.
  - Visual disturbances (halos, floaters, double vision, decreased peripheral vision)
  - Crossing eyes. This is not a condition that will correct itself without treatment. Untreated cross-eyes in young children can lead to a condition called **amblyopia** or loss of vision in the lazy eye.
  - Growths on or near the eyes
  - Discharge or increased tearing
  - Pupil irregularities
- Retinal detachment causing sudden holes in vision without pain requires medical treatment to prevent permanent vision loss.

Table 17-5
Nursing Interventions for a Person with Decreased Vision or Blindness

Possible Problems	Interventions
• Anxiety, depression	• Evaluate acceptance or stage of grieving • Provide careful, unhurried explanations • Facilitate expression of feelings • Announce self when entering or leaving room • Tell person you are present before touching him • Orient person to immediate environment if new
• Decreased sensory stimulation	• Provide diversion • Encourage use of other senses (touch, smell, hearing)
• Potential injury	• Orient to new environment • Clear pathways (rugs, cords, furniture) • Do not rearrange furniture • Leave doors completely open or closed • In hospital, leave bed in lowest position and the call light near • In new environment, assist with ambulation (person grasps your arm, you walk slightly ahead, announce steps, *etc.*)

• Difficulty with activities of daily living	• Increase lighting (except with cataracts, because glare is a problem)
	• Stay in person's field of vision if peripheral vision is decreased
	• Use large print (medications)
	• Refer patient to a teacher of braille
	• Teach techniques for adapting (*e.g.,* folding paper money)
	• Keep environment constant
	• Use clock analogy to describe position of food:
	    Milk at 1 o'clock
	    Bread and butter at 3 o'clock
	• Assist in opening cartons, *etc.,* p.r.n.
	• Orient to surroundings

• Glaucoma, a leading cause of blindness, is best detected by a painless check of intraocular pressure on routine examination in persons over 40 and those designated at risk.

Eye Surgery

The potential for successful outcome from eye surgery has increased markedly in recent years. It is now possible to correct cataract defects with implanted artificial lenses and to repair retinal detachment. The possible problems, of course, vary with the nature of the surgery and the underlying con-

dition. A brief list with possible nursing interventions is presented in Table 17-6.

Hearing Problems

As noted earlier, there are two basic hearing losses: conductive or sensorineural, as well as mixed losses. Temporary hearing losses are likely to be of the conductive nature and are usually due to infections, foreign bodies, or wax buildup. Increased hearing loss may also be noted in persons receiving ototoxic drugs.

Table 17-6
Nursing Interventions Following Eye Surgery

Possible Problems	Interventions
• Temporary or decreased vision	• Same as those described for the person with decreased vision or blindness
• Increased intraocular pressure	• Teach person to avoid lifting, bending, straining at stool, vomiting, sneezing or coughing, falls (assist with ambulation), pushing on eye
	• Show correct positioning: lie on unoperated side in cataract extraction
• Decreased knowledge of self-care activities after discharge	• Wash hands before touching eye or using drops
	• Teach how to put in drops
	• Instruct person to avoid activities that increase intraocular pressure
	• Avoid trauma to eye

Whether the hearing deficit is complete or partial or in one or both ears will affect interventions. Common problems related to hearing deficits and ear surgery, with suggested interventions, are listed in Table 17-7.

Again, the principle of intervention is health teaching to prevent hearing problems. Below we list some points to be included in health teaching for hearing:

- Avoid excessive noise.
- Avoid inserting sharp objects into ears.
- Avoid excessive cleaning of ears.
- Avoid practices that can cause infection; treat infection early.
- Know symptoms of hearing loss.

Touch Problems

The person with altered touch sensation is prone to a variety of potential safety problems. Chapter 18 offers a detailed discussion of decubitus ulcers, which can result when this sensation is absent or severely compromised. Less serious alterations in the sense of touch may involve other kinds of hazards. For example, bruises may occur almost unnoticed, and small particles may be retained in the eye, mouth, or shoe without being realized. Therefore, people with a diminished sense of touch should be forewarned about such possibilities. They should also be alerted to the fact that because sensations to the lower extremities may be altered, solid well-fitting shoes and good foot care are important. At the same time, cautions about possible burns from bath water, cigarettes, and heating pads should be offered. Along the same lines, in cold weather extra protection against frostbite may be needed. Decreased perception of vibration may diminish awareness of safety hazards such as an unsteady ladder or loose footing.

The nurse can help clients anticipate a variety of sensory changes and their implications. Equally important, the nurse assists the client to mobilize strengths, minimize dysfunction, and adapt environment and function to altered abilities.

Adaptation to the Environment

General Considerations

Adapting to the environment is an everyday activity of living that is taken for granted by most persons. Table 17-8 lists the types of injuries which all of us can sustain from environmental hazards. Many of these environmental hazards are present in hospitals. Others are unique to the hospital, such as **nosocomial infections,** which are in essence hospital-ac-

Table 17-7
Nursing Interventions for Persons with Hearing Deficits and Ear Surgery

Possible Problems	Interventions
Anxiety Communication difficulties	Face person, stand on the side of the good ear
	Stand in good lighting
	Do not exaggerate lip movements
	Speak slowly and distinctly, using simple terms
	Use nonverbal techniques (gestures, pointing, writing)
	State major topic, then specific thoughts
	Speak loudly but do not raise pitch of voice
	Decrease background noise (T.V., radio)
	Let person see you before you touch him to avoid startling him
	Consider rephrasing statements (some consonants cause problems for elderly)
Surgery	
Possible nausea or dizziness related to inner ear disturbance	Encourage slow movement
	Keep bed low, side rails up
	Assist with walking
	Provide medications (antiemetics as ordered)
Decreased knowledge about postdischarge care	Instruct about shampoo, shower, and swimming restrictions
	Instruct about avoiding increased middle ear pressure (sneezing, blowing nose, airplane flying)

quired infections. For all hospitalized patients, the nurse accepts individual responsibility for controlling hazards by practicing safely, reporting unsafe practices, and orienting patients to hazards.

As in hospitals, most homes pose general environmental hazards that are often overlooked by persons who have full functional abilities. Such hazards include poorly lighted areas, loose rugs, absence of stair rails, and faulty equipment. Similarly, the hazards posed by risk-taking behavior such as bad driving habits, keeping the doors unlocked, and traveling alone are frequently ignored.

Specific Adaptations Needed for Special-Sense Alterations

Adapting to the environment sometimes involves modifying the environment to facilitate the person's adaptation, especially when an alteration in one of the special senses is involved.

In addition to specific interventions mentioned under nursing process applications, some of the following environmental considerations will be important for those with altered special senses:

- Increased lighting

Table 17-8
Types of Injuries Caused by
Environmental Hazards

Mechanical

Falls

Thermal injury

Burns

Frostbite

Chemical

Too strong chemicals on skin or internally

Drug overdose

Electrical

Current from defective wiring or electrical equipment—may result in burn, shock, or death

Radiational

X-rays

Radium, cesium, cobalt

Isotopes

Bacteriological

Staphylococcal or pseudomonal infections common hospital-acquired, or nosocomial, infections

Allergenic

Drugs

Foods

Human derivatives

Psychological

Sensory deficit

Sensory overload

- Stairs and doors painted clearly, possibly with contrasting-color steps and trim
- No slippery floors or loose rugs
- Clear traffic patterns free of loose electric cords
- Large-print reading material or talking books
- Secure locks
- Emergency means to summon assistance
- Decreased background noises

- Decreased temperature on water heater
- Available bath thermometer
- Protected space heaters or radiators
- Hand rails in tubs and on stairs
- Smoke detectors

In addition to environmental alterations, two other considerations are pertinent to those with impaired vision, hearing, or touch. First, with age, adaptation is slower. That is, the time required for impulses to reach the brain and for reactions to occur is greater. Additionally, a stronger impulse may be necessary to elicit a response (Bozian and Clark, 1980, p. 473). Second, the awareness of being cared for comes to us through a comforting sight, a kind voice, and a tender touch. Those who experience alterations in their special senses may receive fewer reinforcements affirming that they are cared for and regarded as significant persons. Nurses who understand basic human needs will intervene appropriately to circumvent potential problems.

Conclusion

This chapter has considered the concepts of special senses and the environment as they relate to nursing care of the holistic person. Because the person uses special senses to adapt to the environment, any change in special-senses function may threaten this adaptation. A person-centered focus for nursing care suggests, therefore, that both assessment and intervention for sensory alteration be based on individual needs. The factors that affect function of special senses include age, heredity, and both sensory deficit and sensory overload. The nurse often is the first person to recognize a significant sensory alteration. This recognition may prompt both referral for medical treatment and nursing intervention to assist adaptation. Nurses' awareness of normal sensory function across the life span enhances both recognition of and appropriate intervention for altered function. Also, because of their close and continuous contacts with their clients, nurses often have unique opportunities to recognize impending sensory overload and sensory deprivation related to factors in the hospital setting. In the community, nurses have many opportunities to teach persons about the hazards of sensory overload in their work and leisure environments. For the person who experiences altered sensory function, individualized nursing interventions are directed toward modifying activities and the environment to assist optimal adaptation.

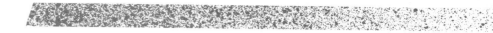

Study Questions

1. What safety precautions are especially necessary for a person who has lost the following senses:
   a. Sight
   b. Hearing
   c. Touch
   d. Taste
   e. Smell

2. Mr. K. is a 78-year-old retired carpenter. He has poor vision and hearing and is isolated in a private room. He is also immobilized and has few family visitors. You notice that the window shades are pulled, he has no reference points, and he is disoriented. Suggest some nursing measures to improve his state of sensory deprivation.

3. Infections are an environmental hazard, especially in a hospital situation. The essential links in the infection chain are as follows:
   The infectious agent or organism
   A reservoir for the pathogens
   A portal or exit from the reservoir
   A means of transmission
   A portal of entry to a new host
   A new host
   Discuss the role of the nurse in breaking this infection chain.

Glossary

Amblyopia: The lazy eye resulting from squint or strabismus.

Anesthesia: The loss of sensation.

Appetite: A psychological response to food.

Astigmatism: An irregularity of the cornea that causes blurred vision and makes lines appear distorted.

Conductive hearing loss: A hearing loss due to a problem with the external or middle ear; it may be related to infection, foreign body, or otosclerosis.

Congenital: Present at birth.

Hyperesthesia: An exaggerated feeling or pain.

Inherited: Genetically determined.

Legal blindness: A functional visual ability of less than 20/200 with corrective lenses.

Myopia: Nearsightedness; occurs when the unassisted eye focuses images in front of the retina.

Nosocomial infection: A hospital-acquired infection.

Oculist: A medical doctor who specializes in eye conditions or diseases; an ophthalmologist.

Ophthalmologist: A medical doctor who specializes in eye conditions or diseases; an oculist.

Optician: A technician who is competent to grind and mount corrective eye lenses.

Optometrist: A person who measures the eye's refractive powers and fits lenses to correct ocular defects.

Paresthesia: A feeling or sensation or tingling or numbness.

Perception: A mental mechanism by which the nature and meaning of sensory stimuli are recognized and interpreted by comparing them with stimuli associated with past experiences.

Presbycusis: The hearing loss of aging.

Presbyopia: A condition of aging in which decreased elasticity of the lens hinders the accommodations to close vision.

Sensation: An awareness of internal and external conditions resulting from the stimulation of sensory receptors.

Sensorineural hearing loss: Hearing loss caused by inner ear or central nervous system problems.

Sensory deprivation: A severe deficit or restriction of a person's usual sensory input; may involve one or more senses; may involve altered function or environment.

Sensory overload: High intense sensory stimulation that may lack meaningful patterns.

Strabismus: An eye disorder due to lack of muscular coordination; also known as squint or cross-eye.

Tinnitus: Ringing, tinkling, buzzing, roaring, or other unusual ear sensations experienced by a person; inaudible to examiner.

Bibliography

Ahrens RA: Sucrose, hypertension, and heart disease: An historical perspective. Am J Clin Nutr 27:403–422, April, 1974

Aspinall JM: Scoring against nosocomial infections. Am J Nurs 78:1704–1707, October, 1978

Bates B: A Guide to Physical Examination, 2nd ed. Philadelphia, JB Lippincott, 1979

Beidler LM, Smallman RL: Renewal of cells within taste buds. J Cell Biol 27:263–272, November, 1965

Boles R: Hearing test without an audiometer. University of Michigan Medical Center J 37, No. 3:156, 1971

Bozian MW, Clark HM: Counteracting sensory changes in the aging. Am J Nurs 80:473–476, 1980

Burnside I: Touching is talking. Am J Nurs 73:2060–2063, December, 1973

Chaffee EE, Greisheimer EM: Basic Physiology and Anatomy, pp 230–234. Philadelphia, JB Lippincott, 1977

Finnerty FA, Linde SM: High Blood Pressure. New York, McKay, 1975

Grzegorczyk P, Jones SW, Mistretta CM et al: Age-related differences in salt taste acuity. Gerontol 34:834–840, November, 1979

Jenny J: What Should You Be Doing About Infection Control? Nurs '76 6:78–79, 1976

Johnson JE, Rice VH: Sensory and distress component of pain. Nurs Res 23:203–209, 1974

Kubuk HM: Safety precautions: Protecting your patients and yourself. Nurs '76 6:45–52, 1976

Lentz JR, Meyer EA: The dirty house. Nurs Outlook 27:590–591, September, 1979

Lindenmuth JE, Breu SS, Malooley JA: Sensory overload. Am J Nurs 80:1456–1458, August, 1980

Lograsso BA: Using words without sound. Am J Nurs 80:2187, 1980

Malasanos L, Barkauskas V, Moss M, Stoltenberg-Allen et al: Health Assessment. St. Louis, CV Mosby, 1981

Morris CG: An Introduction to Psychology. New York, Appleton-Century-Crofts, 1973

Murphy C: The effect of age on taste sensitivity. In Han S, Coons D (eds): Special Senses in Aging: A Current Biological Assessment, pp 21–33. Ann Arbor, University of Michigan, Institute of Gerontology, 1979

Noble MA: Communication in the ICU: Therapeutic or disturbing? Nurs Outlook 27:195–198, March, 1979

Schiffman L: Changes in taste and smell with age: Psychophysical aspects. In Ordy JM (ed): Sensory Systems and Aging in Man. New York, Raven Press, 1979

Waterson M: Hot and cold therapy. Nurs '78 8:46–49, October, 1978

Weinstock FJ: Emergency treatment of eye injuries. Am J Nurs 71:1928–1931, October, 1971

Wesseling E (ed): Symposium on patients with sensory deficits. Nurs Clin North Am 5:449–538, September, 1970

West M: The Salamander. New York, William Morrow, 1973

Integumentary Status

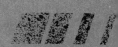

Margaret A. Banning

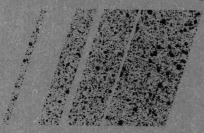

●

Apply principles of anatomy
and physiology to the care of
the person's skin.

●

Identify the functions of the
skin in maintaining the
person's health.

●

Describe the general nursing
assessment of the skin.

●

Describe nursing interventions
for persons with alterations in
skin.

●

Identify the psychological
implications of skin problems.

The skin is the largest organ of the human body, but its normal functioning is often taken for granted. Although many people are greatly concerned about their hearts or digestive systems, they rarely pay such attention to their skin. Even health practitioners may overlook the skin's value as an indicator of general health. Yet the condition of the skin may reflect nutritional status, heart and lung function, and body temperature. Skin irregularities such as jaundice, excessive dryness, decreased elasticity, or unusually warm or cool temperatures may suggest that a person has underlying health problems. Nurses must be able to recognize subtle changes in the skin as possible signs of altered health status.

The skin functions not only as a biological barrier between the person and his environment; it also serves as a psychological mediator between the individual and society. Certain areas of the skin are uniquely adapted for emotional expression. Most of us have experienced social situations that elicited blushing of the face or sweating of the hands and feet. Emotional disturbances may produce skin lesions such as a rash on the chest. Moreover, the person with red, weeping, raw, discolored, or scaling skin may fear that others will see him as unattractive or repulsive and may in fact evoke such feelings in others. This chapter examines the role of the skin in the person's physical and psychosocial adaptation.

Anatomy and Physiology

The skin consists of three basic layers: the epidermis, dermis, and subcutaneous tissue (Fig. 18-1).

Epidermis

The outermost layer of the skin is the epidermis, which consists of a thin layer of stratified epithelium and up to five additional layers, depending on the area of the body. Only the lowest layer is alive and growing. As cells develop, they are pushed to the surface where they flatten and die, forming a fibrous, nearly waterproof shield. This exposed surface of dead cornified cells, the *stratum corneum*, protects against loss of fluid and damage from friction. Its thickness varies according to the need for protection; it is thin in such areas as the abdominal wall but much thicker in areas subjected to pressure, such as the soles of the feet. Cells of this cornified layer are constantly being sloughed off and replaced by cells that move gradually outward from the deepest layer.

Cells called *melanocytes* are located at the junction of the epidermis and dermis. These cells produce the pigment melanin, which helps to shield the body from injurious ultraviolet radiation. In black persons, these skin cells, which are darkly pigmented, may slough off on a washcloth when the skin is washed and may be mistaken for dirt. A nurse who makes this presumption may scrub the skin vigorously, removing more cells and erroneously concluding that the person is hopelessly dirty.

The nails of the fingers and toes consist of epidermal cells which have been converted to keratin.

Hairs are threads of hard keratin that are projected outward through the epidermis from epithelial bulbs located in the dermis.

Dermis

Beneath the epidermis is the dermis, a dense layer of fibrous, elastic connective tissue. It has a rich supply of nerve endings and capillaries. In contrast, the outermost epidermal layer has only a few nerve endings and no direct vascular supply. The nutritional needs of the epidermal layer are met by the capillaries that supply the dermis and come in close contact with the epidermal layer.

The glands of the skin originate in the epidermal layer but grow into the dermis, with the larger glands plunging as deep as the subcutaneous layer. There are two basic types of glands, sudoriferous (sweat) and sebaceous (oily); modifications of these occur in certain areas of the body.

Sebaceous Glands

The sebaceous glands occur wherever there are hairs. The ducts of these glands open into the hair follicles. Sebaceous glands secrete an oily substance, sebum, which coats the hair, keeping it pliable and supple. A shortage or absence of sebum results in stiff, dry hair and dry skin, as is commonly seen in elderly persons. Sebaceous glands exist independently of hair in a few locations such as the genitalia, the areola and nipple of the breast, and the eyelids. The face has a large number of sebaceous glands; when these glands are occluded with debris, blackheads are formed. The size of the sebaceous gland is influenced by hormones, with androgen acting to

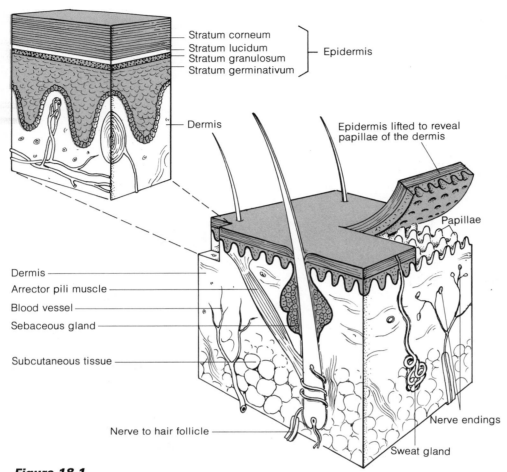

Figure 18-1
Anatomy of the skin.

increase gland size. As we grow older sebum production decreases; therefore, the nurse should limit the use of soap when bathing elderly people.

Sweat Glands. The skin also has 2 to 3 million coiled sudoriferous glands, also known as eccrine (exocrine) sweat glands, which are distributed over the entire surface of the body. These glands secrete sweat, which passes through ducts that open directly onto the surface of the skin. Stimulation of the sympathetic nervous system provokes a discharge of sweat from all of the various sweat glands. Quantities as high as 2 kg to 3 kg of sweat can be delivered to the surface of the body in 1 hour. Excessive sweating (**diaphoresis**) can cause serious fluid depletion and is therefore an important sign to note. In a subsequent section we will explore how sweat helps to maintain normal body temperature.

Apocrine Glands. The largest sweat glands are called apocrine glands and are located in the axilla, areola of the breast, and genital area. They differ from ordinary sweat glands in two ways: they discharge into hair follicles rather than directly onto the skin surface, and their discharge consists of some cell cytoplasm which produces the characteristic odor of sweat. That is why it is necessary to clean the apocrine gland areas carefully while bathing a person.

Modified apocrine sweat glands are located in the external ear canal and are called *ceruminous glands.* The secretion from these glands hardens on exposure to air to form the characteristic cerumen or wax, which prevents foreign matter from entering the auditory canal. The nurse should explain this protective function of the cerumen because many people tend to clean their ears excessively.

Subcutaneous Tissue

Beneath the dermis is a layer consisting mainly of adipose or fatty tissue, which insulates underlying areas from extremes in temperature and also provides a substantial cushion between the skin and the underlying bony prominences. Its size is a contributing factor in the development of pressure sores (ischemic ulcers) and is explored later in the chapter. Subcutaneous tissue contains sweat glands and the remainder of the hair follicles.

Protective Functions of the Skin

The skin acts as a protective barrier against the environment and plays a major role in our ability to adapt to internal and external changes. The protective functions of the skin are many and varied: it acts as a barrier against water loss, infection, and toxic substances; it protects the underlying organs; it regulates temperature; it protects against radiation; it serves special sensory functions; and it is an indication of one's general state of health (Fig. 18-2).

Barrier Against Water Loss or Entry

The skin has probably the lowest water permeability of any biologically produced membrane and prevents dehydration. The skin not only prevents the loss of body fluids but it also slows down the entrance of potentially toxic materials from the environment. The outermost horny layer or stratum corneum is

Figure 18-2
The skin serves many protective functions.

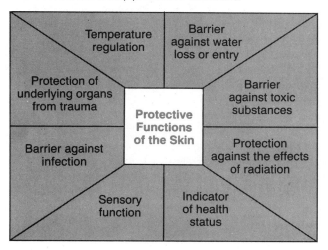

the water-retaining barrier of the skin. Very little water is lost through intact skin, but research has shown that with removal of the horny layer, water is lost by diffusion as fast as if the entire epidermal layer had been removed. Nurses need to be mindful of this phenomenon when caring for persons with burns or large, open wounds. These individuals experience an accelerated water loss through the damaged or absent skin which can cause serious or even fatal dehydration.

Barrier Against Infection

The skin also aids the body in its fight against pathogenic organisms. The stratum corneum acts as an impermeable barrier to bacteria from the outside. Fungi can only live in its outermost layers. Bacteria tend to be the most numerous in moist areas such as the perineum, so the relative dryness of most of the skin operates as a deterrent. It is doubtful, however, whether the skin presents a barrier to viruses.

The constant sloughing of surface cells also acts as a protective mechanism by carrying away a portion of the potential bacterial colonies (Downey and Darling, 1971). Bacteria and fungi are also inhibited by the lipids that are present in the sebum produced by the sebaceous glands. Research has shown that athlete's foot, a fungal infection that occurs in moist areas between the toes, greatly decreases at the time of puberty when increased androgen levels cause sebaceous glands to become more active. On the other hand, increased production of sebum and increased keratinization are factors that contribute to acne, an inflammatory disease that occurs most often in adolescents.

Obviously, any person with a break in the skin is susceptible to invasion by microorganisms. The nurse should observe wounds or other open skin areas for signs of infection and should initiate preventive care, as will be described later in the chapter.

Protection of Underlying Organs

The skin and the musculoskeletal system have some ability to protect underlying organs from injury. Bony encasements such as the ribs, combined with subcutaneous tissue, help protect vital organs such as the kidneys.

Temperature Regulation

The skin regulates body temperature by two mechanisms: the evaporation of sweat and the dilation and constriction of blood vessels allowing either more or less blood to radiate heat to the outside.

When skin temperature reaches 32° to 34° C (89.6°–93.2° F), a sudden outbreak of sweating occurs (Downey and Darling, 1971). Sweat secretion is stimulated by a rise of the temperature of the vascular supply reaching the central nervous system. It is important to recognize that excessive perspiration may indicate health problems such as fever. Excessive sweating can also cause electrolyte disturbances, dehydration, and heat exhaustion, which results from sodium depletion due to profuse sweating in hot weather. Heat is also lost from the skin through the process of radiation as described in Chapter 23. If body temperature rises, vasodilation occurs in the skin to promote heat loss to the environment. This process is evident in the flushed skin tone and warm skin temperature of persons with a fever.

Protection Against the Effects of Radiation

Despite the warnings of dermatologists and cancer specialists, most Americans still equate a deep summer tan with attractiveness and health. Current research documents that long-term indiscriminate exposure to sunlight is a cause of premature aging of the skin (Basler, 1978). People, such as sailors and farmers, with a long history of constant sun exposure show evidence of irreversible solar injury while still young. There also appears to be a causal relationship between sun exposure and lethal malignant melanoma. Nurses can be instrumental in teaching protective measures and moderation in sun exposure to those who sunbathe extensively.

Melanin is the only pigment that acts as an ultraviolet screen. The melanin in a well-tanned or naturally dark-skinned person greatly reduces the amount of ultraviolet radiation reaching the underlying dermis. The events responsible for sunburn are too complex to be described here, but it can be said that in most cases of mild sunburn the cutaneous inflammation (redness, sunburn) abates in 24 to 48 hours, followed by the appearance of a mildly protective tan. More severe sunburn reactions can lead to the formation of vesicles and bullae, followed by epithelial sloughing. Ultraviolet wavelengths that cause sunburn and degenerative damage can be separated from those that cause tanning; tanning products block harmful portions of the ultraviolet spectrum (Basler, 1978).

Nurses can teach their clients to avoid sunlight during midday hours when the rays are most intense. If exposure at this time is unavoidable, sunscreen can be effective in protecting against harmful ultraviolet radiation while only partially inhibiting tanning. Nevertheless, late afternoon exposure is best. Dermatologists suggest that persons with naturally dark pigmentation probably need sunscreen only on facial skin, which is more exposed to the sun. However, each person will need assistance in determining individual needs and appropriate guidelines.

Sensory Function

The skin is abundantly supplied with sensory receptors that transmit impulses of pain, temperature, light touch, and deep pressure to the central nervous system. The skin's function as a sense organ is dependent upon an abundant supply of cranial and spinal nerves. The larger nerve trunks subdivide continuously to form finer and finer networks as they get closer to the epidermis. Hair greatly adds to the sensitivity of skin because each hair follicle is surrounded by a complex of nerve fibers. The survival value of sensory fibers is apparent throughout a normal day's activities. We quickly withdraw our hand from a hot stove, feel pain in shoes that are too tight, determine if the shower temperature is safe, and sense the need for more or fewer clothes when environmental temperatures are excessively cold or hot. Anyone with impaired skin receptor mechanisms is quite vulnerable to injury from burns, cuts, abrasions, and the like. Elderly persons, or those with diabetes, strokes, spinal injuries, or debilitating conditions, are just a few of those who need intensive teaching in ways to assess the safety of their environment and reduce the dangers of sensory loss.

Barrier Against Toxic Substances

The stratum corneum prevents the penetration of many chemicals with which it comes in contact. Any process that damages or destroys this keratinized layer will strip away the skin's impermeability. Some chemicals, such as household bleach or lye, can disrupt the stratum corneum. Burns, abrasions, certain skin diseases, inflammatory processes, and moisture can also remove some of this layer, making it possible for toxins to penetrate the skin. **Abrasion** and maceration from moisture contribute to skin breakdown and the subsequent development of pressure sores, as is described later in the chapter.

Damage to the stratum corneum has a useful aspect, however, because it allows certain medications to be administered topically. Such medications, although unable to penetrate intact skin, can be absorbed through blistered areas of the skin in which the epidermal layers have been peeled away.

In the same way, mucous membranes which do not have a keratinized layer can allow certain substances to be absorbed. That is why aspirin can be administered as a rectal suppository or nitroglycerin, given under the tongue.

On the other hand, certain factors such as increased skin temperature, hyperemia, and a high surface concentration of medication may increase absorption through intact skin, even if to a limited degree. For instance, nitroglycerin can be applied as a paste to the skin to prevent chest pain due to angina. A ribbon of this medication is squeezed from a tube onto a sheet of paper and applied to a small area of the person's skin, providing a high surface concentration. The area is covered with plastic wrap, which promotes absorption by increasing skin temperature.

Indicator of Health Status

As has been indicated earlier, the color, temperature, and texture of the skin may be an indication of the person's health status. For example, nutritional status may be reflected in skin color or texture and may affect wound healing. The adequacy of the blood supply to a body part may be reflected in skin color, capillary filling, hair growth patterns, and skin integrity. Inadequate oxygenation may be reflected in pallor or cyanosis. Hemorrhagic diseases and trauma may produce bruising. Emotions such as embarrassment or fear may be evident through such skin manifestations as blushing or pallor. Likewise, some skin diseases, such as psoriasis, may be related to psychosocial factors. Each factor which is critical to a complete skin assessment is examined in the following section.

Skin Assessment

Overview

The skin is relatively easy to assess because it is so visible and does not require any special tools of evaluation. However, the very simplicity of skin assessment may mislead one into underestimating its importance in evaluating health status. Yet, a patient, systematic examination will offer a great deal of information and provide a good overall picture of the person's condition.

Skin color changes that are easily identified in lightly pigmented persons may not be apparent in darker individuals. Accurate interpretation of skin color requires knowledge of assessment techniques for both types of coloration. Much of the original work in the area of skin assessment for darkly pigmented individuals was done by Lora Roach (1974). Her work, which is cited in this section, describes data collection techniques that are helpful in the assessment of dark-skinned persons.

A thorough skin assessment depends not only on the nurse's physical examination skills but also on the ability to establish a trusting relationship. Such measures as providing privacy and a warm environment, preventing unnecessary exposure, and allowing a free expression of feelings may help in this regard, as will offering an accepting, objective attitude and "talking before touching."

Beginning students are sometimes uncomfortable about examining someone else's skin. Yet in order to set the person at ease, nurses must become comfortable with their own feelings about skin assessment. They should also be sensitive to the fact that some people feel self-conscious about a skin lesion that they may consider to be disfiguring or shameful. Such individuals may conceal a lesion with make-up, clothing, or jewelry and may be reluctant to talk about it or answer questions directly. By being sensitive to such feelings, the nurse may be able to work around evasive answers and help bring such concealed lesions to light (Roach, 1974).

Inspection and palpation are the primary techniques of skin assessment. Inspection of the skin and mucous membranes reveals changes in color, contour, integrity, and hygiene. Adequate lighting, preferably with natural light, is essential. Fluorescent lights have been known to cause people to appear cyanotic (Roach, 1974). Similarly, flashlights and overbed lights are inadequate for noting subtle color changes. Palpation assists in evaluating skin texture, temperature, and sensitivity to touch. Finally, the nurse's sense of smell will often be useful in detecting any odors that emanate from the skin.

It is also important to consider the effects of emotions, cigarette smoking, temperature, and gravity on the way the skin appears and feels. Chilling, anger, fright, and smoking all cause vasoconstriction and may hide pallor or cyanosis (Roach, 1974). Similarly, lying on a cold examination table may cause the skin to blanch. Conversely, the person who is excessively warm or is embarrassed by skin exposure may experience erythema, which can mask skin abnormalities. Positioning during the examination is also a crucial factor. Examining the lower extremities at heart level while the person is in bed may indicate satisfactory blood supply, but when the person sits with legs dangling over the side of the bed, it may become apparent that circulation is impaired. A complete assessment involves examination in both positions.

If the person is hospitalized, a thorough skin assessment may best be done at the time a complete bath is given. In the person's home or in an ambulatory care setting, the nurse usually defers skin assessment until trust has been established and the person is comfortable. Areas to consider in the skin assessment include color, temperature, turgor, texture, odor, intactness (integrity), hair and nails, lesions, and age.

Color

The amount of pigment or melanin in the skin varies according to the person's race, age, and condition. Caucasians have less melanin than dark-skinned persons, but elderly Caucasians often have darker skin because of exposure to ultraviolet light over a lifetime. Albinism means a complete lack of pigment, giving the characteristic white hair and transparent skin color. Skin color is also indicative of oxygenation and nutritional status. For instance, pallor may reflect anemia due to a diet deficient in iron, whereas cyanosis may be a sign of inadequate oxygen due to respiratory distress. The best places to observe color changes are those areas in which the capillary beds are superficial and pigmentation is minimal, such as the nail beds, lips, conjunctiva, hard palate, palms of the hands, and soles of the feet (Roach, 1974).

Pallor

Pallor in a dark-skinned person is noted by an absence of the underlying red tones that normally give the brown or black skin its glow or living color. Thus, the brown-skinned person appears more yellowish-brown and the black-skinned person more ashen-gray (Roach, 1972). Generalized pallor again is noted in the mucous membranes, lips, and nail beds, with the mucous membranes appearing ashen-gray.

Cyanosis

Cyanosis is a diffuse bluish color that occurs when the blood contains 5 g per 100 ml or more of reduced (deoxygenated) hemoglobin. Further assessment and interpretation of cyanosis is found in Chapters 23 and 24. As indicated in the preceding paragraph, cyanosis is very difficult to detect in the darkly pigmented person. The normal assessment sites, the skin around the mouth, cheeks, and ear lobes, often have dark pigmentation that obscures the signs of beginning cyanosis. However, regular close inspection of the person's palms and soles, the lips, nail beds, and conjunctiva usually helps the nurse recognize cyanosis in its early stages of development (Roach, 1972). In addition, the lips and tongue may appear ashen-gray. It is important to become familiar with the person's normal color in order to detect changes which may occur later.

Erythema

Erythema is a reddish color caused by congestion or dilation of cutaneous blood vessels. Erythema is one of the cardinal signs of inflammation, but there are many other causes. If a reddened area is noted on the person's skin, other findings should be checked, such as the distribution of the erythema (general or localized); the presence of hardness, lesions, or itching; and pain produced by touch.

Palpation may be the most important assessment technique for detecting erythema in a dark-skinned person. The presence of warmth might suggest inflammation; induration over a bony prominence suggests a pressure sore; slick, tight skin suggests edema; a bumpy texture of the skin suggests a papular rash. Generalized rashes can be observed in the mucosa of the mouth. In addition, the nurse will need to ask the person about other symptoms, such as pruritis, burning, or pain, in order to detect erythema and analyze its cause.

Petechiae

Petechiae are round, flattened, pinpoint spots of purplish-red resulting from intradermal or submucosal bleeding. These hemorrhagic lesions usually occur in the mucous membranes as well as in the skin. Petechiae occur in health problems that result in low platelet count (thrombocytopenia) or in certain infectious processes that cause small-blood-vessel damage.

In the dark-skinned person petechiae are usually visible in the areas of lighter melanization such as the abdomen, forearms, and buttocks. If the person's skin is especially dark, petechiae are not visible on the skin; however, they can be detected on mucous membranes. Therefore, the nurse should carefully inspect the buccal mucosa and conjunctiva for petechiae (Roach, 1972).

Ecchymosis

Ecchymosis (commonly known as a bruise) can be defined as a purple or blue, nonelevated, rounded, or irregular area in the skin or mucous membrane. Ecchymosis is distinguished from petechiae by its larger size. Large areas of ecchymosis that merge with one another are termed **purpura.**

Ecchymosis is the result of hemorrhage beneath the skin. When a blood vessel is broken, the blood is quickly deoxygenated and seeps into the subcutaneous tissue, causing the characteristic purple-blue color. As the blood cells are reabsorbed, the color usually changes over time in a pattern from reddish-purple to blue-black, to greenish-brown, to yellow. The color can therefore provide information about the age of the lesion (Roach, 1974). Ecchymosis may result from trauma such as falls, venipunctures, or bumps or from systemic problems such as spontaneous internal bleeding (*e.g.,* in hemophilia).

The nurse needs to obtain information from the person about incidents that may have caused ecchymosis since such a relationship might provide a clue to possible coagulation problems. For instance, the person who is taking anticoagulant medication might note bruised areas of his body but not recall having bumped himself in any way that may have caused them. In this instance, the nurse might suspect that the medication is causing abnormal bleeding and would therefore notify the physician.

In the dark-skinned person, bruises may not be as prominent, but a history of trauma and the presence of an area that is painful to touch would suggest the possibility of ecchymosis. It is easy to confuse ecchymosis with hematomas, because both often have the same history and physical findings. However, a **hematoma** also produces swelling that can be detected by palpating the surface of the skin. Ecchymosis is usually large enough to be visible on dark skin; this is in contrast to petechiae, which are difficult to see because of their small size (Roach, 1972).

Jaundice

Jaundice is a yellow skin discoloration that occurs with the excessive accumulation of bilirubin in the tissues. Jaundice is most often noted in the sclera and the skin. Mucous membranes on the other hand, are colored by capillaries and become jaundiced only when serum bilirubin levels are extremely high.

Jaundice is seen in many types of health problems including cardiac, hepatic, and renal abnormalities. Any condition in which there is obstruction of the passage of bile, increased destruction of red blood cells, or disturbances in the function of liver cells can cause elevated levels of bilirubin and thus jaundice. A yellow color can also be created by other conditions, such as high levels of cholesterol, excessive carotene, industrial chemicals, certain drugs (*e.g.,* quinacrine), picric acid, or even a fading suntan (Roach, 1974). Such discoloration may be mistaken for jaundice.

Jaundice may be the only indication of certain health problems, so the nurse should be able to recognize it early. The best area to check for jaundice in both light-skinned and dark-skinned persons is the sclera, because the skin may not become yellow until very late. Jaundice is frequently accompanied by clay-colored stools or dark gold-brown urine, which can confirm its presence.

The sclera of many darkly pigmented persons appears jaundiced because of deposits of subconjunctival fat containing carotene. Inspecting the portion of the sclera that is normally revealed by the lid slit will help the nurse identify true jaundice. If the sclera appears to be jaundiced to the edges of the cornea, inspect the posterior portion of the person's hard palate, where jaundice can often be observed in its early stages. If the palate does not appear yellow, assume that the person is not jaundiced (Roach, 1972).

Temperature

Skin temperature is a reflection of the flow of blood through the cutaneous vessels. These vessels dilate during fever and in hot weather to cool the body by heat loss through the skin. In this instance, the abnormally warm skin temperature reflects an increase in blood flow. In the same way, inflamed tissue is hot to the touch because of vasodilation in the injured area. Abnormally cool skin temperature indicates a diminished flow of blood to the particular body part in question. For instance, the skin of a person in shock feels cool to the touch owing to the shunting of blood flow from the skin to the vital organs.

Unfortunately, the nurse cannot determine that a problem exists on the basis of abnormal skin temperature alone. For instance, if nurse Karen Jones notices that Mr. Smith's right foot feels cold, she might wonder if this is caused by the cold room temperature or by a cast on his right leg that may be too tight. Nurse Jones can make additional observations to analyze the information she already has. She can compare the temperature of the right and left feet; if one is colder than the other, it suggests inadequate circulation in the cool body part. She can also look for other evidence of diminished blood flow, such as pale skin color and slow capillary refill. If she notes these changes she will notify the physician and obtain a cast cutter should the cast need to be released to improve circulation. Two principles help the nurse analyze skin temperature findings:

- Compare temperature of a body part to other areas.
- Make additional observations (Table 18-1).

Turgor

Turgor is defined as "the fullness of tissue" or "resiliency of skin," that is, its ability to bounce back. Turgor provides a quick means of determining tissue hydration. It is assessed by grasping the skin between the forefinger and thumb, pulling upward and then releasing. If the skin fails to resume its normal contour promptly, it may denote decreased hydration. In the elderly, however, poor skin turgor may be due to loss of elastic tissue rather than dehydration.

Turgor is also affected by fluid retention or *edema* that causes swelling, making the skin taut and shiny and obliterating bony prominences and normal contour. Fluid retention or edema can be tested by pressing a forefinger against the person's skin (Fig. 18-3). If the indentation remains after the forefinger is removed, this is termed "pitting edema" and can be indicative of serious fluid retention, as discussed in Chapter 23.

Texture

The term "texture" describes the feel of the skin. By touching the skin, the nurse can observe whether it is smooth, dry, rough, or calloused and whether

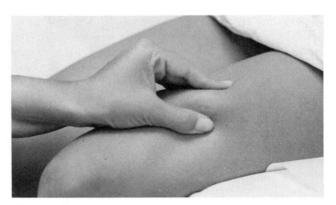

Figure 18-3
Testing skin turgor.

there are corns, wrinkles, scaly skin, and scars. The older person has drier, less elastic skin resulting in coarser skin texture. Rough or coarse texture may indicate dry skin due to inadequate lubrication. Because dry skin is vulnerable to cracking and broken skin is susceptible to infection, the nurse should apply emollient lotion to dry areas. Areas of the skin that are exposed to pressure are often indurated (hard), as is the case with the skin of feet. Inflamed areas may also be indurated.

Odor

The odor of a person's skin may be an indication of personal hygiene and cleanliness. Any hairy region of the body is particularly susceptible to odors because bacteria are more numerous in such areas. The nurse should cleanse these areas well during the bath.

Odors are also associated with infections and lesions. For instance, a musty odor is associated with infections in casted extremities. Characteristic foul

Table 18-1
Analyzing Skin Temperature Changes

Skin Temperature	Associated Findings	Possible Interpretation
Cool temperature	Moist, clammy skin, generalized pale color	Shock
Cool temperature	Absent local pulse, localized pale color, slow capillary filling	Poor arterial circulation to affected part
Warm temperature	Painful area to touch, localized erythema, and edema	Inflammation of affected area
Warm temperature	Diaphoresis, generalized erythema	Fever

odors are frequently associated with *Pseudomonas* and *Staphylococcus* infections, as well as necrotic tissue.

Because skin odors are associated with poor hygiene in our culture, they often cause a sense of shame. Persons with foul-smelling skin conditons may make comments such as, "I don't know how anyone can be around me," or, "I feel so filthy." The diminished sense of self-esteem reflected by these statements is obvious. It is important to maintain an objective and caring attitude when working with these individuals. Commercial deodorants can help mask foul odors and help the person feel less offensive. Other considerations related to low self-esteem are presented at the end of this chapter and in Chapter 15.

Skin Integrity

The skin can serve a protective function only when it is intact. Loss of skin integrity prevents the skin from functioning as a barrier against the environment. Any breaks in the skin surface serve as openings either for the entrance of infection and toxic substances or for the loss of fluids. Pressure sores, burns, lacerations, surgical incisions, and open blisters all break the continuity of the skin.

When assessing the person for breaks in the skin, the nurse should note and chart location, size, symmetry, and distribution, at the same time observing for the presence of inflammation, drainage, and pain.

Hair and Nails

The distribution, texture, condition, and amount of body hair are related to factors such as age, sex, and genetic make-up. It is important to note changes in characteristics of the hair because these may be related to the person's health status. For instance, the woman who diets excessively may note that her hair has become dull and brittle. The young man receiving chemotherapy might experience hair loss. **Alopecia** (hair loss) may also be due to radiation therapy or aging. The nurse should assess the person's grooming patterns so that these can be maintained if he needs assistance with hair care.

Nails can also be indicative of the person's health status. The texture, thickness, configuration, cleanliness, brittleness, and condition must be noted. Poor nutrition can cause brittleness or ridges in the nails. Poor arterial circulation can cause the nails, especially the toenails, to thicken. Elderly persons may have tough, brittle nails that make trimming difficult.

Skin Lesions

Because nurses are the health-care providers who spend the most time with clients, they are often the first to notice skin lesions as well as any daily changes in skin condition. Knowledge of dermatological terminology assists nurses to make relevant observations, note changes, and use appropriate terms in reporting and recording this information. Nurses need to pay close attention to minute details when identifying alterations in the person's skin. Lesions need to be examined for specific type (flat, elevated, depressed), shape or configuration, and possible grouping. Flat lesions are in the plane of the skin, elevated lesions are above the plane of the skin, and depressed lesions are below the plane of the skin. Some lesions can be of more than one type.

Skin abnormalities can be divided into two other groups. *Primary lesions* are those that appear as the immediate result of some initiating factor; *secondary lesions* result only from changes in the underlying primary lesions (Table 18-2).

Assessment of Skin in the Elderly

The effects of aging on the skin are discussed in Chapter 6. In general there is a decrease in effective circulation, decreased subcutaneous tissue, decreased elasticity, wrinkling, thinning, sagging, and increased dryness. There is also an increase in pigmentation from frequent exposure to ultraviolet light. The skin of elderly people is also less sensitive to heat and cold because of decreased nerve sensitivity. The nails thicken, become brittle and tough, and splinter easily. The nurse should be aware of the psychological effects of these changes as they may contribute to altered body image in elderly persons.

Nursing Measures Related to Hygiene

Bathing has traditionally played an important role in human society. Archeologists have uncovered organized provisions for bathing that are at least 6000 years old. In various cultures bathing serves medical, religious or ceremonial, social, and recreational functions, as well as the purpose of physical cleansing. Eastern religions, such as Buddhism and Shintoism, strongly emphasize the religious aspect of bathing; their bathing houses are often constructed

Table 18-2
Types of Skin Lesions

Primary Lesions

Macule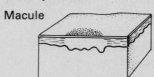

A circumscribed area of color change, usually less than 1 cm in size, with no depression or elevation of its surface in relation to surrounding skin. Macules may be the result of hyperpigmentation or hypopigmentation or may be due to permanent vascular abnormalities of the skin. The small erythematous lesions seen in roseola and secondary syphilis are examples of macules, as are freckles.

Papule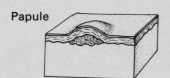

A solid, elevated lesion, less than 1 cm in diameter. Color is important in identifying these lesions and analyzing their cause. Papules may be red and pointed as in acne, red and flat-topped as in psoriasis, copper-colored as in lesions of secondary syphilis, or a variety of other colors.

Plaque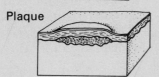

A lesion that may be either macular or papular but that occupies a relatively large surface area (larger than 1 cm in diameter). It can be formed by a confluence of papules such as in psoriasis. Mongolian spots are another example.

Nodule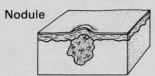

A palpable, solid lesion, less than 1 cm in diameter, which can be located in the epidermis or can extend to the dermis and subcutaneous layers. These raised lesions may indicate systemic disease and result from inflammation, malignancies, or metabolic deposits in the tissue.

Tumor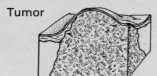

A general term to indicate a large nodule of more than 1 cm in size and it denotes any mass, benign or malignant.

Vesicles and bullae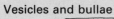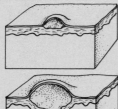

A fluid-filled, circumscribed, elevated lesion of less than 1 cm in size. Often the vesicle walls are so thin or translucent that the accumulation of serum, lymph, blood, or extracellular fluid just beneath the epidermis is visible. These lesions are commonly seen in chickenpox and smallpox. If a vesicle is relatively large (greater than 1 cm), it is then termed a bulla, for example those found in second-degree burns.

Pustule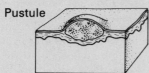

A lesion identical to a vesicle or bulla but containing pus (purulent exudate), such as the lesions seen in acne. These elevated lesions may appear yellow, white, or greenish yellow, depending on the color of the exudate.

Wheal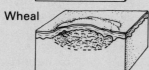

A rounded or irregularly shaped elevation of the skin or mucous membranes, which is characterized by rapid change. It may disappear within hours or shift from the involved to uninvolved, adjacent areas. These lesions result from edema and have a distinctive appearance. A variety of initiating agents, such as insect bites, can cause an allergic response seen as a wheal.

Primary Lesions

Cyst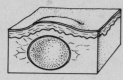
An encapsulated, fluid-filled, or semisolid mass in the dermis or subcutaneous tissue layers. A cyst may contain fluid, cells, or cell products. Unlike a nodule or tumor, a cyst feels resilient. The most common cysts are epidermal or keratinous cysts and sebaceous cysts.

Secondary Lesions

Scales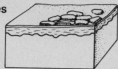
Dry or oily masses of dead tissue from the stratum corneum or horny layer of the skin; for example, the dry and silvery flakes of skin seen in dandruff and psoriasis, or the oily yellow tissue of seborrheic dermatitis. Normally, cells found in the outermost layer of the skin contain cell debris but no nuclei. Desquamative layers of skin including nuclei are termed scales.

Crusts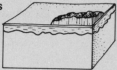
Encrusted exudates that result when serum, blood, or purulent drainage dries on the skin surface. Crusts may be thin, delicate, and friable, or thick and adherent. Crusts are yellow when formed from dried serum, green or yellow-green when formed from purulent exudate, brown or dark red when formed from blood.

Fissures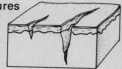
Cracks or deep linear splits through the epidermal layer of the skin into the dermis. These cleavages can be painful and are seen following excessive drying of the skin. Some treatments for conditions such as dermatitis may cause fissures in the hands and feet. Chapping in cold weather is another example, as is the cracking of the skin with athlete's foot.

Erosions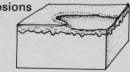
Loss of the outermost layer of the epidermis only; for example, a superficial scratch of syphilitic chancre.

Ulcers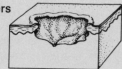
Irregularly shaped excavation in which there has been necrosis of tissue with destruction of both the epidermis and the dermis. Certain features such as the location and borders are helpful in determining the cause of the ulcer. The ulcer usually heals with the production of excess collagen, and a scar results. Venous stasis ulcers due to poor tissue nutrition are most commonly seen on the ankle or lower leg. Ischemic ulcers such as decubitus ulcers or pressure sores may be found at pressure points.

Lesions Common to Darkly Pigmented Individuals

Keloids
Thick, fibrous lumps or scars that occur due to an exaggerated wound healing process. The healing following surgery, trauma, ear piercing, or simply the spontaneous healing process of certain skin diseases may cause a keloid to form.

Pseudofolliculitis
Numerous elevated bumps disturbed on the face or neck due to ingrown hairs. The thick, wooly hair of darkly pigmented individuals makes them susceptible. These lesions can be prevented by not shaving or by cutting the hair on the neck.

close to temples so that purification may precede worship (Aaland, 1978). Saunas or steam baths are integral to cultures as disparate as those of Scandanavia, Turkey, Ireland, Germany, Russia, Mexico, and some American Indians. Public bathing is an integral part of Japanese life. But whether it is communal or private, whether people sprinkle hot water over rocks, jump in ice-cold tubs, roll in the snow, luxuriate in bubble baths, or take brisk showers, bathing frequently involves some kind of custom. Our distinctive bathing practices become part of our individual way of life and help to determine our sense of well-being. Nurses therefore should strive to understand each person's customary bathing habits and incorporate these customs into the person's care whenever possible.

Bathing

The two major purposes of bathing are to cleanse the skin of dirt, bacteria, and dead epithelial cells and to provide comfort. Most persons feel relaxed and refreshed after bathing. "I'm going to take a long, hot bath," is a common saying after a particularly tense or trying day. However, bathing has other benefits that are not as obvious. Vigorous scrubbing during the bath increases circulation to the skin by dilating cutaneous blood vessels. As the person goes through the motions of bathing, he exercises his muscles and joints; thus, bathing may be a means of maintaining joint range of motion and muscle strength for the bedridden person.

When the nurse bathes a client, assessment of the condition of the skin, musculoskeletal system, and circulatory function is easily performed. Bathing a person often promotes rapport and provides an opportunity to uncover emotional needs, assist the client to talk about concerns, and even begin problem solving. However, in order to establish such a relationship, the nurse must feel comfortable about working intimately with a person's body. Many students are apprehensive about bathing a client for the first time. Such feelings reflect discomfort about invading the client's privacy or working intimately with another's body, particularly if the client is of the opposite sex. Talking out such feelings in a group or with a supportive instructor can assist the student to feel more comfortable and thereby help the client to feel relaxed.

The procedure for assisting a person with the bath is not described here. Rather, general considerations concerning ways of assisting the person with hygiene needs are presented (Table 18-3).

Table 18-3
Assisting with a Bed Bath

- Assess the client's routine.
- Offer the appropriate amount of assistance.
- Maintain privacy and modesty.
- Maintain warmth.
- Maintain safety.
- Teach self-care activities as needed.

- Assess the client's routine. Most persons have established bathing practices such as preference for a tub or shower bath, using deodorants or powder, taking morning or evening baths, or bathing with or without soap. The nurse assesses these practices so that they can be maintained as much as possible if the person requires assistance with hygiene.

- Offer the appropriate amount of assistance. Some individuals might be encouraged to participate in bathing as a means of exercise. Others will need the nurse to assume much of the procedure in order to conserve energy for other activities.

- Maintain privacy and modesty. Close the door or draw curtains around the bathing area. If you are bathing the client, only expose the area that you are bathing.

- Maintain warmth. Room temperature should be comfortable because the person is uncovered. Exposing only the area being bathed also helps keep the person comfortably warm.

- Maintain safety. Do not leave dependent persons such as children or unconscious individuals unattended. Leave the call bell within reach if the client is performing some of his own bath.

- Teach self-care activities as needed. For instance, persons taking a bed bath for the first time may need information about how to perform this activity more easily.

Maintaining hygiene includes care of the hair, nails, and mouth. Assess the person's usual routine for these activities and maintain this as much as feasible. If the person is hospitalized, family members or friends may provide special shampoos or hair products. Dark-skinned individuals have hair care needs which are different from those of Caucasians because their hair is thicker, coarser, curlier, and drier. Davis (1977) and Grier (1976) describe step-by-step instructions on ways to comb, braid, and care for the hair of dark-skinned persons.

Massage

Like bathing, massage has been practiced in a wide range of human societies. By instinct, it seems, people resort to pressing and rubbing the body to relieve pain and alleviate certain illnesses (Nichols, 1973). Massage as a method of pain relief has recently been the focus of much research (see Chap. 25). Massage is also an excellent way to promote relaxation and a feeling of well-being and can be a very effective intervention for a person on prolonged bed rest.

Massage may involve either superficial stroking or deep kneading. Stroking—slow, gentle, and rhythmic—can soothe the person and alleviate fatigue. The slight friction of the hand as it slips along the surfaces of the skin also helps to improve the circulation and glandular activity of the skin. Deep kneading—compressing and squeezing the flesh—can stimulate the flow of blood and lymph, thus helping to prevent muscle stiffness following prolonged exertion. Some estimate that blood passes three times more readily through the muscle after massage (Nichols, 1973). The nurse should begin kneading the person's skin lightly, increasing the pressure gradually. Obviously, more pressure can be tolerated over thick, fleshy areas such as the buttocks than over light tissue or bony surfaces. Massaging around bony prominences stimulates circulation to these areas, preventing damage from oxygen starvation. A massage of the back should begin at the buttocks and move up toward the neck, following the fibers of the major muscle groups. Massage of the extremities is not recommended because of the danger of dislodging a thrombus.

Lubricants such as lotions and powders are often used in massage. Lotions should be warmed in the nurse's hand before use. Alcohol is very drying and may chill the person, but it can be used if the skin is particularly oily.

Nursing Process
Applied to Specific Skin Problems

Tissue Injury

Since the skin acts as a protective barrier and is exposed to the outside world, it is often subjected to trauma. The damage can be of several different types:

* Nonpenetrating trauma caused by a blow or by prolonged pressure
* Penetrating trauma from wounds or surgical incisions
* Chemical, thermal, or radiation burns and injuries
* Bacterial injury

Adaptation

Adaptation to such trauma occurs through the processes of inflammation, fibroplasia, and scar maturation and contraction.

Inflammation
Inflammation is the initial biological response of the skin to trauma. Inflammation is a defensive vascular and cellular response that limits tissue damage by disposing of microorganisms, foreign material, and dead or necrotic tissue. It also helps to prepare for the subsequent repair process.

The initial stage is characterized by vascular changes. There is an immediate and brief constriction of the local vasculature lasting between 5 and 10 minutes. Histamine released by injured tissues causes vasodilation and increased blood flow and is responsible for the phenomenon known as **hyperemia** (vessel engorgement). This can be seen as a bright flush on the surface of the skin or edema visible at the injury site. The area feels warm to the touch. Hyperemia floods the damaged area with needed oxygen, nutrients, and antibodies and assists in the removal of toxic waste products. White blood cells engage in phagocytosis of foreign substances, engulfing bacteria and other foreign material.

Histamine action also increases vascular permeability. Exudate is then formed, which is made up of vascular fluid and blood cells, damaged tissue cells, and foreign material such as bacteria. Exudate can be serous (such as the clear sterile fluid seen in blisters), sanguinous (hemorrhagic), or purulent (pus-like) if the wound is infected. Purulent exudate is thick fluid containing necrotic tissue debris plus large amounts of bacteria. Exudate can develop in the absence of bacterial invasion and may in some cases be sterile. Purulent exudate can delay or even prevent wound healing by interfering with epithelialization and fibroplasia. The collection of exudate may also cause swelling, pain, and sometimes loss of function.

Fibroplasia

As most of the foreign material is removed by white cells, the stage of tissue fibroplasia begins. On the surface new epithelial cells—granulation tissue—have begun to cover the defect (epithelialization). Deeper in the area of injury fibroplastic cells begin synthesizing scar tissue, primarily collagen and protein, forming a fibrous network (fibroplasia). The scar that is formed during fibroplasia is an enlarged dense structure of collagen that is highly soluble, making the union very fragile.

Scar Maturation and Contraction

During the last phase of healing, pronounced changes in the form, bulk, and strength of the scar occur (scar maturation). Small blood vessels in the new tissue disappear and the scar contracts or shrinks in size (contraction). This phase may last indefinitely. The connective tissue scar is much stronger than the fragile granulation tissue.

In summary, tissue healing (scar formation) occurs through the processes of inflammation, fibroplasia, and collagen maturation. Although each of these stages has been discussed separately, they are, in fact, a continuum that overlaps and occasionally varies somewhat from the order given.

Assessment

When evaluating an area of injury the nurse should consider the factors described in the assessment of skin integrity found earlier in this chapter. In the stage of inflammation, erythema, edema, and induration may be noted in the area of injury. The injured area is often warm and painful to touch. The amount and type of exudate should be assessed. Granulation tissue, which is bright red and friable, may be noted in the stage of fibroplasia if the wound is open. If the injury has healed to the point of scar formation, the nurse should note its appearance and integrity.

Nursing Interventions

Appropriate nursing interventions to facilitate healing vary greatly depending on the depth and extent of skin involvement, the nature of the condition, and the type of injury. Interventions appropriate for burns, pressure sores, and common dermatological problems are covered in a later section. The following are general interventions requiring adaptation and modification to each individual situation.

Cold applications (ice packs, cold compresses, cold or alcohol sponge baths) are used immediately following contusions, sprains, and strains and for the first 24 hours after injury to limit the accumulation of fluid in body tissue. Cold constricts blood vessels, limiting the vascular stage of the inflammatory process, slowing cellular metabolism, inhibiting microbial growth, and aiding in the control of hemorrhage when necessary. Cold also has an anesthetic effect, preventing edema that causes pain by pressure on nerve endings. However, if edema is already present, cold should not be used because it prevents dilatation and the removal of waste products.

Heat applications (heat lamps, warm compresses, heating pads, sitz baths, hot water bottles) are often used for the relief of congestion (edema), inflammation, and muscle spasms and to promote tissue healing; for instance, heat is commonly applied to relieve edema after an IV infusion infiltration, to reduce the inflammation of thrombophlebitis, and to alleviate muscle soreness. Heat causes vasodilation, increased blood flow which furnishes more oxygen and nutrients, and more rapid removal of toxic products and congesting fluid. Healing is promoted as tissue metabolism improves. However, the danger of burns when heat is improperly used cannot be overemphasized.

Moist compresses are helpful for many persons with skin problems and dermatological lesions. As water evaporates, these dressings have a cooling effect that helps to relieve itching, burning, and inflammation. They are also helpful in the removal of dried exudate resulting from crusting types of skin conditions. If allowed to dry, they will adhere to tissue and can thus be used for manual debridement of necrotic tissue. For this reason they are used in the treatment of persons with burns and infected wounds. However, moist dressings that are left in contact with healthy epithelial surfaces for prolonged periods of time not only soften the skin but can actually cause maceration of the underlying skin. Warm compresses are used in conjunction with wet dressings to add the beneficial effects of heat. When the nurse is applying dressings to open areas of skin, sterile technique should be used to avoid the introduction of pathogens.

Cleansing the skin helps to stimulate circulation, decrease bacterial count, and remove scales or crusts. The person's skin is frequently scrubbed prior to surgery to decrease the bacterial count. Cleansing can also be used to relieve itching and to apply medications. The agents used are as varied as the skin problems and lesions involved. It is beyond the scope of this chapter to outline them all here. However, it is important to recognize that some agents, including soap and water, may be contraindicated in certain instances. The nurse can choose the appropriate intervention only after a thorough assessment has been made.

Irrigation is another form of cleansing that helps to remove debris. The eye, ear, throat, vagina, perineum, and wounds are areas particularly suited to cleansing by irrigation.

Protection is another measure that promotes healing. Mechanical padding, such as a dressing, may be used to protect the area from direct trauma. A shield can be used to prevent fluid loss and microorganism entry. An eyeshield is a light metal plate that is taped over the area surrounding the eye socket.

Common Skin Conditions

Nursing care of the person with a common skin problem such as a rash may be complex. There are not only many causes of such skin conditions but also a variety of signs, symptoms, and treatments. As a beginning nurse you will not be responsible for diagnosing skin problems. However, your observations can be valuable in determining factors associated with the person's problem, such as diet, emotions, or medications. This section emphasizes how the nurse can assist the person with common dermatological problems. A more extensive discussion can be found in a dermatology or medical–surgical textbook.

Assessment

Derbes (1978) feels that the three most common mistakes health professionals make in this area are to: (1) readily attribute skin disruptions to emotional disturbances; (2) brush aside cancers as merely a birthmark or a mole; and (3) assume a lesion is not contagious. Emotional disturbances are not the cause of very many eruptions, although skin diseases such as psoriasis may be exacerbated by stress. A lesion that grows, changes color, or bleeds could be a carcinoma. Although 95% to 98% of all lesions are not contagious, respect the few that are (e.g., any lesion with purulent exudate, warts, chickenpox, herpes zoster, shingles, and lesions on the genitalia).

Nurses are the health professionals most likely to see a hospitalized person's skin. The nurse in the community may also be the first to identify a skin problem. If the nurse notes skin lesions, additional observations should be made in order to interpret findings accurately:

* Location of the lesions (localized, generalized, body parts affected)
* Onset of the lesions (time of occurrence; relationship to activities, medications, food, exposure to infectious conditions)
* Appearance of the lesions (raised, flat, color, exudate) and related signs or symptoms (e.g., itching).

Rashes

Localized rashes are rarely due to systemic diseases, food, or drugs. A person who develops a rash on his skin at the edge of a cast or a person with a rash at his incision site may have contact dermatitis. Approximately 3% of the population is allergic to mercury, which is a frequent component of substances used to prepare a person's skin for surgery (Derbes, 1978). Some individuals are allergic to the terpenes contained in certain balsams that are used as soothing lotions prior to cast application. Also, a rash may simply be a sign of irritation from rough edges of a cast.

Contact Dermatitis

Contact dermatitis usually has an abrupt onset with pruritic, red, oozing, and scaly lesions, primarily in areas such as the face, neck, hands, forearms, genitalia, and lower legs. Contact dermatitis, when seen in women who have new babies and are constantly exposing their hands to soap and cleansing agents, is sometimes known as "housewives' eczema." Nurses are also susceptible to contact dermatitis, as can be seen by the condition of their hands when they are on duty—a condition that clears up during time off. Businessmen may experience the opposite, from hobbies that cause flare-up on the weekend and that clear up during the week. Obviously, this eczema is awkward to treat because of the difficulty in avoiding its cause.

Drug Reactions

Drug reactions are another common cause of skin eruption. Drugs can produce a variety of skin lesions, including baldness and lesions that mimic fungus infections, cancers, psoriasis, measles, or chickenpox. Lesions may even look like acne or ringworm. The most common drug eruption is **urticaria** (hives). If skin eruptions suddenly appear, the nurse must check to see whether the person is taking any new drugs. Large areas of skin may slough off, making the drug reaction life threatening. All drugs, except those necessary for life must be stopped, and the area must be treated.

Nursing Interventions

Nurses carry out both dependent and independent interventions in caring for persons with skin lesions. Dependent functions include administering prescribed medications and treatments. Independent functions are just as important in assisting the person. Such interventions include the following:

- Assessing the person's skin condition in order to evaluate beginning problems and the response to therapy. For instance, the nurse is often the first to note a rash that might indicate an allergic response to a medication.
- Teaching the person about medications and treatments, including their purpose, administration, and side-effects.
- Assisting the person to identify and remove potential irritants from the environment.
- Assisting persons in the community to determine when medical attention is necessary for treat-

ment of their skin condition. Many persons are tempted to treat rashes with over-the-counter preparations, which may be useless or dangerous for their skin condition.

Nurses are also important in assisting the person to cope with the emotional effects of chronic skin conditions. This aspect of nursing care is described later in the chapter.

Pressure Sores

Pressure sores (ischemic **ulcers,** decubitus ulcers, bedsores) are localized areas of cellular **necrosis;** they are usually found over bony prominences that are subjected to pressures in excess of capillary pressure for prolonged periods of time (Kosiak, 1961). The original term, decubitus, came from the Latin meaning lying down and was used because the pressure sore seemed to occur most frequently in the recumbent person. Pressure in any position is now known to be the cause (Fig. 18-4).

The topic of decubitus ulcers is extremely important for nurses because this devastating problem is preventable through appropriate nursing care and extensive patient teaching. One pressure sore can extend the length of hospitalization more than twofold, thus increasing medical care costs by astronomical amounts. Prolonged hospitalization also increases the loss of income, lengthens separation from family and friends, and may delay physical therapy and other programs, not to mention the tremendous psychological cost to the individual. Being restricted to bed rest, dependent on others for care, and conscious of an unsightly pressure sore

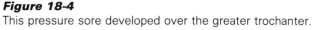

Figure 18-4
This pressure sore developed over the greater trochanter.

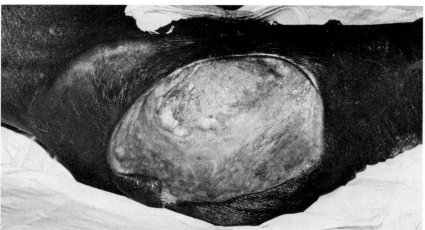

greatly threatens any feelings of being an intact and attractive person.

Many other problems are associated with pressure sores, including chronic infection, septicemia, protein and electrolyte loss, osteomyelitis, and secondary amyloidosis. *Secondary amyloidosis* is the accumulation of fibrous material in tissue that accompanies prolonged inflammatory or infectious diseases and is a cause of death in paraplegics and quadriplegics with either decubitus ulcers or urinary tract infections.

The nurse is frequently the first to notice potential breakdown areas while doing routine nursing care such as bathing or turning the person or carrying out range-of-motion exercises. Physicians and allied health-team members look to the nurse as the expert in prevention and management.

Physiological Effects of Pressure

The average capillary pressure is 32 mm Hg. Considering that on the average sitting in a regular straight-backed chair exerts at least 300 mm Hg against the body surface, it is easy to see how circulation to an area can be impaired. Normally an individual experiences discomfort or pain when the tissues become anoxic (deprived of oxygen). We unconsciously squirm and shift our position, restoring the blood supply to a given area.

Bony prominences of the body, such as the ischium or the trochanter, are covered by multiple layers of soft tissue that vary in thickness depending on their location and on a person's nutritional intake. Normal cell metabolism in these areas is dependent on blood flow for the receipt of oxygen and nutrients and the removal of metabolic waste and carbon dioxide. Pressure from sitting or lying down is transmitted to the underlying bone, compressing overlying tissue. Pressure is greatest directly over the bone and diminishes progressively in peripheral areas (Shea, 1975). (See Fig. 18-5.) Thus body weight is concentrated on small peak-pressure areas in which this high pressure collapses blood vessels and blocks blood flow. If one could see this area, it would appear ischemic, looking much whiter than the surrounding skin.

Severe or prolonged circulatory interference eventually leads to the death of the cell. Intense pressure of short duration is less injurious to the skin than lower pressures exerted for longer periods of time. Research on animals demonstrates a critical period of 1 to 2 hours prior to pathological change. This finding is the physiological basis for a turning schedule of every 2 hours. However, each person should be assessed to determine his individual skin tolerance.

Factors Causing Pressure Sores*

- *Shearing force* is the angular force and compression placed on sacral tissue when the head of the bed is raised more than 30 degrees. As the person's torso slides toward the foot of the bed, the skin tends to remain in the same spot due to friction against the bed while the sacrum and firmly attached deep fascia do not, leading to compression of the vascular supply in this area (fig. 18-6).

- *Moisture* from perspiration or incontinence of urine and feces can macerate the skin and reduce its resistance.

*Current research is exploring the possibility that impoverishment, together with one or more of the factors noted, increases the susceptibility of persons to pressure sore development.

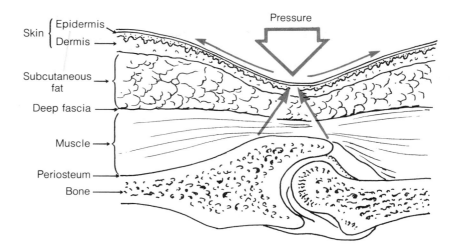

Figure 18-5
Pressure over a bony prominence compresses overlying soft tissue and causes ischemia. *(Shea DG: Pressure sores: Classification and management. Clin Orthop 112:89–100, Oct 1975)*

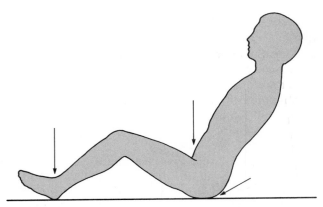

Figure 18-6
Shearing force exerts a downward and forward pressure.

- *Friction* results in a loss of epithelial cells. Any break in the integrity of this surface reduces the protective barrier and predisposes to infection, edema, and increased moisture. Friction may result from sheet burns, poor transfers, and spasticity. The person should always be lifted and not slid across the sheets and should be taught to lift his body when transferring to a stretcher or wheelchair.

- *Poor general nutrition* can also contribute to pressure sore formation. A person in negative nitrogen balance is susceptible to edema in the dependent parts of the body because osmotic pressure is insufficient to hold fluid in the vascular system (see Chap. 23). This edema decreases the rate of diffusion of oxygen and metabolites.

- *Negative nitrogen balance* decreases protein needed for new cell growth. The person with poor general nutrition often has marked loss in subcutaneous tissue and muscle bulk, leading to a decrease in mechanical padding between the skin and underlying bone and an increased susceptibility to pressure.

- *Anemia* further diminishes cell oxygenation due to a decreased quantity of hemoglobin. Thus, anemia increases the chances of tissue necrosis.

- *Disuse atrophy* is the reduction in muscle mass that occurs in persons experiencing prolonged bed rest and muscle disuse. Muscle atrophy decreases the protective padding over bones and increases pressure effects on the skin.

Assessment

Phases of Pressure Sores

To protect itself from pressure-related injury, the body has certain adaptive mechanisms. Thus, if changes are detected at an early stage, any damage is still reversible with good nursing care.

Grade I

Ischemia (lack of oxygen to the tissues) of short duration is immediately followed by the inflammation response and hyperemia, which floods the area with needed oxygen and nutrients and removes toxic waste products (grade-I pressure sore). This process was described earlier in the chapter. Hyperemia prevents damage to deprived areas if pressure is removed sufficiently soon. A bright flush that blanches to the touch may be seen on the surface of the skin. Blanching with a quick circulatory response indicates the process is still reversible.

Grade II

If pressure persists, there will be an irregular area of soft-tissue swelling associated with induration, heat, and erythema (grade-II pressure sore). The area may or may not blanch to the touch and takes up to an hour to clear or partially clear. Recognition at this stage is essential because the process is still reversible with the total removal of any pressure and other general supportive measures.

Grade III

In a grade-III pressure sore there is definite circulatory and cellular damage. Adaptive mechanisms now become insufficient and irreversible changes occur. Initially, superficial layers of skin may suffer **excoriation** and blistering, but soon there is progression through the dermis involving the subcutaneous fat. Here extensive and rapid undermining occurs. Any wound contamination matures rapidly to infection and a draining, foul-smelling, infected necrotic area of tissue with skin rolled at the edges and undermining in all directions is apparent.

Grade IV

A grade-IV pressure sore penetrates the deep fascia and muscle and eliminates the last barrier to extensive spread. Deep undermining now progresses rapidly to involve bone. With osteomyelitis profuse drainage and necrosis are seen. This is an extremely toxic situation that can be fatal. As much as 50 g of protein can be lost each day from a large open pressure sore. Some have said that there are cases in which exudate from a pressure sore is so severe that the person cannot eat fast enough to replace the protein lost and to maintain a positive nitrogen balance.

Population at Risk

Many individuals are susceptible to pressure sores: the elderly or debilitated, persons with sensory disturbances and altered awareness, persons subjected to prolonged surgery, and individuals who are paralyzed and unable to shift their own weight. Many of these persons have a lack of response to, or an inability to feel, painful stimuli originating from the skin.

Areas Most Frequently Involved

The areas most frequently involved reflect the position the person is in at the time of damage. The sitting position most frequently involves the ischial tuberosity areas; the side-lying position affects the greater trochanter and malleoli; the supine position involves the sacrum and heels. Other areas less frequently affected are the knees, elbows, scapula, and occiput. The ischial sore has the greatest effect on mobility because the person must maintain complete bed rest in order for healing to take place (Fig. 18-7).

Pressure sores may occur where tubes such as Foley catheters or nasogastric tubes press against the skin. They may also occur if pressure points develop inside casts. This is common with children who drop small objects into their casts.

Nursing Interventions

Prevention of Pressure Sores

Pressure sores are a preventable problem with meticulous nursing care. The following interventions should be individualized to each person's needs:

- Eliminate pressure at regular intervals throughout the day and night by establishing a turning schedule. Assist the person to turn in as many directions as possible: side to back to side to prone position. Even small shifts in weight are helpful. Pillows are helpful to separate bony areas that rub or lie against each other, for example, a pillow between the knees.
- Eliminate shearing forces, assist the person to avoid slumping or sliding.
- Closely inspect the person's skin several times a day during turning, bathing, or dressing.
- Control incontinence, keeping the person clean and dry as much as possible.
- Keep sheets clean, dry, and wrinkle free. Check linen frequently for any crumbs or foreign objects that may have fallen into the bed.
- Help the person to resume active mobilization as soon as possible. Physical activity, recreation, activities of daily living, ambulation, or wheelchair mobility may help in this endeavor.
- Provide for adequate bathing and proper skin hygiene, thereby reducing the bacterial population of the skin and decreasing the chances of infection.
- Provide a proper wheelchair, including footrests and armrests, which distribute weight over posterior thighs. If footrests are too high, a greater proportion of weight is shifted to the ischial tuberosities.
- Assist the person in maintaining a high-calorie, high-protein intake. This may be supplemented by iron and vitamins if anemia exists.
- Provide resilient surfaces for weight bearing such as cushions, air mattresses, egg-crate mattresses, and supplemental foam mattresses, which help to distribute weight over a larger area.
- After a person has been on bed rest, increase his sitting tolerance slowly with frequent weight shifts, lifting the person up for a full minute at least every hour.
- Educate the person in preventive measures. Assist persons who have decreased ability to detect pain in identifying what is hot, such as floorboards and mufflers of cars, heat lamps, heating pads, and hot water pipes. They must be aware of their bodies and possible physical agents that may harm it. They should understand the causes of skin breakdown and early interventions.

Management of Pressure Sores.

Persons with existing pressure sores should not bear any weight on the ulcerated area. The ulcer will not heal and will enlarge rapidly if subjected to pressure. However, if the person stays off the pressure sore but stays too long on another site, a second pressure sore will form; the nurse must not allow this common mistake to occur. If there are several ulcers, leaving no safe position, a special bed with a mud or sand mattress becomes mandatory.

A pressure sore must be clean in order to heal. **Debridement** is the removal of all necrotic or foreign tissue from a wound. This can be done by using dressings or techniques such as sharp debridement with scissors or scalpel, chemical debridement, or

Figure 18-7
Common sites for pressure sores: (*A*)
side lying, (*B*) sitting upright on chair,
(*C*) supine, (*D*) sitting in bed.

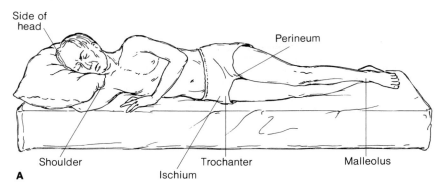

Side of
head

Perineum

Shoulder

Ischium

Trochanter

Malleolus

A

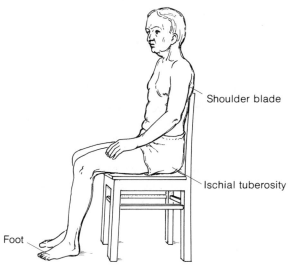

Shoulder blade

Ischial tuberosity

Foot

B

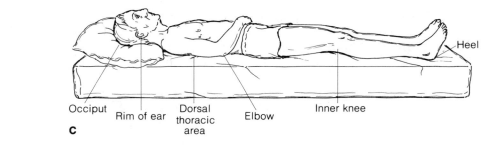

Heel

Occiput

Rim of ear

Dorsal
thoracic
area

Elbow

Inner knee

C

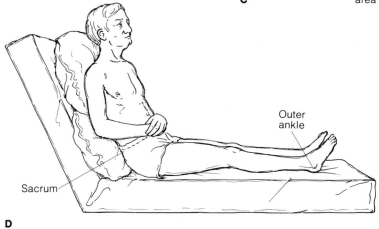

Outer
ankle

Sacrum

D

mechanical debridement in a whirlpool. The physician determines the method. The nurse can perform any technique except sharp debridement (Table 18-4).

Almost every concoction imaginable has been placed on ulcers with the intention of promoting wound healing (Table 18-5). Kosiak (1961) said that the rationale behind all of these treatments seems to be that if there is a hole, then you stick something in it; he feels that you can put anything you want on a pressure sore except the person himself. Each of the special agents in Table 18-5 was felt to have value by its researcher. What they all have in common is good nursing care, elimination of pressure, and cleansing of the wound by the application and removal of topical agents.

Electrical lamps to promote drying, ultraviolet light to kill the surface bacteria, hyperbaric oxygen to increase the oxygen to granulation tissue, sawdust beds, and water beds have also been used. However, rubber rings and "doughnuts" must never be used because they actually decrease circulation to the area around the sore.

Tissue healing and scar formation were previously discussed under nursing care of the person with tissue injury. We shall only repeat here that prevention and treatment of infection, protection of the traumatized tissue, and good nutritional intake promote wound healing. In addition to the suggested management strategies, nurses will want to assess and intervene concerning the person's possible impoverishment, basic need fulfillment, and resolution of developmental tasks.

Some pressure sores are so large and undermined that surgical management is indicated. If bone is involved, the area will not heal by itself, take too long to heal, or heal poorly with a fragile and adherent scar. This makes the person susceptible to future breakdown, because the skin has minimal padding and protection over bony prominences. The excessive loss of proteins, fluids, and electrolytes may also be an indication for surgery. Surgical intervention (closure, skin graft, or skin flap) prevents reoccurrence by removing all compromised tissue and bone and resurfacing the ulcer with multiple layers of soft tissue (padding). Individuals are kept prone for several weeks following surgery.

Burns

Burns continue to be a leading cause of disfigurement, disability, suffering, and death. The elderly are more seriously affected by burns than younger per-

Table 18-4
Nursing Interventions to Prevent Pressure Sores

- Eliminate pressure at regular intervals throughout the day and night by establishing a turning schedule.
- Eliminate shearing forces; help the person to avoid slumping or sliding.
- Closely inspect the person's skin several times a day during turning, bathing, and dressing.
- Control incontinence, keeping the person clean and dry as much as possible.
- Keep sheets clean, dry, and wrinkle free.
- Encourage active mobilization as soon as possible.
- Provide for adequate bathing and proper skin hygiene to reduce bacteria on skin and avoid infection.
- Provide a proper wheelchair with footrest and armrest to distribute weight over posterior thighs.
- Encourage a high-calorie, high-protein diet.
- Provide cushions, pillows, or air mattresses to help distribute weight over a larger area.
- Educate the person in preventive measures.

Table 18-5
Selected Topical Agents Used in Pressure Sore Treatments

Charcoal	Starch
Vitamin C paste	Aspirin
Sugar	Acetic acid
Cod-liver oil	Boric acid
Aluminum, silver, gold	Dried blood plasma
Poultices of carrots, turnips, bread	Antibiotics
Brine baths	Enzymes
Maalox	

sons even when the percentage of body surface burned is the same. Burns can be thermal, chemical, or electrical. Thermal burns are caused by dry or moist heat (as from steam), fire, hot metals, or grease. Chemical burns may be caused by strong acids or caustic materials. Electrical burns vary in severity depending on the type and voltage of the current.

Frequently, burns result from carelessness or inadequate knowledge of safety precautions. The nurse's role in teaching safety measures cannot be overemphasized. Education can be done in schools, through any form of media, in the home, clinics, or hospitals. Emphasizing first aid may also be helpful. In this chapter we examine the classification of burns and initial first aid. The hospital treatment of burns can be found in any medical–surgical textbook.

Assessment

Health-care providers classify a burn in order to determine what treatment is needed. Severity of a burn can be appraised by determining the size and depth of the burn (Fig. 18-8). A quick method for determining the size of a burn is the "rule of nines,"

which divides the body into multiples of 9% (Fig. 18-9):

Head and neck	9%
Anterior trunk	18%
Posterior trunk	18%
Upper extremities	9% each
Lower extremities	18% each
Perineum	1%

This method is convenient but somewhat inaccurate, particularly when used with children. However, other more precise methods require the use of tables and take longer to calculate.

There are several methods for determining the depth of a burn. In general, the greater or more extensive the contact with the burn source, the greater the damage. Crews' classification describes the depth of a burn based on its visual characteristics (1967, p. 8):

* A first-degree burn has redness of the skin without blister formation.

* A superficial second-degree burn causes blisters to form with redness in and around the blistered areas. This is usually caused by contact with a hot or boiling liquid.

Figure 18-8
A cross-section of the skin shows the relative depths of the types of burn injury.

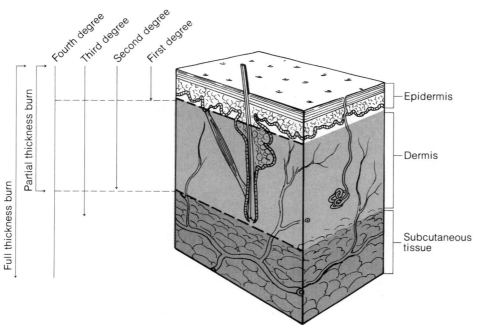

- A deep second-degree burn is one in which all but the deeper layers of the dermis are destroyed.
- A third-degree burn causes complete destruction of the skin. The burned skin has a brownish leathery appearance.
- A fourth-degree burn has not only destroyed the full thickness of the skin but structures underneath the skin as well.
- A char burn is a destruction of the body area involved by charring. The area is black. Deep electrical burns are char burns and they usually produce toxins that endanger life.

Crews' method is no longer preferred by health professionals, but nurses should be familiar with it because it is still widely used by the lay public.

Another more recent method of differentiating depth is to distinguish between partial thickness burns and full thickness burns (Feller and Archambeault, 1974, pp. 5–6).

- *A partial thickness burn* involves only the epidermis or portions of the dermis. Such a burn heals without grafting. The burned area is erythematous, blanches when pressure is applied followed by return of erythema, and may give rise to vesicles. Partial thickness burns are equivalent to first- or second-degree burns.
- *Full thickness burns* involve the entire epidermis and dermis and may extend to subcutaneous tissue, muscles, and bones. Burns of this type require skin grafting to heal. Full thickness burns are white, tan, brown, black, or red and leathery in appearance. Reddened areas do not blanch with pressure and pain sensation is absent. Full thickness burns are equivalent to third- or fourth-degree burns.

Nursing Interventions

Minor burns are treated by immediate immersion of the burned area in cool water. The burn should be washed with soap and water daily. The physician may prescribe dressings, topical medications, or analgesics. Clients often need instruction on how to perform these treatments at home. The nurse should also describe signs of infection and instruct the client to observe the burned area daily for indications of this problem (Feller and Archambeault, 1974).

In the case of severe burns, the less done, the better. Clothing should not be removed, no ointments or salves should be applied, and no pain relievers or sedation given. If medical treatment is indicated,

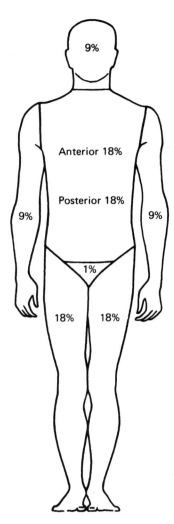

Figure 18-9
The "Rule of Nines" is a convenient method for calculating the size of a burn. According to this method, the entire head is 9% of the body surface area; each entire arm is 9%; each entire leg is 18%; the genital region is 1%; the front torso is 18%; and the back torso is 18%. However, individualization is necessary to account for differences in body size, for example, in children.

the individual should be wrapped in clean sheets and a blanket and sent to the hospital.

Psychological Effects of Skin Abnormalities

The skin has been described as a psychological mediator between a person and society. However, the individual with skin abnormalities may fear that he looks unclean or unattractive and that others will not want to be near him. These feelings may have a foundation of truth, if those around him do not know the causative factors of skin disease. Ancient writers often associated skin abnormalities with moral impurity and internal disharmony. Leper colonies isolated large numbers of people from their families and friends. History books write of those excluded from communal life because of a rash which had the stigma of impurity.

Medical technology, education, and increased communication have largely erased these moral overtones, but publicly visible skin disease, particularly if severe, can arouse strong negative feelings, causing others to withdraw emotionally and physically. Even those closest to the person may have mixed feelings toward him or her. The individual may feel helpless and hopeless, searching everywhere for a cure. One nurse who works with psoriasis patients found that some of them had suicidal thoughts. Death to them was the ultimate escape from the physical and psychological burden of their skin disease.

Skin disease can lead to marked disturbances in body image and impaired self-esteem as a result of impaired social interactions and family life. Such problems can occur at all stages of development. A child with eczema may not be held or fondled. An adolescent with acne fears rejection by his peers. A middle-aged woman with an open, infected surgical wound may feel repulsive to others.

The nurse's role involves assisting the person to develop a positive body image and a sense of self-esteem. Verbalizing acceptance of the person and touching him can be of central importance to the individual's self-esteem. The nurse can encourage the person to express his feelings and fears in a supportive environment. Casual touch during care and treatment reassures the person that you do not find him or her repulsive. Education of the client and the family about the cause and care of skin conditions may improve self-esteem by increasing self-care abilities and dispelling misinformation. Other interventions related to body image are discussed in Chapter 15.

Conclusion

Because the skin is easily visible it provides an excellent means of assessing the person's overall health. A person's skin reflects his psychological as well as physical status. Conversely, the condition of the skin can have implications for the person's body image and thus his emotional well-being. This chapter has considered both aspects of a person's skin.

Pressure sores are one of the most common skin problems encountered in the hospital, yet they are usually preventable with good nursing care. Nursing interventions are directed toward eliminating pressure over bony prominences, providing skin hygiene, promoting good nutrition, and teaching preventive care. Other skin problems include inflammation due to injury, rashes, and burns. Ongoing assessment is important because the nurse's observations provide a basis for determining initial care and evaluating the person's response to therapy. Additionally, nurses implement prescribed therapy such as topical medications and applications of heat and cold. Finally, health education is a nursing responsibility that assists persons to participate effectively in the care of their skin condition. Throughout their interventions nurses are sensitive to body image changes which accompany changes in skin appearance.

Two general nursing measures that promote healthy skin are bathing and massage. These actions not only maintain hygiene; they also promote relaxation and often are a demonstration of the nurse's caring attitude. Nursing care that maintains or restores healthy skin is an important means of assisting the person to attain optimal physical function and of enhancing self-esteem.

Study Questions

1. What modifications in the skin assessment would you make when observing for skin color changes in a darkly pigmented person?

2. Mr. D. is an 82-year-old man who is confined to bed following a fracture of his right hip. He has been eating poorly since his admission to the hospital. What factors make Mr. D. susceptible to pressure sores? What assessment should the nurse make to

identify this problem early? What preventive actions should the nurse take?

3. Susie H. is a 5-year-old girl whose mother brought her to the clinic with a skin rash over her entire body. Describe how you would assess this client. What interventions would be appropriate?

4. Your neighbor injured his ankle while running 5 hours ago. The area is edematous and painful to touch. What physiological processes are taking place? Would you apply heat or cold to the ankle? Why?

5. Describe the first aid treatment of a minor burn.

6. Mrs. G. is a 54-year-old woman who is hospitalized with an open, infected surgical wound. She often comments on the odor from the wound and states that she feels disgusting to others. You notice that she is becoming more withdrawn and takes little pride in her appearance. What nursing interventions might be appropriate?

Glossary

Abrasion: Skin injury caused by friction or rubbing.

Alopecia: Hair loss.

Bulla: A large vesicle, more than 1 cm in size.

Crust: Exudate that results from dried serum, blood, or purulent drainage on the skin.

Cyanosis: A diffuse bluish color of skin and membranes due to deoxygenated hemoglobin.

Cyst: Encapsulated, fluid-filled, or semisolid mass in the dermis or subcutaneous tissue.

Diaphoresis: Excessive perspiration.

Debridement: Removal of necrotic or foreign tissue from a wound.

Ecchymosis: Purple or blue, nonelevated, rounded, or irregular area in the skin or mucous membrane; commonly, a bruise.

Edema: Presence of abnormally large amounts of fluid in the intercellular tissue spaces.

Erosion: Loss of the outermost layer of the epidermis.

Erythema: Reddish skin color caused by congestion or dilation of cutaneous vessels.

Excoriation: Rubbing or wearing away of skin; abrasion.

Fissure: Cracks or deep linear splits through the epidermal layer of the skin into the dermis.

Hematoma: Tumor or swelling that contains blood.

Hyperemia: Process of blood vessel engorgement resulting from vasodilation and increased blood flow.

Jaundice: Yellow discoloration of the skin.

Keloid: Thick, fibrous lump or scar due to an exaggerated wound healing process.

Macule: Circumscribed area of color change, not depressed or elevated from the skin surface, and less than 1 cm in size.

Necrosis: Localized tissue death.

Nodule: Palpable, solid lesion, less than 1 cm in size, located in the epidermis, or extending to the dermis and subcutaneous layers.

Pallor: Deficiency of color, paleness.

Papule: Solid, elevated lesion, less than 1 cm in size.

Petechiae: Round, flattened, pinpoint spots, purplish-red in color, resulting from intradermal or submucosal bleeding.

Plaque: Macular or papular skin lesion that occupies an area larger than 1 cm.

Pseudofolliculitis: Area of numerous elevated lesions distributed on the face or neck due to ingrown hairs.

Purpura: A large area of ecchymosis.

Scales: Dry or oily masses of dead tissue from the stratum corneum layer of the skin.

Shearing Force: The angular force and compression placed on sacral tissue when the head of the bed is elevated more than 30 degrees.

Tumor: Large nodule, greater than 1 cm in size, may be benign or malignant.

Turgor: Elasticity or resiliency of the skin.

Ulcer: Irregularly shaped excavation of the skin in which there is necrosis destroying both the epidermis and dermis.

Urticaria: An allergic skin disorder marked by raised edematous patches of skin or mucous membrane and intense itching.

Vesicle: Fluid-filled, circumscribed, elevated lesion of the skin, less than 1 cm in size.

Wheal: Rounded or irregularly shaped elevated area of the skin or mucous membrane, caused by an allergic reaction.

Bibliography

Asland M: Sweat. Santa Barbara, Capra Press, 1978

Anderson TP, Andberg MM: Psychological factors associated with pressure sores. Arch Phys Med Rehabil 60:341–346, August, 1979

Basler RSW: Damaging effects of sunlight on human skin. Nebr Med J 63:337–340, October, 1978

Berecek KH: Etiology of decubitus ulcers. Nurs Clin North Am l0:157–170, March, 1975a

Berecek KH: Treatment of decubitus ulcers. Nurs Clin North Am 10:171–210, March, 1975b

Brunner LS, Suddarth DS: Textbook of Medical-Surgical Nursing, 4th ed. Philadelphia, JB Lippincott, 1980

Crews ER: A Practical Manual for the Treatment of Burns, 2nd ed. Springfield, IL, Charles C Thomas, 1967

Davis M: Getting to the root of the problem. Nurs '77 7:60–65, April, 1977

Derbes VJ: Rashes, recognition and management. Nurs '78 8:54–59, March, 1978

Downey JA, Darling RC: Physiological Basis of Rehabilitation Medicine. Philadelphia, WB Saunders, 1971

Feller I, Archambeault C: Nursing the Burned Patient. Ann Arbor, Institute for Burn Medicine, Braun-Brumfield Press, 1974

Fitzpatrick TB, Eisen AZ, Wolff K et al: Dermatology in General Medicine. New York, McGraw-Hill, 1979

Fitzpatrick TB, Haynes HA: Interpretation of alterations in the skin. In Harrison's Principles of Internal Medicine. New York, McGraw-Hill, 1977

Grier ME: Hair care for the black patient. Am J Nurs 76:1781, November, 1976

Gruis, ML, Innes B: Assessment essential to prevent pressure sores. Am J Nurs 76:1762–1764, November, 1976

Guthrie RH, Goulian D: Decubitus ulcers: Prevention and treatment. Geriatrics 28:67–71, August, 1973

Hannigan L: Nursing assessment of the integument system. Occup Health Nurs 26:19–22, January, 1978

Harlin VK: How we do it. J Sch Health 47:365–367, June, 1977

Hollinshead WH: Textbook of Anatomy. Hagerstown, MD, Harper & Row, 1974

Johnson T, Miller T: The Sauna Book. New York, Harper & Row, 1977

Kosiak M: Etiology of decubitus ulcers. Arch Phys Med Rehabil 42:19–29, January, 1961

Luckmann J, Sorensen KC: Medical-Surgical Nursing: A Psychophysiologic Approach. Philadelphia, WB Saunders, 1974

Miller ME, Sachs ML: About Bedsores: What You Need to Know to Help Prevent and Treat Them. Philadelphia, JB Lippincott, 1974

Nichols F: Theory and Practice of Body Massage. New York, Milady, 1973

Prior JA, Silberstein JSS: Physical Diagnosis: The History and Examination of the Patient. St Louis, CV Mosby, 1977

Roach LB: Color changes in dark skins. Nurs '72 2:19–22, November, 1972

Roach LB: Assessing skin changes: The subtle and the obvious. Nurs '74 4:64–67, March, 1974

Roberts SL: Skin assessment for color and temperature. Am J Nurs 75:610–613, April, 1975

Schell VC, Wolcott LE: The etiology, prevention and management of decubitus ulcers. Mo Med 63:109–119, February, 1966

Shea DG: Pressure sores: Classification and management. Clin Orthop 112:89–100, October, 1975

Viherjuuri HJ: Sauna: The Finnish Bath. Brattleboro, Vermont, Stephen Greens Press, 1965

Mobility Status

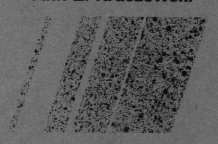

Ann Z. Kruszewski

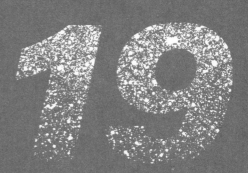

The ability to walk and move about with ease is so often taken for granted by healthy people that they rarely consider its importance. Yet mobility is so intimately related to our human needs that even a minor impairment can cause alterations in self-concept. Anyone who has ever sprained an ankle or a wrist is aware of the changes in life-style that these injuries required. Eating, dressing, getting to and from work or school, and participating in sports or social activities—all were more complicated. Most people can recall a sense of helplessness and dependence during this time. If small impairments have so much impact, imagine the effects of a major mobility problem!

In order to give holistic care, nurses need both an appreciation of the impact that changes in mobility have on a person's life-style and self-concept and an ability to intervene with the problem itself. This chapter presents information about common mobility problems and explores their effects on a person's biological and psychosocial functioning.

Mobility in Relation to Human Needs

Chapter 2 introduced the concept of human needs in terms of Abraham Maslow's hierarchy. Each of Maslow's five levels of human needs has a relationship to mobility.

Physiological needs, the most basic level, include such needs as food, water, pain avoidance, and elimination. It is easy to see how the ability to move about is essential to obtaining adequate food and water, escaping from pain-producing situations, and meeting other basic needs. Without mobility we are in a very vulnerable and dependent position, much like the infant who must rely on his parents for food and protection.

Safety and security needs are also affected by mobility. Protection of the physical self depends on the ability to move away from threatening situations. Imagine the vulnerability of the person confined to a wheelchair when a threat of fire exists or even when it is necessary to cross a busy street. *Psychological security* also depends on mobility. Motor status impairment often means a change in roles and expectations that can threaten established patterns of interaction with friends and family. For example, picture the reactions of a 50-year-old truck driver who has had a leg amputation. Certainly this must require major changes in his role as provider and head of the family. Imagine the feelings of insecurity brought about by the new behavior patterns he must develop.

The need for love and belonging may also be threatened by motor status impairments. Although some mobility problems are accompanied by changes in physical appearance, all result in changes in physical abilities. Both types of alterations may result in fear of rejection by one's family and friends. A young man paralyzed in an auto accident may fear that he will lose his former friends and be unattractive to women. The teenager who cannot participate in sports because of a motor status problem may fear rejection by his peers. Unfortunately these fears are often realized, leading to increased feelings of isolation.

Self-esteem or self-worth, as part of Maslow's hierarchy, depends in most individuals on a sense of independence and a feeling of usefulness or "being needed." Mobility is crucial to independence and certainly affects our ability to participate in useful activities. For example, impaired ambulation or fine motor skills due to arthritis may affect an elderly woman's ability to live independently or to cook, clean, and sew. The sense of uselessness she experiences leads to diminished self-esteem.

Self-actualization needs, as defined by Maslow, involve the need to fulfill oneself by developing all the potential elements one has. Achievement of self-actualization depends on having other human needs met. Because mobility problems can interfere with lower level needs, they may also impair the achievement of self-actualization. Since the goal of nursing is facilitating the person's highest level of functioning, mobility needs are a very important area of nursing care.

Mobility and Self-Concept

The ability to meet our human needs is closely related to self-concept. Because mobility affects human needs, it also influences self-concept. It is easy to see how a person with a motor impairment may feel helpless, useless, or like a burden to others (Fig. 19-1). The importance of mobility to the person's sense of safety, belonging, and self-esteem affects the degree to which self-concept is threatened by motor impairments. For instance, a leg cast may be more anxiety-producing to a professional football player than to a middle-aged homemaker.

Body image is a component of self-concept and is often adversely affected by mobility problems. Sensations that are received through movement contribute to the formation of body image (Murray, 1972). Conversely, impaired sensation could result in a depersonalized view of the body part involved. For instance, a person with a paralyzed arm may call it by a name (*e.g.*, "Harold"), indicating that since it cannot be felt, it is really not a part of him. Or consider the instance of a woman who was paralyzed on one side and complained that someone else was in bed with her. The nurses worked hard to help her realize that it was her own left arm and leg which she could not feel and which she perceived as belonging to someone else.

One's life experiences, the reaction of significant others, and social or cultural values also affect body image. Because health and wholeness are important values in our society, people may react with fear or disgust to mobility impairments such as paralysis or amputation. Such responses invariably contribute to negative body image. Since the affected person also holds the same cultural values, he may feel a self-loathing if he perceives himself as useless or no longer "whole."

Motor status impairments frequently alter a person's functional abilities. As the body's abilities change, so will the feelings about the physical self. Body image alterations often cause a great deal of anxiety as well as grieving for lost functions or body parts. Communication skills will help the nurse identify the feelings of loss the person is experiencing. Nursing interventions for those who are grieving, as well as those with body image alterations are discussed in Chapter 15.

Factors Affecting Motor Function

Because mobility is so closely related to human needs, we can expect other functional abilities to affect motor status. Factors that can influence mobility include developmental level, psychological and mental functioning, environmental factors, oxygenation, nutrition, and the structural integrity of the neuromuscular and musculoskeletal system.

Developmental Level. Crawling and walking are important skills leading to successful resolution of the developmental task of autonomy in the very young child. More complicated motor abilities progress further as the person matures. (For detailed

Figure 19-1
Mobility problems affect our ability to meet basic needs.

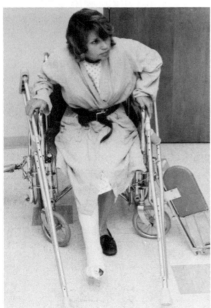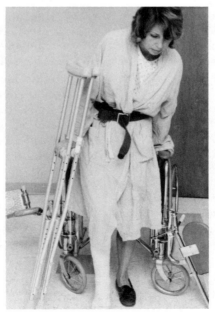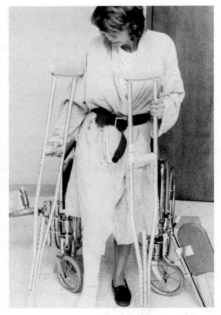

information on development of motor skills, see Murray and Zentner, 1979.)

Psychological and Mental Function. Motor activity often reflects the person's emotional state. Movements can serve as nonverbal communication in reflecting emotions such as anxiety, depression, and hostility. Slumped posture, slow purposeless movement, and feelings of muscle fatigue may indicate depression. Rapid movements, tightly contracted muscles, and clenched fists may show anger or hostility. Astute nurses are alert to the person's movements and relate them to other data regarding his emotional state.

Because all motor activity is integrated and controlled by the central nervous system, motor function can give important clues about the person's mental status. Decreased motor response to stimuli may indicate altered level of consciousness. Purposeless movements, impaired balance, and weakness of an extremity are other signs of a central nervous system impairment.

Environment. The person's environment can have a major effect on his mobility. For example, stairs may pose a physical barrier to an elderly person with arthritis. If bathing, sleeping, and kitchen facilities are on different levels of the home, it will be difficult for him to carry out normal daily activities. Even items such as throw rugs may be an environmental hazard for someone on crutches or for a person who has a shuffling gait.

Nurses need to be mindful of environmental effects on mobility, particularly when doing hospital discharge planning, when preparing a home assessment for a person with motor problems, or when adapting the hospital environment to the person's needs.

Environment and mobility also interact through our sense of **proprioception.** Proprioception is the term for position sense, that is, the ability to detect the position of body parts in relation to the environment. Adequate environmental stimulation, which is partly achieved through movement, is important to normal central nervous system control of mobility. Persons who are immobilized in bed sometimes develop impaired proprioception, which leads to vague sensations of floating and a decreased ability to perform motor tasks. This problem is a result of decreased information about the environment due to diminished body movement.

Oxygenation. Oxygen is necessary for the formation of adenosine triphosphate (ATP), the energy source for muscle activity. Persons with cardiac or respiratory disorders such as anemia or chronic bronchitis often have hypoxia, which can result in feelings of fatigue or muscle weakness. Some individuals with cardiac or respiratory disorders experience dyspnea (difficulty in breathing) with mild-to-moderate activity. These persons often must limit their activity in order to breathe comfortably. Nurses caring for these persons need to explore the effects of fatigue or dyspnea on their life-style and assist them to plan and prioritize their activities within their limitations.

Nutrition. Adequate nutrition supplies both glucose for the formation of ATP and vitamins and minerals that are essential for normal bone and muscle function. Generalized poor nutrition may cause muscle weakness or fatigue. Inadequate calcium intake in the elderly may make them susceptible to fractures. By assisting these persons to improve their nutrition, nurses can also promote healthy motor function.

Structural Integrity of the Neuromuscular and Musculoskeletal System. Intact neuromuscular and musculoskeletal systems provide structure and motion to the body, giving it the ability to perform purposeful, independent activity. Health problems that affect these systems can limit mobility and disrupt many of the person's functional abilities. Some degree of independence in self-care is often lost, making it necessary to alter life-style temporarily or permanently. The effects of mobility limitations are described later in this chapter.

General Assessment of Mobility Status

In order to identify actual and potential mobility needs, the nurse must be able to collect appropriate data. When assessing motor status it is important to consider not only the status of individual muscles and joints but also how effectively the person's motor abilities enable him to perform his daily activities. The motor status assessment as described here emphasizes general functional abilities as well as specific motor functions.

General Movements and Gait

Quite often it is possible to observe a person's general movements before any other observations are made. The way the person walks through the door of the clinic, the way he greets the nurse at his hospital bedside, or the manner in which he welcomes the nurse into his home all constitute helpful clues in assessing motor status.

Points to note include whether movements are coordinated and purposeful or repetitive and tremulous and whether movements are quick and sure or slow and deliberate. Such observations can help determine the person's ability to perform his daily activities. For example, the slow, deliberate movements of an elderly person may indicate that he needs to be given extra time for morning hygiene. General movements also can indicate the person's emotional state. For instance, rapid body motions and shaking hands might be a clue that the person is anxious.

If the person is able to walk, his gait should be described. Normal gait consists of two phases: stance and swing. *Stance* begins when the heel of one leg strikes the ground and ends when the toe pushes off and leaves the ground. In the *swing* phase, the foot leaves the ground and the leg moves from behind to in front of the body. It ends when the heel again touches the ground. While one leg is in the stance phase, the other is in the swing phase (Fig. 19-2.)

Some common gait abnormalities such as ataxic gait, scissors gait, Parkinson's gait, and steppage gait are listed in Figure 19-3. Other gait abnormalities include stooped posture, looking at the feet when walking, leaning to one side, or limping. It is better to try to describe elements of the gait because the labels presented in Figure 19-3 do not cover every type of alteration that can occur.

Any gait abnormality may indicate a potential safety problem because unsteady ambulation makes the person susceptible to falls. For instance, a person who shuffles his feet is prone to tripping over throw rugs or other objects on the floor.

If the person uses any aids for ambulation such as a cane, walker, or crutches, these devices should be noted and his ability to use them, described. It is also important to describe whether these aids are adequate for mobility. If not, then the method the person uses for mobility should be recorded (wheelchair, stretcher). In addition, any medical restrictions on mobility such as complete bed rest or limited stair climbing should be listed.

Endurance

Endurance is defined as the ability of muscles to continue a particular task. Assessing endurance involves describing how much and what type of activity the person can perform before feeling fatigued. The person's own statements are most helpful: "I can do almost anything without getting tired," or "I've noticed that I seem to get tired just getting dressed in the morning." Pulse rate is another indicator of endurance and should be checked at rest as well as during and after activity. If moderate activity such as walking causes tachycardia (heart rate greater than 100) or a rate increase greater than 20 beats per minute, the person is probably exceeding his endurance (Gordon, 1976). Dizziness, dyspnea, frequent pauses in activity to rest, or marked increase in respiratory rate after moderate activity may also indicate limited endurance that most likely interferes with daily activities.

Figure 19-2
Normal gait.

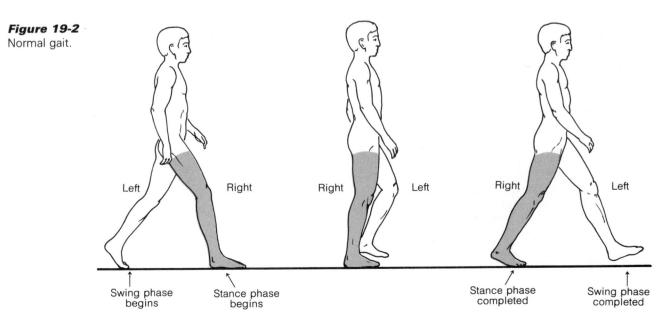

Left   Right   Right   Left   Right   Left

Swing phase begins   Stance phase begins   Stance phase completed   Swing phase completed

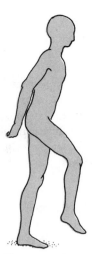

Steppage gait

Steppage gait is associated with footdrop usually secondary to lower motor neuron disease. The feet are lifted high, with knees flexed, and then brought down with a slap on the floor. The patient looks as if he were walking up stairs.

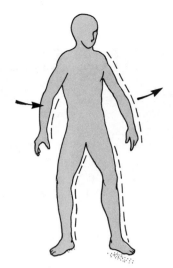

Cerebellar ataxia

Cerebellar ataxia is associated with disease of the cerebellum or associated tracts. The gait is staggering, unsteady, and wide-based, with exaggerated difficulty on the turns. The patient cannot stand steadily with feet together, whether eyes are open or closed.

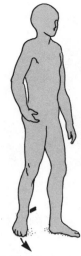

Spastic hemiparesis

Spastic hemiparesis is associated with unilateral upper motor neuron disease. One arm is flexed, close to the side, and immobile; the leg is circled stiffly outward and forward (circumducted), often with dragging of the toe.

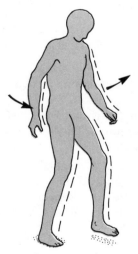

Sensory ataxia

Sensory ataxia is associated with loss of position sense in the legs. The gait is unsteady and wide-based (the feet are far apart). The feet are lifted high and brought down with a slap. The patient watches the ground to guide his steps. He cannot stand steadily with feet together when his eyes are closed (positive Romberg test).

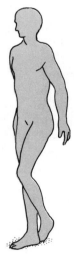

Scissors gait

Scissors gait is associated with bilateral spastic paresis of the legs. Each leg is advanced slowly and the thighs tend to cross forward on each other at each step. The steps are short. The patient looks as if he were walking through water.

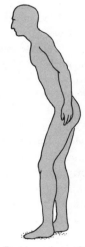

Parkinsonian gait

Parkinsonian gait is associated with the basal ganglia defects of Parkinson's disease. The posture is stooped, the hips and knees slightly flexed. Steps are short and often shuffling. Arm swings are decreased and the patient turns around stiffly—"all in one piece."

Figure 19-3
Gait abnormalities. (*Adapted from Bates B: A Guide to Physical Examination. Philadelphia, JB Lippincott, 1980*)

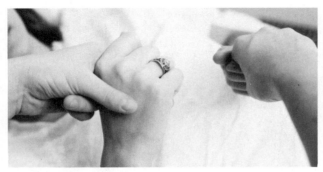

Figure 19-4
Test motor strength by noting the client's ability to squeeze your hands. *(From: Decision Audiovisual Media. Neurological Care Series. Philadelphia, JB Lippincott)*

Muscle Tone, Mass, Strength

Muscle tone is the degree of muscle tension that is present even at rest. It is assessed by palpating muscle groups. Healthy muscles should feel firm to the touch. Decreased tone (called **flaccidity**) may be the result of lack of conditioning, disuse, or neurological impairment. Greatly increased tone that interferes with movement is called **spasticity;** this is caused by neurological abnormalities.

Muscle tone is reflected in muscle strength. The strength of various muscle groups can be tested by asking the person to perform a task against resistance. For example have the person push his foot against the palm of your hand. Grasp strength can be assessed by having the person grasp two fingers of your right hand with his left hand and two left fingers with his right hand. Note any differences between left and right hand strength (Fig. 19-4). More important, observe the person's abilities to do daily activities. Is muscle strength adequate for pulling himself up in bed, climbing stairs, or getting from the bed to the chair? The person's own statements related to muscle strength are also significant. For instance, if the person says that muscle weakness is interfering with job performance or recreational activities, this should be noted.

Muscle mass, meaning muscle size, is noted in general and then in comparision of one muscle group to another. Decreased muscle mass is termed "atrophy." **Atrophy** may result from neurological impairment or from disuse. An area of suspected atrophy can be most accurately assessed by comparing tape measurements of a muscle with its pair (e.g., right and left calf measurements). **Hypertrophy** is the term for increased muscle mass; it is the result of forceful muscle activity such as exercise or training.

Posture or Alignment

Note the person's posture in various positions (sitting, standing, lying in bed) and compare with correct posture as illustrated in Figure 19-5. Indicate whether the person is able to maintain adequate alignment on his own.

Joint Assessment

Joint assessment includes noting a joint's range of motion as well as its appearance. The majority of joints are freely movable and are termed **diarthroses** or **synovial joints.** There are several types of freely movable joints:

- *Hinge joints* allow movement in two directions only, flexion and extension. The elbow, the two distal joints of the fingers and the distal joint of the toes are hinge joints. The knee is a complex type of hinge joint.

- *Pivot joints* consist of a ringlike structure that turns on a pivot (usually a bony prominence). A good example is the joint between the first and second vertebrae, which allows rotation of the head.

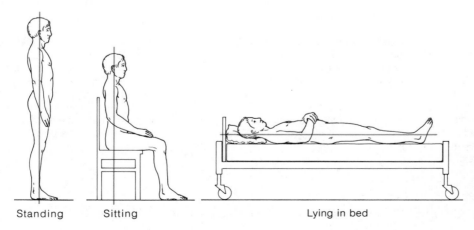

Standing   Sitting   Lying in bed

Figure 19-5
Adequate posture. Note that in sitting and standing positions a straight line can be drawn from the ear through the shoulder and hip. In bed, the head, shoulders, and hips are aligned.

- *Condyloid joints* consist of an oval head of one bone, which fits into a shallow cavity of another bone, allowing movement to occur in four directions. Examples are the wrist and the most proximal joints of the fingers and toes (metacarpal–phalangeal and metatarsal–phalangeal joints).

- *Saddle joints* have a bone surface that is convex on one side and concave on another. The two sides form a right angle. The articulating bone is reciprocally concave and convex. The proximal thumb joint is a saddle joint.

- *Ball and socket joints* consist of a globe-shaped head on one bony surface that fits into a cuplike socket of another bone. Examples include the shoulder and hip joints.

- *Gliding joints* contain two flat surfaces of bone which interface. The vertebral column contains gliding joints. Diarthroses permit a variety of movements.

The types of joint movement are described in Table 19-1.

Range of motion (ROM) is the degree of movement permitted by a joint and varies according to the type of joint (Fig. 19-6). Range of motion may be *active*, meaning the person is able to initiate movement, or *passive*, meaning someone else must move the joint. Range of motion can be observed directly by asking the person to move various joints to the extent of their motion or by assisting him to do so. Limited range of motion is present if joints resist full motion. Pain is produced at the point of resistance. ROM may also be checked indirectly by observing the person's self-care activities and noting whether joints are sufficiently mobile to permit him to carry out his normal daily routine.

While range of motion is being observed, the appearance of the joints should be noted including any signs of redness, warmth, or swelling. These findings indicate inflammation due to physical injury, infection, or joint disease such as gout and rheumatoid arthritis. Inflammation is often accompanied by joint pain and limited range of motion.

(Text continues on p. 360)

Table 19-1
Types of Motion of Synovial Joints

Motion	Description
Flexion	Decreases the angle between bones
Extension	Increases the angle between bones
Abduction	Movement away from the median plane of the body; with the fingers and toes, movement away from the third digit
Adduction	Movement toward the median plane of the body; with the fingers and toes, movement toward the third digit
Internal rotation	Movement along a central axis turning a body part inward
External rotation	Movement along a central axis turning a body part outward
Special Movements	
Pronation	Movement turning the palm of the hand downward (occurs at the elbow joint)
Supination	Movement turning the palm of the hand upward (occurs at the elbow joint)
Inversion	Turning the sole of the foot inward (occurs at the ankle)
Eversion	Turning the sole of the foot outward (occurs at the ankle)

Figure 19-6
Range of motion of selected joints.

Neck

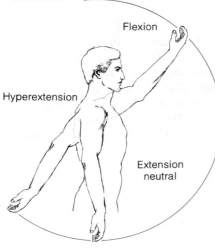

Extension
neutral

Flexion

Rotation

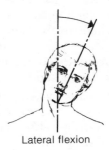

Lateral flexion

Shoulder

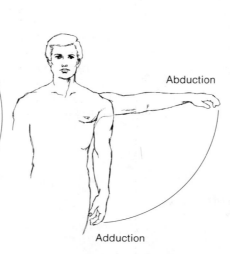

Flexion

Hyperextension

Extension
neutral

Abduction

Adduction

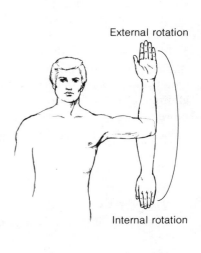

External rotation

Internal rotation

Elbow

Flexion

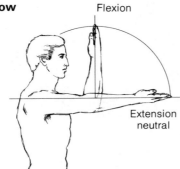

Extension
neutral

Supination

Pronation

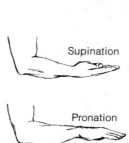

Wrist

Hyperextension

Extension
neutral

Flexion

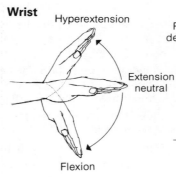

Radial
deviation

Ulnar
deviation

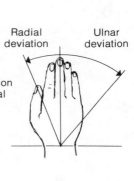

Fingers

Flexion

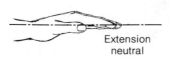

Extension
neutral

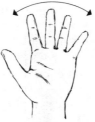

Abduction

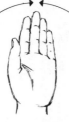

Adduction
neutral

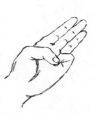

Opposition of
thumb to finger

Hip

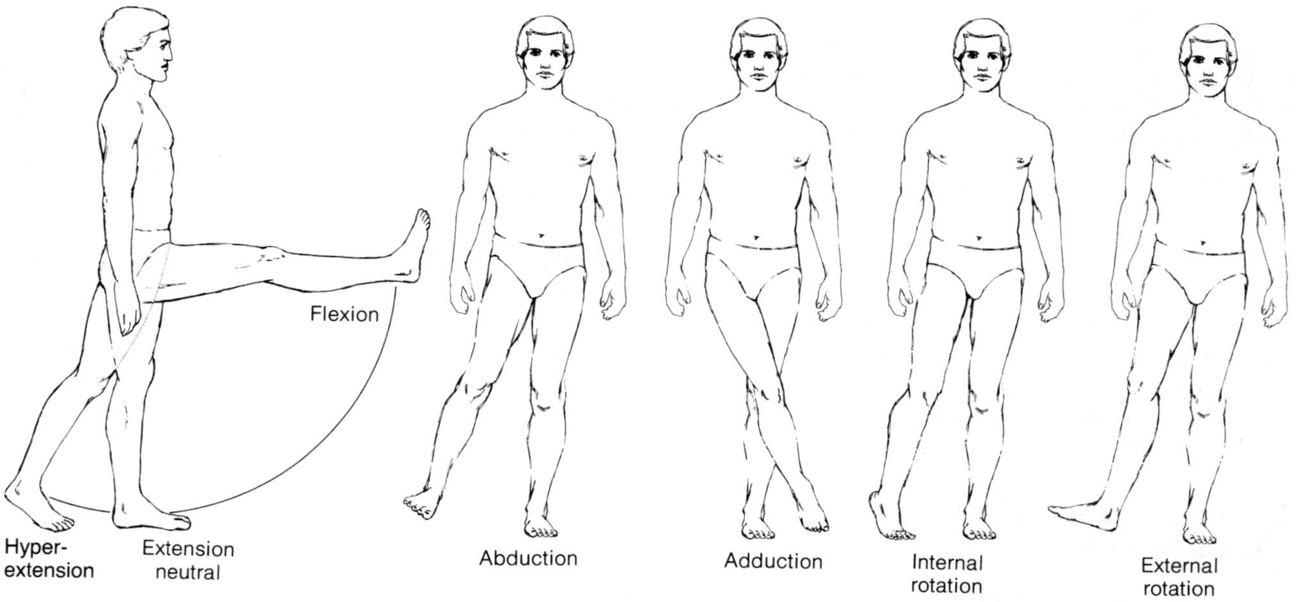

Flexion

Hyper-extension Extension neutral Abduction Adduction Internal rotation External rotation

Knee

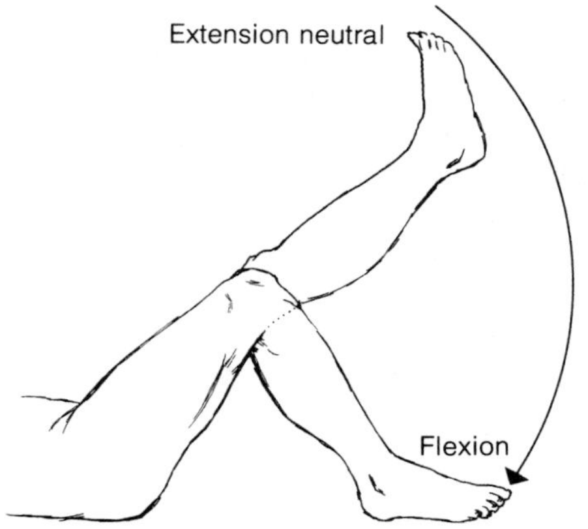

Extension neutral

Flexion

Ankle

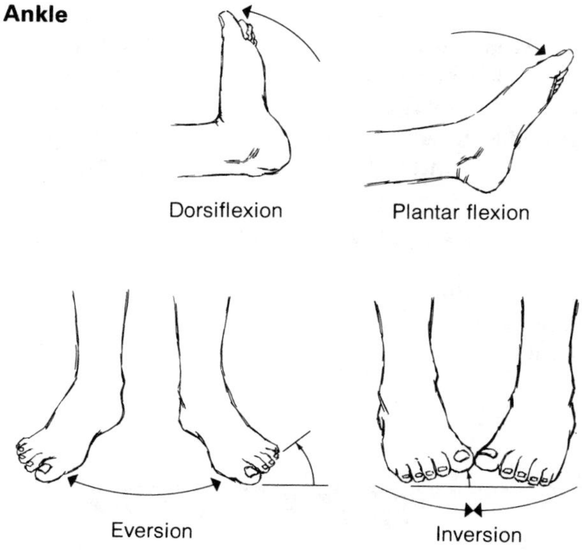

Dorsiflexion Plantar flexion

Eversion Inversion

Toes

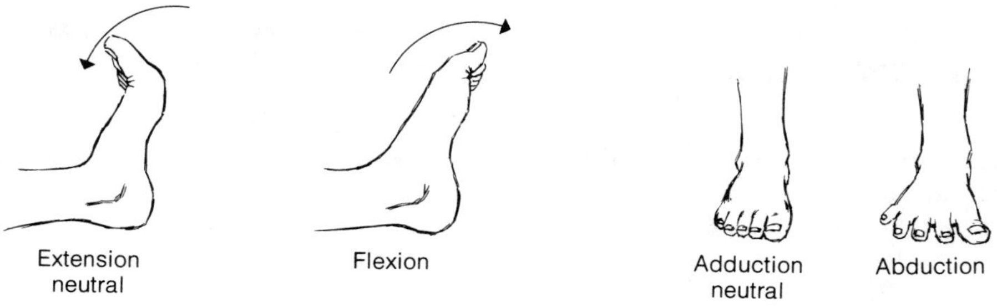

Extension neutral Flexion Adduction neutral Abduction

Joint appearance can also be altered by the presence of nodules, which look like knobs and frequently affect hand joints. They can occur in gout or other types of arthritis. If a nodule is noticed, joint pathology may exist, possibly limiting mobility. It is especially important to carefully assess range of motion and ability to perform daily activities in these individuals.

Handedness

Handedness may be determined by direct observation or by asking the person which hand he uses predominantly. Handedness may have implications for nursing care. For instance, a right-handed person whose right arm is immobilized probably needs assistance with many of his daily activities.

Deformities or Abnormal Muscular Innervation

The presence of an amputation or fracture should be indicated, along with the body part affected. Abnormalities of innervation such as *paralysis* (inability to move a body part) or *paresis* (partial paralysis causing weakness) should also be noted. **Hemiplegia** is a term for paralysis that affects one side of the body. Paralysis of the lower half of the body is termed **paraplegia.** It is important to describe the body parts involved and the effect on the person's mobility.

Activities of Daily Living

Activities of daily living (ADL) encompass all of the activities the person engages in, including those at home, at work, and in the community. These activities involve functions such as eating, dressing, walking, and personal hygiene, as well as job-related skills and recreational activities. Because each person's activities of daily living are unique, mobility impairments do not affect equally every individual's abilities to perform daily activities. The nurse first needs to identify the person's daily routine as well as recreational or job activities. Then the effect of health problems on ADL performance should be determined. This can be assessed both by interviewing the person and by observing how ably he performs self-care.

There are certain common activities that can be assessed for every person experiencing a health problem. These include bathing, brushing the teeth, grooming, eating, dressing, walking, sitting, and climbing the stairs. The areas that are unique to the person's life-style should also be assessed. For instance, does the young mother's generalized muscle weakness interfere with her ability to care for her child? Is the carpenter's joint pain causing difficulty with his job performance?

Remember that what the person is able to do for himself in the hospital may be quite different from what he can do in his home. As an example, an elderly man may have been very independent in his home, which was arranged to suit his needs. However, in the hospital he is unable to bathe himself because of the IV in his right hand and because he needs help to get to the bathroom. A new ADL assessment should be done whenever the person moves from the home to a health-care facility. It is also important to consider the effects of decreased independence in ADL performance on body image and self-esteem. Nursing interventions related to ADL are discussed later in the chapter.

Nursing Process
Applied to Specific Mobility Problems

Problems Related to Musculoskeletal Disuse

It is a physiological principle that tissues that are not used begin to atrophy. Both structure (composition) and function (abilities) of bones and muscles are altered through disuse. The consequences of disuse include diminished muscle tone, mass, and strength, loss of joint mobility, and loss of bone mass.

Diminished Muscle Tone, Mass, and Strength

A certain amount of contraction is necessary in order to maintain muscle fiber size and strength. In normal muscles there is a continuous slight contraction called muscle *tonus* which is activated by nerve impulses. If nerve supply to a muscle is destroyed, tonus is lost and the muscle atrophies rapidly. This can be seen in a paralyzed limb. Atrophy also occurs if muscles are used only for very weak contractions. Prolonged bed rest can result in muscle atrophy for this reason.

Both the size of individual muscle fibers and the quantity of contractile protein are diminished in muscle atrophy. Another change is proliferation of fat and connective tissue between muscle fibers. The decrease in muscle tone, mass, and strength caused by atrophy is a direct result of the loss of muscle protein and decreased fiber size. Loss of strength is hazardous because it begins a vicious cycle of muscle weakness, further disuse, continued atrophy, greater muscle weakness, and so on.

Evidence of atrophy may be seen even after a short period of disuse. One study of immobilized leg muscles in rats showed a 20% weight loss in the first week of disuse (Jarvinen, 1977). Many of us are familiar with the feeling of general weakness that follows 2 or 3 days of bed rest when we are ill. It is estimated that it takes 4 to 6 weeks to recover from 6 weeks of bed rest (Browse, 1965).

Loss of Joint Mobility

Muscles that are not stretched through their full degree of motion begin to stiffen and shorten. This is due to a natural tendency of muscle fiber protein to assume a shortened length. The result is limited range of motion in the affected joint, called a **contracture.** If disuse lasts for only a few days, the joint may be restored to normal mobility by stretching exercises. However, contractures eventually become irreversible because connective tissue proliferates and adhesions form within the joints. Surgery is often the only treatment that will release permanent contractures.

Muscle weakness and atrophy favor the formation of contractures. Weakness contributes to contractures because it promotes diminished use. Atrophy may cause an imbalance between flexor and extensor muscle groups so that the stronger muscles dominate. Because the flexors are often stronger than extensor groups, flexion contractures are more common.

Persons on prolonged bed rest are prone to contractures, particularly if they are very ill or weak. Those with paralyzed limbs are also susceptible to this problem. Bed rest favors contractures for several reasons. The legs tend to roll outward when a person is in a supine position, which can result in an external rotation contracture of the hip. Feet tend toward plantar flexion because of gravity and the weight of bedcovers, causing a flexion contracture at the ankle called *footdrop.* Decreased shoulder use results in frozen shoulder. If the head of the bed and the knee gatch are constantly elevated, flexion contractures may develop at the hips and knees. This can also occur if the person spends most of his day sitting up in a chair.

Loss of Bone Mass

Bone is constantly being renewed by the activity of osteoblasts and osteoclasts. Osteoblasts deposit bone matrix whereas osteoclasts reabsorb it. Weight bearing and muscle pull on bones favor osteoblastic activity so that bone develops in proportion to the work it must perform. On the other hand, inactivity increases osteoclastic activity, causing bone to become thinner and more porous. Dietrick, in his classic study of immobility, found that bone reabsorption was demonstrated by increased urinary calcium levels as early as the third day of complete bed rest (Dietrick *et al,* 1948).

Continued disuse results in **osteoporosis,** a condition in which bone matrix and minerals are depleted. As a result, bones become structurally weaker making the person more prone to fractures. Osteoporosis can result from prolonged bed rest or immobilization of a joint. It is felt that inactivity is one of the factors that contribute to osteoporosis in the elderly. The high incidence of fractures in the elderly is evidence of the problems that osteoporosis can cause.

Causes of Disuse

Musculoskeletal disuse has a variety of causes, including those below:

- Promotion of healing (*e.g.,* casts or traction applied to fractures)
- Relief of pain (*e.g.,* rest prescribed to alleviate discomfort from back injuries or joint inflammation)
- Reduction of energy (*e.g.,* bed rest prescribed to reduce energy needs of the ill person)
- Self-imposed restrictions (*e.g.,* decreased activity in elderly, depressed, or ill persons)

Although rest is often therapeutic, prolonged immobility may have the harmful effects just described. Certain individuals are susceptible to the problems of musculoskeletal disuse, including those with fractures who are immobilized in casts or traction, those on bed rest, and those with paralysis, painful musculoskeletal disorders, or muscle weakness. Very ill persons are at risk because of reduced activity. The elderly may be prone to disuse problems due to normal aging changes, which cause some degree of muscle weakness and atrophy. These changes include diminished neuron function and nerve-impulse transmission and decreased circulation to muscles. The nurse should be aware of persons who are at risk for potential problems and begin preventive actions as soon as possible after the onset of disuse.

Assessment

The nurse needs to assess any of the individuals described in the preceding section for the potential problems of disuse. Nursing assessment of muscles and joints can be carried out as described in an earlier section of this chapter. Muscle atrophy can be detected by measuring arm or leg girths with a tape measure. It is helpful to compare the circumferences of both extremities and to repeat measurements over a period of time to detect trends.

The early signs of contractures can be recognized by the presence of resistance to movement. When attempts are made to move the affected joint, it feels stiff and has limited range of motion. Attempts to move the joint to its fullest extent result in pain. Never force the joint to move beyond the point of pain because this may cause permanent injury. Figure 19-7 illustrates common contracture sites.

Unfortunately, signs and symptoms of bone changes are not usually present before damage is severe. Bone pain and pathological fractures are indications of osteoporosis. This emphasizes the need to begin preventive action as soon as possible after the onset of disuse.

Nursing Interventions

The consequences of disuse can severely incapacitate the person. Picture how contractures, osteoporosis, and muscle weakness affect the ability to move about, perform a job, or carry out other daily activities. Treating these problems may be complex and costly. Nursing interventions should be directed toward maintenance of structure and function rather than treatment of disabilities.

There are four categories of nursing interventions that maintain musculoskeletal function: exercise, positioning and body alignment, supportive devices, and consultation or referral.

Exercise

There are several types of exercise that prevent the problems of musculoskeletal disuse. Table 19-2 summarizes the effects of three types of exercise—isotonic, isometric, and passive—and gives examples of each.

Figure 19-7
Common contracture sites.

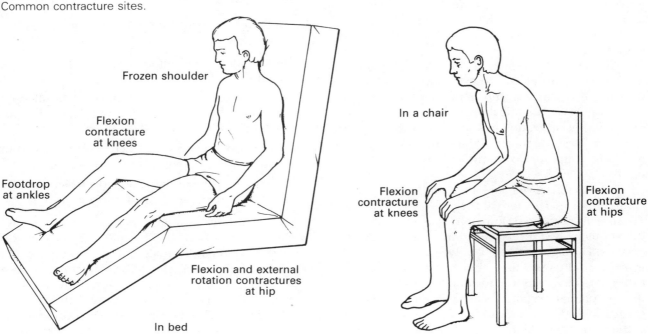

Frozen shoulder

Flexion contracture at knees

Footdrop at ankles

Flexion and external rotation contractures at hip

In bed

In a chair

Flexion contracture at knees

Flexion contracture at hips

Table 19-2
Summary of Isotonic, Isometric, and Passive Exercise

Exercise	Effects	Possible Contraindications	Examples
Isotonic exercise (involves muscle shortening, active movement, and mechanical work)	Increased muscle tone, mass, strength Improved joint mobility Increased osteoblastic activity Increased circulation to exercised body part Improved cardiac and respiratory function	Cardiac or respiratory pathology Exercise involving injured or inflamed muscles and joints Exercise involving immobilized body parts	Performing ADL Performing active ROM (see Table 19-3); should be performed at least 2 times daily; each motion should be performed several times during an exercise period. Sports, walking, jogging
Isometric exercise (involves muscle contraction without shortening; no movement or mechanical work performed)	Increased muscle tone, mass, strength Increased circulation to exercised body part Increased osteoblastic activity	Cardiovascular pathology Exercise involving injured or inflamed muscles and joints	"Setting exercises" (may be done in supine or sitting position; allow a 2-minute rest between contractions) Gluteal setting: pinch buttocks together and tighten gluteal muscles; hold for 6 seconds Quadriceps setting: dorsiflex the feet and push the knee(s) downward into the mattress; hold for 6 seconds Abdominal setting: tighten abdominal muscles; hold for 6 seconds Biceps setting: raise arms to shoulder height and interlock fingertips of both hands; try to pull hands apart using arm muscles; hold for 6 seconds Triceps setting: raise arms to shoulder height; make a fist with one hand and place against the palm of the other hand; push hands together as hard as possible for 6 seconds *Note,* caution person not to hold his breath during these exercises as this places strain on the heart.

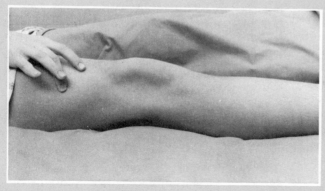

Example of isometric exercise—quadriceps setting

(Continued)

Table 19-2 (continued)
Summary of Isotonic, Isometric, and Passive Exercise

Exercise	Effects	Possible Contraindications	Examples
Passive exercises (involves exercise performed for the person; body part does not exert effort)	Improved joint mobility Increased circulation to exercised body part	Exercise involving injured or inflamed muscles and joints Acute cardiac pathology	Passive range of motion exercises (see Table 19-3); can be incorporated into nursing care such as bathing, turning, and positioning; Passive ROM should be performed 2 times daily; each motion should be performed at least 2 times during the exercise period

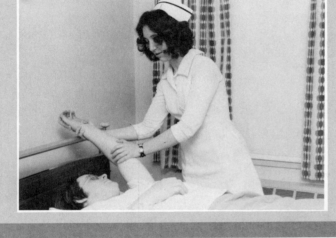

How does the nurse determine which type of exercise is best suited to the person's needs?

1 Look at the goal to be achieved. If the goal is to maintain muscle strength for eventual crutch-walking, either isotonic or isometric exercises are appropriate. If the goal is to maintain range of motion for the person on complete bed rest, isotonic or passive ROM exercises would be useful. Many times combinations of different types of exercises are used.

2 Look at the person's general level of functioning including endurance, strength, cardiorespiratory status, and ability to move independently. A certain type of exercise may be more appropriate to the person's functional abilities. For instance, almost any well person can benefit from isotonic exercises since many of us lead sedentary lifestyles. However, isotonic exercises tax the cardiac and respiratory systems and may be harmful to persons with oxygenation problems. Passive exercises are the least strenuous although they do cause an initial increase in respiratory rate due to stimulation of proprioceptors in skeletal muscles (Guyton, 1976, p. 567).

The nurse should consult with the physician before initiating exercise programs for persons with known cardiorespiratory problems and before exercising an immobilized body part or inflamed or injured joints. Persons over the age of 35 should have a physical examination before beginning a strenuous exercise program.

Nurses not only teach persons how to perform exercises and assist them in doing them but also explore how these activities can be incorporated into their life-style. For instance, consider the nurse who is teaching a woman who recently experienced a breast removal how to exercise her arm and chest muscles to rebuild their strength. This nurse not only gives information on range of motion exercises for the shoulder but also determines what this woman's normal activities are and demonstrates how the exercises can be performed during her daily routine (e.g., while hair brushing or dressing).

Position Changes and Body Alignment

The healthy person shifts position frequently in response to sensations of discomfort or pressure. Weak or very ill persons may have difficulty changing their position and maintaining good alignment. Paralysis also favors poor positioning because the person is unable to feel discomfort and thus is often unaware of an awkwardly positioned body part. Paralyzed limbs cannot support their own weight; consequently they are "heavy" and pull the person out of good alignment.

One consequence of infrequent position change and poor alignment is the development of contractures. These most frequently affect the hip, knee, ankle, shoulder, and elbow joints. The common types of contractures were described earlier in this chapter.

In order to help the person avoid this problem, the nurse should assist him in changing his position every 2 hours (Fig. 19-8). Position changes stretch

muscles and keep joint tissues elastic. The nurse should also assist the person to maintain good body alignment. This means that the head, shoulders, and hips are positioned in a straight line (see Fig. 19-5). If the person is sitting, flexion should occur at the hips, not the spine (Fig. 19-9).

To avoid plantar flexion, the bedcovers should not be tucked in so tightly that they pull the feet down. A principle to remember is that good body alignment maintains joints in a physiological position. This prevents fatigue and muscle aches that occur with abnormal joint positions.

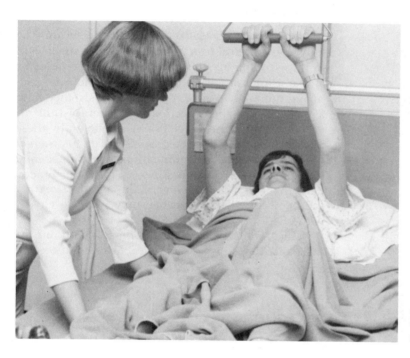

Figure 19-8
Position changes prevent the development of contractures.

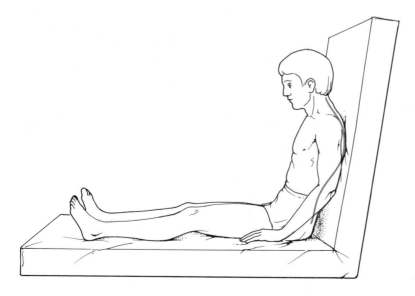

Figure 19-9
Flexion of the spine in bed.

Figure 19-10
Supportive devices.

Trochanter Roll

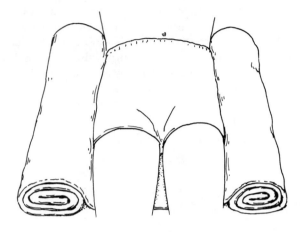

Bed Cradle
(bed covers are draped over the cradle)

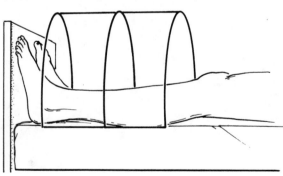

Footboard

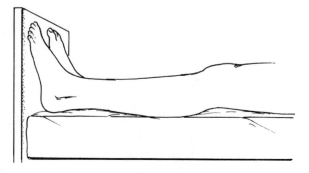

Supportive Devices

Supportive devices, such as trochanter rolls, footboards, and bed cradles, are useful in maintaining proper joint position. A trochanter roll placed along the hip joints prevents external rotation contractures, and a footboard maintains the ankle in a neutral postion and prevents footdrop. A bed cradle is also useful for this purpose because it relieves the pressure of bedcovers from the feet. Figure 19-10 shows these commonly used supportive devices.

Consultation and Referral

A person with specialized mobility needs may be helped by referral to a professional who specializes in these problems. Persons who have experienced a stroke, a fracture, paralysis, or any serious or permanent mobility problem may need assistance from a physical therapist, occupational therapist, or orthotist. Some of the special services offered by these professionals include exercise therapy, instruction in crutchwalking or ambulation, techniques and devices for ADL, and prostheses, splints, or braces. Remember that nurses may be the first to recognize the need for referral because they work so closely with clients.

A sample care plan for the person with musculoskeletal disuse is shown in Table 19-3.

Fatigue and Decreased Endurance

Endurance was defined earlier in the chapter as the ability to continue a task. Several factors affect endurance, the most obvious being the condition of the muscles. If the muscles have become weakened through disuse, the person tires easily. Another factor is cardiac and respiratory status. The heart and lungs must work harder during activity in order to meet the increased oxygen needs of the tissues. Cardiac or respiratory problems may interfere with the ability to perform daily activities; strenuous activity may even be hazardous. Nutritional status also affects endurance because inadequate nutrient intake limits the fuel available for muscular work. This accounts for the tired feeling that frequently accompanies fad diets. Most health problems that affect nutrition are accompanied by fatigue (diabetes or cancer, as examples). Finally, emotions can affect energy levels, as evidenced by the feeling of fatique that commonly

Table 19-3
Sample Nursing Care Plan for the Person with Musculoskeletal Disuse

The following is a care plan for W.B., a 60-year-old woman who experienced right-sided hemiparesis resulting from a stroke. W.B. has difficulty using her right side because of weakness.

Potential Problems	Goals/Expected Outcomes	Interventions
Loss of muscle strength and atrophy	Client will maintain muscle strength and mass	Assist client to ambulate to chair b.i.d.
Decreased joint mobility (contractures)	Client will maintain full ROM of all joints	Active or passive ROM to all joints b.i.d. —Explore how to incorporate into ADL (bathing, grooming)
Decreased bone mass (osteoporosis)	Client will maintain bone composition	—Trochanter roll to both hips —Apply footboard to bed —Turn q 2 hr and check body alignment; reposition as necessary —Consult physician about PT referral for muscle strengthening exercise and transfer techniques

occurs with depression and anxiety. Nurses should be alert to possible emotional needs in persons with unexplained chronic fatigue.

Limited endurance and fatigue are common symptoms which accompany physical and emotional stress. Most of us recall the feeling of tiredness that occurs when we are ill or the sensation of exhaustion after we have completed a difficult examination in school. This fatigue is protective in that it limits activity and so conserves energy for coping with stressors. Nurses should recognize that any client in crisis, whether with a physical illness or emotional stress, may have limited endurance.

Assessment

Identifying endurance problems was described in the earlier section on motor assessment. To review briefly—it is important to be alert for subjective statements of fatigue as well as for objective data such as frequent pauses to rest, shortness of breath, or elevated vital signs after mild activity. A complete assessment includes evaluation of cardiorespiratory, nutritional, and emotional statuses, as well as motor status, to identify possible causes for fatigue.

Nursing Interventions

Nursing interventions are directed toward assisting the person to conserve energy and improve activity tolerance. If the person has underlying cardiac, respiratory, or nutritional needs, the nurse should intervene for these problems as well.

The first step is to determine the person's activity tolerance level. How much activity brings on fatigue? For one person this may be a walk of 50 feet; for another it may be climbing the stairs or performing light housework.

Conserving Energy. The nurse can use the information about activity tolerance to plan with the person ways to conserve energy. Together they may decide that the activities which are especially tiring can be assumed by the nurse or family members. For instance, the nurse might bathe the client, while a family member might perform housework. It is also important to help the person to space his daily activities and allow frequent rest periods. For example, if the hospitalized person experiences fatigue after walking in the hall, a rest period before and after ambulation may prove helpful. The nurse may need to help the person prioritize daily activities and omit those that are less important or have another assume them. For instance, the nurse might bathe the postoperative patient in order to help him conserve energy for the important activities of ambulation and respiratory exercises. Finally, the nurse can help the person identify more efficient methods of performing daily activities. As an example, the housewife might conserve energy by sitting to prepare meals or do ironing. Rearranging the environment to eliminate the need for stair climbing or other inefficient activities may be helpful. It is essential to remember that the purpose of the nursing intervention is to assist the person to conserve energy, not to limit all of his activity. This is an important difference, because inactivity only causes decreased muscle tone and strength, which limit endurance even further.

Exercise and Endurance.　Endurance level may be gradually increased through exercise. A person with limited activity tolerance should probably begin with isometric exercises since these require less energy. Otherwise mild isotonic exercises can be started. Walking is an excellent method of improving endurance. Increasing the distance walked each day improves muscle strength and tone as well as cardiorespiratory capacity.

At the same time the person should be helped to find ways to avoid overexertion. Signs of limited endurance, as discussed under assessment of motor status, can be taught to the client. One must be particularly cautious when working with persons who have cardiac or respiratory problems because overexertion could lead to dangerous hypoxia. It is best to consult with the physician before planning exercise programs with these persons. In some instances fatigue is rooted in emotional origins. This type of fatigue is more successfully dealt with by psychological interventions. The nurse can use communication skills to assess the cause of fatigue, to assist the person to explore his feelings, and to offer support. Table 19-4 shows a sample nursing care plan for the person with limited endurance.

Decreased Ability to Perform Activities of Daily Living

Assessment

Many persons with motor status problems experience some difficulty in performing ADL. An important area of nursing assessment is to determine what specific daily activities the person is unable to perform for himself. The reader may wish to review material on data collection in the area of ADL, which was described earlier in the chapter.

Nursing Interventions

Nursing interventions are directed toward assisting the person to perform activities which he cannot do and to increase his independence in ADL. If the impairment is only temporary, as might be the case

---

Table 19-4
Sample Nursing Care Plan for the Person with Limited Endurance

The following is a care plan for M.L., a client with chronic respiratory disease. His oxygen deficiency has limited his activity tolerance.

Problems	Goals/Expected Outcomes	Interventions
Limited endurance due to hypoxia	Client will perform ADL within limits of endurance Client will increase activity tolerance	Identify specific activities that cause fatigue. Have nurse or family assume very tiring activities. Prioritize activities and limit those that are least important. Identify efficient methods of performing activities. Begin mild exercise program. Avoid overexertion. Intervene for respiratory needs.

with a fracture or extreme fatigue due to illness, the nurse supports the person by assuming some of his activities, such as bathing or feeding him.

Such support is also appropriate in the early stages of permanent injury (*i.e.*, paralysis due to stroke or spinal cord injury). But unless the person is to remain permanently dependent on others for his care, he needs to learn new methods of performing his own ADL. The occupational therapist is the usual referral source for planning a learning program. The therapist may teach the client ways of doing ADL and provide devices that assist him in eating, dressing, or carrying out other activities. Examples of devices include long-handled brushes or eating utensils with looped handles that fit over the hand (Fig. 19-11).

The nurse's role is to support, encourage, and supervise the person as he performs self-care and to coordinate the nursing plan with the therapist's activities. Often special forms are used to record the client's progress in ADL, making it easier for all professionals who work with the client to be aware of his current abilities. It is very important to assist the person to do as much as he is capable of doing for himself. "Doing for" the person rather than assisting him to "do for himself" encourages dependence. Although this may meet the nurse's need to nurture, it does not promote maximum function of the client's ability nor does it allow him control over his situation. A sensitive nurse assesses the client's abilities and helps him to perform as much as he is capable of doing, not more or less.

Relearning ADL can be a frustrating experience, because lowered self-esteem occurs with loss of independence. The nurse can help the person maintain a positive attitude by giving encouragement and supporting his efforts. Empathy skills are an impor-

Figure 19-11
Assistive devices for eating.

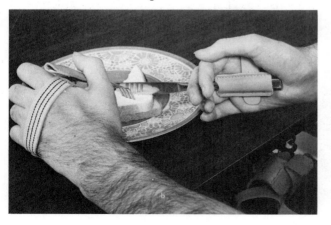

tant part of this process. ("It must be very frustrating when you feel you're progressing so slowly.") Keeping a chart of the person's progress in a visible spot helps him feel that he is moving toward independent function.

Another nursing intervention is to teach exercises to strengthen body parts that will eventually be used in self-care. For instance, teaching isotonic exercises for arm muscles is an aid in crutchwalking. It is imperative that disuse complications such as contractures or atrophy be prevented before the person begins learning ADL. Range of motion and other exercises maintain functional abilities for eventual ADL performance. Table 19-5 shows a sample care plan for the person with decreased ability to perform ADL.

Nursing Care of the Person Immobilized by Bed Rest

The effects of musculoskeletal disuse resulting from immobilization of a particular body part were explored in the first part of this chapter. This section discusses the effects of immobilization due to bed rest. However, because bed rest affects every body system as well as the psychological status, much of the information presented here is also discussed within the other chapters that describe the specific statuses of the person. This section integrates that information and applies it to the special needs of the immobilized person.

Bed rest has several purposes. It conserves energy for persons with minimal energy reserves such as those with cardiac conditions or serious illness. It allows immobilization of body parts for treatment of health problems and promotion of healing (*e.g.*, traction for a fractured femur, radium implant to treat cancer of the cervix). Finally bed rest may be imposed by a functional disability such as a nervous system disorder or severe pain.

Unfortunately, bed rest also is associated with potential complications. Many of these complications were identified by Dietrick and his associates who were intrigued by the finding that World War II soldiers, when mobilized rapidly after their injuries, seemed to experience fewer complications than patients who had been treated with prolonged bed rest in the traditional manner (Dietrick *et al*, 1948). In essence nearly every body system is affected by prolonged bed rest. These effects and related nursing interventions are presented in the following pages.

Table 19-5
Sample Nursing Care Plan for the Person with Problems Performing ADL

The following is a care plan for J.B., a 25-year old client whose lower legs were paralyzed following an automotive accident.

Problems	Goals/Expected Outcomes	Interventions
Decreased ability to perform ADL –Transferring between bed and wheelchair –Dressing –Bathing	Client will be able to –Transfer between wheelchair and bed independently –Dress and bathe independently	Identify the person's current abilities. Assist with ADL as needed. Refer to occupational therapy. Supervise the person while he performs ADL; give suggestions, encouragement, and support. Allow client to do what he can for himself. Keep a chart of current abilities. Exercise body parts that will be used in self-care.
Anger due to loss of functional ability and slow progress in learning ADL skills	Client will experience decreased anger	Facilitate verbalization of feelings. Stress the progress being made toward goals.

Respiration

The person who is confined to bed is susceptible to respiratory infection and *atelectasis* (collapse of all or part of a lung).

Respiratory infection is favored because respiratory secretions pool or collect in dependent areas of the bronchioles when the person is supine (Fig. 19-12). This effect allows the remaining portions of the mucous membranes lining the bronchioles to become dry. Such drying leads to impaired function of the cilia (tiny hairlike projections that move mucus toward the large airways). As mucus pools in the lungs, bacteria grow readily. The respiratory infection that may eventually develop is termed *hypostatic pneumonia*.

Atelectasis is caused by factors that decrease pulmonary ventilation (air moving into and out of the lungs). In the person on bed rest these factors include decreased activity, which reduces the stimulus for deep breathing; muscle weakness due to age or illness; decreased chest expansion caused by resistance of the bed; and increased respiratory secretions (described above), which limit air move-

Figure 19-12
The effect of gravity on the distribution of mucus within a bronchus. *(Browse NT: The Physiology and Pathology of Bedrest, p. 60. Springfield, Illinois, Charles C. Thomas)*

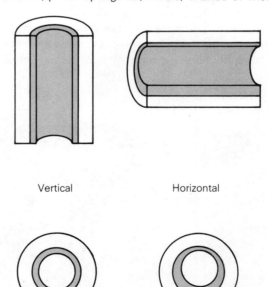

Vertical   Horizontal

ment through affected bronchioles. When ventilation is reduced the production of pulmonary surfactant decreases. Surfactant is a substance that reduces the natural tendency of alveoli to collapse. The result of alveolar collapse may be atelectasis.

Nursing Interventions

The nursing interventions which can prevent alveolar collapse and atelectasis are aimed at reducing pulmonary secretions and increasing pulmonary ventilation. Coughing and deep breathing exercises and frequent position changes prevent pooling of mucus and encourage ventilation of all areas of the lungs. More information about these and other nursing interventions can be found in Chapter 24.

Circulation

Bed rest increases cardiac workload, decreases exercise tolerance and may lead to venous thrombosis (presence of blood clots in the veins) or orthostatic hypotension. Each of these complications is a potentially serious problem of persons confined to bed, particularly those with existing cardiac or vascular problems.

Cardiac Workload

At first it may seem more likely that bed rest would decrease the workload of the heart. However, research has shown that the opposite is true. Coe (1954) found that cardiac workload is 30% greater in the recumbent position than when sitting, and subsequent studies confirmed this finding. The explanation behind this finding is that blood which normally pools in the extremities when the person stands returns to the heart when he is supine. This increases the volume of blood that must be pumped, thereby increasing cardiac workload. Because heart-rate falls and cardiac output increases when the person assumes the supine position, it follows that the heart pumps more blood with each ventricular contraction. This means that the heart performs more work per contraction when the person lies in bed.

Valsalva Maneuver

Increased use of the *Valsalva maneuver* by persons in bed contributes to the cardiac workload. The Valsalva maneuver involves holding the breath and straining against a closed glottis, thereby increasing intrathoracic pressure. We often do this while lifting heavy objects or straining to have a bowel movement. Persons in bed use this maneuver frequently when changing positions. During a Valsalva maneuver, venous return is reduced. When the maneuver stops, the volume of blood returning to the heart suddenly increases, increasing cardiac workload. Considering that persons in bed perform Valsalva maneuvers 10 to 20 times per hour, the stress placed on the heart becomes obvious (Browse, 1965).

Exercise

Although cardiac workload increases with bed rest, there is a progressive decrease in exercise tolerance. This is evidenced by tachycardia, which occurs during periods of strenuous activity (Kottke, 1964). It takes 4 to 6 weeks of conditioning to return the heart to its former abilities after prolonged bed rest.

Nursing Invervention

Nurses can assist the person on bed rest to reduce cardiac workload by teaching him to avoid Valsalva maneuvers while moving. "Breathe through your mouth whenever you change positions," is a helpful reminder that prevents straining against a closed glottis. Straining during bowel movements can be minimized by preventing constipation and by assisting the person to a sitting position before defecation. The person should sit in a chair, if possible, rather than lie in bed because sitting decreases cardiac workload.

Orthostatic Hypotension

Orthostatic hypotension is a problem which is more likely to occur the longer the person remains on bed rest. Normally, peripheral and splanchnic blood vessels constrict when we move from a lying to a standing position. The person on bed rest becomes less able to produce this postural change as immobility continues. When he first attempts to stand, blood pools in the extremities and the splanchnic area causing a rapid drop in blood pressure which can result in fainting.

Nursing Intervention

Hypotension produces increased sympathetic nervous system activity and thus provides important clues to impending fainting by the person's pale, cool, moist skin, by the presence of tachycardia, and by his statements of feeling "dizzy" or "shaky." If these occur, the person should be assisted to bed immediately. As a means of avoiding orthostatic hypotension, elastic bandages or stockings may be worn to prevent venous blood from pooling in the legs. If the person is able to sit in a chair or dangle his legs over the edge of the bed, he should be assisted to do so throughout the period of immobilization. This preserves postural mechanisms that maintain blood pressure.

Thrombosis

Venous thrombosis, discussed more fully in Chapter 23, is another potential hazard of immobility. The person on bed rest has increased risk of developing this problem for several reasons. Decreased activity allows blood to pool in the leg veins (*venous stasis*), promoting thrombus formation. Certain bed positions (such as elevating the bed gatch under the knees) put pressure against vein walls and lead to damage of the intima layer. Platelets collect in these areas, initiating clotting. The tendency of the blood to clot may increase with bed rest because of increased serum calcium levels due to bone resorption. Calcium is a factor in the clotting mechanism (Olson and Johnson, 1967).

Nursing Interventions

Nurses can prevent thrombosis by promoting venous return. Elevating the foot of the bed and assisting the person to perform leg exercises will increase the blood flow from the lower extremities to the heart. Chapter 23 presents other interventions including teaching plans for clients at risk for thrombophlebitis.

Skin: Pressure Sores

More often than necessary *pressure sores* are a problem for persons confined to bed. Two factors that favor the development of these lesions are friction, such as rubbing the skin against bed sheets, and pressure on the skin from bony prominences. Friction can wear away skin layers creating denuded areas that are prone to infection. Pressure from bearing weight on the bony prominences causes inadequate blood flow to affected tissue, depriving these areas of oxygen and nutrients. Eventually the tissue dies and sloughs, creating open lesions. Treatment of decubitus ulcers can be psychologically, physically, and financially costly. It is important that nursing care emphasizes prevention of this problem.

Nursing Interventions

The most important nursing interventions are directed toward relieving pressure from the skin and reducing friction. Persons who are most at risk of developing pressure sores are those who cannot move or reposition themselves readily or those with diminished pain sensation. These persons need nursing assistance to turn every 2 to 3 hours and to position themselves so that pressure points are minimal. Chapter 18 contains specific information about positioning persons to achieve these goals.

Other measures include padding friction areas such as elbows and heels to maintain intact skin and prevent denuding; massaging the skin overlying bony prominences to increase blood flow and bring oxygen and nutrients to these areas; and using alternating pressure mattresses to relieve pressure from tissue over bony prominences.

Bowel Elimination

Constipation is a problem for many persons confined to bed. Several factors may contribute to this complication. For one thing, it is difficult to assume a normal position for defecation when lying in bed. Even if the head of the bed is elevated, it is difficult to flex the knees in bed, which normally assists with defecation. If the person is in a hospital, there is the added stress of diminished privacy during bowel movements, which violates an American cultural value. Finally, illness or age may weaken abdominal and levator ani muscles which are used in defecation. These factors may decrease the person's ability or urge to move his bowels. As feces remain in the colon for longer periods, water reabsorption continues. This causes stools to harden, making it difficult to pass them through the anal sphincter. As a result, fecal impaction may occur.

Nursing Interventions

Nurses can assist their clients with bowel elimination by providing as much privacy as possible in an unhurried atmosphere. If possible, the person should get out of bed for bowel movements; a bedside commode may be useful to conserve energy while allowing a normal position for defecation. If the person cannot get out of bed, elevating the head of the bed to a comfortable level makes defecation easier. The person should also be warned that the urge to defecate must be heeded or it will diminish. It is also helpful to plan for increased dietary intake of bulk and other natural laxatives the person normally uses (*e.g.*, prune juice or morning coffee). Finally, the nurse should watch for deviations from the person's normal pattern of bowel elimination so that the potential constipation can be detected and treated as early as possible.

Urinary Elimination

Urinary elimination is altered during bed rest in two ways: the act of micturition is more difficult to perform, and urine pools in the kidney pelvis. It is difficult to relax perineal muscles and the external sphincter in the supine position. Lack of privacy may also inhibit micturition for those who are hospitalized.

Stasis of urine is favored by the supine position as indicated in Figure 19-13. Drainage of the renal pelvis occurs by gravity when the person is standing. When the person is lying on his back, urine collects in the dependent areas of the renal pelvis making it difficult for urine to enter the ureters. Urinary stasis allows any crystals contained in the urine to remain in the urinary tract long enough to form the nucleus for stones. Urinary calcium is elevated and urine becomes more alkaline during bed rest (Dietrick, 1948); both of these conditions favor the formation of stones.

Nursing Interventions

Nurses can aid their clients to maintain normal urinary elimination during immobility by assisting them to a normal position before voiding. If possible, males should stand; females should sit. It is important to provide privacy and adequate time during micturition. Some helpful ideas that encourage relaxation for the person who is unable to void are listed in Chapter 21.

Urinary stasis can be prevented by providing adequate fluid intake, helping the person to change positions frequently, and assisting him to ambulate or sit in a chair if this is possible. An acid ash diet (one which is metabolized to acid end products) inhibits the formation of renal calculi, because stones composed of calcium salts do not enlarge readily in acid urine. Foods which promote acid urine include meats, cereals, and cranberry juice. The nurse should observe the person frequently for signs of urinary retention or renal calculi to detect problems early.

Nutrition

Dietrick (1948) identified increased urinary nitrogen excretion in his immobilized subjects 5 or 6 days after bed rest began. This indicates that persons on bed rest develop negative nitrogen balance. Protein catabolism (breakdown) exceeds synthesis, eventually causing possible protein deficiency and tissue wasting. This problem is often compounded by anorexia (diminished appetite). Appetite changes in

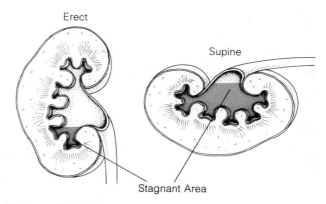

Figure 19-13
The effect of posture on the drainage of the kidney.
(Browse NT: The Physiology and Pathology of Bedrest, p. 83. Springfield, Illinois, Charles C Thomas)

the immobilized person may be caused by factors such as surgery on the gastrointestinal (GI) tract, fatigue, boredom, depression, or a disease process. Negative nitrogen balance favors muscle atrophy and muscle fatigue, which may cause further immobility. Negative nitrogen balance also inhibits tissue repair, such as wound healing, and makes the person more susceptible to decubitus ulcers.

Nursing Interventions

Nitrogen balance is favored by a diet that contains adequate protein and carbohydrate. The nurse needs to plan meals with the person to include foods that are both nutritious and appealing. This is especially important if anorexia is present. Smaller, more frequent meals are sometimes more acceptable than large servings. Nutritious liquids such as milkshakes or eggnogs may appeal in these instances. Chapter 20 contains additional information on caring for the person with anorexia.

Sensory and Emotional Functions

Sensory alterations in immobilized persons are well documented by research. Decreased sensory stimulation is a common problem, particularly in the hospital. The sights and sounds that are present in the environment such as beeping monitors, unfamiliar hospital equipment, and colorless walls are either monotonous or meaningless for the person. Sensory deprivation is a serious potential problem. It is compounded by reduced movement, which further decreases incoming sensory messages. Downs (1974) found that immobility alone can cause sensory

---

Table 19-6
Nursing Care of the Immobilized Person

Status	Problem	Goals/Expected Outcome	Intervention
Motor	Loss of muscle strength		
	Decreased muscle mass	See Tables 19-4 and 19-5	See Tables 19-4 and 19-5
	Decreased joint mobility		
	Decreased ability to perform ADL		
Respiratory	Increased respiratory secretions	Client will have lungs clear to auscultation.	Teach and support deep breathing and coughing.
	Decreased ventilation		Assist with position change.
			Support use of incentive spirometer.
Circulatory	Increased work of heart	Client will maintain vital signs within normal limits.	Avoid prolonged supine position.
	Orthostatic hypotension		Avoid straining while moving or defecating.
	Venous thrombosis	Client will maintain adequate venous return.	Exhale through mouth during bed exercises.
			Change position (relative to gravity) gradually.
			Elevate legs.
			Perform leg exercises.
Integumentary	Pressure areas (decubitus ulcers)	Client will maintain intact skin.	Turn and position every 2 hours.
			Check pressure areas and bony prominences for skin condition.
			Cleanse and dry skin surfaces when moist.
			Provide alternating-pressure mattress.
			Provide sheepskin.

---

deprivation. Motion stimulates kinesthetic receptors, providing a form of stimulation that seems to be as important as sights or sounds for normal processing of information from the environment. Because immobility decreases the amount and relevance of sensory information, the person receives less information about the environment, which in turn decreases his ability to to interpret environmental cues correctly. Time distortion, anxiety, hallucination,

"floating sensations," decreased ability to think coherently, and inability to concentrate may all be experienced.

Nursing Interventions

The symptoms of sensory deprivation are often frightening. The person may fear he is losing his mind, particularly if hallucinations occur. Preventive

Status	Problem	Goals/Expected Outcome	Intervention
Elimination	Constipation	Client will have regular bowel movements.	Provide privacy.
			Assist to sitting position if possible.
	Urinary retention	Client will maintain urine output of at least 1500 ml/day.	Encourage roughage in diet.
			Provide privacy.
			Maintain normal voiding position, if possible.
	Renal stones	Client will maintain normal constitution of urine.	Encourage fluid intake.
			Avoid prolonged supine position.
			Give an acid ash diet.
Nutrition	Negative nitrogen balance	Client will maintain appropriate calorie intake for height and weight.	Ensure adequate protein and carbohydrate in diet.
	Anorexia		Create an attractive environment and servings.
			Assess client's preferences.
			Give small, frequent feedings.
Sensory	Sensory deprivation	Client will identify time, person, and place appropriately.	Provide variety in the environment (T.V., radio, conversation).
			Provide social contact.
			Provide reference points (clocks, calendars, *etc.*).
Psychological	Altered body image Powerlessness	Client will verbalize positive body image.	Assist client to express feelings.
		Client will demonstrate appropriate control of environment.	Assist client to work through loss.
			Encourage client to participate in self-care activity to limits of ability.
			Provide opportunities for decision making.

nursing action can alleviate this emotional distress. Providing meaningful environmental stimulation, such as familiar objects from the person's home, is therefore essential. In addition, clocks, calendars, T.V.s, and radios help orient the person to time. Kinesthetic information is provided through movement; therefore exercises and self-care activities increase stimulation of kinesthetic recepters. Taking the person for a ride in a wheelchair out of doors or at least out

of the room also provides new sensory information. Additional discussion of sensory deprivation can be found in Chapter 17.

Emotional effects of immobility have been described throughout the chapter. Feelings of dependence, powerlessness, and low self-esteem are common and may be expressed through signs of anxiety, depression, anger, or withdrawal. The true meaning of these expressions first needs to be identified before beginning to work with the person to meet the specific emotional need. For instance, if the nurse identifies that the person's hostility is rooted in a feeling of powerlessness, interventions can be directed toward restoring control to the client. Increasing the person's involvement in his health care and related decisions is a helpful approach to restoring control. Preventing harmful emotional effects of bed rest is as important as preventing physiological complications.

Table 19-6 summarizes potential problems of the immobilized person and provides related goals and nursing interventions.

Conclusion

Mobility is essential to a person's ability to function in his normal daily activities and is intimately related to human needs. Mobility is also a determinant of a person's sense of wholeness and self-concept. Nurses work with a variety of people with mobility needs, both in the hospital and in the community. Some of the most common mobility problems are related to musculoskeletal disuse.

Nursing interventions that prevent the problems resulting from disuse are exercise, position changes, proper joint alignment, supportive devices, and referral to physical or occupational therapists. Nursing interventions for two other common mobility problems—decreased endurance and decreased ability to perform ADL—include exercise, teaching self-care, assisting the person to function within his disabilities, and supporting his abilities. Immobility due to bed rest has consequences not only for the musculoskeletal system but also for every other body system. Because the problems of bed rest can cause needless physical, emotional, and financial harm, nursing interventions are directed toward preventing such problems before they occur.

Person-centered care involves consideration of the emotional, physical, and social consequences of mobility problems. This is true whether the person has a minor mobility impairment or is completely immobilized in bed. Nurses have the skills to assess motor function, identify needs, and plan with clients to implement appropriate interventions. In this way nurses can often make a major contribution to the person's attainment of maximum level of functioning.

Study Questions

1. Why is mobility so important to the person? Describe its relationship to human needs.

2. What are the components of a mobility assessment?

3. What are the physiological effects of disuse on bones, muscles, and joints?

4. Describe nursing interventions that prevent the consequences of musculoskeletal disuse.

5. Describe some causes of decreased endurance. List nursing interventions for the person experiencing this problem.

6. Describe the relationship between ambulation difficulties and the person's safety needs. What nursing interventions help the person maintain safety?

7. Describe the emotional responses that the person who has limited ability to perform ADL might experience as he relearns ADL skills. What nursing interventions would assist this person?

8. Why might a person with a musculoskeletal health problem have an altered body image? What are the behavioral responses to altered body image? What nursing interventions help this person adapt to altered body image?

9. What potential problems accompany prolonged bed rest? How can the nurse assist the person to avoid these dangers?

10. Describe the differences between isotonic, isometric, and passive exercise. What are the effects of each on the musculoskeletal system? How does the nurse determine which type of exercise best meets the person's needs?

Glossary

Activities of daily living: Activities in which the person engages, including those done at home, at work, and in the community.

Atrophy (muscle): Decreased muscle mass due to diminished size of individual fibers.

Contracture: Condition in which fibrosis of tissues surrounding a joint causes muscular resistance to passive stretching.

Diarthrosis: A joint in which adjoining bones are freely movable.

Endurance: The ability of muscles to continue a particular task.

Flaccidity: A state of decreased or absent muscle tone.

Hemiplegia: Paralysis of one side of the body.

Hypertrophy (muscle): Increase in size of a muscle structure due to increased size of individual fibers.

Isometric exercise: Muscle activity involving muscle contraction without muscle shortening, movement of a body part, or performance of mechanical work.

Isotonic exercise: Muscle activity involving muscle shortening, active movement of a body part, and performance of mechanical work.

Muscle tonus: A degree of muscle contraction that is present even when the muscle is at rest.

Orthostatic hypotension: A drop in blood pressure following movement from supine to erect position.

Osteoporosis: A condition in which bone matrix and minerals are depleted.

Paraplegia: Paralysis of the lower portion of the body including both legs.

Passive exercise: Activity in which the moving body part does not exert any significant effort.

Proprioception: The sense of awareness of position and movement of body parts and changes in equilibrium.

Range of motion: The degree of movement permitted by a joint.

Spasticity: A state of increased muscle tone resulting in muscular rigidity.

Synovial joint: Articulation containing a membrane that lines the joint capsule and secretes fluid.

Bibliography

Basmajian J: Therepautic Exercise, 3rd ed. Baltimore, Waverly Press, 1978

Brower P, Hicks D: Maintaining muscle function in patients on bedrest. Am J Nurs 72:1250–1253, July, 1972

Browse N: The Physiology and Pathology of Bedrest. Springfield, IL, Charles C Thomas, 1965

Burns L, Johnson P: Health Assessment in Clinical Practice. Englewood Cliffs, NJ, Prentice-Hall, 1980

Coe S: Cardiac work and the chair treatment of acute coronary thrombosis. Ann Intern Med 40:42–47, January, 1954

Dietrick J, Whedon GD, Shorr E et al: Effects of immobilization upon various metabolic and physiologic functions in normal men. Am J Med 4:3–36, January, 1948

Downs F: Bedrest and sensory disturbances. Am J Nurs 74:435–438, March, 1974

Gordon M: Assessing activity tolerance. Am J Nurs 76:72–75, January, 1976

Guyton A: Textbook of Medical Physiology, 5th ed. Philadelphia, WB Saunders, 1976

Hirschberg G, Lewis L, Vaughan P et al: Promoting patient mobility. Nurs '77 7:42–47, May, 1977

Jarvinen M: Immobilization effect on the tensile property of striated muscle. Arch Phys Med Rehabil 58:123–127, March, 1977

Kottke F, Blanchard R: Bedrest begets bedrest. Nurs Forum 3, No. 3: 57–72, 1964

Murray R: Foreword: Symposium on concept of body image. Nurs Clin North Am 7:593–595, December, 1972

Murray R, Zentner J: Nursing Assessment and Health Promotion Through the Life Span, 2nd ed. Englewood Cliffs, NJ, Prentice-Hall, 1979

Nutter D, Schlant RC, Hurst JW et al: Isometric exercise and the cardiovascular system. Mod Concepts Cardiovasc Dis 41:11–15, March 1972

Olson E: Hazards of immobility. Am J Nurs 67:780–796, April, 1967

Olson E, Johnson B: Hazards of immobility: Effects on cardiovascular function. Am J Nurs 67:781–782, April, 1967

Snyder M, Baum R: Assessing station and gait. Am J Nurs 74:1256–1257, July 1974

Nutritional Status

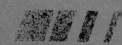

Mary L. Hunter

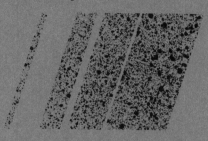

- Apply principles from the
sciences of nutrition, anatomy,
and physiology in promoting
the client's nutritional health.

- Assess the nutritional status
of self and clients.

- Use the factors that affect the
nutritional status to provide
person-centered care.

- Describe several health
problems related to alterations
in the normal nutritional state.

- Design nursing care plans to
assist persons with special
nutritional needs.

A person's sense of health and well-being is
closely associated with his nutritional status. Being well nourished,
having healthy eating habits, and maintaining a comfortable weight
are essential for optimum health. Related factors such as proper rest
and exercise combine with nutrition for healthy living. Good nutrition
is achieved when the food supply is adequate in quantity and quality,
the person is physiologically and psychologically capable of eating,
and his body cells use food in the proper physiological manner.

Principles from the sciences of nutrition and anatomy and physiology are the basis from which the nurse practices nutritional health
care. The nutritional status embodies much of the very persons we
are with regard to life-style, cultural and religious practices, emotional states, and communication with others. The purpose of this
chapter is to help students consider these factors and understand
how health is influenced by the utilization of nutrients and the
mobilization of strengths.

Anatomy and Physiology

The gastrointestinal tract, or alimentary canal, is a continuous tube extending from the mouth to the anus. It is lined with an extremely thin and wet epithelial mucous membrane. The thinness of the lining allows for **absorption** of digested food into the blood and lymph streams for transportation to all the cells of the body. The auxiliary structures and organs of digestion include the teeth, tongue, salivary glands, gallbladder, pancreas, and liver. The mechanical process of digestion consists of breaking up food by chewing and propulsion of food along the tract by peristalsis. The chemical process breaks the food into simpler components through the action of enzymes and acid which enter the tract at strategic points from the auxiliary digestive organs and from the cells of the tract itself.

The swallowing reflex is an essential part of the physiology of digestion. It is initiated when the tongue forces the food to the rear of the mouth and pressure receptors in the walls of the pharynx are stimulated. These receptors send afferent impulses to the swallowing center in the medulla which coordinates the swallowing process. The swallowing center inhibits respiration, raises the larynx, and closes the glottis, thereby keeping food from entering the trachea. The swallowing reflex may be inhibited as a result of inadequate innervation of the pharyngeal muscles or radiation therapy for a tumor. The swallowing reflex is also diminished by the administration of local anesthesia to the oral cavity or throat for dental work or diagnostic procedures such as bronchoscopy.

After food is swallowed and absorbed, the anabolic phase of metabolism occurs. Absorbed foodstuffs such as simple sugars, free fatty acids, and amino acids are used to synthesize body carbohydrates, fats, and proteins. The total digestive system must be intact and functioning properly to achieve a healthy nutritional state. Figure 20-1 illustrates the anatomy of the digestive system.

Factors that Affect Nutrition

Protective Mechanisms

The digestive system protects our bodies through a variety of adaptive mechanisms, including the swallowing reflex, appetite, the gag reflex, and vomiting. The swallowing reflex, as previously mentioned, protects the respiratory tract. A diminished appetite, **anorexia,** indicates to the person that his body will not tolerate food or fluids. The gag reflex protects against unpalatable food or fluids and can be stimulated to produce vomiting when a harmful substance has been ingested.

Vomiting, as a protective mechanism, may occur spontaneously or be induced by digital stimulation to eliminate irritating or harmful substances from the upper portion of the gastrointestinal tract. Vomiting may also be helpful if over-distention of the stomach or duodenum occurs from eating. It may also occur as a result of certain disease processes.

The sphincters, present at the ends of each portion of the gastrointestinal tract, such as the stomach and duodenum, open according to pressure

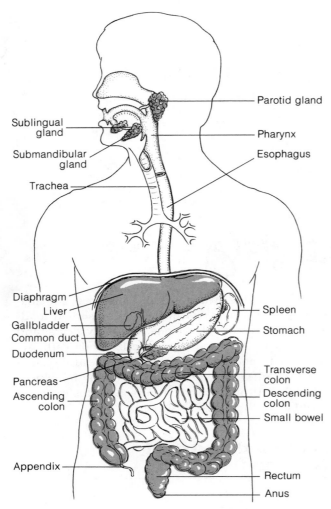

Figure 20-1
Anatomy of the gastrointestinal tract.

gradients and allow an appropriate amount of food to enter the next portion of the tract, thereby preventing distention.

Basic Needs

Our ability and desire to eat is easily affected by other physiological processes. For example, the need for oxygen in a person in respiratory distress dominates the need for food and thus leads to a diminished sense of hunger and appetite. A diminished energy level, may result from inadequate nutrition as well as from a struggle for oxygen. Alterations in elimination may cause constipation and flatus, thereby reducing the desire to eat. Some persons find the need for rest or the need to avoid pain more important than the need to eat.

Love and safety needs are often associated with altered eating patterns. Some people lose their appetite or enthusiasm for food when they become sad or depressed. Others may use food to replace that which they perceive as missing in their lives. In some instances when alcohol or drugs are used in an attempt to meet basic needs, appetite can be affected adversely.

Cultural Patterns

One notable authority on foods and cooking states, "Man's social structure has always revolved around food and its presentation. The basis of hospitality, yesterday and today, is the sharing of food and drink with friends and acquaintances" (Vic, 1968, p. 8). According to a well-known fictional detective, if we know what a particular society eats, we can deduce a great deal about its culture, philosophy, morals, and politics (Stout, 1955). In other words, much of what we are is reflected in our nutritional practices.

Countries or societies of people have developed nutritional practices based on regional characteristics such as climate, soil conditions, and proximity to the sea. Ethnic inheritances, historical background, and religious beliefs have also influenced the role that food plays in a culture. For example, the Italians are a hearty, hospitable people who use food as a means of communicating with their family and friends. The fact that they are close to the sea has made fish an important part of their cuisine. The same is true of the Japanese, who have made an art out of preparing food and have developed an elaborate sense of manners and etiquette in association with their nutritional practices. In America, the nutritional practices are influenced by geographical regions, religious background, and the customs of people who emigrate from other lands.

Religious Factors

Religious practices sometimes impose dietary restrictions on persons of particular groups. Orthodox Jews exclude pork and shell fish from their diet. Catholics used to eliminate meat on Fridays and certain other days of penance. Some religious groups practice vegetarianism or eliminate other foods from their diets at certain times of the year. Small children, elderly, ill, or hospitalized persons are often exempt from these practices, especially if acceptable substitutions for essential nutrients cannot be found. However, elderly, or ill persons who have practiced these restrictions for a long time may find it difficult to change and may wish to continue with their usual customs.

Finances

Persons with limited finances often cannot afford foods such as meats, fresh fruits, or vegetables and may subsist on diets high in carbohydrate and fat. This causes problems for children with growth needs, and for anyone who has recently undergone surgery. Persons with diabetes also have difficulty staying on a planned diet if they are unable to afford the proper foods.

We are all aware of underdeveloped areas of the United States and other countries where financial resources are inadequate to feed whole segments of the population. The media often depict starving children and make appeals for monetary contributions to help with the world hunger problem. There are a few services in the United States for persons who have a limited income. Programs such as Government Food Stamps or Motor Meals, which serve handicapped or elderly persons in their homes, are often available.

Motor Status

Persons with mobility alterations may find it difficult to shop for and prepare food. Those with quadriplegia or arthritic joint problems may even be unable to eat without assistance. These limitations have less effect on the person's nutritional status when there are family members or friends available to assist. The following clinical example describes the effect of mobility on nutritional status.

Example ☐ Mr. Thomas, a bachelor with diabetes, was to return home from the hospital following the amputation of his left leg. He was to use crutches and a wheelchair until the suture line on the stump healed and a prosthetic leg could be fitted. He planned to drive a car to go grocery shopping but could not manage the grocery cart while using crutches. Plans were made for his sister to go shopping with him. She would push the cart and pick up the items, and Mr. Thomas would make the decisions on which foods he needed for his diabetic diet.

At home, he prepared meals from his wheelchair, and a community nurse assisted him in planning nutritious, easily prepared foods. This conserved his energy and prevented him from becoming discouraged with food preparation. He returned to his former independence after the prosthetic leg was fitted. ☐

Growth Needs

Infants, children, and young adults have growth needs that should be considered when planning nutrition. Young people because they grow at irregular rates, may eat heartily on one occasion and poorly on another. Growth needs also occur when new tissue is developing after a surgical procedure or burn. The diet for these persons should be high in calories to cover energy expenditure and high in protein to assist with the growth of new tissue.

Atmosphere During Meals

Companionship and pleasant conversation among friendly people offer an ideal way to pass a mealtime. Many families use the time for positive communication and leave grievances behind. Other families have unhappy and disruptive experiences at mealtimes, using them to air grievances. Persons who are depressed or have many somatic ailments can sometimes trace their problems back to stressful mealtimes. Elderly persons and others who live alone often do not have family or friends close by for mealtime companionship. This may result in altered nutritional patterns and inadequate nutrition to meet daily activity needs.

General Assessment of Nutritional Status

Bodily Dimensions

Height, weight, and body build, together with age and sex, are data to consider early in the assessment phase. Standardized charts can be used as guidelines and serve as a basis of comparison with an established norm. Ideally, however, each person's body weight is that which pleases him in terms of how he looks and feels. The nurse also wants to consider normal alterations, such as individual growth patterns in children, density of muscle tissue in athletes, and changes in bone structure in the elderly. These alterations may make a person look heavier or lighter than his actual weight.

Anthropometric measurements are another means of assessing nutritional status (Fig. 20-2). The measurements are determined by means of a caliper and provide an estimation of muscle mass and fat stores. They can be especially helpful in assessing the severely ill or those who are obviously undernourished. However, the calipers used for measurement are not always available, and the measurement procedure has not been standardized. Students may refer to Salmond (1980) in the bibliography for instructions on how to take anthropometric measurements.

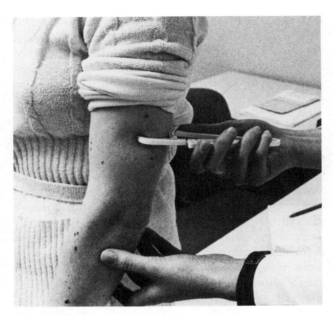

Figure 20-2
Anthropometric measurements. Skinfold calipers for measurement of skinfold thickness. *(Photo by Doug Herdman/Kettering Medical Center)*

Some basic observations can help determine a person's nutritional status in terms of obesity, emaciation, and cachexia:

- **Obesity** is generally thought to be a weight 20% to 30% higher than normal for a person of a given age, sex, and body build. It is characterized by large amounts of fat on the body.
- **Emaciation** is the state of being extremely lean.
- **Cachexia** is a state of severe emaciation, which becomes most obvious in those areas of the body that normally contain prominent deposits of fat, such as the buttocks, and muscle masses, such as the thighs and back. The fat or muscle mass waste away allowing the bones to protrude. The skin becomes thin and loose owing to the wasting away of underlying muscle tissue. The skin also becomes dry, pale, and cold and loses resiliency. The hair is dry and dull and falls out easily; the eyes are sunken. The person often becomes apathetic, the heart rate slows, the blood pressure drops, and respirations decrease in rate and efficiency.

Patterns of Weight Gain and Loss

A significant weight gain or loss may indicate a health problem or it could be a result of dieting. A significant gain in a person who was previously underweight could be a healthy sign. On the other hand, weight gain may be associated with overeating or edema related to alterations in cardiovascular or renal function. Weight loss may also be healthy, although it could be associated with an inability to obtain food, poor eating patterns, or physiological alterations in the use of food, such as may occur in cancer.

Emotional factors can alter eating habits and may cause anorexia and weight loss or overeating and weight gain. Persons who are ill or fatigued, or are taking medications that suppress the appetite may lose weight rapidly. If the weight change has occurred recently and was unplanned, assess for physical or psychological stressors that may be implicated. If patterns of weight gain and loss have occurred over a lifetime, assess factors that affect nutrition. For example, the assessment of love and safety needs may be very helpful in determining the reason for alterations in weight patterns.

Patterns of Daily Food Intake

In order to make use of healthy eating practices as well as specific food preferences, the nurse should assess foods the person eats and his usual daily schedule of meals and snacks. Assessment should include a typical day's pattern of food intake, the amounts eaten, and the usual times for eating. Remember to look at work schedules and how various work shifts affect the person's nutritional patterns. Evaluate the adequacy of nutrients the person receives in a typical day (Fig. 20-3).

Appetite

Appetite is a psychological response to food related to our past experiences with food, the cultural implications of eating, the esthetics of the food placed before us, and other individual factors. **Hunger** is a basic physical need. Usually as hunger diminishes, so does appetite. However, occasionally a person is hungry yet has little appetite, or does not feel hungry but eats because the food tastes good. Sometimes a certain food may quiet hunger pangs but not appeal to the appetite.

The nurse should assess factors that affect both hunger and appetite in the individual person: his food preferences and those items he dislikes; medications he takes that alter appetite, and the effect of stress on appetite.

Risk-Taking Behavior

Although overeating and undereating are at times linked to self-destructive impulses, for the most part people practice poor nutritional habits for conven-

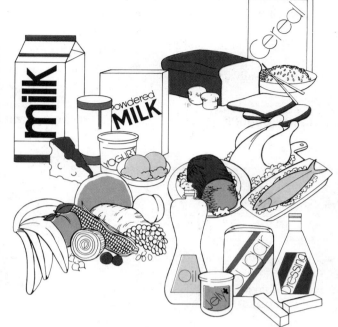

Milk Group
Some milk for everyone
Children under 9 . . . 2 to 3 cups
Children 9 to 12 . . . 3 or more cups
Teenagers . . . 4 or more cups
Adults . . . 2 or more cups

Vegetable Fruit Group
4 or more servings
Include—
A citrus fruit or other fruit or
vegetable important for vitamin C
A dark-green or deep-yellow
vegetable for vitamin A—at
least every other day
Other vegetables and fruits,
including potatoes

Bread Cereal Group
4 or more servings
Whole grain, enriched, or
restored

Meat Group
2 or more servings
Beef, veal, pork, lamb, poultry,
fish, eggs
As alternatives—dry beans, dry
peas, nuts

Other Foods
To round out meals and meet
energy needs, most everyone
will use some foods not
specified in the Four Food
Groups. Such foods include
breads, cereals, flours, sugars,
butter, margarine, other fats.
These often are ingredients in a
recipe or added to other foods
during preparation or at table.
Try to include some vegetable
oils among the fats used.

Figure 20-3
An adequate diet consists of foods from each of the four basic food groups. Food for Fitness: A Daily Food Guide *(Modified from Leaflet 424, U.S. Department of Agriculture, Institute of Home Economics)*

ience or to lose weight or because of inadequate information. Of the numerous ways that people can take nutritional risks, perhaps one of the most prevalent is fad dieting. Because dieting is so popular, new diets are always being developed. To ensure proper nutrition, persons need help in looking at these plans objectively and altering them as necessary.

Persons with health problems may frequently engage in nutritional risk-taking behavior. For example, those with hypertension or diabetes may continue to eat foods that are high in sodium or carbohydrate. When risk-taking behavior is apparent, consider that this may represent the person's attempt to satisfy other needs.

Level of Nutritional Knowledge

Assessment of the person's knowledge of basic nutrition serves as a guide in determining the kind of diet-related instruction the nurse offers. Because food is so frequently discussed in the media, most adults and many children and adolescents have some knowledge about good nutritional practice. The nurse may often find that although persons have basic nutritional knowledge, they need help in making food a more meaningful experience and in applying nutritional knowledge to their own situation.

The nurse should determine whether the person had some previous diet instruction and should assess if it was helpful or relevant. Sometimes nurses, doctors, or dietitians do not formulate mutual plans with the person but instead dictate diets and give instructions that do not fit the individual's needs and life-style. Information about useful past instruction helps the nurse plan a more relevant diet with the person.

Condition of the Oral Cavity

A functional oral cavity contributes greatly to our sense of well-being. An intact oral mucosa and an adequate salivary flow facilitate both nutrition and communication. If our breath is pleasant we are more comfortable talking and relating to others. A healthy oral mucosa is also an important defense against infection in the oral cavity.

Although secretion of saliva has a number of functions, it is also a part of the protective system within the gastrointestinal tract and is necessary in maintaining a healthy oral mucosa. The average adult secretes from 1 to 2 liters of saliva each day. Nearly all of this is swallowed and reabsorbed, thereby preventing the loss of large amounts of fluid and salt through the gastrointestinal tract. The content of the saliva is primarily water; a small percentage consists of various salts and a few proteins.

Persons who may have a decreased salivary flow include the following:

- Those in an environment of low humidity

- The elderly, whose salivary secretions diminish as a part of the aging process
- Those with fever
- Those who are inadequately hydrated
- Those receiving radiation therapy
- Those unable to take anything by mouth; they may experience diminished salivary secretions even if intravenous fluids are adequate

Table 20-1
Assessment of the Oral Cavity

Observation	Function	Healthy	Deficient
Salivary flow	Moistens and lubricates mucosa	Smooth, moist, resilient, coral-colored mucosa	Statements indicating dry mouth; clicking or smacking of lips and tongue
	Protects against ulceration and bacterial invasion		Dull, flat, brownish appearance of oral mucosa
	Moistens and lubricates food		Tongue dry with white or brownish crusting
	Secretes enzyme ptyalin which begins breakdown of starch		Lips dry, flaky, rough
	Assists in tasting process		Cracks or fissures in mucosa
	Protects against swallowing foods that taste as if they may be harmful		
	Together with jaw movements, assists with the removal of food, decreases acidity of mouth, both of which help in the prevention of tooth decay		

Color:
  Lips
  Gingiva
  Oral mucosa
    (inner lip,
    buccal)
  Tongue
		Variations of coral pink shading	Dull flat, pale pink, or brownish mucosa
			
			Shiny, beefy-red coloration

Palates and pharynx		Dark pigmented person: deeper coral to brown Very darkly pigmented person: splotchy or	In order to distinguish between healthy and deficient in the darkly

- Those losing fluids in other ways: nasogastric tube, large draining wounds, respiratory distress, mouth breathing, joggers, athletes
- Those experiencing anxiety or fear

Table 20-1 indicates the areas to assess in the oral cavity and describes findings that are healthy or deficient.

Abdominal Assessment

There are several important reasons why the nurse should carry out an abdominal assessment:

- To recognize the basic characteristics of a person's abdomen in order to differentiate normal from abnormal findings
- To observe for signs of bowel obstruction

Observation	Function	Healthy	Deficient
		diffuse bluish coloration; spots of brown pigmentation	pigmented person, the nurse needs to consider all observations together.
		Tongue well papillated	
Teeth		Smooth, white enamel	Brownish-yellow stains from tobacco, tea, coffee, tetracycline, poor oral hygiene
Integrity: Mucosa	Protection against bacterial invasion	Smooth, soft, resilient Free from lesions	Bleeding tendency: Person's description of bleeding while brushing teeth Spongy, edematous, beefy-red, shiny Cracks, fissures, ulcerations
Teeth	Chewing: Begins digestive process Release taste substances that stimulate salivation Detect materials that are potentially harmful to the digestive tract	32 teeth In good repair Firmly in place No cracked, broken, or carious teeth Properly fitted dentures	Missing, cracked, loose, dental caries Improperly fitted dentures; edentulous
Movement of soft palate Swallowing reflex	Continue moving food along the tract	Place tongue blade on middle of tongue and ask person to say "ah." Uvula will rise up on the midline.	Uvula which rises up and deviates to the left or right; immobile uvula; these findings indicate inadequate innervation of pharyngeal muscles and related difficulty in swallowing.

- To identify areas of pain or tenderness
- To determine the person's readiness or need to have a change of diet:
    - The return of the intestine to normal functioning after surgery is one important factor in determining the person's readiness to begin oral feedings and progress to a general diet.
    - Feelings of hunger and a desire for food are other data that indicate a readiness to eat.
    - In instances of chronic nausea and vomiting, absence of appropriate bowel sounds signal the need for a change to clear liquids or cessation of oral intake.

As you begin your assessment, divide the abdomen visually into four quadrants. Imagine lines running horizontally and vertically and crossing at the umbilicus (Fig. 20-4). There are four quadrants: the upper right (URQ), the lower right (LRQ), the upper left (ULQ), and the lower left (LLQ). The boundaries of the adbomen include the following:

- Xyphoid process—The lowest portion of the sternum is the upper border of the abdomen.
- Costal margins of the ribs—Follow the rib cage from the xyphoid process to the sides of the body. The soft tissue is considered the abdomen, although parts of the abdominal organs are included: liver, spleen, intestine, and stomach are under the lower portion of the rib cage.
- Iliac crests—These mark the lower boundary of the abdomen.

Table 20-2 describes the assessment of the abdomen, based on observations that can be made for people in healthy and deficient states. These observations are based on the techniques of inspection, ausculation, and palpation.

General Inspection

Persons who have an inadequate nutritional status display signs and symptoms in other status areas. For example, the skin may be very dry; turgor may be poor; breaks may occur in skin integrity; pressure sores may develop and areas of ecchymosis may be

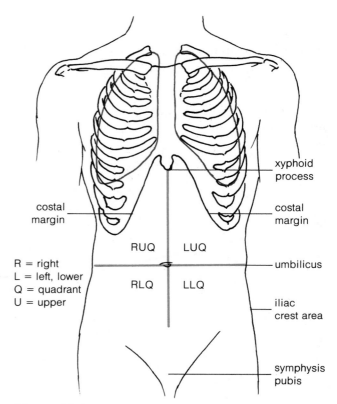

Figure 20-4
Boundaries of the abdomen.

noted. In addition, surgical wounds may take a long time to heal. Hair becomes sparse and loses its sheen. The eyes may be dry and bloodshot, and visual disturbances, especially blurring of vision, may occur.

Therapeutic Dietary Needs

Special dietary needs should be assessed. The nurse needs this information to secure the proper diet for the hospitalized person and to understand the learning needs for the person in the community. The use of food supplements and vitamins also constitutes necessary data. If the person is receiving nutrition through a feeding tube or the intravenous route, assess the reason, the kind of feeding, and its ingredients, as well as amount and times administered.

Table 20-2
Assessment of the Abdomen

Tool	Observation	Healthy	Deficient

Observation and inspection	Four quadrants
	  URQ
	  LRQ
	  ULQ
	  LLQ		

	State of skin		
	Color	Flesh tones from various skin colorations	See Chapter 18
	Integrity	Smooth, soft	Current surgical incision, trauma, old scars; ostomies
	Hydration	Elastic skin turgor	Dehydration: loose, wrinkled, dry, and flaky Overhydration: tense, pale, shiny
	Contour	Flat or concave	Obese: rounded, or convex Distended: tense, convex; umbilicus protruding, bulging over iliac crests
	Peristaltic waves	None observable	Observable
Auscultation	Listen with stethescope to all 4 quadrants	5 to 12 low gurgling sounds per minute	High-pitched tinkling sound Borborygmus Decreased sounds Absence of sound
Percussion	Sounds on percussion	Hollow, resounding sound over most of abdomen; dull thud over areas of density such as liver and spleen.	Dull thud over areas of abdomen that should sound hollow and resounding
Palpation (light)	Turgor of the skin	Elastic	Tense or flabby
	Underlying structures	Not palpable on *light* palpation; abdomen soft.	Tense, rigid, palpable hard organs or masses
	Areas of tenderness or pain	No tenderness or pain	Areas of tenderness or pain

Nursing Process
Applied to Problems of Nutritional Status

Dry Mouth

Assessment

Dry mouth or **xerostomia** is a common problem that accompanies many conditions, both mild and severe. It is easily assessed by observation and a few questions. (Refer to Table 20-1 and the discussion on salivary flow earlier in the chapter.)

Nursing Interventions

Oral hygiene maintains the integrity of the oral cavity mucosa and protects the mouth from bacterial invasion. Toothbrushing helps clear the mouth of food, bacteria, and **dental plaque,** a gluelike substance consisting of mucus and microorganisms. Dental plaque adheres to the teeth, provides a medium for bacterial growth, and is implicated in tooth decay and inflammation of the gingivae.

Jaw movements and the flow of saliva, together with oral hygiene, cleanse the cavity, reduce the acidity of the mouth, and thereby assist in the prevention of tooth decay. A well-balanced diet that includes fibrous foods cleans the mouth and stimulates the gingivae. Finishing the meal with a fruit rather than a concentrated carbohydrate dessert also assists in cleansing the teeth.

A bristle toothbrush with a soft rounded tip provides the best cleaning results and is unlikely to damage the mucosa. Because mechanical action is the essential part of oral hygiene, a dentifrice is not necessary but may be used as a mouth and breath freshener. Mixtures such as salt with bicarbonate of soda, or hydrogen peroxide combined with equal parts of water or saline, can also be used. When hydrogen peroxide is used, continued assessment is important because this substance may be irritating to the oral mucosa.

Oral hygiene for the dependent person should be provided in the morning, at midday, and in the evening. Mouthwashes and swabs or toothettes are useful temporary measures. Prolonged use of mouthwash in a debilitated person could lead to tissue irritation and the overgrowth of yeast microorganisms in the mouth. Moreover, the necessary mechanical action from the brush, which stimulates

salivary flow and decreases oral bacteria, will be missing. When either the toothbrush or mouthwash is used, forceful rinsing should follow.

Lemon–glycerin swabs can be used between brushings. The glycerin coats the surface of the oral mucosa and keeps it soft and moist. Lip care is also important since the skin over the lips is thin and dries out quickly. A water soluble jelly, petrolatum (Vaseline), or a chapstick can be used to cover the lips and help them retain moisture.

Increasing fluid intake when possible and adding flavorings such as drink ades, bouillon, or tea when water is unpalatable can also alleviate a dry mouth. Providing citrus fruits or juices and appetizing foods, as well as assisting with a planned schedule of oral hygiene, are all ways the nurse can help the person to improve salivary secretions.

The Overweight Person

Overeating, overweight, and obesity are complex, frustrating problems. Research has been done on the subject, and diet aids, exercise plans, and weight reduction programs have been developed to cope with it; yet people have great difficulty losing weight and keeping it off. Techniques such as strict dieting or behavior modification with reward systems have been helpful to some persons. However, the majority of overweight persons struggle for years with the problem. Those who are successful in losing weight frequently regain it.

To some people there is a stigma attached to being overweight, similar to that associated with mental illness or epilepsy. Although overeating is only one of the reasons for overweight problems, it is often assumed that the overweight person has no willpower and cannot control his impulses. One man reported that the label on his diet prescription read, "This medication is not a substitute for willpower." The overweight person suffers added indignities when he discovers that he is evaluated by his weight rather than his abilities or achievements.

Undoubtedly, many overweight people do overeat. Some do so secretly, carefully dieting when others are around. Research indicates that the roots of overeating are often found in childhood problems that no longer exist. Sometimes relatively uncomplicated feelings associated with the past can be resolved using supportive nursing intervention. More complex problems may require long-term counseling.

The nurse's approach to the overweight person varies, depending on each individual's particular needs. The following discussion suggests total person-centered nursing care which can help in coping with some of the underlying emotional implications of being overweight.

Assessment

- Consider the person as an individual with a unique personality.
- Assess his health and strengths.
- Assess the person's basic needs and try to help him meet those needs first. Many persons can memorize nutritional information but cannot follow a diet because they are using food to meet love and safety needs.
- Establish readiness. Determine whether the person perceives his weight as a problem and can state that he wishes to diet. Be aware that many overweight persons know the cardiovascular risks involved but are still unable to cope with the process of losing weight.
- Assess the nutritional status. Assess the person's daily food patterns and how these practices may vary on weekends or other unscheduled times. Writing this down can help the person identify problem areas.
- Assess knowledge of basic nutrition. Persons often have some knowledge but are unaware of many useful points.

Nursing Interventions

- Develop a trusting relationship. The person will feel comfortable discussing the overweight problem with the nurse if he is valued on the basis of his personality and not judged by his size.
- Help the person identify the stimulus or antecedent to eating. Have him look for factors that influence the patterns of eating behavior such as frustration, anger, or loneliness. Does he omit lunch and then binge later in the day? For example, consider the mother with teenagers and a full-time job. She may respond to the stress of the day by snacking as she cooks dinner and listens to her children. Perhaps she could

change the snacking behavior if she took a few minutes to rest before she began her family work.

- Begin diet planning. Incorporate personal preferences and cultural or ethnic foods and practices into the diet plan. Suggest ways to experiment with foods that are meaningful to the person, such as eating dessert on special occasions. Identify foods with minimal calories for snack suggestions.
- Help the person plan goals with an emphasis on good nutrition rather than pounds lost.
- Help the person incorporate an exercise program into his life-style.
- Help the person resolve guilt feelings about former eating behavior. This can be a cyclic problem. Persons who feel guilty about eating often eat more, in an attempt to ignore uncomfortable feelings. Helping the person explore some of those feelings encourages his ability to resolve them.
- Accept the fact that some persons will never want to lose weight.

Adjustment in Self Concept. At times it is necessary to help the person revise his self-concept as he begins to lose weight. This important point is often overlooked. Consider the concept of loss described in Chapter 29. Loss, even when positive, can produce a grieving response. This may be one reason why persons who lose weight sometimes have difficulty maintaining weight loss. At the same time they must struggle with certain expectations of behavior that are often involved in weight gain and loss. For example, sometimes a person who loses weight no longer belongs with his group of other overweight people. Yet he is not accepted by others who still think of him as fat. Young women may feel self-conscious in clothes they have wanted to wear for years. The wife who helps her husband lose weight may become jealous when he is more attractive to other women and so withdraw her attention from him.

This interesting example was offered by a student nurse, "You might be surprised to hear that I never had a date in high school. I was 30 pounds overweight, had braces on my teeth, and wore pigtails. When my braces were taken off, I started losing weight and curling my hair. People told me I was pretty and guys started asking me out. I couldn't believe that guys found me attractive because I still pictured myself fat with pigtails."

The Underweight Person

Persons are underweight for many reasons, some of which are related to personal preference. Being underweight is frequently caused by anorexia, which results in the inability to take in adequate food. However, underweight may also be caused by difficulty in obtaining food or by improper physiological use of food. Anorexia is frequently associated with the person's emotional status. The condition known as *anorexia nervosa* is an extreme state of inability to eat, associated with emotional problems. Students may read more about this condition in texts dealing with abnormal psychology.

Some persons may find they are unable to eat properly before exams or other events that demand a certain level of performance. This usually results in a temporary interruption of proper nutrition. Distressing problems such as marital difficulties, financial concerns, or school pressures may affect the person's ability to eat over a long period of time.

Elderly persons and others who live and eat alone may feel isolated and have little desire to eat. Eating is a social activity, and eating alone often causes a decrease in feelings of dignity and self-worth. For example, when a woman who has cooked for a large family finds herself widowed and her children grown, she may not bother to cook for herself alone. The decrease in mobility and activity that often accompanies aging may affect the person's ability to obtain food, his hunger level, and his interest in eating.

Assessment

Persons who are underweight because of various states of inadequate nutrition can be found in the home, the hospital, or extended-care facilities. Assessing the cause is the nurse's first concern. Anorexia may be associated with lack of companionship and feelings of isolation. Further data may indicate a medical problem as well. Moreover, factors such as financial status, mobility, and food preferences may be contributing to the problem.

Nursing Interventions

It is important to plan goals with the person in order to give him ultimate control over decisions about his diet. These goals should emphasize nutrition rather than pounds gained. Remember that trying to gain weight can be just as discouraging as trying to lose weight.

Help the person identify friends or family who can provide occasional companionship and assist with food shopping and preparation. Suggesting nutritious meals or foods that require minimal preparation is another userful intervention. Such foods might include peanut butter, nuts, powdered instant breakfasts, raw vegetables and fruits, cottage cheese and other cheeses, ice cream, and meats that can be broiled such as steaks, chops, or hamburgers. If the person likes casseroles, perhaps large portions could be made, divided, and frozen for future use. Certain frozen meals from the supermarket can also be used if attention is given to the amount of calories, sodium, carbohydrate, and fat content in them. Table 20-3 gives suggestions for nursing care of the underweight person.

Nutrition for the Severely Ill Person

It is a nursing challenge, when working with the severely ill person, to provide hydration and nutrition which will help him remain comfortable and alert for as long as possible. Remember that even with physical limitations, the person's feeling of hopefulness and self-esteem directly affect his ability to participate in his care, especially in the nutritional aspect.

Assessment

The most common severe illness that causes nutritional problems is cancer. The person with cancer experiences weight loss, impaired digestion and absorption, competition between the host and the tumor for nutritional elements, and an increased basal metabolism rate (BMR) resulting in an increased energy expenditure. Frequently the person also has increased **gluconeogenesis,** a decrease in insulin secretory capacity, and abnormal glucose tolerance curves. He often has an increased desire for sweet foods but a decreased physiological capacity to metabolize the carbohydrate.

Persons with tumors may also experience a **negative nitrogen balance.** This is a state that indicates that tissue is breaking down faster than it is being replaced. Nitrogen balance can be determined in the following way: total nitrogen excretion is obtained by taking the value of the 24-hour urea nitrogen and adding to it a value (usually 3.5) of nitrogen to account for stool and cutaneous nitrogen losses. This quantity is compared to the total nitrogen

Table 20-3
Nursing Care for the Underweight Person

Assessment Considerations	Intervention Considerations
Height, weight, body build, age	Develop goals that are related to nutrition rather than weight gained
Causes of underweight and anorexia	Help person plan how to use available resources such as food stamps or motor meals.
Financial status	
Mobility status	
Resources available such as family, friends, facilities, and services	Leave decisions in the hands of the person so that he retains control.
Food preferences	Suggest foods high in nutrition which require a minimum of preparation.
Nutritional knowledge	
Other areas necessary in individual situations	

intake as determined by the calorie count (Salmond, 1980). Rapidly growing tumors tend to be nitrogen traps that take up the available nitrogen and reduce the body's supply. At the same time there is a decreased tolerance for some protein products, especially red meat, and an acute awareness of foods with any bitter, salty, or acidic tastes.

Persons who are treated with radiation in the area of the head and neck experience very sore mucous membranes, a reduced salivary production together with excessive mucous, and a condition known as **dysgensia,** or mouth blindness, which produces a change in taste buds and food tastes. Surgery or radiation may occur at various points along the gastrointestinal tract. The person may experience pain from resulting mucosal changes, malabsorption of digested food, and a decrease in digestive enzymes from the various auxillary organs. If the disease is not closely associated with the gastro-intestinal tract, nutritional problems may still exist, although digestion itself may not be impaired.

Nursing Interventions

One major aim of nursing care is to help the person with cancer remain comfortable and alert, while preventing the development of cachexia. Diet planning should be mutual and should include frequent assessment of those foods the person desires since these preferences change each day. The person may also experience **early satiety,** a state which causes

him to feel full after a few bites. In such instances, it is rarely possible or even desirable to achieve complete nutrition. Helping the person to eat enough to gain some energy permits him to do a few of his former activities. He may talk with friends or family, read, write letters, perhaps go on an outing, and do much of his own care.

To improve oral intake, six small meals are preferable to three larger ones. It is best to limit the use of low or noncaloric drinks such as coffee, tea, and sugarless soda because these beverages are filling but not nutritious. The texture and consistency of the food should be smooth and soft in order to prevent irritation to possible ulcerated areas of the gastrointestinal tract and to make it easier for persons with low endurance to chew or swallow. Other suggestions include experimenting with flavorings or spices until food is more palatable. For the most part, food should be of moderate temperature because hot or cold foods are not easily tolerated. Try substituting protein sources, such as cheese or milkshakes, for meat. Puddings or custards with fruit added can be very nourishing and smooth. A local anesthetic such as Xylocaine Viscous for painful oral mucosa or an **antiemetic** drug for those who are chronically nauseated might also be useful measures, although both measures require a physician's order. Table 20-4 lists nutritional problems and nursing interventions for the severely ill person.

Former Vice President Hubert Humphrey provided an excellent example of a person severely ill

Table 20-4
Nutritional Planning for the Severely Ill Person

Nutritional Problems	Nursing Interventions
Negative nitrogen balance	Assess nutrition status on a planned schedule.
↑ BMR and ↓ energy	Promote hydration and nutrition.
Diminished appetite	Promote alertness and ability to communicate.
Early satiety	Plan periods of rest prior to meals.
Weight loss	Assess food preferences.
	Provide six small meals.
↓ tolerance for red meat	Avoid red meats and provide alternate protein sources.
↓ tolerance for bitter, salty, or acidic tasting foods	Provide smooth, soft foods.
	Provide foods cool in temperature.
	Consider tastes of foods offered.
↑ gluconeogenesis	Avoid concentrated carbohydrates.
↓ insulin secretory capacity	
↓ salivary production	Plan a schedule of mouth care.
	Provide adequate fluid intake.
Tenacious oral mucous secretions	
Painful oral mucosa	Obtain physician's order for local anesthetic agent or antimetics as needed.
Nausea	

with cancer who used these ideas. Just days before his death he was still going to meetings and activities that were important to him. In an interview, he described his program of rest, activity, and nutrition which gave him the energy he needed to engage in these activities. He was able to "finish his business," which Erikson has described as the final developmental task of life.

Another example is that of Mrs. Henderson, a 56-year-old woman with cancer. The student nurse who cared for her toward the end of her life describes her experience.

Example □ She was so ill that she could no longer get out of bed, and we could hardly keep her pressure sores under control. She was very meticulous about her skin care and her nutrition. She took bits of milkshake or custard throughout the day even though she had to force herself. She said, "If I can take a little food it gives me enough energy to talk to my husband and daughters. In a few days my nephew is coming and I want to be able to hear about his trip to England." She was so calm, but I felt discouraged and dreaded going back the next day. I returned because I decided that if she could keep her composure and feel hopeful, then so could I! □

The examples of Hubert Humphrey and Mrs. Henderson represent much more than meeting nutrition needs. They identify the healthy aspect of two people in the face of severe illness. They also demonstrate the total person concept and the importance of providing care that incorporates all facets of a person's being.

Vomiting

Vomiting is defined as the expulsion of the contents of the stomach and upper intestinal tract through the mouth. It occurs as a result of a complex reflex mechanism coordinated by the vomiting center located in the medulla of the brain. Vomiting is protective, in that it can remove irritating and harmful substances from the gastrointestinal tract, although it may result in the loss of valuable fluid and electrolytes as well. Most episodes of vomiting are relatively short-lived and not harmful. However, if the person is already dehydrated and malnourished, or if the vomiting continues unchecked for longer than 24 hours, fluid and electrolyte disturbances may result.

Vomiting is generally preceded by feelings of nausea, an increase in salivation, a very hot feeling, diaphoresis, and an increased heart rate. This grouping of symptoms is the result of a discharge from the autonomic nervous system.

Vomiting is an exhausting experience and, if prolonged, can lead to generalized weakness and fatigue; aching muscles in the abdomen, thorax, and throat; and fluid and electrolyte disturbances.

Vomiting occurs as the result of input to the vomiting center in the medulla from a number of sensory receptors in the gastrointestinal tract, the brain, and other areas of the body such as the heart, uterus, kidneys, and the semicircular canals of the ears. The following are some of the ways in which the vomiting reflex can be stimulated:

* Tactile stimulation to the back of the throat
* Overdistention of the stomach or duodenum
* Increased intracranial pressure. Vomiting from this cause is often projectile and may occur without nausea.
* Rotating movements of the head, or motion sickness. This may occur in cars, in persons with orthostatic hypotension, and in those walking after prolonged bed rest.
* Intense pain
* Anxiety
* Inflammatory conditions of the gastrointestinal tract from microorganisms or ulcerative conditions

Assessment

The nurse should identify persons at risk for vomiting and attempt to determine the cause, helping them avoid episodes whenever possible. Factors such as foods, position changes, coughing, pain, or anxiety are often implicated. Persons who have just had surgery and those receiving certain chemotherapy are also likely to have episodes of vomiting.

Nursing Interventions

Most persons can assume a position that is comfortable for vomiting. However, weak and dependent persons, namely those who are paralyzed, in traction or body casts, or in a coma, need the nurse's assistance. It is especially important to prevent the aspiration of vomitus into the respiratory tract. The unconscious person should be turned onto his side and the head of the bed lowered slightly below level during a vomiting episode. The muscles of the thorax and throat are likely to be relaxed and the vomitus will flow out easily in this position. Drainage from the tracheobronchial tree will also be facilitated if any vomitus has been aspirated.

For a conscious person, the head of the bed should be elevated as high as possible. If this is problematic because of restrictive traction, casts, or limited tolerance, turn the person on his side and elevate the head of the bed slightly.

Aspiration is a life-threatening situation. If it should occur, the nurse's responsibility is to call for help and then attempt to establish an airway (see Chap. 24). An alert nurse can identify those persons at risk for aspiration and prevent it by using proper positioning and by instructing the person to report feelings of nausea immediately. The nurse should also become aware of available emergency equipment and procedures in the agency or community.

Additional interventions to help provide safe care for anyone susceptible to vomiting include the following:

* Prevent further episodes of vomiting. Identifying the cause can assist the nurse to plan prevention.
* Identify and remove irritating items from the environment.
* Attend to the cleanliness of the person and the environment and provide mouth care after each episode.
* Instruct the person in abdominal breathing exercises: Take a deep breath, push the diaphragm outward on inspiration, hold the breath for a few seconds, and then let it out slowly. These exercises relax the person physically by reducing

the irritability of the gastrointestinal tract, and psychologically by distracting him from feelings of nausea as he concentrates on breathing. If the person is nauseated because of pain, the deep breathing exercises may also help by diminishing the pain sensation.

- Have the person swallow. A voluntary initiation of swallowing depresses the vomiting reflex. Use this intervention with caution because swallowing of air may distend the stomach.

- Cool the person's forehead, neck, and wrists with a damp cloth. Remember that persons feel hot and diaphoretic just prior to vomiting. This cooling measure is especially helpful in managing nausea and vomiting during ambulation after surgery or prolonged bed rest.

- Position the person comfortably, darken the room, and keep stimulation at a minimum.

- Limit food and fluids until nausea has subsided. Resume oral intake slowly using clear liquids such as apple or grape juice, bouillon, jello, tea, or soda. Clear means free from residue rather than colorless. Ask the person to choose the liquid that sounds palatable.

- Antiemetics are often ordered as needed by the physician. The nurse and the person together can assess the nausea and vomiting and plan how these medications should be used. If nausea and vomiting remain severe, gastric decompression and intravenous therapy are instituted. The nursing interventions for this plan of care are discussed later in the chapter.

Table 20-5
The Person with Glucose Imbalances

Imbalance	Causes	Symptoms	Nursing Interventions
Hyperglycemia	Undiagnosed insulin deficiency	Polyuria	Assist the person to identify his own symptoms of hyperglycemia.
	Physiological stress—fever, infection	Polydipsia	Listen carefully to person's statement of how he feels when hyperglycemia occurs.
	Psychological stress—worry, anxiety, fear, loss	Polyphagia	Help person reestablish a proper diet.
	Improper insulin dose	Alterations in weight—either gain or loss	Identify cause or precipitating factors.
	Improper administration of insulin—inability to obtain insulin, decision not to take insulin, increase in carbohydrate ingestion	Severe fatigue	Teach good skin care (see Chap. 23).
		Visual changes	Identify need for knowledge and do appropriate health teaching.
		Nausea	Identify psychological needs and intervene as appropriate with supportive nursing care.
		Poor wound healing	Help person to replan his therapeutic program according to his own value system. Use referral to other professionals as needed.
Hypoglycemia	Improper balance of food, insulin, and exercise	Acute, severe hunger	Provide carbohydrate (use one):
		Weakness and fatigue	—One fruit exchange
		Headache	

Problems of Glucose Imbalance

Although glucose imbalances are generally thought of in relation to diabetes mellitus, they are discussed here as common health problems. Hypoglycemia and hyperglycemia are described separately but the student should note that either state can be present in the same person at different times. A normal blood glucose range is 80 mg to 110 mg%.

Hyperglycemia

In the person with normal pancreatic function, the insulin secreted is adequate for carbohydrate ingestion. If the pancreas does not produce enough insulin, glucose is not properly absorbed by the cells and continues to circulate in the blood causing **hyperglycemia.** The cells may also be prevented from utilizing blood glucose when excessive amounts of hormones that are antagonistic to insulin are present or when insulin receptors at the cell level are inadequate. The effects of hyperglycemia are serious; however, it may take many weeks for the level to reach dangerous proportions. It is also possible for the state to develop in a matter of hours.

Assessment

Table 20-5 lists some of the common causes as well as the major symptoms of hyperglycemia. Note that alterations in weight is considered a major sign.

Imbalance	Causes	Symptoms	Nursing Interventions
Hypoglycemia *(continued)*	Ingestion of meal high in carbohydrate Omission of meals	Dizziness Numbness and tingling Diaphoresis Shakiness Restless, nervousness, irritability Double vision Confusion and disorientation Fear or free-floating anxiety Unconsciousness	—2 to 4 large or 3 to 5 small sugar cubes —Clear, hard candy, about two pieces —Soda, about 8 oz —Dextrose tablets, two or three —Honey, corn syrup, or dextrose jelly Follow with protein, either the next meal or a snack with peanut butter or meat. Help the person reestablish a diet. Assess nutritional status as suggested under hyperglycemia and intervene as appropriate.
Both			Suggest wearing of identification stating health problem. For insulin-dependent person, suggest wallet card stating insulin dosage and usual treatment for hypoglycemia. Provide health education. Support all healthy behaviors toward continued and effective self-care.

Frequently persons, especially younger ones, lose weight if insulin secretion is inadequate even though they may take in large amounts of food. Because glucose cannot enter the cells for use or storage, large amounts of glucose are eliminated in the urine. The remaining glucose stays in the circulating blood and does not add to the person's weight.

On the other hand, in older people there may be a weight gain that precedes the hyperglycemic state. It is postulated that obesity decreases the receptor sites to insulin, resulting in a relative insulin deficiency and hyperglycemia. The nurse will want to help the person identify exactly how he feels when his blood sugar is elevated. Persons who have experienced hyperglycemia for some time usually know when it is occurring.

Hyperglycemia becomes serious when the glucose load exceeds the reabsorptive ability of the renal tubules, resulting in the excretion of glucose in the urine. Since it takes 10 ml to 20 ml of water to excrete each gram of glucose, the person can become dehydrated quickly and lose sodium and eventually potassium as well.

In order to meet energy needs in the hyperglycemic state, the cells engage in an activity that also may have serious side-effects. Adipose tissue begins to release fatty acids for energy. As fatty acids are used by the liver, ketone bodies accumulate. Because the ketones are acids, they cause an increase in the hydrogen ion concentration and result in *metabolic ketoacidosis* (see Chap. 22). Ketones also require water for excretion, which further contributes to dehydration.

Nursing Interventions

In an emergency situation the person is usually hospitalized and the physician orders insulin, fluids, and electrolytes. When oral intake can be resumed, the nurse assists the person to reestablish the proper diet. As the situation becomes less urgent, the nurse considers some of the general concerns of the nutritional status. Assessment and intervention should center on such factors as basic needs, financial concerns, mobility status, nutritional knowledge, and so forth (see Table 20-5).

At least one nursing study is currently looking at the needs of persons with altered blood glucose levels. The study is based on the premise that appropriate nursing support helps persons resolve developmental tasks, develop and strengthen their coping mechanisms, and alter their response to stress. As persons cope adaptively with stress, it is hypothesized that their own insulin supply may be more effective and the need for exogenous insulin

may decrease. The results of the study have not yet been tabulated, but individual subjects have demonstrated a positive psychophysiological response to the nursing interventions.*

Hypoglycemia

Low blood glucose may result when insulin levels or energy needs exceed glucose availability. **Hypoglycemia,** however, is not always associated with exogenous insulin and may be the result of a high carbohydrate diet. Persons eating this kind of diet may overstimulate insulin production from the pancreas, leaving an excess of circulating insulin. Persons who skip meals, especially breakfast, often experience symptoms of hypoglycemia. Persons who are used to functioning on a certain level of blood glucose may feel hypoglycemic if their level falls slightly but still remains within the normal range. This is *relative hypoglycemia*. The symptoms are annoying but can usually be remedied with a piece of fruit or cheese. Candy and soda may also help but are not nutritious and have a shorter effect. The symptoms of absolute hypoglycemia, in which the blood glucose level is below the normal range, are similar but often more severe.

Assessment

Table 20-5 lists the symptoms of hypoglycemia. It can be noted, these symptoms are similar to those of hyperglycemia, making it difficult to distinguish between the two states. Generally, the hypoglycemic reaction occurs quickly and reaches a problematic state shortly after the first symptoms appear. The hunger symptoms may be different in the two states. Hyperglycemia may cause a constant need to eat, whereas the hypoglycemic state often causes a sudden acute hunger. Persons who have experienced these glucose imbalances frequently know which state is occurring.

Nursing Interventions

If the person is hospitalized the nurse should assess which symptom of hypoglycemia occurs first. Some people experience dizziness first, but others experience diaphoresis or headache. Occasionally persons report confusion. This symptom is dangerous because the person may lose consciousness and injure himself in a fall. Persons who are unable to

*Health Promotion Among Diabetics: Comparing Nursing Systems. The Department of Health, Education and Welfare: The Division of Nursing, Grant No. Nv00658-03, Mary Ann Swain, Principal Investigator, September 1978–September 1981.

walk straight or who faint are often thought to be drunk or suffering from a drug overdose. This is very distressing to the person who experiences hypoglycemia. The nurse should be aware that appearances are deceiving and that hypoglycemia must be considered when a person demonstrates confusion or ataxia.

The hospitalized person's symptoms of hypoglycemia should be written on the nursing care card. The nurse should also determine how the person manages a hypoglycemic reaction and whether he needs assistance in planning his management. Nutritious food is the most effective way of managing hypoglycemia. Commercial products such as dextrose tablets and dextrose gel are also available and are easily carried in pockets or purses.

If the person is unable to take food during hypoglycemia, honey, corn syrup, or dextrose jelly can be applied to the oral mucosa, which is very vascular. These items are thick and adhere readily to the mucosa reducing the potential for aspiration. Injections of glucose are also used at home by persons with frequent, severe hypoglycemia, if there is a reliable person to administer them. For further detail on planning interventions for a person in a hypoglycemic state, see Table 20-5.

If hypoglycemia is not treated the person may lose consciousness and then gradually awaken within 20 minutes to a half hour. He may feel weak but is not likely to suffer ill effects except possibly injury from a fall. This spontaneous remission of the hypoglycemic state may occur because the decrease in plasma glucose concentration stimulates the hypothalamus and, by means of a reflex chain, creates a rise in plasma epinephrine. This process stimulates the liver, muscle, and adipose tissue to release glucose, thereby raising blood glucose. In spite of this adaptive mechanism, hypoglycemia should be treated whenever possible. Loss of consciousness can result in injury, and frequent and prolonged sttacks of hypoglycemia may cause mental or neurological impairment.

Self-Care and Problems of Glucose Imbalance

Health education related to the problems of glucose imbalance, such as diet instruction, care of the skin, or administration of insulin, is important. In addition, the nurse also wants to suggest that persons with glucose imbalances wear identification bracelet or neck tags. These tags can be purchased in drug stores and some jewelry stores and simply indicate the name of the disease or health concern. In addition, insulin-dependent persons may want to carry a wallet card providing information about their insulin dose.

Assisting the person to understand himself and to become aware of how he feels physically during health or illness capitalizes on his strengths and helps him to take much better care of himself. This intervention can be as important as health teaching because it increases the person's self-esteem and sense of control. A clinical example may serve to emphasize this point.

Example □ Debby, a college student with diabetes, underwent an appendectomy. After surgery her wound did not heal well and she experienced blood glucose imbalances. Her physicians did not agree with her suggestions on insulin dosage. Finally, in desperation she pleaded to be allowed to regulate her own insulin. She told the nurse, "The doctor looked at me for awhile and then said, 'Okay, Debby, you win; we'll manage your wound and you manage your blood glucose.' " After that Debby watched her diet and blood and urine glucose levels carefully and decided on the amount and type of insulin she needed. Her blood glucose finally came under control again. □

Persons who have lived with diabetes and other long-term conditions, while requiring help at times, often know their needs better than anyone else. This is the basis for the self-care philosophy.

Nasogastric Tube for Decompression

The term **decompression** means the removal of flatus and fluid from a body cavity. This is accomplished with a tube such as a urinary catheter or a tube connected to a suction machine. Gastric decompression is accomplished by inserting a tube through the nose and throat into the stomach (Fig. 20-5). Sometimes the tube is extended as far as the ileum for intestinal decompression.

Normally the digestive tract secretes approximately 2 liters of fluid in a 24-hour period. This fluid, together with secretions of several more liters of fluid from the liver and pancreas, is used to digest food substances and lubricate the tract for smooth passage of the food products. Much of this fluid is absorbed along with the digested products, and any excess is excreted. Because secretions are stimulated to enter the tract by the need for digestion and absorption, secretions diminish when a person does not eat. However, even then some fluids enter the tract, along with any air that is swallowed. If decreased gastrointestinal motility or a bowel obstruction prevents fluids and air from passing through the tract, de-

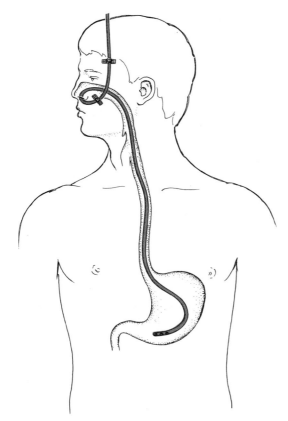

Figure 20-5
Nasogastric tube.

compression is necessary. The person is then given nutrition through the intravenous route.

The presence of accumulated material in the tract also becomes a medium for bacteria; thus any absorption that does occur may carry bacterial toxins into the circulation. Moreover, the continued presence of distention eventually disrupts circulation and causes ischemia and tissue necrosis. In extreme cases, if treatment is not instituted gangrene can develop.

The following are some common reasons for decompressing the gastrointestinal tract:

- Removal of potentially harmful or poisonous substances that have been ingested. This is often called the *stomach pump.* Because quick removal of the stomach contents is essential, a syringe is used, rather than a suction machine which is meant to provide decompression over a period of days.

- Removal of the stomach contents for the purpose of analysis and diagnosis. Analysis of gastric contents assists in the diagnosis of certain gastrointestinal diseases. Swallowed respiratory se-

cretions can also be analyzed to diagnose certain respiratory diseases.

- Prevention or treatment of bowel distention or obstruction. A nasogastric tube is sometimes inserted prior to surgery. Decompression helps prevent the accumulation of flatus and secretions that could create distention of the tract, severe vomiting, and bowel obstruction. A bowel obstruction may also be caused by a paralytic ileus or tumor. Decompression assists the person with these problems. (See Chap. 21 for a discussion of flatus and decreased gastrointestinal motility.)

Nursing Interventions

Anyone who must undergo decompression with a nasogastric tube requires specialized nursing care planning. In order to increase comfort and provide freedom of movement and self-care, the nurse will first want to consider the psychological and mobility needs of these persons. The presence of a nasogastric tube can cause an altered body image and a decreased sense of self-worth, because it is unsightly and presents a constant reminder that one cannot eat in the usual manner.

In addition to these concerns, the presence of a nasogastric tube causes dryness of the oral and pharyngeal mucosae and the lips, pharyngeal irritation, and an unpleasant taste in the mouth. The tube may also cause friction on the skin of the nares and thus a potential pressure sore. Because the tube is connected to a suction machine, mobility becomes a problem as well. Moreover, if the tube and machine are not monitored carefully, abdominal distention, irritation to the gastric mucosa, and fluid and electrolyte disturbances can result. Interventions related to psychological needs, oral cavity and skin care, mobility, and fluid and electrolyte balance must also be considered. Table 20-6 describes nursing care problems and interventions for persons with these needs. Descriptions of the tubes and suction machine used for gastrointestinal decompression can be found in the nursing procedures manual accompanying this text.

Altered Feeding Methods

Tube Feedings

Some persons are unable to eat in the usual manner and must be fed through a tube placed in the gastrointestinal tract through which formula is in-

Table 20-6
Nursing Care Planning for the Person
with Gastrointestinal Intubation for Decompression

Needs/Problems	Nursing Interventions

Psychological needs
  Emotional distress related to the passage of the tube
  Alterations in body image and self-concept related to the presence of the tube
  Diminished feelings of self-worth related to the inability to carry out normal functions or to eat in the usual fashion
	Establish rapport and a trusting relationship, explain the procedure for passage of the tube and how one functions with the tube.
	Provide an opportunity for discussion and verbalization of concerns while the tube is in place.

Oral and pharyngeal needs
  Dryness of oral and pharyngeal mucosa and lips
  Unpleasant taste
	Assess the oral cavity once each day.
	Use toothbrush and a dentrifice for mouth care three times each day.
	Apply water-soluble lubricant to lips.
	Use saline gargle as needed.
	Provide cracked ice, throat lozenges, popsicles, hard candy, or gum. (Check with physician first.)

Potential breakdown of nares skin at point of friction from the tube	Provide skin care around the nares. Keep the area clean and dry. Lubricate the skin lightly with petroleum jelly. Change the tape that secures the tube when it is wet or soiled. When retaping, move the tube slightly on the nares and secure it in a different position.
Altered mobility related to presence of equipment	Institute a regular schedule of activity; include range of motion exercises. Disconnect the tube from the machine for short periods four times a day. (Check with physician first.) Place the person in semi-Fowler's position to prevent reflux of stomach contents into the esophagus.
Potential abdominal distention	Observe the amount, color, consistency, and odor of the drainage. Observe the abdomen for distention; measure abdominal girth around the middle of the abdomen and over the umbilicus. Assess for nausea, pain, or a sense of fullness. Check the suction pump. Is the setting (low or high) as ordered? Is it plugged in and turned on? Is the tube unclamped and free from kinks or compression? Check the tube for patency. See nursing procedure manual.

(Continued)

Table 20-6
Nursing Care Planning for the Person
with Gastrointestinal Intubation for Decompression *(Continued)*

Needs/Problems	*Nursing Interventions*
Irritation to gastric mucosa	Assist the person to turn from side to side at frequent intervals.
	Assess for pain in the upper left abdominal quadrant.
	Advance or retract the tube 2 to 3 inches if the person experiences pain. (Check with physician first.)
Inability to eat	Consider interventions discussed under psychological needs.
	For discussion of intravenous nutrition, see Table 20-8.
Potential fluid and electrolyte disturbances	Assess for adequate hydration and electrolyte balance.
	Examine laboratory reports on electrolytes.
	Use normal saline when irrigating the tube to help replace the sodium washed out by the irrigation procedure.
	Refer to Chapter 22 for further interventions.

stilled. A tube placed through the nose and into the stomach is the most accessible and comfortable approach. However, if there is disease or injury in the upper part of the tract, the tube may be inserted through the abdominal wall and directly into the stomach. This approach is called a **gastrostomy.** Tubes can also be placed at several other points along the gastrointestinal tract, namely the esophagus, the duodenum, or the jejunum. If nutritional substances are introduced below the stomach, formulas known as **elemental diets** are used. These are nonresidue formulas that supply nutritional requirements in a predigested, soluble form. They are readily absorbed in the small intestine and require minimal digestive action.

Some common reasons why a person might need nutrition provided by nasogastric tube include the following:

- Wired jaws
- Tumors of the head and neck
- Coma
- Inability to swallow
- Esophageal stricture or trauma

There are a variety of commercially prepared tube feeding formulas available. These consist of planned nutrition with a definite number of calories and nutrients per volume. Some use soy protein instead of milk and animal protein; different kinds of fat are used, and some have lactose. Commercial formulas can be stored, unopened, for long periods of time and are labor saving devices, although they are expensive.

Certain agencies, as well as persons using formulas at home, still prepare the feedings using blender food that is pureed and thinned sufficiently to go through the tube. This approach can provide adequate calories and nutrients for total nutrition. The following is a list of ingredients contained in a typical formula: strained liver, eggnog mix, strained applesauce, strained carrots, frozen undiluted orange juice, skim milk powder, brewer's yeast, and water. Many other foods may also be blended and used for formula.

Most medications are available in liquid form and can be instilled through the tube. Powder or crushed tablets with water added are not satisfactory for tube instillation. Powder rarely dissolves completely and often adheres to the tubing. The liquid form of medication may alter absorption rates, and then the effects of certain medications may be experienced more quickly than usual. Medications should be given prior to or following the feeding, depending on drug specifications. Medications should not be placed in the formula unless specified, because if the person does not tolerate the total feeding, the amount of medication absorbed cannot be determined.

Nursing Interventions

Nursing responsibilities include helping the person and his family adapt to the new feeding method. If the person is using tube feedings at home, the nurse can help him plan how to participate in family mealtimes. He may wish to take the formula during mealtime or just join the family for conversation. Experimentation should be encouraged until a comfortable approach is found. It is nearly impossible to shield the person from the realities of food preparation and eating. A successful adaptation, therefore, requires that he learn to cope with these activities. The length of time that tube feedings are necessary makes a difference in the planning.

In addition to some of the problems already mentioned, the person who is receiving nutrition through the nasogastric tube has several of the same needs as the person who is undergoing decompression with the nasogastric tube. Both share psychological needs related to the presence of the tube; physical discomfort due to dry, irritated mucous membranes in the mouth and throat; potential skin breakdown associated with friction from the tube on the skin of the nose; and possible fluid and electrolyte disturbances.

Other problems that sometimes arise include the danger of aspiration of the feeding, a possible intolerance for the feeding, and bacterial growth in the tube and gastrointestinal tract if the tube is not properly flushed with water. Persons being tube fed may experience feelings of hunger and thirst and need to be observed closely to be certain that they reach and maintain an appropriate weight.

Mouth care and skin care needs are similar to those encountered in gastrointestinal decompression. In addition, the nurse will want to assess carefully the psychological, respiratory, nutrition, elimination, and fluid and electrolyte statuses on a regular schedule (Table 20-7).

Intravenous Nutrition

Certain persons must be given part or all of their nutrition by the intravenous route. Those who have undergone surgery may need this support for a short period of time. Anyone who has suffered extensive burns requires such support together with oral intake to meet tremendous caloric needs. Persons with disruptions of the gastrointestinal tract may need complete support and for a longer period of time. There are two basic ways to provide intravenous nutrition: the peripheral venous route and the central venous route.

The Peripheral Venous Route. Veins located on the outer portions of the body, namely arms, legs, and sometimes scalp veins, are used for peripheral administration of intravenous fluids. Because peripheral veins are small and become inflamed easily, isotonic solutions, which cause the least vascular damage, are often used. Dextrose 5% in water is isotonic and provides about 200 calories per liter of solution. Because the average adult can tolerate about 3 to 4 liters of fluid in a 24-hour period, this nutritional approach will provide 600 to 800 calories per day, hardly enough for an adult even at the resting state. Moreover, this solution provides only carbohydrate, and no protein or fat, although vitamins can be added. Dextrose 10% provides twice the calories, but again, no protein or fat. The average male adult in good health requires 2400 to 2800 calories a day, and the average female adult in good health requires 1800 to 2400 calories a day (Williams, 1977). In the resting state these calorie requirements may be reduced to 1500 for the male and 1000 for the female (Salmond, 1980). However, critically ill persons who cannot eat or persons who have just experienced major surgery are not in the resting state, even though they are in bed. Energy expenditure in the critically ill person with cancer is high, and the person who has had surgery needs extra energy to aid wound healing and repel infection. Fever, stress, certain drugs, extensive burns, and trauma create further caloric needs.

It is important to recognize that carbohydrates that are stored in the liver as glycogen may not supply energy needs beyond several hours. After carbohydrate depletion, gluconeogenesis begins. This converts amino acids into glucose for energy and depletes the body's protein stores. Finally muscle protein is used to meet energy requirements, and the person may develop cachexia. Remember that adipose tissue also releases free fatty acids for energy which are utilized by the liver causing the development of ketone bodies; metabolic acidosis and dehydration may result, compounding the nutrition problems.

The intravenous therapy following surgery, trauma, or an acute illness consists of 5% dextrose sometimes combined with 0.2% or 0.45% saline. As the person begins to take liquids and demonstrates ability to

Table 20-7
Nursing Care for the Person Receiving Nutrition Through the Nasogastric Tube

Problem/Need	Nursing Interventions
Psychological needs	See Table 20-6.
Potential respiratory distress (potential aspiration)	Check placement of tube before starting the feeding. See nursing procedures manual for instructions.
	Assess respiratory status during feeding.
	Position person in semi-Fowler's.
Intolerance to feeding	Aspirate gastric contents before beginning the formula; if more than 50–75 ml is aspirated, allow the person time to digest the amount remaining in the stomach before adding more.
	Assess for intolerance: cramping, nausea, vomiting, diarrhea, constipation, abdominal distention.
	Record accurate intake and output.
	Measure the formula accurately. Follow package instructions for administration.
	Regulate temperature of the feeding according to individual person's needs. A colder formula is less likely to develop bacteria.
	Regulate the flow of the feeding according to the person's tolerance and any fluid restrictions.
Bacterial growth in tube and GI tract	Following ingestion of feeding, flush tubing with at least 50 ml of tap water to provide patency, cleanliness, and prevention of bacterial growth in the tube. Extra fluids may be given according to specific needs.
	Detach the tube from the gavage bag and clamp; cover the proximal end.
Oral and pharyngeal needs	See Table 20-6.
Nasal skin breakdown	See Table 20-6.
Potential fluid and electrolyte imbalance	See Table 20-6.
Maintenance or promotion of appropriate weight	Assess weight daily.
	Assess energy level and feelings of hunger.
	Plan with the person, the physician, and the dietitian to change calories as needed.

reestablish his former diet, the intravenous therapy can be discontinued.

Persons who are unable to eat for long periods of time and those who cannot eat enough to maintain a positive nitrogen balance must be given an intra-venous solution that can fulfill all nutritional requirements. Five- or ten-percent solutions require a large fluid volume to meet these requirements and would result in circulatory overload. Solutions that are hypertonic might provide enough calories without causing hypervolemia but they are not well tolerated by the peripheral vessels of the body. The person, therefore, is provided nutrition by the central venous route.

The Central Venous Route. The jugular or the subclavian veins are used for entry into the central venous system. A catheter is threaded through one of these veins into the superior vena cava. These veins are much larger than peripheral veins. The large volume of blood flowing through them immediately dilute's the hypertonic solution so that it may be more readily tolerated by the smaller vessels of the body. This form of intravenous nutrition is known as **hyperalimentation** or **total parenteral nutrition** (TPN). The solution is usually 25% dextrose for carbohydrate and caloric needs and 4% amino acids for protein needs. It provides one calorie per milliliter and 3000 to 4000 calories in a 24-hour period. For persons who require an even higher caloric content, the concentration of the solution can be raised somewhat. Vitamins and electrolytes can also be added.

Candidates for TPN include those persons who cannot eat enough to maintain a positive nitrogen balance, such as those with chronic fatigue from disease; cachexia; excretion of protein-laden body fluids such as in burns, weeping skin disease, or large open wounds from surgery or trauma; and emotional distress causing severe anorexia. TPN is also used for persons whose gastrointestinal tract cannot maintain nutrition, namely those with prolonged paralytic ileus, bowel obstruction, malabsorption syndrome, or other digestive organ disorders such as ulcerative colitis and gastrointestinal ulcerations or fistulae.

In certain circumstances, the pancreas may have difficulty adjusting to the heavy glucose load from this solution and may not secrete enough insulin, causing hyperglycemia and glycosuria to result, at least temporarily. Insulin may be added to the solution to help utilize all glucose supplied. Ten to forty units of regular insulin have been effective in alleviating hyperglycemia. Occasionally, instead of hyperglycemia, the person may experience hypoglycemia. The concentrated glucose solution may stimulate the pancreas to produce more insulin than necessary. The maintenance of appropriate blood glucose levels can be a complex problem. This should be explained carefully to the person and his family because the addition of insulin to the solution may make it appear as if he has diabetes in addition to his other health concerns. Heparin is another possible additive to TPN. Clots form easily at the tip of

the catheter and heparin can prevent this from occurring.

Fat emulsion solutions are not routinely part of TPN. They are expensive to administer and are not always readily available. Since fatty acid deficiency does not occur quickly in adults, a clear indication for need is warranted before intralipid infusions are administered. When TPN is used for extended periods, a fatty acid deficiency must be prevented or reversed. Fat emulsion can be used when it is desirable to provide nutrition through the peripheral route. Intralipid 10% solution provides one calorie per ml and is isotonic. It is concentenated enough not to overload the circulation and does not cause inflammation of peripheral veins.

Infection at the infusion site and systemic infection are of concern with the use of TPN. Entry into the central venous circulation makes it imperative that very careful aseptic technique is followed at all times. Skin irritation from tape at the catheter site is an additional concern.

The person can be maintained for months on TPN because the nutrients are sufficient to achieve tissue synthesis and to maintain a normal weight or gain the weight desired. Table 20-8 describes nursing care of the person receiving TPN.

Psychological Implications of Altered Feeding Methods

People who are unable to eat as usual may experience a psychological need for food. This may be associated with complex needs related to oral satisfaction, which include chewing and tasting, the need for companionship and communication with family and friends, the need for the continuation of usual lifestyle, and needs related to body image, self-concept, and self-worth. Change in usual functioning and the presence of a disfiguring tube can be disruptive to psychological well-being. Temporary therapy may be tolerable, but long-term or permanent therapy may cause difficult adaption. Careful assessment of needs associated with the person's psychological status is essential in order for the nurse to give appropriate support.

Persons frequently experience the stages of grief over the loss of self-concept and life-style. Family members may experience similar feelings of grief and loss for the person and for the changes his problems create in their own lives. As questions are answered and routines established, both the person and his family will begin adapting to the changes and searching for solutions to many of their problems. Supportive and caring assistance from the

Table 20-8
Nursing Care of the Person Receiving Intravenous Nutrition
(Central or Peripheral Venous)

Problems/Needs	Nursing Interventions
Underweight	Assess the person's weight daily.
	Assess nutritional status daily.
Hyperglycemia or hypoglycemia	Explain the alterations in blood glucose.
	Explain that this is generally a temporary problem that resolves itself as the pancreas adapts.
	Observe for signs of glucose imbalance.
	Test urine for glucose and acetone every 4 hours.
	Monitor intake and output carefully.
	If the proper solution is temporarily unavailable, the nurse may hang a container with 10% dextrose to maintain an open vein for nutritional solutions.
Hunger	Explain that hunger is not unusual and that it diminishes as one adapts to the new way of obtaining nutrition.
	Consider data from the nutritional assessment to determine whether adequate nutrition is being administered.
	If the person can eat at all, hunger will not be a problem. Check care plan for Gastric Decompression.
Psychological need for food	See Table 20-7.
Infection at the infusion site or systemic infection.	Observe for signs and symptoms of infecton at the infusion site, such as pain, erythema.
	Maintain complete sterility during changing of the tubing.
	Maintain sterile, airtight dressing over the catheter site.
	Tape securely around all four sides of the catheter.
	Tape connecting sites to avoid possibility of disconnection.
	Use hyperalimentation line only for nutritional solution.
	Do not use line for adding medications, drawing blood, or monitoring central venous pressure.
	Hyperalimentation solution, with its high glucose content, is a medium for bacteria.
Skin irritation from tape at catheter site	Inspect the skin carefully at each dressing change.
	Use hypoallergenic tape if necessary.
Dry oral mucous membranes	See Table 20-7.
Potential fluid and electrolyte imbalances	See Chapter 22.

nurse aids this adaptation and helps persons return to many of their former activities.

Inadequate Nutrition in the Hospital

It should not be assumed that anyone in the hospital on a general diet receives proper nourishment. In most hospitals today, people can select from a menu and decide whether or not to eat the food. Often no one assesses whether the four basic food groups have been met. If persons are on a special diet, the nutritional intake is checked more carefully.

Butterworth (1974) has described hospital malnutrition as one of the most serious health problems induced by the hospital today, and he cites several factors that contribute to the problem. Of those identified, there are some which the nurse may influence directly:

- Failure to assess and record height and weight. Without baseline height and weight information, the person is deprived of the most readily available means of assessing his nutritional status.
- Failure to continue to assess weight changes on a planned schedule.
- Failure to observe the person's food intake. This, together with assisting the person to choose a nutritious menu, are essential to maintain good nutrition.
- Use of tube feedings without proper understanding of the amount, composition, and conditions under which the feeding should be administered.

Careful assessment of the following situations and appropriate professional communication with the physician may help alleviate certain nutritional inadequacies.

- *Prolonged use of glucose and saline intravenous feedings.* The physician makes the decisions about the use of this therapy. However, if the nurse has assessed the person's nutritional status on a continuing basis, communication with the physician can provide objective data and influence the course of treatment.
- *Withholding meals prior to diagnostic tests.* This practice is difficult for the nurse to influence because of scheduling with other specialized units. However, often both breakfast and lunch are missed, and it may be difficult to obtain food between meals in some settings. Nurses should be aware of food policies in the particular insti-

tutions where they work, especially whether there are facilities to save meals and what sort of food can be ordered between meals.

- *Unwarranted reliance on antibiotics and other medications,* together with the lack of appreciation for the role of nutrition in the prevention of infection and the promotion of wound healing. Although the nurse does not make medication decisions, appropriate observations and nursing care related to infection, healing, and nutrition may decrease the amount of medication necessary (Butterworth, 1974).

Role of the Dietitian

Because this chapter has discussed primarily the nurse's role in nutritional planning with clients, students may wonder about the role of the dietitian. The dietitian is the professional person most directly involved in planning regular meals or therapeutic diets for those who are hospitalized or eating in institutions where many meals are served. The dietitian's involvement in a particular setting may depend upon budgeted positions and availability of trained personnel in the area. Large medical centers usually have many dietitians on their staffs, but smaller hospitals and care facilities may employ only a few. In such instances, the nurse is frequently called upon to do the diet planning and carry out client instruction. In county health departments nutritional counselors are available on a limited basis. However, in most settings the nurse needs to provide guidance in the selection of appropriate foods and the principles of good nutrition.

Because nurses practice from a total person perspective, it is appropriate that they provide certain nutritional counseling. In those agencies which use a team arrangement, the nurse and the dietitian work together, combining the expertise of both health professions and thereby promoting better nutritional care. Students should recognize that as graduate nurses they will have the knowledge and skills necessary to assist with nutritional needs and can seek the expertise of the dietitian when necessary.

Conclusion

The state of our health is very much related to our nutritional status. This in turn is affected by a wide range of factors, including the integrity and functioning of our digestive system, the level at which basic needs such as love or self-esteem are met, our cultural and religious practices, financial resources, mobility, individual growth needs, and the atmosphere established during meals.

Common problems related to nutrition which were explored in this chapter include excessive or inadequate weight, inadequate nutrition related to severe illness, vomiting, glucose imbalance, altered feeding methods through tubes or hyperalimentation, and gastric decompression. Nursing interventions for each of these problems involves assessing how the person is meeting basic needs and assisting him to make alterations in life-style and diet while preventing secondary problems such as fluid and electrolyte imbalance. Because many nutritional problems have psychological implications, such as those related to altered body image, the nurse is responsible for giving appropriate support.

Inadequate nutrition in the hospital, unfortunately, can be a serious health problem for some. Through communication with the physician and ongoing assessment of diet, possible weight changes, and the effects of diagnostic tests and medical therapy, nurses can promote optimal nutrition for those who are hospitalized. By assisting persons both in and out of the hospital in achieving good nutrition, nurses can promote general physical and emotional adaptation.

Study Questions

1. Describe the ways in which the digestive system protects the person from injury.

2. Mrs. G. is a Mexican-American woman, aged 68, who lives alone in an apartment. Her income is a monthly social security check. Her height is 5′1″ and her weight is 168 pounds. Mrs. G. has several daughters and a son, who live nearby with their families. They visit her occasionally but not as often as Mrs. G. would like. Mrs. G. can walk to the neighborhood grocery store but finds the items there very expensive. She must take insulin and often has problems with both hypoglycemia and hyperglycemia. The community health nurse who visits Mrs. G. believes she has inadequate knowledge about glucose alterations and proper diet.
   a. Identify the factors in these data that may be affecting Mrs. G.'s nutritional status.
   b. Develop a nursing care plan for Mrs. G. Consider her age, obesity, and blood glucose alterations.

3. On assessment, you note that your hospitalized patient has a diminished salivary flow.
   a. What data did you obtain that indicated this?
   b. Describe how a decreased salivary flow affects the nutritional status.

4. State the principles to consider when developing an oral hygiene care plan for the dependent person.

5. Match the interventions on the left with the correct choice on the right.
   a. Prevent aspiration.
   b. Elevate head of bed.
   c. Lower head of bed below level.
   d. Identify cause of vomiting.
   e. Analgesic
   f. Antiemetic

   ___ Intervention for the conscious vomiting person
   ___ General intervention
   ___ Intervention for the unconscious vomiting person
   ___ Nurse's prime concern for vomiting person

g. Jello, tea, ginger ale
h. Cocoa, milk, orange juice
i. Prevent further episodes of vomiting.

____ Diagnostic intervention
____ Appropriate examples of liquids for the nauseated person
____ Medication to relieve nausea and vomiting

6. Your patient has a nasogastric tube for decompression. He tells you he is beginning to feel nauseated. Explain the areas you would assess to help you identify the cause of this problem.

7. You are working with Mrs. Jones and her family so she can leave the hospital to return home on tube feedings. Develop a care plan to help this woman and her family cope with tube feedings at home.

8. Describe the differences between the peripheral and central venous routes for providing fluids for nutrition. Under what circumstances would you expect to see these different routes used?

Glossary

Absorption: The entry of digested food into the blood and lymph streams for transportation to all the cells of the body.

Anorexia: Diminished appetite.

Antiemetic: A drug that decreases nausea.

Appetite: A psychological response to food.

Cachexia: A state of severe emaciation, malnutrition, and wasting of adipose and muscle tissue.

Decompression: The removal of flatus or fluids from a body cavity.

Dental plaque: A gluelike substance consisting of mucus and microorganisms, which adheres to the teeth.

Dysgensia: Mouth blindness; a state that produces a change in the taste buds and food tastes.

Early satiety: A state which causes the person to lose hunger and appetite and to feel full after eating only a small amount of food.

Elemental diet: Nonresidue formula that supplies nutritional requirements in a predigested soluble form.

Emaciation: A state of being extremely lean.

Gastrostomy: An opening in the wall of the stomach to the external surface of the abdomen.

Gluconeogenesis: Hepatic synthesis of glucose from several sources, which increases blood glucose concentration.

Hunger: A basic physical need for food.

Hyperalimentation: Feeding the person in a way other than the alimentary canal or gastrointestinal tract, namely, feeding through the circulatory system.

Hyperglycemia: A high blood glucose level.

Hypoglycemia: A low blood glucose level.

Negative nitrogen balance: A state in which tissue breaks down faster than it is synthesized.

Obesity: A weight approximately 20% to 30% higher than the normal weight for a person given his height, age, sex, and body build.

Total parenteral nutrition (TPN): A hypertonic solution administered through the circulation, which provides total nutrition.

Vomiting: The expulsion of the contents of the stomach and upper gastrointestinal tract through the mouth.

Xerostomia: Dry mouth.

Bibliography

Abrams B: Helping pregnant teenagers eat. Nurs '81 11, No. 3:46–47, March, 1981

Arlin M: Controversies in nutrition. Nurs Clin North Am 14, No. 2:199–213, June, 1979

Beck C: Dining experience of the institutionalized aged. J Gerontol Nurs 7, No. 2:104–107, February, 1981

Biermann J et al: Emotional aspects: The patient's view. Diabetes Educ 6, No. 4:16–19, Winter, 1980

Borgen L: Total parenteral nutrition in adults. Am J Nurs 78, No. 2:224–228, February, 1978

Buergel N: Monitoring nutritional status in the clinical setting. Nurs Clin North Am 14, No. 2:215–227, June, 1979

Butterworth E: The skeleton in the hospital closet. Nutr Today 9, No. 2:4–8, March/April, 1974

Butterworth CE, Blackburn GL: Hospital malnutrition. Nutr Today 10, No. 2:8–18, March/April, 1975

Colley R, Wilson J: Meeting patients' nutritional needs with hyperalimentation. Nurs '79 9: No. 5:76–83, May, 1979a

Colley R, Wilson J: Meeting patients' nutritional needs with hyperalimentation. Nurs '79 9: No. 6:57–63, June, 1979b

Colley R, Wilson J: Meeting patients' nutritional needs with hyperalimentation. Nurs '79 9: No. 7:50–53, July, 1979c

Colley R, Wilson J: Meeting patients' nutritional needs with hyperalimentation. Nurs '79 9: No. 8:56–63, August, 1979d

Colley R, Wilson J: Meeting patients' nutritional needs with hyperalimentation. Nurs '79 9: No. 9:62–69, September, 1979e

Craft CA: Body image and obesity. Nurs Clin North Am 7, No. 4:677–685, December, 1972

Davenport HW: Physiology of the Digestive Tract, 4th ed. Chicago, Year Book, 1977

Didrich FM: Gauging abdominal girth accurately. Nurs '81 11, No. 7:32–33, July, 1981

Garber R: The use of a standardized teaching program in diabetes education. Nurs Clin North Am 12, No. 3:375–391, September, 1977

Greene HL: Nasogastric tube feeding at home: A method for adjunctive nutritional support of malnorished patients. Am J Clin Nutr 34, No. 6:1131–1138, June, 1981

Griggs BA, Hoppe C: Nasogastric tube feeding. Am J Nurs 79, No. 3:481–485, March, 1979

Groer M, Pierce M: Guarding against cancer's hidden killer: Anorexia-cachexia. Nurs '81 11, No. 6:39–43, June, 1981

Hoppe M: Your patients are what you feed them. Nurs '80 10, No. 3:79–85, March, 1980

Hutchison MM: Administration of fat emulsions. Am J Nurs 82, No. 2:275–277, February, 1982

Kagawa-Bushy KS, Heitkemper MM, Hansen BC et al: Effects of diet temperature on tolerance of enteral feedings. Nurs Res 29, No. 5:276–280, September/October, 1980

Kiser D: The Somogyi effect. Am J Nurs 80, No. 2:236–238, February, 1980

Korczowski MM, Van Coevern S et al: Strengthen the nurse's role in nutritional counseling. Nurs Health Care 2, No. 4:210–213, April, 1981

Kornguth ML: Nursing management. Am J Nurs 81, No. 3:553–554, March, 1981

Kubo WM, Grant M, Walike B, Wong H et al: Fluid and electrolyte problems of tube-fed patients. Am J Nurs 76, No. 6:912–916, June, 1976

Langford RW: Teenagers and obesity. Am J Nurs 81, No. 3:556–559, March, 1981

Mahan LK: A sensible approach to the obese patient. Nurs Clin North Am 14, No. 2:215–227, June, 1979

McCarthy J: Somogyi effect: Managing blood glucose rebound nursing. Nurs '79 9, No. 2:39–41, February, 1979

McConnel EA: Ten problems with nasogastric tubes . . . and how to solve them. Nurs '79 9: No. 4:78–81, April, 1979

McConnel EA: Overeaters anonymous: A self help group. Am J Nurs 81, No. 2:560–563, March, 1981

Rains BC: The non-hospitalized tube-fed patient. Oncol Nurs Forum 8, No. 2:8–13, Spring, 1981

Rose JC: Nutritional problems in radiotherapy patients. Am J Nurs 78, No. 7:1194–1196, July 1978

Salmond SW: How to assess the nutritional status of acutely ill patients. Am J Nurs 80, No. 5:922–924, May, 1980

Schweiger JL, Schweiger JW, Lang JW: Oral assessment: How to do it. Am J Nurs 80, No. 4:654–658, April, 1980

Smith CE: Abdominal assessment, a blending of science and art. Nurs '81 11, No. 2:42–49, February, 1981

Stout R: The Final Deduction. New York, Viking Press, 1955

Tribble NM, Hollenberg EE: The impact of a quality assurance program on diabetes education. Nurs Clin North Am 12, No. 3:365–373, September, 1977

Troupe CF: Don't give up on the hopelessly obese. RN 44, No. 4:71–86, April, 1981

Vander AJ, Sherman JH, Luciano DS: Human Physiology, The Mechanisms of Body Function, 3rd ed. New York, McGraw-Hill, 1980

Vic T: Trader Vic's Pacific Island Cookbook. New York, Doubleday, 1968

Volden C, Grinde J: Taking the trauma out of nasogastric intubation. Nurs '80 10, No. 9:64–67, September, 1980

Wedman B: Use and abuse of food exchangers. Diabetes Educ 5, No. 4:21–23, Fall, 1979/1980

White JH, Schroeder MA: Nursing assessment. Am J Nurs 81, No. 3:550–552, March, 1981

Williams SR: Nutrition and Diet Therapy, 3rd ed. St Louis, CV Mosby, 1977

Wineman NM: Obesity: Locus of control, body image, weight loss and age-at-onset. Nurs Res 29, No. 4:231–237, July/August, 1980

Yen PK: Nutrition: How can you lower sodium intake. Geriatr Nurs 2, No. 3:228–230, May–June 1981

Elimination Status

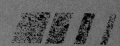

Mary L. Hunter

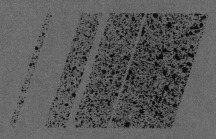

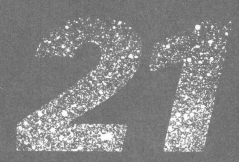

In the holistic view of man, all physiological systems of the body, together with the psychosocial and spiritual systems, need to function at an optimal level if we are to have a sense of health and well-being. We can identify critical functions in each of our systems, without which we could not sustain life. However, four specific areas may quickly create a sense of discomfort and illness when they are not functioning well. These include the abilities to take in food and fluids, to rest and sleep well, to move about freely, and to eliminate wastes from the body. It is the purpose of this chapter to discuss how a person's health is influenced by the elimination of both urinary and bowel waste from the body. We will also consider how the nurse facilitates elimination and helps persons with problems of this nature to move toward adaptable patterns of elimination.

Returning to the Maslovian framework presented in Chapter 2, we recall that elimination is a first-level, or physiological need. However, the need to eliminate affects other level needs as well. For example, consider how your ability to learn in a lecture is affected when you have an urgent need to go to the bathroom. Or perhaps you can remember your reaction when you wet your pants as a small child. The embarrassment and loss of self-esteem, even if temporary, was probably excruciating. If you were scolded for the accident, your feelings of love and safety may have been affected as well. Imagine how you would feel if, as an adult, you still had difficulty controlling your elimination status.

The ads we often see on television for laxatives describe rather accurately the discomfort and irritability associated with constipation, even if the product being advertised is not the best solution for the problem. Some persons suffer for years from chronic problems such as bladder infections, diarrhea, or constipation. Other persons only encounter these problems when they become ill, have surgery, or experience some of the processes of aging. We usually think of the area of the body involved in elimination as private, potentially unclean, and one that must be kept under control. Because of this thinking, nurses sometimes have difficulty assessing and intervening with elimination problems. Successful nurses are those who feel comfortable with their own bodies and physiological processes and who use techniques of empathy and general communication with skill.

Part One: Principles of Urinary Elimination

Micturition

Urine is produced in the kidneys and flows to the urinary bladder through two long conduits from each kidney, called *ureters*. The ureters are lined with smooth muscle that propels urine along to the bladder by peristaltic contractions. Micturition is basically a local spinal reflex which is influenced by higher brain centers (Vander *et al*, 1980, p. 377). When approximately 300 ml of urine has entered the bladder, the stretch receptors in the bladder wall become stimulated. This causes a contraction to occur, which squeezes the walls of the bladder inward and increases the pressure of the urine in the bladder. As the bladder contracts, urine enters the urethra. The external sphincter and the perineal muscles then relax, and **micturition** or **voiding** occurs. See Figure 21-1 for an anatomical representation of the urinary tract.

Micturition is basically an involuntary process upon which voluntary control can be imposed. We begin teaching the child early in life to make the voiding process a voluntary or controlled act. Delay of micturition is accomplished by means of descending pathways from the cerebral cortex. This inhibits the bladder parasympathetics and stimulates the motor neurons to the external sphincter, thereby overriding the opposing sympathetic input from the bladder stretch receptors (Vander, 1980, p. 378). Figure 21-2 describes the sequence of steps leading to micturition. You will want to consider this mechanism when we discuss the problems of incontinence and retention of urine.

Factors that Affect Urinary Elimination

Patterns of urinary elimination are individual and affected by many factors as indicated below.

• **Alterations in fluid intake cause alterations in urinary output.**

Under normal conditions, fluid loss exactly equals fluid gain and no net changes of body fluid occur (see Chap. 22). You will remember times when taking in large amounts of fluid caused you to eliminate more urine than usual. This also happens when persons receive intravenous fluids, especially if they are already well hydrated. Some fluids, such as coffee, colas, and cocoa, have diuretic properties and cause more urine to be eliminated from the body.

At night we generally take in less fluid and tend to void less. Physiological changes in the concentration of the urine, which occur during sleep, also cause less urine to be produced.

• **Dietary intake alters urinary output.**

Persons with high or low salt intake eliminate precisely the amount of salt required to maintain sodium balance and the proper internal physiological environment. When salt is eliminated, water is eliminated with it.

An increase of diet protein increases urinary output. This occurs because urea, the by-product of protein breakdown, requires fluid to help eliminate it from the body.

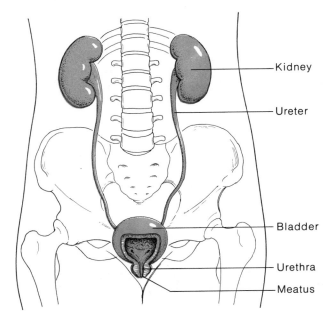

Figure 21-1
Urinary tract.

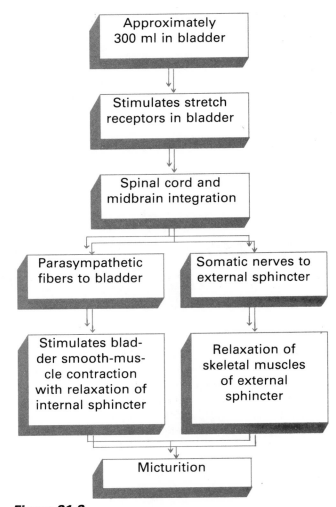

Figure 21-2
The reflex of micturition.

- *Excretion of fluid through other systems causes a decrease in urinary output.*

Fluid may be lost through the skin from perspiration or from large open wounds associated with surgery or trauma. Fluid is also lost through the respiratory tract, in some cases in large amounts, in the athlete or the person in respiratory distress. As fluid leaves the system through these and other routes, less fluid is eliminated from the urinary tract.

- *An increase in abdominal pressure may cause an escape of urine.*

Increased abdominal pressure is caused by such activities as coughing, sneezing, or laughing. Loss of small amounts of urine during these activities is known as **stress urinary incontinence (SUI).** We've all heard children say, "I laughed so hard I almost wet my pants." The "almost" is important because it rarely happens. SUI does occur in persons, usually women, who have diminished tone of the pelvic-floor muscles. Increased abdominal pressure causes them to lose small amounts of urine involuntarily, to their distress and embarrassment.

- *Different emotional states alter urinary elimination.*

Fear may cause involuntary loss of urine. This phenomenon is more common in small children but can occur in adults if the fear is extreme.

The more common emotional state that affects alteration in urinary elimination is anxiety or embarrassment. These states may cause difficulty in relaxing the muscles around the urinary tract structures and thus lead to an inability to void. Inadequate privacy such as occurs during hospitalization is a common cause of this problem. If the person has had surgery on or near the urinary tract, the combination of the strange hospital environment and discomfort in the surgical area may cause both muscle and emotional tension and difficulty in voiding.

- *An irregular body position may cause difficult urinary elimination.*

Most of us stand or sit to void. When we are unable to assume the position most natural to us, we often find it difficult or impossible to void. Persons who are asked to use a bedpan or urinal as they lie or sit in bed often find elimination difficult or impossible.

- *Certain diseases may cause changes in urinary elimination.*

At this point, let us distinguish between urinary production and urinary elimination. If the kidneys are not functioning properly, less urine is produced, resulting in reduced urinary output. This is very different from the state in which urine is produced and flows to the bladder, but cannot be eliminated. Some conditions that may result in inadequate urine production include dehydration, renal disease, and shock from various causes. Adequate production of urine but inadequate elimination may result from urinary tract infection, spinal cord lesions due to disease or trauma, and obstructive disease such as urinary calculi (stones) or tumors.

Certain renal diseases and a condition known as diabetes insipidus may cause an overproduction and elimination of urine.

- *Certain drugs cause changes in urinary production and elimination.*

Diuretics are designed to cause **diuresis,** an increase in production and elimination of urine. Diuril and Hygroton are two such drugs. Urecholine is a cholinergic stimulator that increases bladder tone, causing bladder contractions strong enough to initiate micturition. Other drugs may create a decrease in urine production as a side-effect. Consider carefully the effect on the urinary tract of all drugs you administer.

General Assessment of Bladder Function

Assessing bladder function includes collecting data on differences in the person's elimination patterns at home as well as in the hospital setting. Assessment also involves trying to learn how a person's current health problem has affected his patterns of elimination.

Voiding Patterns

The healthy adult usually voids five or six times in a 24-hour period, for a total of 1200 ml to 1700 ml. Voiding is generally less during sleeping hours than for a similar number of hours during the waking state. To determine voiding patterns, the following alterations in elimination should be assessed:

- **diuresis (polyuria)**—excessive production and elimination of urine

- **oliguria**—scanty elimination of urine caused by retention or inadequate urine production
- **nocturia**—voiding during the night. Nocturia may occur as a result of increased fluid intake, urinary tract infection, or an excessive elevation of blood glucose. An increased production of urine at night may also indicate that the kidneys are not concentrating the urine. This could be an early sign of renal failure.

Changes in voiding patterns that occur in relation to a health problem or under other specific circumstances are of greater concern than the amount and frequency of voiding. Because most people do not measure their urine or count their voidings, suggesting familiar units of measurement may help with data collection. For example, the nurse might ask, "Do you void about a cup each time?" When a person is hospitalized for surgery or for a specific renal or urinary tract problem, careful records of urinary output should be kept.

History of Urinary Tract Disease

Assessment of common urinary tract problems assists the nurse in interpreting observations and developing individualized care plans. Two conditions to consider are **cystitis** or inflammation of the bladder and urinary **calculi** or stones. Both can be painful, distressing, and obstructive and are likely to cause kidney damage if not properly treated. The severe pain associated with these conditions is protective because it demands immediate intervention. **Benign prostatic hypertrophy,** the enlargement of the prostate gland at the base of the bladder, is also an obstructive disease state. This problem, common in men over 50, can cause urinary retention, pain, and infection. The problem of cystitis is discussed later in the chapter.

Characteristics of Normal Urine

Urine consists of 95% water and 5% solids. The solids include urea, uric acid, creatinine, ammonia, sodium chloride, potassium chloride, calcium, magnesium, and phosporus.

Sterility

Because the urinary system is essentially a closed system, urine is usually sterile. At times there may be small amounts of bacteria in the urine but generally not enough to cause infection. Bacteria may enter the urinary system through blood circulating to the urinary tract or more likely from *E. coli* present in fecal material, which may gravitate to the urinary meatus and enter the system. Detecting bacteria in the urine requires laboratory analysis.

Color

Urine should be clear and a medium yellow color. A lighter, straw-colored urine from a healthy person may indicate dilute urine due to a large fluid intake. In the ill person, urine that is straw colored or very light could mean that the kidneys are not adequately concentrating the urine. As urine becomes more concentrated, it deepens to an amber color. Dark urine could indicate an inadequate fluid intake. If dark urine persists, renal disease may be a possibility.

Clarity

Urine should be clear. However, urine left in a collection bottle and allowed to cool becomes cloudy. Particles, sediments, or cloudiness in freshly voided urine may indicate bacteria or renal problems.

After inspecting the urine for color and clarity, the nurse may use specially treated lab sticks or paper strips to determine urinary *p*H and the presence of protein, blood, glucose, and ketones. There are a variety of products on the market for testing urine. Package directions are explicit and easy to follow.

Urinary pH

Urinary *p*H measures the hydrogen ion concentration in the urine. The *p*H can vary greatly and still be within normal limits. The range may be as wide as 4.5 to 8.0, but the usual *p*H of a pooled urine sample from a 24-hour period is around 6.0. Persons on a vegetarian diet may have a more alkaline urine.

Protein

Proteinuria is usually indicative of infection or renal disease. However, vigorous exercise can cause protein to appear in the urine of a healthy person.

Blood

Although there may be three or four red and white blood cells present in urine on laboratory examination, none should be detectable when the lab stick is used. Blood in the urine, or **hematuria,** is not necessarily detectable with the naked eye. The nurse should check for the presence of blood if the urine appears concentrated, smoky, or smoky pink. Actual blood may appear when there is infection or calculi present, following surgery on the lower urinary tract, or in serious disease states such as bladder tumor or leukemia.

Glucose

In the healthy person, glucose is filtered through the glomeruli of the kidney and reabsorbed by the tubules. Although the kidney is responsible for maintaining the composition of body fluids, it does not regulate plasma glucose. This function is performed by the liver and the endocrine system. Normally the renal tubules reasbsorb all the glucose that is filtered from the plasma. However, if the filtered load of glucose exceeds the ability of the tubules for reabsorption, glucose is excreted in the urine. Several instances in which **glycosuria** may occur are discribed in Chapter 20.

Ketones

There are small amounts of ketones present in the urine, but these should not be detectable unless examined by laboratory analysis. When urine is positive for ketones as determined by lab sticks, ketoacidosis is present to some degree. This may occur in such states as diabetic ketoacidosis or starvation.

Specific Gravity

The **specific gravity** of the urine is the ratio of the weight of the urine to the weight of an equal volume of distilled water. The weight of distilled water is represented by 1.000. The specific gravity test evaluates the ability of the kidneys to dilute and concentrate the urine and thus to maintain body fluid and osmolar balance (see Chap. 22).

The normal range of specific gravity varies according to the reference or laboratory values being used. Some texts describe it as ranging widely from 1.003 to 1.030; however, it is more commonly described as 1.010 to 1.025. The student is referred to the nursing procedures manual accompanying this text for instructions on how to measure specific gravity.

Urine specific gravity varies throughout the day. The amount and type of solids we ingest influence the concentration of the urine. For example, diets high in protein or sodium cause a more concentrated urine with a higher specific gravity, whereas diets low in those substances yield a more dilute urine with a lower specific gravity.

The amount of fluid the person drinks also influences the concentration of the urine. Early morning specimens are usually more concentrated (closer to 1.025) than specimens checked later in the day after more fluids have been taken. Noting this difference helps the nurse to assess the person's state of hydration. Voiding small amounts of highly concentrated urine may indicate a state of dehydration, whereas voiding large amounts of dilute urine could mean overhydration. In renal failure, the specific gravity of the urine may register 1.010 to 1.012, which is within the normal range. However, this reading remains fixed and does not fluctuate according to the amount of fluid ingested, indicating that the person's kidneys are not concentrating or diluting the urine during periods when there is an alteration in fluid intake.

Nursing Process
Applied to Problems of the Urinary Tract

Urinary Incontinence

Incontinence means involuntary voiding, or, as Yeates describes it, "the passage of urine in an undesirable place" (Yeates, 1976, p. 29). There are several types of incontinence that will be described briefly. Stress urinary incontinence, or the loss of small amounts of urine with an increase in abdominal pressure, was described earlier.

Urge incontinence is the inability to control bladder and urethral functions voluntarily. The bladder contracts involuntarily and large amounts of urine are lost. This may occur following episodes of stress incontinence, at times of chronic inflammatory conditions of the urinary tract, or in certain elderly persons. It may also accompany obstructive disease, tumors, or congenital anomalies.

Neurogenic incontinence is the result of neurological disease or trauma. The person loses the sensations in the bladder and is not aware of the need to void.

The problem of incontinence occurs in small children who are still learning toilet training; in some confused persons, especially if they are in an unfamiliar environment; in certain elderly persons; and in persons with neurological deficits. Occasionally persons who have had surgery on the lower urinary tract experience a few episodes of incontinence.

Assessment

As small children we are taught that to be good, clean, and grown-up we must learn to use the toilet and control our bowel and bladder functions. Mercifully we remember little of the effort and struggle associated with learning these important skills. As adults, however, some of the emotions from this effort may come back to us. One wonders if the extreme difficulty some persons have with using the bedpan is associated both with the unnatural position and with a fear of wetting the bed. For example, Mrs. L., a woman who was seriously ill with cancer, had a commode at her bedside which she used frequently. As the fatigue associated with her illness became greater, she asked for an indwelling catheter. The nurse suggested she might prefer using a bedpan, but her response was, "I'd rather have a catheter. I might wet the bed using a bedpan, and I couldn't stand that."

The first step, then, is to assess what incontinence means to the person. In the case of an elderly person, it may represent social isolation, which is often self-imposed, and loss of one's status in the family. This leads to feelings of guilt and depression and may result in institutionalization if the problem is not managed properly. In the person with a neurological deficit, incontinence may mean expending energy on a bodily function rather than on personal adaptation in the interest of better living.

A complete assessment of the person, especially an elderly person, is the next step in data collection. Frequently, there is an underlying cause which, if corrected, greatly relieves the problem of incontinence. For example, elderly persons may be taking diuretic drugs for hypertension. These drugs cause an increase in the production of urine which, when added to decreased muscle tone in older persons, may contribute to urgency and incontinence. Decreased mobility can prevent a person from reaching the bathroom in time, whereas diminished eyesight may make it more difficult to find restrooms in unfamiliar environments.

After information specific to the problem of

incontinence has been collected, a general assessment of bladder function should be reviewed and the data completed. Data about voiding patterns are especially important at this stage because they provide a base for altering the pattern to a more satisfactory state.

Nursing Interventions

Because a variety of interventions are possible, depending on the cause of incontinence, the nurse needs to rely on personal judgment in many instances when implementing care. Persons who are incontinent of urine are often those with decreased mobility. These two problems combine to promote conditions for skin breakdown. Therefore, careful skin care is essential at the same time that attempts are being made to solve the problem of incontinence.

The decreased self-esteem that incontinence often causes is frequently the result of soiling one's clothes or the bed linen and feeling embarrassed by the odor. A sensitive nurse finds ways to protect the privacy of the person and dispel the odor by cleaning up and using deodorizers.

At some point, the person, his family, and care givers must make a decision about what approach should be used in managing the incontinence. Both an indwelling catheter and intermittent self-catheterization are possibilities but each has limitations, as is discussed later in the chapter. A bladder-retraining program is often helpful. This approach consists of establishing the person's readiness and ability to participate, providing a measured amount of fluid intake at specific times of the day, and planning regular toilet times at set intervals following intake. Intermittent catheterization is sometimes used as part of this approach.

Some persons, particularly those with stress incontinence, may benefit from **Kegel exercises** of the perineal muscles. (Kegel exercises are often suggested as measures to improve perineal muscle control after childbirth.) These exercises are done by squeezing or contracting the perineal muscles while in a sitting position. For example, imagine that you are urinating and then attempt to stop the stream quickly. The exercise is repeated ten times, at least four times a day. The knees should be spread apart and the feet firmly planted to ensure contraction of the correct muscles. Another technique for controlling stress incontinence is to try to stop the urinary stream when voiding.

There are many products on the market to help manage the problem of incontinence, including incontinence pants, pads, sheets, and external cathe-

ters (condom drainage for males). As yet, there is no satisfactory external catheter for females. Some of these aids can be quite helpful if used after careful assessment and for the right person. The pants especially may provide a feeling of security. However, it is important to remember that these devices may discourage any attempts at regaining continence. That is, padding may suggest that it's all right to void because clothing and furniture are protected. It is much more beneficial to establish a feeling of positive expectations.

Whatever techniques are used, it is important to maintain proper fluid balance. The nurse will want to be alert for persons who limit their intake in the hope of decreasing their output. Although a bladder-retraining program may necessitate some manipulation of fluid intake, it is always important that the person receive the needed fluids.

Urinary Retention

Urinary retention refers to the state in which urine is produced but cannot be eliminated. A full bladder may cause extreme discomfort and an urgency for relief. However, under certain circumstances, the bladder may fill gradually, allowing the person to adapt to the sense of fullness without discomfort. He may not be aware of the fullness except by observing a distended lower abdomen or a change in voiding patterns.

Urinary retention may be caused by obstructive urinary disease, such as infection, calculi, tumors, or benign prostatic hypertrophy. Surgery on, or in the area of, the lower urinary tract may also cause retention. Women who undergo surgery to repair pelvic-floor muscles often have difficulty voiding for several days postoperatively. This also occurs in males after lower abdominal surgery. Surgical discomfort and concern that one may be unable to void contribute to the problem. The women, moreover, usually have a catheter in place postoperatively for several days, causing a temporary diminishing of bladder tone, which contributes to retention.

Assessment

Assessment of urinary retention requires that the nurse use several tools of data collection and then synthesize the data to determine that urinary retention actually exists.

- Interview—Ask the person to describe his voiding patterns and any feelings of discomfort he is experiencing in the lower abdomen.

- Observation—A full bladder is often difficult to observe unless it is very distended. However, if the midportion of the abdomen is swollen as in pregnancy or ascites (an accumulation of fluid), this may accentuate the fullness and aid observation.

- Inspection—Careful records of intake and output are essential to note discrepancies (a greater intake than output) in those persons likely to experience retention. If the bladder becomes very full and the person is unable to void, the excess urine may overflow, resulting in frequent small voidings (20–30 ml every half hour). If the person cannot feel the sensation of a full bladder or is unable to reach the toilet without help, there may also be dribbling and incontinence.

- Palpation—The symphysis pubis, the bone in the lower midportion of the pelvic region, is superficial and easily palpated by placing two fingers behind this bone. However, a full bladder causes resistance and makes it impossible to palpate the bone in this manner.

  The person should also be examined for a fecal impaction, in which collection of feces in the rectum obstructs the urethra and interrupts the normal flow of urine. Discussion of fecal impaction appears later in the chapter.

- Percussion—Percussing over the area of a full bladder should produce a dull thud, sometimes described as a kettle-drum sound.

Nursing Interventions

If urinary retention causes acute discomfort, catheterization may be necessary. Generally, however, the catheter is not left in place unless it is needed to maintain a patent urethra in cases of obstruction. After the discomfort has been relieved, other measures to encourage voiding can be instituted. Such old fashioned remedies as putting the person's hand in water, running the water so it can be heard, or pouring warm water over the perineum all have some effectiveness. They are worth a try and are preferable to using a catheter or resorting to drug therapy.

Persons experiencing pain or tension of the muscles in the perineal area, may find it helpful to sit for 20 minutes several times a day in a tub of warm water to relax those muscles. This procedure is known as a **sitz bath.** A program of ambulation and exercise is often effective as well.

Proper fluid balance should again be mentioned. Whereas the incontinent person may limit his fluid intake for fear that it will come out, the person experiencing retention may limit fluid for fear that it won't! Careful assessment of your client's needs is essential. Although he should not be encouraged to take in large amounts of fluid that will lead to a full bladder, his fluid needs must be met. Urinary bladder problems should not be dealt with through fluid restriction.

Infection of the Lower Urinary Tract

Bacteriuria, or the presence of bacteria in the urine, is a relatively benign and transient condition in persons who are moving about with ease and are properly rested, nourished, and otherwise in good health. Its presence might not even be detected as long as the resistance of the host exceeds the threat of pathogenic organisms. However, if the bacteria begin to multiply and the person is unable to resist the process, the tissue of the urinary tract may become infected, resulting in such conditions as **cystitis, urethritis,** or **ureteritis.**

These conditions occur most commonly in the female, both child and adult. A number of reasons for this have been suggested by researchers who have studied the problem. Some investigators believe that the short female urethra, together with the close proximity of the urinary meatus to organisms from the rectal area, may be an important factor. Others believe that overdistention of the bladder, the real cause of urinary tract infection, is more likely to occur with the female than the male. Reasons advanced for this include inconvenience for the female to void because of the need to remove clothing or because of modesty in certain situations. Public facilities are often hard to find and are frequently undesirable to use, especially for the female. Both sexual intercourse and childbearing have also been implicated in female urinary tract infection. Men also experience urinary tract infections, especially as they grow older and become more susceptible to obstructive diseases such as benign prostatic hypertrophy, which causes urinary retention and bladder distention.

The work of Dr. Jack Lapides, a well-known researcher of urinary tract infection, indicates that bladder distention and the resulting compromised blood supply to the bladder are the most likely causes of infection. He states, "Thus the key to prevention of urinary tract infection is the maintenance of a good blood supply to the urinary tract"

(Lapides, 1973, p. 109). The mechanism for this may be described as follows: if urine is retained, the bladder attempts to empty, resulting in strong bladder contractions. These contractions cause an increase of pressure inside the bladder, a cessation of blood circulation to bladder tissue, and a resulting ischemia. Even though this may occur for only a moment, it still decreases the delivery to the bladder of leukocytes and antibacterial agents necessary for defense. If this occurs frequently and over a period of time, the tissue becomes invaded by any bacteria that are present in the blood, urine, or at the site of the urinary meatus. In other words, the host is no longer able to resist the pathogenic organisms. Figure 21-3 outlines the sequence of events leading to urinary tract infection through urinary retention.

Assessment

Although low-grade urinary tract infections may be asymptomatic, more commonly an infection is excruciatingly painful and demands immediate atten-

Figure 21-3
Urinary retention and urinary tract infection.

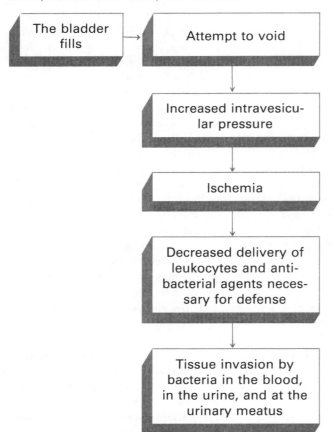

tion. When clients are assessed for this problem, the following signs and symptoms may be helpful:

- **Dysuria**—painful urination; may be present as a burning sensation throughout the voiding process or may follow a comfortable voiding in the form of an extremely painful contraction ascending up the urethra
- Frequency and urgency—the frequent, urgent feeling to go to the bathroom; may occur as often as every 20 minutes
- Hesitancy to initiate stream—despite the urgent need to void, the stream may take several seconds longer to start than usual.
- Lower abdominal pain—contractions of the bladder causing pain in the lower abdomen
- Blood—occasionally blood appears on the toilet tissue or in the urine specimen. If not obvious, it is usually detectable when treated lab sticks are used.
- Appearance—the urine has a cloudy, concentrated appearance.

Other areas to assess are the history of urinary tract infections and the person's usual way of managing them. A number of nursing interventions to assist this person are described below. Determine whether your client has tried any of these ideas and incorporate useful ones into your plan for prevention and care.

Nursing Interventions

Urinary tract infections are exasperating and frustrating experiences. Moreover, persons having one infection are likely to have others. Some women and older men are plagued with them for years. The interventions suggested here, while helpful, by no means cover all aspects of the problem. Careful assessment and plans to develop self-care management according to specific needs are the most helpful interventions that can be provided. Persons with chronic urinary tract infections are themselves their own true care givers.

The interventions listed in Table 21-1 are suggested as a teaching plan.

Catheterization

The placement of tubes into any portion of a person's body is an invasive procedure. Some tubes even require an incision and suturing in order to hold

---

Table 21-1
Self Care Teaching for Urinary Tract Infection

- Prevention is the first part of treatment.
  - Assess your own voiding patterns and plan a regular schedule of fluid intake and elimination as a permanent part of your daily routine.
- Proper nutrition and rest help maintain optimal health and assist you to resist infection.
- Be aware of your own mind–body relationship.
  - Assess the kinds of stressful events that upset your total system and precipitate urinary tract infection.
  - Plan new ways of coping.
- If you experience frequent infections, keep testing sticks on hand to check your urine when you suspect an infection.
  - Arrange with your doctor to have extra medication or a current prescription available for use at inconvenient times such as during weekends and when traveling.
- Avoid situations that increase the bacterial count in the perineal area. (This is especially true for women.)
  - Avoid nylon underwear, panty hose, wet bathing suits, very tight slacks, and extensive bike riding.
  - Empty your bladder and wash the perineum before and after sexual intercourse.
- Avoid harsh substances that may irritate the urinary meatal area.
  - Bubble bath, harsh bath soaps, douching without sound reasons, and laundry detergents and fabric softeners may cause irritation. (The last two areas [*i.e.,* situations that increase the bacterial count and harsh substances] are usually considered of little importance by scientific investigation. However, women who experience infections often find avoidance of them helpful for prevention.)
- Be aware of your first symptoms and begin planning care immediately.
  - Begin medical treatment as well as your own management as soon as possible.
  - The physician may prescribe antibacterial agents such as Gantrisin or Macrodantin, to treat the infection and decrease the possibility of bacteria invading the renal area.
- During an infection, increase your fluid intake in order to irrigate the bladder and decrease pain during urination.
  - Be aware, however, that retention and distention precipitate and aggravate infection.
  - If the fluids you consume are not eliminated, you may need additional medical intervention.
- If the burning sensation or lower abdominal pain persists between voidings, sitting in a tub of warm water can be very comforting.
  - Sometimes a mild analgesic such as Tylenol is helpful.
- You may feel tired during an infection.
  - Conserve your physical resources to combat the infection.
  - Rest frequently to add to your strength.
- The symptoms of infection should begin to diminish gradually after medication is begun.
  - If you are not feeling better within 2 days, the medication may not be right for you.
  - Return to your physician.
  - Remember to take all prescribed medication, even after symptoms have subsided.

---

them in place. The urinary catheter, although relatively easy to insert, with a minimum amount of discomfort to the person, is nonetheless an invasive device from both a physical and a psychological standpoint. The perineal area is a part of our body that we have been taught to keep private, clean, and within our own control. Therefore, having a catheter inserted into this very private area can be extremely distressing. The presence of an unsightly drainage bag also contributes to these uncomfortable feelings.

One woman who was required to retain a catheter for about 3 days after a vaginal hysterectomy expressed feelings that reflected an altered body image when she stated that the catheter made her feel unlike herself and unfeminine. In the same vein, a 10-year-old boy who had had a catheter following heart surgery stated that once the catheter was removed, he "felt himself again" and could "do things now." Although he still had an IV, which could also be considered invasive and restricting, it was the catheter with its added emotional impact that made him feel more dependent. Regardless of its negative psychological effects, the catheter is a fairly common piece of equipment that health-care workers often treat in a casual manner. The sensitive nurse takes care to preserve privacy and provide the person with an opportunity to express his feelings about the catheter.

Types of Catheters

When the urinary bladder must be drained artificially, a straight or an indwelling catheter may be used.

The *straight catheter* is a rubber tube about 16 to 18 inches long, which can be inserted into the bladder through the urethra. The bladder is then drained and the tube is removed. The purposes for this kind of drainage may include the following:

- To determine the amount of residual urine in the bladder after the person has voided
- To drain the bladder to relieve a person who is temporarily unable to void
- To obtain a sterile urine specimen for analysis. (This procedure is rarely used now because a clean voided specimen is a safer and more adequate means of collecting a specimen for analysis.)

The *indwelling catheter* is a tube similar to the straight catheter, except that it has two lumens at the distal end. One lumen is connected to the drainage tubing, and the other is used to instill 5 ml of fluid. The fluid serves to inflate the small balloon at the proximal end of the catheter, which then holds the catheter in place. (The student is referred to the nursing procedures manual for instructions on placing and irrigating a catheter and collecting a specimen.) The indwelling catheter may remain in the bladder for many days, according to the person's needs. Purposes for placing the indwelling catheter may include those below:

- To prevent obstruction: after surgery on the lower urinary tract, which may cause swollen tissues or clots to obstruct the passage of urine; in the presence of urinary calculi or tumor
- To monitor urinary output during shock or following surgery

- To manage incontinence in some persons with neurological deficits
- To assure urinary drainage during most surgical procedures.
- To relieve urinary retention when the person is unable to void for long periods of time
- To assure urinary drainage in certain critically ill persons

Danger of Infection

The urinary catheter, particularly the indwelling type, is a potential source of urinary tract infection. It is an established fact that the most common site of nosocomial infection is the urinary tract and that the great majority of these infections involve the use of an indwelling catheter. In the healthy person, urinary tract infections are treated fairly successfully with antibiotics. However, the person with health problems may have added difficulty coping with an infection. Moreover, persons who have indwelling catheters may not experience the pain that is usually associated with cystitis, allowing the infection to go unnoticed and untreated for some time. The result of this could be kidney infection or even septicemia.

Assessment

Although a physician's order is necessary to catheterize a person, many physicians establish a standing or p.r.n. order based on the nurse's assessment of the need for catheterization. Asking yourself the following questions may help you to make this assessment:

- If the person is a male, would condom drainage (an externally applied drainage system) be as effective?
- If a sterile specimen is needed, would a clean voided midstream specimen be adequate?
- If the person is unable to void after surgery, is he properly hydrated?
- Have all possible means of assisting normal voiding been instituted?
- Has the proper assessment been done to determine whether the bladder is distended or not?
- Is it reasonable to try a single straight catheterization for relief of immediate retention and then to institute other measures to help the person void normally, rather than placing an indwelling catheter prematurely?

- If the person is incontinent, how great is the potential for skin breakdown and other management problems if he is not catheterized?

Nursing Interventions

The nurse should institute the following measures when giving care to the person with an indwelling catheter:

- Instruct the person in the proper care and positioning of the catheter to allow him to participate in self-care whenever possible.
- Follow the principles of sterile technique when inserting the catheter and when changing the dependent drainage system.

  - Assess each person individually to determine when the catheter and collection system should be changed.
  - Changes should not be done routinely.
  - Observe for the presence of sediment in the transparent tubing or roll the catheter between the fingertips to feel for sandy particles.
  - A foul odor from the urine may indicate infection and require a system change.
  - A change is also needed if the system leaks or becomes contaminated.
- Prevent the catheter from undermining the tissue integrity of the urinary meatus, the urethra, and the bladder.
  - Keep the catheter taped in place to prevent movement and trauma to the urethra.
  - Tape to the inner aspect of the thigh on the female (Fig. 21-4); for the male, raise the penis upward and tape catheter to the abdomen.

Figure 21-4
Catheter taped to inner aspect of thigh.

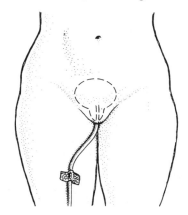

- Allow slack when taping to prevent pressure from the inflated balloon on the urethra or the bladder.
- Encourage fluid intake. Remember that the best method of catheter irrigation is fluid intake.
- Position the collection bag below the level of the bladder at all times. This provides continuous flow of urine and prevents backflow of stagnant urine from the drainage system into the bladder.
  - Position the person carefully to prevent compressions and loops in the tubing.
  - Instruct the person to keep his arm fully extended when ambulating and carrying the bag.
  - Instruct him to inform others as to the correct position of the bag when ambulating or transferring him.
  - The person on a stretcher or in a wheelchair should have the bag attached to the equipment and not placed on the abdomen or lap.
- Separate persons with catheters from each other geographically. Close proximity of potential contaminating agents contributes to the development of infection.
- Maintain a closed urinary drainage system.
  - Persons with indwelling catheters frequently develop bacteriuria within 4 days.
  - If the bacteria count becomes high enough it may invade the bladder and cause infection.
  - The development of bacteriuria is reduced if a closed drainage system is maintained.
  - Consider the total system: person, catheter, drainage tubing, collection bag.
  - There are three areas where bacteria may enter this system: the catheter–meatal junction, the catheter–tubing junction, and the mouth of the spigot. Proper care as described in Table 21-2 reduces the possibility of infection through these routes.

Intermittent Self-Catheterization

Persons with neurological deficits, partially obstructed urethras, or a temporary inability to void normally are candidates for **intermittent self-catheterization (ISC).** ISC promotes adaptation and more self-control for persons with long-term problems and provides needed relief in persons with short-term problems.

A great deal of research on ISC has been done by Lapides and his associates. The results have proven that this procedure is a great aid in assisting people to regain health, independence, and control over their lives. Aside from the use ISC has for cleanliness, dryness, skin integrity, and the like, it provides another significant service. In the past, persons with neurological deficits often underwent surgery for urinary diversion. This procedure can take several forms, but its purpose is to redirect the

---

Table 21-2
Maintaining a Closed Drainage System

- The catheter–meatal junction:
  - Wash hands thoroughly before handling the catheter.
  - Carry out perineal care twice a day and after each bowel movement.
  - Baths or showers may be taken.
  - The catheter may be cleaned with an antibacterial solution such as peroxide or betadine.
- The catheter–tubing junction:
  - To maintain a closed system, do not disconnect the catheter from the drainage tubing.
  - Keep the system connected during ambulation or transference by stretcher or wheelchair. An intact system minimizes the amount of bacteria that can enter and avoids the use of plugs and clamps that obstruct urine flow, cause bladder distention, and increase the potential for infection.
  - Irrigate the catheter only when necessary to maintain patency.
  - Use the closed procedure for irrigation.
  - The open procedure should be used only when the catheter is impatent and pressure is needed. However, be aware that even minimal pressure can be painful and may undermine tissue integrity.
  - Use the closed method of obtaining a urine specimen. The specimen should be taken from the tubing that contains urine most directly from the bladder, rather than from the pooled collection in the drainage bag.
- The mouth of the spigot:
  - Do not remove the spigot from the sheath except when emptying the drainage bag.
  - Wipe the spigot with two or three alcohol swabs before and after emptying the bag. Figure 21-5 shows the drainage system.

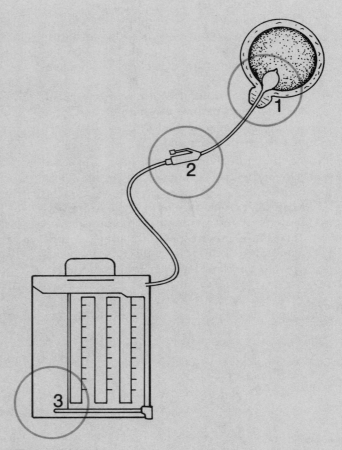

Figure 21-5
Urinary drainage system: (*1*) the catheter–meatal junction; (*2*) the catheter–tubing junction; (*3*) the mouth of the spigot.

flow of urine out of the body, usually by means of an opening in the abdomen. ISC has relegated this procedure to the last resort (Lapides, 1975, p. 17).

The general plan for ISC is to have the person catheterize himself on a definite schedule throughout the 24-hour period. Frequently, the schedule calls for the person to eliminate every 2 or 3 hours and engage in purposeful waking once or twice during the night for elimination. This procedure is done using clean, rather than sterile, technique because it is a more practical method to use at home. Clean technique is acceptable because ISC is based on the premise that the single most important factor in the development of urinary tract infections is an overdistended bladder and not bacteria.

The idea may be puzzling to students who have just read the importance of using sterile technique for the placement of catheters. It should also be stated that not everyone agrees with the unsterile ISC method. However, the following ideas may help reconcile these differing points of view and underscore the importance of using assessment to determine the person's physical, psychological, and social capabilities for participating in this kind of program.

- Persons who need an indwelling catheter often have many health problems so that their resistance to bacteria is low. Persons using ISC are usually out in the community and generally are in better health, making their resistance to bacteria higher.

- Persons who need an indwelling catheter are often in the hospital or nursing home and are being exposed to a variety of organisms to which they have not developed resistance.

- The emotional impact of the indwelling catheter may cause the person to have less resistance to infection.

- Persons involved in self-care activities such as ISC feel more independent and in control of their lives and thus are more resistant to complications.

- When nurses provide care to a person needing an invasive procedure they use the most sterile technique possible.

These ideas indicate the importance of using sterile technique when the catheter is inserted by the nurse. On the other hand, when the person is inserting the catheter for self-care purposes, the emphasis is on emptying the bladder and avoiding retention.

Part Two: Principles of Bowel Elimination

Defecation

The colon, or large intestine, forms the last 4 feet of the gastrointestinal tract. It consists of three fairly straight segments, known as the ascending, transverse, and descending portions, which end with the sigmoid colon, the rectum, and the anus. There are no digestive enzymes secreted in the colon, and only a very small amount of absorption takes place there. The primary function of the colon is to store and concentrate fecal material prior to defecation. Feces are stored in the sigmoid colon and enter the rectum only when it is time for expulsion.

The process of **defecation** begins when chyme—containing water, electrolytes, undigested cellulose, cell debris from intestinal epithelium, and bile pigments—enters the colon through the ileocecal valve. As these substances move through the colon, sodium chloride and water are absorbed and the stool becomes solid. The movement of feces along the colon is accomplished by brief, strong waves of peristalsis, which occur after each meal.

The movement of feces along the colon is involuntary. Feces in the rectum distend the walls of the rectum causing the urge to defecate. A reflex response occurs, which consists of a contraction of the rectum, relaxation of the internal and external anal sphincters, and increased peristaltic activity in the sigmoid colon which pushes the feces through the anus. The external anal sphincter is under voluntary control. If this sphincter is voluntarily contracted when the rectum is filled, the urge to defecate eventually subsides. It returns again only when more feces are pushed into the rectum.

The person normally assists defecation by taking a deep breath which is followed by a closing of the glottis and contraction of abdominal and chest muscles. This causes a marked rise in intraabdominal pressure that assists in the elimination of the feces. An understanding of this physiological mechanism is helpful in the following discussion of bowel elimination.

Occasionally, particularly in the elderly person, straining to eliminate may cause a stroke or coronary occlusion. This is the result of increased abdominal and intrathoracic pressures during the Valsalva maneuver (*i.e.,* closed glottis and contraction of chest muscles on full lungs). The consequences of this maneuver are a rise in arterial pressure, a stoppage of venous return with a rise in peripheral venous pressure, a fall in stroke output, and a subsequent fall in arterial pressure. The nurse will want to assess carefully the bowel elimination patterns of the person at risk for stroke or heart attack. The discussion on constipation later in this chapter provides suggestions for assessment and interventions.

Factors Affecting Bowel Elimination

Although the factors affecting bowel function are described here separately, they should be considered in combination. For example, diet combined with exercise, rest, fluid intake, and so forth creates the overall effect of health and well-being.

Diet. The bowel may well provide a more immediate response to the food we eat than does any other structure of the body. The various effects that nutrition can have on bowel elimination are discussed in more detail with specific problems.

Fluid Intake. Adequate fluid intake is essential for comfortable elimination. When diarrhea occurs, fluid intake, whether oral or intravenous, is necessary to replace the fluid lost through the stool.

Exercise. Regular exercise has long been known to maintain or improve intestinal motility. In addition, purposeful exercising of the abdominal muscles strengthens them and enhances the actual process of defecation. Persons whose mobility has decreased or who are bedridden often report serious difficulty with bowel elimination.

Position. As with urinary elimination, assuming a position that is natural for defecation facilitates the function. Leaning forward from the hips in a squatting or sitting position is usual.

The immobilized or bedridden person is again at a disadvantage. Thiroloix writes, "Bed patients can't go to the bathroom and must use this barbaric device [the bedpan] that must have been created solely for the discomfort and humiliation of the bedridden. It is easy to understand why their unconscious reflex is not to move their bowels" (Thiroloix, 1976, p. 29). We do need the bedpan, but it is not conducive to the best elimination process.

Defecation Reflex. If the person does not respond to the urge to defecate, the muscles of the rectum relax and the urge subsides. At a later point when more feces enter the rectum, the defecation reflex again is initiated. Water from unexpelled feces remaining in the rectum is reabsorbed, causing them to become dry, hard, and difficult to pass.

Regular Pattern for Defecation. Patterns of elimination are many and vary among individuals. The bowel can be trained to evacuate at a certain time each day, or every 2 or 3 days, depending on the person's need. Bowel elimination at a specified time and place is more convenient and relaxing for most persons.

Pregnancy. Pregnant women commonly have altered bowel elimination. One reason is the change in body contour that creates difficulty in assuming the usual position for evacuating the bowel. Another cause is the increased secretion of progesterone, which causes smooth muscle relaxation.

Travel. Traveling can disrupt our usual bowel patterns very quickly. This may be associated with such factors as a change in food and fluid consumption, the need to suppress the defecation reflex until a toilet becomes available, and the inconvenience of using public facilities.

Sociocultural Factors. Miller (1978) has written that the English are obsessed with their bowels, while others state that America is a bowel-conscious nation. People in general often believe that a bowel movement every day is essential, although there is no valid research to prove this. Social opinion varies as to when and how children should be toilet trained, but most parents feel distressed if their children are still having "accidents" by age 3. Other social considerations include the availability and cleanliness of public restrooms, the ease of removing clothing, and shyness about creating an odor.

Emotional Factors. The classic work by Walter B. Cannon, *Bodily Changes in Pain, Hunger, Fear, and Rage,* describes how our emotions affect each of our body systems. He states, "... the peristalsis and the kneading movements (segmentation) of the small intestine, and the reversed peristalsis of the large intestine all cease whenever the observed animal shows signs of emotional excitement." He also states, "Mild affective states, such as worry and anxiety, can ... check the activity of the colon and thus cause constipation" (Cannon, 1929, pp. 14–15; 338). The sympathetic nervous system provides the responses that lead to "fight or flight," one of which is a decrease in the motility of the gastrointestinal tract. In other instances persons are known to have an increase in gastrointestinal tract motility and diarrhea in response to stress.

Drugs. Many drugs cause alterations in gastrointestinal motility resulting in some degree of constipation or diarrhea. Drugs also affect the coloration of the stool. Some common drugs and their effects on stool color are listed in Table 21-3.

General Assessment of Bowel Function

Defecation Patterns

As with urinary elimination, assessment includes an attempt to collect data about bowel elimination patterns both at home and in the hospital. Infor-

mation about changes in these patterns related to health concerns or some of the factors affecting bowel function would also provide helpful baseline data.

Patterns of bowel elimination are even more individualized than those of urinary elimination. The important factor in assessment is not how frequently one has a bowel movement but whether the person's own pattern of elimination is comfortable for him.

Characteristics of Stool

The fecal mass is generally 75% to 80% water and 20% to 25% solids that are derived from food residues, secretions from the small intestine, bacteria, and the desquamation of old intestinal cells.

Color

Bile pigments are responsible for the characteristic brown color of stool. The absence of these pigments causes a grayish-white or clay coloration that may be indicative of liver or gallbladder disease. This is known as an **ACHOLIC stool.** A tarry black stool may indicate occult (hidden) blood, usually from the upper part of the gastrointestinal tract. It could also indicate that the person takes iron, which produces the same tarry, black appearance. Blood from the

---

Table 21-3
Drugs and Fecal Color Changes

Drug	Color Change
Antacids	Whitish discoloration or speckling
Antibiotics	Green-gray due to impaired digestion
Anticoagulants	Pink to red to black due to GI bleeding
Barium	White to gray
Indocin	Pink to red to black due to GI bleeding
Iron salts	Black due to oxidation of iron
Azo Gantanol, Azo Gantrisin, Pyridium	Orange-red due to dye
Aspirin	Pink to red to black due to GI bleeding
Tetracyclines in glucosamine-potentiated syrup form	Red

From Bradley GM: Fecal analysis: Much more than an unpleasant necessity, Diagnostic Medicine, 64–72, March/April, 1980

lower portion of the gastrointestinal tract may appear as streaking in the stool. Stool can be tested for occult blood by means of the guaiac test. Any time blood is suspected, the stool should be checked by this means. The products for testing come with instructions.

The color of stool may be altered by certain food or drugs. For example, beets and certain berries may give a reddish appearance whereas rhubarb may cause a yellow to brown stool. When an unusually colored stool occurs, all medications the person has been receiving should be checked along with any possible change in diet over the preceding few days.

Consistency and Form

Stool is usually soft, but formed and cylindrical in shape. Very hard, small stools occur when the person is constipated, and watery stools indicate diarrhea. Although it is not abnormal to find occasional pieces of undigested food in the stool, especially in small children, such an occurrence if frequent could indicate inadequate hydrochloric acid in the stomach. This problem is often accompanied by large, mushy stools. Persons with shreds of mucus in the stool often have inflammatory conditions of the bowel. Narrowed or pencil-like stools could indicate a bowel obstruction. For further infomration on assessing this problem, see Chapter 20.

Odor

Stool odor, although difficult to describe, is characteristic and well known to all. The products of bacterial action give the stool its odor. Unusual odors may occur from certain foods, drugs, or diseases.

Nursing Process
Applied to Problems of Bowel Elimination

Diarrhea

Diarrhea is the frequent passage of loose, watery stools. The contents of the intestine pass more rapidly than usual because of increased intestinal motility. This prevents adequate absorption of fluids and digested food products. The additional fluid volume in the colon creates more distention and thus an increase in the need to defecate. Because the ingested food is propelled rapidly through the intestine, there is not sufficient time for digestion and absorption, and undigested pieces of food often appear in the stool.

If diarrhea persists beyond 24 hours, fluid and electrolyte losses, primarily sodium, potassium, and bicarbonate, can become severe. In chronic diarrhea states, vitamin and iron deficiencies, as well as depletion of tissue proteins and decreased serum protein levels, may also occur. Potassium loss is one of the most serious problems because potassium is needed to maintain adequate tone of gastrointestinal smooth muscle.

Diarrhea can be caused by bacterial or viral invasion of the gastrointestinal tract; ingestion of spoiled, disagreeable, or spicy foods; foods that are unusual in the person's diet and therefore cause intestinal mucosal irritation; psychogenic factors; and certain drugs. Diarrhea can also be caused by more serious underlying problems such as celiac disease, dysentery, or ulcerative colitis. However, diarrhea, especially the acute type, is basically a protective mechanism. It is the body's attempt to rid itself of harmful or irritating substances.

Assessment

Assessment of the person's usual bowel elimination patterns provides a comparison with what he is experiencing now. The frequency and amount of the diarrheic stools are important, along with any associated factors such as drugs, foods, or psychogenic factors that might be causing the problem. Remember that a diarrheic stool is primarily fluid and should be measured and added to the person's output records.

Other symptoms might include abdominal pain and cramping, generalized weakness and fatigue, and perhaps even fever and vomiting. The pain and cramping may be related to the increased intestinal motility. However, the other symptoms are more likely to be the effect of the diarrhea on the body. For example, loss of vitamins, iron, and fluids as a result of diarrhea contributes greatly to weakness and fatigue. If the diarrhea continues unchecked, severe dehydration, weight loss, acid–base imbalance, and shock could occur. The nurse should be alert to those persons who are especially susceptible to the serious consequences of diarrhea, including the debilitated patient, the small child, and the elderly adult.

Nursing Interventions

Acute diarrhea from relatively benign irritants such as food or certain infectious agents is usually self-limiting and not serious. Treatment includes primarily the replacement of fluid loss and quiet, restful activities that calm the intestinal tract. Initially the diet may be limited to clear liquids. However, if food is taken, it should be soft and of low fiber to decrease intestinal motility and irritation. Foods with pectin, such as applesauce and bananas, are sometimes helpful. Milk and milk products, extremes of temperature, and concentrated sweets should be avoided.

If diarrhea persists, it may be necessary to give the intestinal tract a complete rest. Clear liquids only can be given, but if this approach does not help, oral intake may have to be stopped and intravenous fluid and electrolyte therapy instituted. In addition, vitamin and iron supplements may be given. The physician makes the decision about when this kind of therapy must be initiated. However, careful assessment by the nurse and communication with the physician are essential for the teamwork necessary to make appropriate decisions.

Continued assessment throughout the period of diarrhea should include evaluation of the nutritional, fluid and electrolyte, and psychological statuses. Skin and perineal care should also be attended to because diarrhea can cause severe irritation.

Constipation

Constipation is the infrequent passing of hard, dry stool by means of a characteristic, involuntary, ineffectual straining movement known as **tenesmus.** The intestinal and colonic motility is considerably slower than usual, resulting in increased absorption of fluid from the fecal mass and thus the hard, dry stool. Unlike chronic diarrhea, chronic constipation is generally not considered potentially serious. Rather it is primarily an uncomfortable state and can contribute to such conditions as hernias, hemorrhoids, and varicose veins. There are a few authorities, however, who suggest the possibility that poor dietary and bowel habits cause constipation, which is a contributing factor to more serious diseases such

as diverticulitis, appendicitis, and even colonic cancer.

Occasionally people worry that not having a bowel movement every day and retaining large amounts of fecal material and bacteria in the body will result in toxicity and poisoning. However, Vander states, "Attempts to isolate such toxic agents from intestinal bacteria have been totally unsuccessful" (Vander *et al*, 1980, p. 438).

Constipation is frequently caused by diets low in fiber, inadequate fluid intake, and poor bowel elimination habits. Flath observes, "Among primitive peoples, who consume nothing but unrefined natural foods and empty their bowels whenever and wherever it suits them best, constipation is virtually unknown. But among the presumably civilized peoples of the twentieth century, constipation is one of the most common ills" (Flath, 1975, p. 1). He believes that our diets, consisting of highly refined and often artificially created foods, may be the reason for this occurrence.

Other causes of constipation include poor muscle tone of the intestine, inadequate exercise, and severely decreased mobility found in persons confined to bed, those who have arthritis, or the elderly. Ingestion of drugs such as sedatives, opiates, and ganglionic blocking agents, and organic disorders such as diverticulosis or obstructive tumors may also be implicated in constipation.

Assessment

The first thing to determine is whether the person is really constipated or not. Reminding him that one bowel movement a day is not necessary may help clarify this point. Of prime importance, however, is his ability to pass a comfortable stool of appropriate consistency. Additional signs to consider include headache, feelings of tiredness and lassitude, anorexia, low back pain, and irritability. There may sometimes be a "gassy," bloated feeling.

Nursing Interventions

Philip Roth's hero in *Portnoy's Complaint* made the following comment about his father, "He drank . . . mineral oil and milk of magnesia; and chewed on Ex-Lax; and ate AllBran morning and night; and downed mixed dried fruits by the pound bag. He suffered—did he suffer!—from constipation . . . I remember that when they announced over the radio the explosion of the first atom bomb, he said aloud. "Maybe that would do the job" (Roth, 1967, p. 4–5).

Health Teaching. Persons with chronic constipation do suffer a great deal. Those with problems resulting from an organic cause require some medical intervention as well as nursing measures. Persons with the more typical constipation resulting from poor dietary and bowel habits would benefit from the suggestions listed in Table 21-4.

Laxatives. There may be an occasional time when a mild laxative assists with an episode of constipation. Such episodes may occur when usual bowel elimination and diet patterns have been disrupted, such as during traveling or after surgery. However, using laxatives generally causes more difficulty than it resolves. For example, laxatives create problems by eliminating more fecal material than the bowel intended at any one time. Consequently, when the person does not have another bowel movement the next day, he concludes he is still constipated and takes more laxative. Gradually the bowel becomes sluggish and loses the muscle tone that assists with natural control. It may then be necessary to take a laxative in order to have a bowel movement. The added danger of laxatives is the tendencey to take them when the problem is not constipation but a more serious complication such as appendicitis. Table 21-5 provides some examples of laxatives.

Enemas. Enemas are primarily designed to evacuate the lower bowel and rectum, although "high" enemas evacuate more of the colon. Enemas stimulate peristalsis by creating distention or by providing chemical irritation or lubrication. One of the main reasons enemas are given is to prepare the bowel for diagnostic studies and surgery. A clean bowel makes it more possible for the physician to see clearly during a procedure. Enemas may also be used to introduce a substance such as barium, which aids in diagnosis during an x-ray exam. At times sedatives, stimulants, and even nutritional elements can be administered by means of an enema, although this type of therapy is not commonly used because the enema solution usually does not rise high enough in the bowel to allow absorption.

As a method of treating constipation, enemas often create the same problems as laxatives. In addition, the invasive nature of the procedure can irritate or undermine the intestinal mucosa and cause psychological distress.

Flatus

Flatus or **flatulence** is gas that occurs in the stomach and intestines. It occurs normally as a result of swallowed air, diffusion of gases from the blood-

---

Table 21-4
Health Teaching to Avoid Constipation

- Determine the cause of constipation, if possible.
- Establish a regular pattern of food intake and elimination.
- Eat breakfast and take a warm liquid with it.
- Plan a diet with high fiber or roughage:
  - Consult a nutritional source for full dietary suggestions.
  - Consider the addition of bran to the diet.
- Eat foods with naturally occurring laxative qualities such as prunes.
- Increase your fluid intake.
- Plan regular exercise and activity. After surgery or a period of time in bed, plan to walk as much as possible. This helps increase gastrointestinal motility.
- Assume a comfortable position on the toilet and try relaxing measures such as reading or listening to music.
- Abdominal muscle strengthening exercises might be helpful. Try sit-ups or a series of abdominal muscle contractions.
- Avoid use of laxatives, cathartics, and enemas.

Table 21-5
Laxatives

Type of Laxative	Example	Brand Names and Sources
Bulk producers	Dietary fiber	Bran, wholemeal bread
	Mucilaginous poly-saccharides	Metamucil, Perdiem
	Methylcellulose	Hydrolose
Stool softeners	Synthetic surface ac-tive agents	Colace, Surfak
Lubricants	Mineral oil hydrocar-bon mixtures	Agoral, Mineral Oil
Osmotic agents	Sodium, potassium, magnesium salts	Magnesium sulfate, epsom salts, milk of magnesia
Chemical stimu-lants	Anthracene com-pounds	Senna, Senokot
	Polyphenolic com-pounds	Bisacodyl, Dulcolax
	Castor oil	

stream into the gastrointestinal tract, and bacterial fermentation in the tract. Flatus is normally passed occasionally throughout the day through the mouth or anus and sometimes in conjunction with a bowel movement.

Excessive flatus, which can be uncomfortable, may be caused by eating rich or spicy foods and gas-producing vegetables, such as onions, beans, and cucumbers. Other contributing factors include drinking soda or other carbonated beverages, drinking with a straw, swallowing excessive amounts of air during periods of anxiety or nausea, eating rapidly and chewing gum or sucking on hard candy. Iced beverages have also been implicated in flatus production. Persons often experience flatus during periods of immobility or following surgery that requires general anesthesia. These have the effect of decreasing intestinal motility. Another serious cause of flatus is intestinal obstruction, which was discussed in more detail in Chapter 20.

Assessment

The person with flatus feels bloated and may even have a swollen or distended abdomen. Measurement of abdominal girth can sometimes be helpful in determining any change in distention. Identifying the cause of the flatus may point to a fairly easy solution, especially if it is due to swallowing excess air or eating foods that do not agree with the particular person's digestive tract. Flatus that creates true distention causes cramping pain both in the abdominal area and occasionally in the rectal area close to the anus.

Nursing Interventions

The following suggestions may be offered as a means of alleviating the discomfort of flatus.

- Help the person identify what foods or possible behaviors are causing the gas so that these foods and activities can be avoided in the future.

- Suggest mild exercise or walking after meals. Especially avoid reclining after meals.

- Suggest a decrease in the fat content of meals.

- Help the person plan regular exercise and activity to increase peristalsis and encourage movement of flatus through the intestine. The flatus can then be expelled through the anal sphincter.

- Suggest massaging the abdomen from the umbilicus toward the perineal area.

Fecal Impaction

Fecal impaction is the presence in the rectum of a mass of hard stool which the person is unable to pass. It is generally the result of an accumulation of feces in the sigmoid colon and rectum. Although fecal impaction can be a result of chronic constipation, it generally does not occur in the person who moves about freely. It most commonly occurs when mobility is severely decreased. Thus, comatose persons and those who have neurological deficits are at risk for this problem.

Assessment

Bowel elimination patterns in persons at risk for forming an impaction constitute an essential part of assessment. Other symptoms to observe include feelings of fullness or bloating, severe rectal pain, everted anus, and occasionally tenesmus. In addition, a digital rectal examination reveals a hard mass just beyond the anus. Remembering that fecal impaction can cause urinary retention, the nurse may also consider patterns of urinary elimination to assist with assessment. The unsuccessful attempt of the defecation reflex to remove the stool often creates increased intestinal motility and results in the formation of liquid stool above the fecal mass. This stool leaks out around the impaction and it appears that the person has diarrhea. Impaction should always be suspected if diarrhea occurs in an immobilized person.

Nursing Interventions

Since fecal impaction ought always to be prevented, careful and continued assessment in persons at risk is the most important intervention. Attention to the interventions suggested for constipation wherever possible would be useful.

If an impaction occurs, the following procedure is usually carried out:

* Give the person an oil retention enema to help soften the stool.
* Follow this with a mild soapsuds enema 2 to 3 hours later.
* Repeat these two steps once if they are not successful at first.
* If the stool is not expelled, try breaking it up by digital manipulation.
* The final step is manual extraction if necessary.

Anal Incontinence

Anal incontinence is the inability of the anal sphincter to control voluntarily the expulsion of feces. As with urinary incontinence, those who suffer from this disorder experience embarrassment, loss of self-esteem, and often self-imposed social isolation. Although anal incontinence is probably less common than urinary incontinence, it does occur in persons with inadequate muscle tone of the anal sphincter, possibly as a result of hemorrhoids; rectal surgery for polyps, cysts, or tumors; age; and occasionally severe diarrhea. Difficulty in controlling the anal sphincter may also be a problem for persons with neurological deficits from disease or trauma. These people frequently experience at one time or another a whole range of bowel and bladder problems, including infection, incontinence, retention, and impaction.

Assessment

When assessing for anal incontinence, it is important to consider both bowel and bladder elimination. Remember that urinary incontinence in the older person is often related to decreased mobility or vision or other environmental factors for which adaptations can be made. The same is true of bowel incontinence. Remember also the chain of events: immobility → constipation → impaction → diarrhea. In certain persons the diarrhea may be difficult to control and incontinence can result.

When assessing anal incontinence in the person with a newly acquired neurological deficit, it helps to assess previous bowel patterns. These data provide a point from which to start a bowel retraining program. Assessment of nutritional status may provide data for altering dietary patterns, an important step in coping with incontinence.

Nursing Interventions

A *bowel retraining program* can be instituted successfully in many instances of anal incontinence. Because feces are stored in the sigmoid colon rather than the rectum, the rectum is generally empty or nearly so until just prior to defecation. The internal anal sphincter is in a state of tonic contraction which prevents the loss of small amounts of stool. Normally, the external sphincter is constantly contracted until we choose to relax it. However, when the nerve supply is interrupted, as in the case of spinal cord injury, external sphincter control is lost. Thus, even though internal sphincter control is still intact, the person is unable to control the loss of a sudden expulsion of stool. It is possible, however, to plan a program of regular bowel evacuation, which will keep the stool from moving suddenly and unexpectedly into the rectum and thus being expelled. Vigliarolo observes, "The purpose of a daily regimen is to habituate the colon to empty daily at the same time. Complete emptying minimizes the possibility that enough fecal material will accumulate to cause a reflex relaxation of the internal sphincter and cause bowel accidents during the day" (Vigliarolo, 1980, p. 105).

There are various ways of approaching a bowel retraining program, depending on the cause of the anal incontinence. Some of the points suggested here may not be useful for all persons. The nurse and the person must plan goals together and choose the aspects that would be most helpful. A general goal would probably be as follows: "The person will develop stool which is formed but soft and easily passed."

- The readiness and ability of the person to participate in the program must be assessed.

- It is important to be alert to perineal skin care needs as attempts are made to solve the problem of incontinence.

- A diet of high fiber foods and an adequate fluid intake should be planned.

- The physician may order a stool softener such as surfak or colace, a bulk-producing medication such as metamucil, and a local stimulant or suppository. These medications can be helpful when regulating bowel evacuation. Irrigation or enemas may be used in certain instances, especially at the beginning of the program.

- Food, fluids, and other aids such as medications should be taken on a planned time schedule. Either hot or cold liquids tend to stimulate peristalsis and can be helpful if administered 10 to 15 minutes prior to inserting the suppository.

- Whenever possible the person should sit on the toilet or the bedside commode to provide a more normal position for defecating. If he must remain in bed, lying on the left side is the most natural position possible.

- Abdominal massage from the cecal area, following the course of the large intestine in clockwise fashion may help stimulate peristalsis.

- The program may take time to become effective. Help the person to express his concerns, but express your belief that a positive outcome is expected.

Artificial Openings for Bowel Diversion

Persons who have obstructive or inflammatory conditions of the intestine may be treated with diet and medication, or with surgery. When surgery is necessary, portions of the small or large intestine, and sometimes the rectum, are removed. In order to create an alternate method of bowel elimination, the surgeon makes an incision into the intestine and draws the severed ends of the bowel through the abdominal wall to the outside of the body. This open portion of bowel is called a **stoma.** If the opening is created in the small intestine, usually the ileum, it is called an **ileostomy.** If the opening is in the large intestine, it is called a **colostomy.** The person then wears a bag, attached to the abdomen over the opening, to catch the feces. The degree to which the bowel elimination process can be regulated depends on the portion of intestine that has been altered.

Assessment

Persons about to undergo ostomy surgery have the usual preoperative concerns, and many others as well. They may believe that the ostomy will be obvious to others because of the bag and possible odor. They may have financial concerns, knowing they must buy ostomy equipment for the rest of their lives. They may be struggling with changes in body image and self-concept and worrying about the ways the ostomy might affect their jobs, recreation, sexual relationships, and so forth. Young women may be afraid that they will not be able to have children.

Assessment in all these areas of concern is essential if the nurse is to provide information and give support. The facts are that the bag is not obvious, even when the person wears a bathing suit, and that odor can be dealt with in many ways. Financial concerns may be very real, but social service agencies and ostomy associations can provide resources. Women with ostomies can have children, and sexual relationships can be resumed according to former patterns when the person is ready. For the most part, common recreational and athletic activities can be resumed, although contact sports are not advised.

Preoperative nutritional patterns and urinary and bowel elimination patterns are important areas to assess. This information can be used later when helping the person plan for the adaptations he must make. Information about family relationships and levels of support provide the nurse with data about the amount of help available at home. If the person has cancer, concerns about serious illness and death must also be considered.

Nursing Interventions

The interventions the nurse plans depend on the physiology of the involved bowel portion, the person's diagnosis, and the amount of family support available. The approach taken depends on the person's ability to alter his body image and adapt to change. The dynamics of grief and loss that are a part of this change are discussed in Chapter 29. It might well be that the person will need the nurse's support in order to proceed through the stages of loss in an adaptive manner. Such adaptation, although it requires time, is essential for health and well-being. Moreover, the person's basic needs of safety and security, love and belonging must be met before he can become a candidate for learning about new diets, skin care, and appliances. An important point to remember is to establish a trusting relationship and then proceed at the client's pace.

Expressing positive expectations about the outcome and helping the person mobilize his strengths will create an atmosphere of hope about his future. At the same time, it is important to avoid any negative connotations about the presence of the stoma. A positive outlook is important because it can make the difference between an atmosphere of hope and one of despair.

Although the literature may refer to the person with an ostomy as an ostomate or stoma patient, we suggest that these expressions not be used. Such labeling tends to depersonalize the individual and emphasize the adverse aspects of the situation.

The following suggestions may constitute a plan of care for the person with an ostomy.

Diet and Fluid Intake. The person's needs depend on the physiology of the affected bowel portion, which could result in diarrhea or constipation. Assess your client's problems and refer to the appropriate section earlier in the chapter for ideas on proper food and fluid intake.

Skin Care and Hygiene. The skin around the stoma and the stoma itself need careful skin care. Many products are available for this purpose. The skin should be kept clean, dry, and free from irritation. The bag should be washed carefully and specially designed deodorizers, used to help with the odor problem. The location of the stoma is also important because of bowel physiology. The higher the ostomy, the more excretion of digestive enzymes will occur, causing irritation to the skin.

Regulation of the bowel depends on the area involved. Colostomies in the descending colon can be regulated rather easily; others may be much more difficult to manage. Although irrigation can be used when the person is first attempting regulation, it is better not to irrigate on a continuing basis, because it diminishes muscle tone and reduces the possibility of the bowel's regulating itself.

Family Relationships. Family members need to be included in the plan of care. They need general information and suggestions of how they can help the person. They also need an opportunity to discuss their feelings about the ostomy with the nurse. A sensitive nurse encourages the person and his family to express their feelings to each other as well.

Sexual Counseling. A careful assessment indicates whether sexual counseling is necessary. The nurse can participate in discussion and provide information. If there is need for further assistance, the nurse can refer the person to a specialist in sexual counseling.

General Support. The United Ostomy Association has chapters in cities throughout the United States.* Members of this group will visit persons with new ostomies to give additional help and support. The organization also provides teaching aids for the person with an ostomy.

Conclusion

Normal elimination is essential to our sense of well-being and to our ability to maintain optimal health. Elimination is a first level or physiological need in Maslow's hierarchy; thus, altered bowel and bladder function affects the ability to meet higher level needs. Nurses who deliver care from a holistic philosophy consider the needs for love, belonging, and self-esteem as well as principles of anatomy and physiology when assisting persons with elimination problems.

Common problems of elimination include incontinence, urinary retention, infection of the lower urinary tract, diarrhea, constipation, and flatus. Nursing interventions are directed toward providing adequate fluids, assisting the person to plan appropriate diet and programs of exercise or rest, and offering guidance through health teaching. Individuals with special elimination problems such as indwelling

* United Ostomy Association, Inc., Dept. N81, 2001 W. Beverly Blvd., Los Angeles, Calif. 90057.

catheters and ostomies require nursing support in the form of hygiene and skin care, prevention of secondary problems such as infection, and teaching related to self-care. Nursing care for any individual with elimination problems includes promoting self-esteem through measures such as odor control, hygiene, and emotional support. By facilitating bowel and bladder function, the nurse assists persons to return to adaptive elimination patterns and to attain or maintain wellness.

Study Questions

1. List signs and symptoms that might indicate a person has a distended bladder. What nursing interventions might be utilized to induce voiding?

2. You are asked to visit an elderly woman in her house. You discover that she is often incontinent of urine.
   a. List the data you would need before developing a plan of care.
   b. Identify factors affecting urinary elimination that might apply to this person.

3. Mrs. Jones tells you she feels pain on urination and sometimes sees a spot of blood on the toilet tissue.
   a. Which problem of urinary elimination might you suspect?
   b. What other data would you need to assess for this problem?

4. You are caring for a person with an indwelling catheter. Develop a list of nursing interventions designed to prevent infection in this person.

5. Your client has paraplegia. Together you are deciding whether he should begin a program of intermittent self-catheterization or continue to use an indwelling catheter. Identify some areas you would consider before making this decision.

6. You have a client who is generally healthy but has been constipated for many years. List several factors that predispose a person to constipation. Identify some nursing interventions that might assist her.

7. Your patient is comatose and has not had a bowel movement for 5 days. On the sixth day she has several episodes of diarrhea.
   a. Identify the bowel elimination problem you suspect.
   b. How will you assess for this problem?
   c. Identify nursing measures to correct the problem.
   d. How will you prevent it from reoccurring?

8. Your client tells you she is having black tarry stools. What are the possible causes of this and how would you assess for them?

9. Your client is going to surgery for an ileostomy.
   a. Describe the psychological implications of this alteration in body structure and function.
   b. What would you expect the stool to be like, considering the portion of the bowel affected?
   c. Describe a nursing care plan for a person with an ileostomy.

10. Describe several ways that urinary and bowel elimination might be affected in
   a. The small child.
   b. The elderly person.
   c. The severely ill person.

Glossary

Acholic stool: A stool without bile pigments; one that is grayish-white or clay colored indicating liver or gallbladder disease.

Bacteriuria: Bacteria in the urine.

Benign prostatic hypertrophy: The enlargement of the prostate gland.

Calculi: Stones, such as kidney stones.

Colostomy: A surgical opening into the colon for drainage of colonic contents.

Constipation: Infrequent passage of hard dry stool.

Cystitis: Inflammation of the bladder.

Defecation: The act of eliminating feces from the rectum.

Diarrhea: Frequent passage of loose, watery stools.

Diuresis: An increase in production and elimination of urine; polyuria.

Dysuria: Painful urination.

Fecal impaction: A mass of hard stool in the rectum which the person is unable to pass.

Flatus or flatulence: Gas that occurs in the stomach or intestines.

Glycosuria: Glucose in the urine.

Hematuria: Blood in the urine.

Ileostomy: A surgical opening into the ileum for drainage of intestinal contents.

Incontinence (urinary): Involuntary voiding.

Intermittent self-catheterization (ISC): The process of catheterizing oneself on a specific schedule.

Kegel exercises: Exercises that strengthen the perineal muscles.

Micturition: Voiding; emptying the bladder of urine.

Neurogenic incontinence: Inability to control bowel and bladder function, related to neurological disease or trauma.

Nocturia: Voiding during the night.

Oliguria: Scanty elimination of urine; caused by retention or inadequate urine production.

Polyuria: An increase in production and elimination of urine; diuresis.

Proteinuria: Protein in the urine.

Sitz bath: A warm therapeutic tub bath.

Specific gravity: The ratio of the weight of the urine to that of an equal volume of distilled water.

Stoma: An artificially created opening such as in a colostomy or ileostomy.

Stress urinary incontinence (SUI): Loss of urine involuntarily during activities that cause an increased abdominal pressure, *i.e.,* sneezing, coughing, laughing.

Tenesmus: An involuntary, ineffectual straining at stool or micturition.

Ureteritis: Inflammation of the ureter(s).

Urethritis: Inflammation of the urethra.

Urge incontinence (urinary): Inability to control the bladder and urethral functions voluntarily.

Urinary retention: The state in which the person is able to produce urine but is unable to eliminate it.

Voiding: Micturition; emptying the bladder of urine.

Bibliography

Altshuler A, Meyer J, Butz MKJ: Even children can learn to do clean self-catheterization. Am J Nurs 77, No. 1:97–101, Jan 1977

Aman RA: Treating the patient, not the constipation. Am J Nurs 80, No. 9:1634–1635, Sept 1980

Bates R: A trouble shooter's guide to indwelling catheters. RN 44, No. 3:62–68, Mar 1981

Battle EH, Hanna CE: Evaluation of a dietary regimen for chronic constipation. J Gerontol Nurs Vol 6, No. 9:527–532, Sept 1980

Beber CR: Freedom for the incontinent. Am J Nurs 80, No. 3:482–484, Mar 1980

Belfy L: Be Aware of the Urinary Catheter, 2nd rev ed. Ann Arbor, Renal Disease Control Program, Towsley Center for Continuing Medical Education, University of Michigan, 1975

Bielski M: Preventing infection in the catheterized patient. Nurs Clin North Am 15, No. 4:703–713, Dec 1980

Bradley GM: Fecal analysis; Much more than an unpleasant necessity. Diagn Med March/April: 64–72, 1980

Brink C: Urinary continence/incontinence, Assessing the problem. Geriatric Nurs 1, No. 4:241–245, 275, Nov/Dec 1980

Bromley B: Applying Orem's self-care theory in enterostomal therapy. Am J Nurs 80, No. 2:245–249, Feb 1980

Bond JH, Levitt MD: Gaseousness and intestinal gas. Med Clin North Am 62, No. 1:155–164, Jan 1978

Butts PA: Assessing urinary incontinence in women. Nurs 79 9, No. 3:72–74, Mar 1979

Cannon WB: Bodily Changes in Pain, Hunger, Fear and Rage, 2nd ed. New York, Appleton, 1929

Chalifoux P: Recognizing warning time: A critical step toward continence. Geriatric Nurs 1, No. 4:254–255, Nov/Dec, 1980

Demmerle B, Bartol MA: Nursing care for the incontinent person. Geriatric Nurs 1, No. 4:246–250, 275, Nov/Dec 1980

Field MA: Urinary incontinence in the elderly: An overview. J Gerontol Nurs 5, No. 1:12–19, Jan/Feb 1979

Flath CI: The Miracle Nutrient. New York, M Evans, 1975

Gallagher AM: Body image changes in the patient with a colostomy. Nurs Clin North Am 7, No. 4:669–676, Dec 1972

Johnson JH: Rehabilitative aspects of neurologic bladder dysfunction. Nurs Clin North Am 15, No. 2:293–307, June 1980

King RB, Dudas S: Rehabilitation of patients with spinal cord injury. Nurs Clin North Am 15, No. 2:225–243, June 1980

Kinney AB, Blount M: Effect of cranberry juice on urinary pH, Nurs Res 28, No. 5:287–290, Sept/Oct 1979

Kinney AB, Blount M, Dowell M: Urethral catheterization. Geriatric Nurs 258–263, Nov/Dec 1980

Kroner K: Are you prepared for your ulcerative colitis patient? Nurs 80 43–49, Apr 1980

Lapides J: Pathophysiology of urinary tract infections. J U of M Med Center J, Ann Arbor, Mich 30, No. 3:103–112, 1973

Lapides J: Neurogenic bladder: Principles of treatment. J Urol Clin North Am 1, No. 1:81–97, 1974

Lapides J, et al: Clean, intermittent self-catheterization in the treatment of urinary tract disease. J Urol 107, No. 3:458–461, Mar 1972

Lapides J, Diokno AC, Lowe BS et al: Followup on unsterile, intermittent self-catheterization. Trans Am Assoc Genitourin Surg 65:44–47, 1973

Lapides J, Diokno AC, Gould FR et al: Further observations on self-catheterization. Trans Am Assoc Genitourin Surg 67:15–17, 1975

Mandelstam D: Special techniques: Strengthening pelvic floor muscles. Geriatric Nurs 251–254, Nov/Dec 1980

Matseshe JW, Phillips SF: Chronic diarrhea, A practical approach. Med Clin North Am 62, No. 1:141–153, Jan 1978

Mendeloff AI: Dietary fiber and gastrointestinal diseases. Med Clin North Am 62, No. 1:165–171, Jan 1978

Miller J: The Body In Question. New York, Random House, 1978

Mowad J: Pyuria: Guide to management. Hosp Med 15, No. 12:34–37, Dec 1979

Oberst MT, Graham D, Geller NL et al: Catheter management programs and postoperative urinary dysfunction. Res Nurs Health 4, No. 1:175–181, Mar 1981

Reinarz JA: Nosocomical Infections. Clin Symposia (Ciba) 30, No. 6:2–32, 1978

Robinson CH, Lawler MR: Normal and Therapeutic Nutrition, 15th ed. New York, Macmillan, 1977

Roth P: Portnoy's Complaint. New York, Random House, 1967

Stamm WE: Guidelines for prevention of catheter-associated urinary tract infections. Ann Intern Med 82:386–390, 1975

Suitor CW, Hunter MF: Nutrition: Principles and Application in Health Promotion. Philadelphia, JB Lippincott, 1980

Thiroloix J: Constipation: Its Causes and Cures. New York, St Martin's Press, 1976

Thomas B: Problem solving: Urinary incontinence in the elderly. J Gerontol Nurs 6, No. 9:533–536, Sept 1980

Turck M: Urinary tract infections. Hosp Pract 15, No. 1:49–58, Jan 1980

Vander AJ, Sherman JH, Luciano DS: Human Physiology: The Mechanism of Body Function, 3rd ed. New York, McGraw-Hill, 1980

Vigliarolo D: Managing bowel incontinence in children with meningomyelocele. Am J Nurs 80, No. 1:105–107, 1980

Watt RC: Colostomy irrigation, Yes or no? Am J Nurs 77, No. 3:442–444, Mar 1977

Wells T, Brink C: Helpful Equipment. Geriatric Nurs 1, No. 4:264–267, Nov/Dec 1980

Wells T: Promoting urine control in older adults, Scope of the problem. Geriatric Nurs 1, No. 4:236–240, 275, Nov/Dec 1980

Wichita D: Treating and preventing constipation in nursing home residents. J Gerontol Nurs 3, No. 6:35–39, Dec 1977

Wilpizeski MD: Helping the ostomate return to normal life. Nurs 81 11, No. 3:62–66, Mar 1981

Wu Y, Hamilton BB, Boyink MA et al: Reusable catheter for long-term sterile intermittent catheterization. Arch Phys Med Rehabil 62, No. 1:39–42, Jan 1981

Sepsis Associated with Indwelling Urinary Catheters, Clin Symposia (Ciba) 30, No. 6:

Yeates WR: Normal and abnormal bladder function in the incontinence of urine. In Willington FS (ed): Incontinence in the Elderly, p 29. London, Academic Press, 1976

Fluid and Electrolyte Status

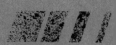

Ann Z. Kruszewski

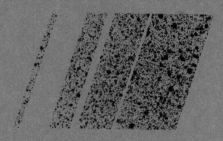

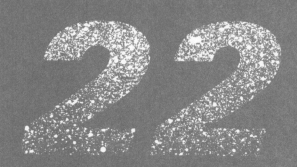

22

Because water is as essential as air for our survival, maintaining fluid and electrolyte balance is an important factor in our health status. Stressors that affect body water and body chemistry surround us. Even simple acts such as eating a salty meal or perspiring heavily can function as stressors to fluid and electrolyte balance. Imbalances can affect a wide range of people, from the small child who is vomiting to the adult who takes diuretic medications, as well as almost any seriously ill person.

Because so many persons are potentially affected by fluid and electrolyte problems, nurses must be knowledgeable about the means of promoting and restoring balanced body chemistry. They must also be able to teach preventive measures to persons with potential fluid and electrolyte needs. This chapter presents the basic adaptive mechanisms that maintain balanced body chemistry and describe common imbalances. It also assists beginning nurses in using the nursing process to assess and intervene in meeting a person's fluid and electrolyte needs.

After completing this chapter, students will be able to:

- *Identify the normal composition and distribution of body fluid.*

- *Identify the function of electrolytes.*

- *List normal routes by which fluid and electrolytes are gained and lost.*

- *Identify adaptive mechanisms that maintain fluid and electrolyte balance.*

- *Assess the person's fluid and electrolyte status using interview and physical examination skills.*

- *Use laboratory values to analyze fluid and electrolyte status.*

- *Use nursing process to assist persons with fluid and electrolyte imbalances.*

- *Describe nursing care of persons receiving intravenous therapy.*

Basic Principles of Fluid and Electrolyte Balance

Body Water

Water is the principal constituent of the body, composing approximately 60% of an adult's weight. There are two major compartments for body water: extracellular and intracellular. The intracellular compartment is located inside the body cells and contains intracellular fluid (ICF), which consists of water and dissolved substances and is important for cellular metabolism. The extracellular compartment is located outside of body cells and contains the extracellular fluid (ECF). The ECF compartment can be subdivided into the plasma compartment (containing fluid within the blood vessels) and the interstitial fluid compartment (containing fluid surrounding the cells). Interstitial and plasma fluid have the same electrolyte composition; however, plasma fluid has significantly more protein.

Adaptive Mechanisms for Water Balance

Mechanisms that maintain water balance are listed in Table 22-1. These mechanisms not only control fluid gain and loss but also maintain balance between the fluid compartments. Only a brief explanation of the mechanisms is included here; for more information the reader should consult a physiology textbook.

Osmosis. One of the principal mechanisms which controls fluid distribution is osmosis. **Osmosis** is the passage of water through a semipermeable membrane from an area of low concentration of dissolved molecules to an area of high concentration of dissolved molecules. In other words, water moves toward its concentration gradient, passing through a membrane to the area of lower water concentration. Cell membranes and capillary walls act as semipermeable membranes in the body. In the extracellular fluid the dissolved molecules that exert **osmotic pressure** are chiefly sodium and protein. Water moves across the body's semipermeable membranes depending on the relative osmotic pressure of the intracellular, plasma, and interstitial compartments. This process is referred to in discussions of sodium imbalances and intravenous therapy.

Filtration. The cardiovascular system has a major effect on fluid distribution between the plasma and interstitial fluid compartments. **Filtration** force, also known as capillary hydrostatic pressure, is exerted by the force of fluid within the capillaries against the vessel walls. This force moves fluid out of the capillaries and into the interstitial compartment. If capillary hydrostatic pressure rises and is not compensated for, edema results.

ADH and Thirst. The kidneys are able to adjust urine volume to meet the body's needs through the action of antidiuretic hormone (ADH). Another important mechanism regulating fluid volume is thirst. Often we take this process for granted because it is so natural for us to respond to thirst by drinking. However, certain individuals, such as those who are unconscious or elderly, may not be aware of thirst or may be too helpless to respond to thirst by drinking. These persons can easily become dehydrated if nurses are not alert to their fluid needs.

Table 22-1
Adaptive Mechanisms for Water and Electrolyte Balance

	Mechanism	*Function*
Water Balance	Osmosis	Influences water movement between the three fluid compartments
	Filtration	Influences water movement between the plasma and interstitial compartments
	Antidiuretic hormone (ADH)	Affects osmolality of ECF; increased ADH secretion causes the kidneys to conserve water
	Thirst	Regulates water intake; thirst center in the hypothalamus responds to increased ECF osmolality by producing thirst sensation
Electrolyte Balance	Diffusion	Influences distribution of electrolytes among the three fluid compartments
	Active transport	Affects distribution of electrolytes between ICF and ECF
	Aldosterone	Affects sodium balance
	Parathyroid hormone	Affects calcium balance

Electrolytes

An **electrolyte** is a substance that has an electrical charge when dissolved in water. Electrolytes have three important functions. First, they exert osmotic pressure and thereby influence the distribution of water among the three fluid compartments. Secondly, they play an important role in neuromuscular function. The concentrations of sodium, potassium, and calcium affect resting membrane potential in nerve and muscle cells. Finally, electrolytes are important in metabolic functions within the cell. For instance, potassium and phosphorus are crucial to metabolism of carbohydrates and amino acids.

Adaptive Mechanisms for Electrolyte Balance

The mechanisms that contribute to total electrolyte balance are listed in Table 22-1 and consist of diffusion, active transport, and the effects of aldosterone and parathyroid hormone. Each is discussed here briefly.

Diffusion and Active Transport
Electrolytes, like water, are able to move between the fluid compartments. This is accomplished by the process of **diffusion,** in which random movements of ions cause them to be distributed equally as they move from areas of high concentration to areas of low concentration.

In spite of diffusion, the extracellular and intracellular compartments are very different in their electrolyte composition. This difference occurs because certain ions (chiefly sodium and potassium) are moved across cell membranes by **active transport.** This process involves movement from areas of low concentration to high concentration, just the opposite of diffusion. Active transport is responsible for sodium being the chief **cation** in the ECF, whereas potassium is the chief cation in the ICF. These differences are important for normal nerve and muscle function.

Aldosterone and Parathyroid Hormone
Aldosterone and parathyroid hormone affect the balance of sodium and calcium, respectively, by influencing renal reabsorption of these electrolytes. Aldosterone, the hormone that regulates sodium balance, also indirectly affects water and potassium balance as well.

Routes of Fluid and Electrolyte Gain and Loss

Normal fluid intake and output averages about 2500 ml daily. The sources of fluid intake include oral fluids, solid foods, and oxidation. Fluid output occurs through urine, lungs, feces, and skin. The average daily value for each of these routes is listed in Table 22-2.

Fluid intake from solid food and metabolism cannot be detected easily, so it is sometimes called *insensible gain*. Fluid that is eliminated through the lungs, gastrointestinal tract, and perspiration is sometimes called *insensible loss*. Notice that in health, fluid intake from insensible routes is nearly equal to insensible loss. This usually allows us to assess fluid balance by measuring oral fluid intake and urinary output.

Electrolytes are taken in through solid food and liquids and eliminated through perspiration, urine, and the gastrointestinal tract.

In illness, any of the routes of insensible loss can become a significant source of fluid or electrolyte depletion. For instance, diarrhea can cause a significant amount of water, bicarbonate, sodium, and potassium to be lost through the gastrointestinal tract. There may also be unusual routes of fluid and electrolyte gain or loss in illness, such as through intravenous therapy, wound drainage, and vomiting. It is therefore important to note any unusual sources of loss or gain when analyzing a person's potential risk for fluid or electrolyte disturbances.

Acid and Base Balance

Before beginning a discussion of acid–base balance, let us review the following definitions.

- **Acid**—any molecule or ion that can donate a proton or hydrogen ion
- **Base**—any molecule or ion that can accept a proton or hydrogen ion

- **pH**—negative logarithm of the hydrogen ion concentration (*e.g.*, H+ concentration of .0000001 = *p*H of 7; *p*H greater than 7.0 is basic; *p*H less than 7.0 is acidic)

pH. Acid–base balance means regulation of hydrogen ion concentration of body fluids. Hydrogen ion concentration is expressed in terms of *p*H. The body maintains a very narrow *p*H range. Normally *p*H of body fluids ranges from 7.35 to 7.45. A *p*H of less than 6.8 or more than 7.8 can result in death. Because careful maintenance of hydrogen ion balance is so essential to life, there are several adaptive mechanisms that regulate *p*H. These are the **Buffer** systems, the lungs, and the kidneys. Let us discuss each of these mechanisms briefly.

Buffer Systems. The buffer systems are the body's first line of defense against changes in *p*H. They react within seconds to alterations in hydrogen ion concentration. Buffers act like chemical sponges to release or absorb hydrogen ions depending on the body's needs. Buffer systems consist of a weak base and a weak acid. The body has several buffer systems, but the one that is used in the clinical laboratory to assess acid–base balance is the bicarbonate–carbonic acid buffer pair.

Bicarbonate (HCO_3^-) is a weak base. Most bicarbonate is found in the form of sodium bicarbonate. Carbonic acid is a weak acid. It is a "carrier" for carbon dioxide because carbon dioxide combines with water to form carbonic acid under the influence of carbonic anhydrase.

$$H_2O + CO_2 \rightarrow H_2CO_3$$

How does the bicarbonate–carbonic acid buffer system work? First, imagine that a strong acid,

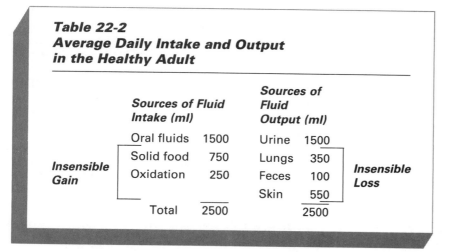

Table 22-2
Average Daily Intake and Output in the Healthy Adult

	Sources of Fluid Intake (ml)		Sources of Fluid Output (ml)		
Insensible Gain	Oral fluids	1500	Urine	1500	**Insensible Loss**
	Solid food	750	Lungs	350	
	Oxidation	250	Feces	100	
			Skin	550	
	Total	2500		2500	

hydrochloric acid, is introduced into the body. The base, sodium bicarbonate, combines with the hydrogen ions released by the strong acid. This results in a weak acid, carbonic acid, and a salt, sodium chloride.

$$NaHCO_3 + HCl \rightarrow H_2CO_3 + NaCl$$

Carbonic acid, as a weak acid, releases fewer hydrogen ions, causing a less drastic change in pH. In this way the body is protected from a dangerously low pH.

Respiratory Mechanism. The lungs are the body's second line of defense against changes in pH. They react within minutes of alterations in hydrogen ion concentration. The lungs can adjust pH by conserving or excreting carbon dioxide. In acidosis, bicarbonate (base buffer) combines with hydrogen ions to form carbonic acid. The formation of carbonic acid is adaptive because it takes up hydrogen ions. Carbonic acid then dissociates to form carbon dioxide and water. The lungs eliminate carbon dioxide, thus raising the pH. The equation below illustrates this process.

$$Excess\ H^+ + HCO_3^-\ (base\ buffer) \rightarrow$$
$$H_2CO_3 \rightarrow CO_2 + H_2O$$

Hydrogen ions stimulate the respiratory center, causing the lungs to eliminate carbon dioxide through rapid, deep respirations.

If body fluids become more alkaline, the lungs conserve carbon dioxide. This reverses the equation shown above and makes more hydrogen ions available, lowering the pH. The bicarbonate produced is excreted by the kidneys.

$$CO_2 + H_2O \rightarrow H_2CO_3 \rightarrow HCO_3^- + H^+$$

Renal Mechanism. The kidneys are the third line of defense against changes in pH. The kidneys can conserve or excrete hydrogen and bicarbonate ions. In the case of a low pH, hydrogen ions are excreted and bicarbonate conserved. If the pH begins to rise, the kidneys save hydrogen ions and excrete bicarbonate.

Henderson–Hasselbach Equation. Let us now pull together what we know about the body's adaptive mechanisms by looking at the Henderson–Hasselbach equation.

$$pH = pK + \log \frac{(HCO_3^-)}{(H_2CO_3)}$$

This equation tells us that pH of body fluid depends on the ratio of bicarbonate to carbonic acid. The pK is the negative logarithm of the dissociation constant for carbonic acid. Because it is constant, it does not affect the relationship between pH and carbonic acid or bicarbonate.

The ratio of bicarbonate to carbonic acid is normally 20:1

$$Normal\ pH\ depends\ on\ \frac{(HCO_3^-)}{(H_2CO_3)} = \frac{20}{1}$$

As long as this ratio stays the same, the serum pH remains normal. For instance, the concentration of bicarbonate may increase, but as long as the concentration of H_2CO_3 increases proportionately, the 20:1 ratio is preserved and the pH remains normal. Bicarbonate concentration is regulated by the kidneys. Carbonic acid (in the form of CO_2) is regulated by the lungs. The regulation of acid–base balance is referred to later in the chapter when acid–base disturbances are discussed.

General Assessment of Fluid and Electrolyte Status

Assessment is one of the most important functions the nurse performs for anyone with fluid and electrolyte needs. Data collection involves nearly all of the body systems because imbalances affect most other functions. Here are some general areas to examine when assessing a person's fluid and electrolyte balance. Specific signs and symptoms associated with fluid and electrolyte problems are described in the next section.

Illnesses, Drug Therapy, Abnormal Routes of Fluid Loss or Gain. Certain fluid or electrolyte imbalances are associated with particular health problems or therapy. For instance, diuretic therapy can lead to potassium depletion; heart failure is associated with fluid overload.

Lab Values. Values for sodium, potassium, chloride, bicarbonate, or other significant electrolytes should be noted. Consult the normal ranges of the laboratory because these values vary among institutions. Another laboratory value, **Specific gravity,** reflects the concentration of urine and is a measure of the kidneys' ability to adjust output to meet the person's fluid needs. The healthy kidney excretes more concentrated urine when fluid depletion occurs. Chapter 21 (Elimination) offers further explanation of urine specific gravity.

Level of Consciousness. Since fluid and electrolyte disturbances affect neurological function, apathy, confusion, or stupor may occur in certain imbalances.

Muscle Tonus. Fatigue, muscle spasms, or flabby muscle tone may be indications of electrolyte disturbances. Normal concentrations of sodium, potassium, and calcium are essential for normal muscle function.

Tissue Hydration. Thirst, edema, dry oral mucosa, or poor skin **turgor** are signs to note as indications of fluid imbalance.

Intake and Output or Body Weight Changes. Intake and output was mentioned earlier in the chapter as a means of assessing fluid balance. The importance of accurate measurement of intake and output cannot be emphasized enough. Unfortunately, amounts are often estimated; this practice does not provide reliable information for assessing fluid balance. If it is difficult to measure intake and output precisely, the person should be weighed daily, a more accurate method of detecting fluid loss or gain. Body weight is especially useful if fluid loss or gain occurs from insensible routes such as profuse perspiration or a draining wound. A weight change of 2 pounds represents approximately 1 liter of fluid.

Respiratory Rate and Depth. Altered respirations may be seen in acid or base disturbances. This assessment is discussed in more depth later in the chapter.

Other Vital Signs. Pulse, blood pressure, and temperature may be affected by fluid and electrolyte disturbances, since body temperature regulation is related to fluid balance, and myocardial function is influenced by electrolyte imbalances, which can alter the pulse or blood pressure.

Nursing Process
Applied to Specific Fluid and Electrolyte Problems

There are so many potential causes of fluid and electrolyte disturbance that almost any one is susceptible to these problems. Often we are concerned about fluid and electrolyte problems in those who are seriously ill, such as persons with cardiac, respiratory, or renal disease or patients recovering from surgery. However, the woman receiving diuretics, the teenager on a fad diet, the infant with diarrhea, or the elderly person who is not eating or drinking properly are also potential candidates for possible fluid and electrolyte disturbance.

Since nurses are often the health-care providers who spend the most time with the person, they are often the first to detect changes that may indicate the early stages of a problem. Although the treatment of fluid and electrolyte problems is usually determined by the physician, the importance of nursing assessment in the prevention of serious disturbances and the analysis of the person's response to therapy cannot be overemphasized.

General Nursing Interventions

This section presents only the more common fluid and electrolyte disturbances along with specific nursing interventions for each. However, the general nursing care for persons experiencing fluid and electrolyte imbalances is the same, no matter what the specific problem. The following suggestions may be used in planning nursing care (see also Table 22-3).

* Determine whether any factors are present that can alter fluid or electrolyte balance (*e.g.*, medications, disease processes).

* Assess signs, symptoms, and laboratory values for indications of fluid or electrolyte needs, including signs that an existing problem is worsening or improving.

* Communicate with the physician about abnormal labaoratory values or findings. Many times the nurse is the first to detect these changes.

* Monitor intravenous or medication therapy carefully. Be alert for opportunities to teach the client self-care abilities (*e.g.*, diet or medication teaching).

* Be alert to nutrition in clients with fluid and electrolyte needs. Some problems can be prevented by adequate fluid intake or nutritional planning.

Table 22-3
Nursing Intervention for Fluid and Electrolyte Problems

- Determine whether any factors are present that can alter fluid or electrolyte balance (*e.g.,* medications, disease processes).

- Assess signs, symptoms, and laboratory values for indications of fluid or electrolyte needs, including signs that an existing problem is worsening or improving.

- Communicate with the physician about abnormal laboratory values or findings. Many times the nurse is the first to detect these changes.

- Monitor intravenous or medication therapy carefully. Be alert for opportunities to teach the client self-care abilities (*e.g.,* diet or medication teaching).

- Be alert to nutrition in clients with fluid and electrolyte needs. Some problems can be prevented by adequate fluid intake or nutrition planning.

- Monitor intake and output carefully. This is an independent nursing function and should be done for any person with potential fluid imbalances.

- Monitor intake and output carefully. This is an independent nursing function and should be done for any person with potential fluid imbalance.

Extracellular Fluid Volume Deficit

Extracellular fluid volume deficit results from an **isotonic** fluid loss, or loss of both water and electrolytes in the same proportion as they occur in extracellular fluid. ECF deficit is commonly called *dehydration* or *hypovolemia;* these terms are often used interchangeably.

Certain clues from the person's history may suggest a possible fluid deficit. Dehydration can develop when there has been insufficient fluid intake such as may occur with nausea, loss of appetite (**anorexia**), or restricted intake. It can also develop when there is abnormal body fluid loss, such as from vomiting, diarrhea, prolonged fever, profuse perspiration, or surgical drainage. Age may also be a contributing factor to dehydration. Confused elderly persons may not drink enough water to meet their needs, compounding the fluid depletion that normally occurs with age when the percentage of total body water decreases. In addition, the ability of older people to conserve water by concentrating urine is also decreased. Thus, older persons are especially prone to dehydration. Infants and young children may also become easily dehydrated because they may not be able to communicate thirst.

Assessment

The nurse must be able to recognize early signs of dehydration. A rapid weight loss is often due to fluid depletion rather than reduced body fat. **Oliguria** (decreased urine output) can also be a sign of dehydration as a result of the kidney's attempt to conserve water in order to balance fluid lost through other routes. Thus the urine is more concentrated as indicated by its dark amber color and its high specific gravity. The person may have dry oral mucous membranes and experience thirst. The skin may also be dry and less elastic and there may be an elevation in temperature reflecting a decrease in total body fluid (Grant and Kubo, 1975).

In severe dehydration the person may feel weak and lethargic and appear gaunt and drawn. The loss of fluid from facial tissue makes the eyes appear sunken and the face look drawn. In its most serious stage fluid deficit leads to shock or renal failure due to severely decreased blood volume.

Hemoglobin and hematocrit may be higher in the dehydrated person because of a change in the concentration of red blood cells. Recall that hemoglobin and hematocrit are expressed as concentrations of hemoglobin or red cells in relation to total blood volume. As blood volume shrinks due to dehydration, erythrocytes become more concentrated. This phenomenon is known as *hemoconcentration*. The BUN (amount of urea nitrogen in the serum) may also be elevated for the same reason (Grant and Kubo, 1975).

Nursing Interventions

The nurse's first responsibility is prevention of dehydration. This means careful assessment of any person who is prone to fluid deficit. As indicated in the preceding section, any susceptible person in the hospital should be monitored for intake and output or weighed on a daily basis. Urine specific gravity should also be assessed to allow early detection of any trends indicating fluid loss. For instance, large fluid loss from gastric suctioning accompanied by scanty output of dark, concentrated urine is a good indication of dehydration.

Encouraging oral fluid is an important intervention in preventing dehydration or restoring fluid balance (Fig. 22-1). Including the person in planning by determining what kinds of liquids he likes (within diet restrictions) and asking when he would like to receive them will result in more successful outcomes. However, if the person is vomiting, oral fluids should not be encouraged, especially plain water, which would wash electrolytes from the stomach during a vomiting episode and thereby cause hyponatremia (discussed further under Sodium Deficit).

Intravenous infusions may be an important part of fluid replacement therapy as prescribed by the physician. Nursing responsibilities for persons receiving intravenous infusions are discussed in a later section.

Mouth and skin care are also important in the presence of a fluid deficit. Dry oral mucous membranes are prone to cracking and thus are susceptible to infection, especially if fluid intake is restricted by an NPO order or if the person is breathing through his mouth. To help lubricate the oral mucous membranes, the person should brush his teeth twice daily and rinse the mouth between brushing. Lemon and glycerine swabs or swabs dipped in a peroxide and saline solution may also help moisten the mouth, depending on the individual's preferences. If the skin is dry, an emollient lotion can be applied several times daily.

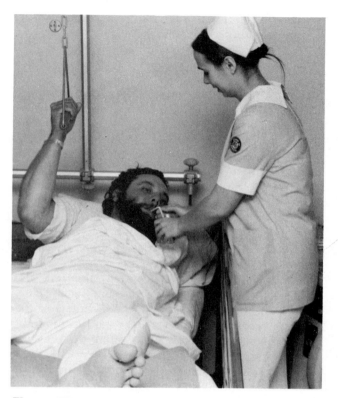

Figure 22-1
Assisting with fluid intake.

Extracellular Fluid Volume Excess

Extracellular fluid volume excess is an isotonic fluid gain; that is, both water and electrolytes are increased in the same proportion as they occur in body fluids. ECF excess is commonly called *overhydration*. Circulatory overload is a form of extracellular fluid excess.

ECF excess is caused by an increased intake or decreased output of fluid. Increased intake may be the result of excessive intravenous fluids, such as may occur when IV therapy is given to someone who has decreased kidney or heart function or to an elderly person with diminished renal and cardiac reserve due to aging. Small children are also susceptible to this problem because extracellular volume is small compared to that of adults and they cannot tolerate volume increases as easily as adults.

Decreased fluid output may also cause overhydration. This condition may occur in renal disease in which the kidneys are unable to excrete sufficient urine volume. It may also occur in cardiac disease such as congestive heart failure in which decreased cardiac output initiates a chain of hormone activity causing sodium and water retention.

Assessment

The most obvious sign of fluid overload is **edema,** that is, accumulation of fluid in the interstitial space. As blood volume increases (*e.g.,* in cardiac or renal disease) capillary hydrostatic pressure rises. In this state there is greater force moving fluid out of the capillaries than the tissue forces moving fluid into capillaries; the net result is fluid accumulation in the tissues. Assessment of edema is described in Chapter 23.

Edema may also occur in pulmonary tissue from fluid accumulating in the lungs. Pulmonary edema interferes with oxygen and carbon dioxide exchange in the alveoli, resulting in **dyspnea.** As a reflection of this condition, the person may state, "I can't catch my breath," or may wake up in the night feeling that he can't breathe. The presence of fluid in the lungs can be detected as **rales** or by noting the presence of a moist-sound cough.

Even before edema is evident, a rapid weight gain may indicate that the person is retaining fluid. An alert nurse would note any such gain as a possible clue to fluid retention because an increase in weight of 10 pounds or 5 kg (representing 5 liters of fluid) may occur before edema is visible. Another sign of fluid gain is distended neck veins (Fig. 22-2). The jugular veins enter directly into the superior vena cava, which in turn empties into the right atrium.

Figure 22-2
Distended neck veins in ECF excess.

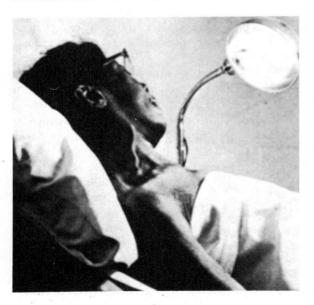

Pressure from excessive fluid volume is transmitted backward from the heart into the jugular veins, which then become enlarged.

Severe fluid gain may also cause increased blood pressure, as well as changes in hemoglobin and hematocrit. The latter values may decrease because of hemodilution, because excess fluid volume results in a lower percentage of red blood cells per unit of plasma.

Nursing Interventions

Ongoing Assessment. As with fluid deficit, nursing interventions are vital in preventing fluid overload. Assessment skills are crucial in detecting early changes of fluid gain. Intake exceeding output over several days with a consistent weight gain of ½ to 1 pound daily may indicate overhydration. Persons who are susceptible to fluid overloads should be monitored carefully for the signs and symptoms just discussed.

The chances of fluid overload in persons receiving intravenous infusions can be reduced by monitoring carefully the flow rate of the solution and by being alert to signs or symptoms of too rapid infusion (Fig. 22-3). Since fluid overload develops quickly in this situation, signs of pulmonary edema may be evident. Pulmonary edema can be a life-threatening problem, a fact which underscores the importance of careful management of intravenous therapy.

Diuretics. Persons who are in a state of fluid overload are often managed with diuretics. Assessing intake and output or body weight is one way of monitoring response to this treatment. Some diuretics cause increased potassium loss, so the person may need instruction on dietary sources of this electrolyte.

Fluid Restriction. The physician may decide to restrict oral fluid intake. Including the person in planning fluid intake is essential if these restrictions are to be acceptable. Informing him of the purpose of the restriction and identifying the amount of the fluid allowed in terms of cups or glasses of liquid per day, and then determining when he would like to have fluids, what type he enjoys, and how he would like them served—all serve as a means of promoting self care and enhancing an understanding of the regimen.

Sodium Restriction. Sodium restrictions in the diet may also be part of treatment. Therefore, the person may need information about which foods are

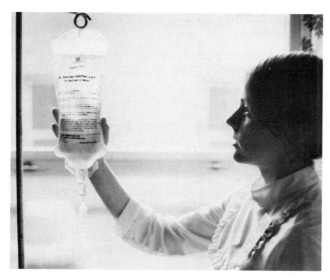

Figure 22-3
Monitoring IV therapy. Nurse carefully checks solution label on plastic parenteral solution container.

high in sodium (*i.e.,* most snack foods, lunchmeat, pickles, catsup, and mustard). He may also need support to eliminate high-sodium foods and table salt from his diet. Suggesting herbs or spices that add taste to unsalted food or referring him to resources in the community that teach low-sodium meal preparation constitute helpful nursing measures to ensure adherence. However, before recommending one of the salt substitutes on the market, check with the physician. These products are high in potassium and may be contraindicated if the fluid overload problem is due to renal disease.

Hyponatremia

Hyponatremia is a sodium deficit in the extracellular fluid. Sodium, as the major cation of the extracellular fluid, is an extremely important electrolyte. Some basic facts about sodium may help explain the physiological mechanism underlying hyponatremia.

- Intake occurs through natural sodium content in food and table salt. Normal adult sodium requirement is 2 g to 6 g/day.
- Output occurs through urine, feces, and perspiration. Bile, pancreatic secretions, and gastric secretions contain significant amounts of sodium.
- Aldosterone regulates sodium balance.
- Normal serum sodium ranges from 137 to 147 mEq/liter.

- Sodium is essential for the normal function of nerve and muscle cells.
- Sodium maintains extracellular osmolarity; as sodium is excreted, so is water.
- Sodium affects fluid balance between extracellular and intracellular compartments; as sodium is lost from the ECF, osmolarity decreases causing water to move into cells.
- Sodium maintains acid–base balance together with bicarbonate.

Sodium deficit can be caused by decreased sodium intake and increased sodium loss. It can also come about through gains in water without a corresponding increase in sodium. This occurs because excessive water dilutes existing sodium, causing decreased sodium concentration. The concentration of body sodium, rather than the amount, determines whether an imbalance exists.

Causes. Clinical conditions which can cause hyponatremia include the following:

- *Heat exhaustion.* Profuse perspiration followed by drinking large amounts of plain water causes sodium deficit. Sodium lost through sweat is not replaced.
- *Brain injury or tumor.* Inappropriate secretion of ADH by the injured brain causes water retention in excess of sodium.
- *Repeated tap water enemas or irrigation of nasogastric tubes with water.* Water is gained through GI absorption without corresponding gain in sodium. Sodium is also drawn from the mucosa and lost through the nasogastric tube or as the enema is expelled.
- *Prolonged administration of dextrose and water intravenous solution.* This causes water gain in excess of sodium.
- *Trauma or major surgery.* The physical stress of surgery or trauma increases ADH secretion, causing water retention in excess of sodium.

Assessment

Signs and symptoms of hyponatremia should be assessed in any susceptible person, in order to detect this imbalance as early as possible. The findings in hyponatremia include the following:

- Apprehension, anxiety, restlessness, confusion
- Convulsions
- Anorexia

- Nausea
- Diarrhea
- Oliguria
- Serum sodium less than 137 mEq/liter
- Pitting edema

Hyponatremia results in many neuromuscular symptoms because sodium is necessary for normal nerve and muscle function. When sodium is lost, there is greater concentration of water in the ECF than in the ICF. Water moves toward its concentration gradient into the cells. Thus, hyponatremia causes cells (including brain cells) to swell. This phenomenon causes behavior changes and pitting edema. Decreased extracellular sodium stimulates aldosterone secretion, causing sodium and water retention by the kidneys and decreased urine output.

Nursing Interventions

Sodium Intake. The physician determines medical treatment and may prescribe that sodium chloride be given orally or intravenously, depending on the severity of the imbalance. As a preventive measure in athletes, salt pills may be given to prevent hyponatremia from excessive perspiration. Water intake may be restricted if the problem resulted from water gain in excess of sodium.

Fluid Intake. Because hyponatremia is a possible complication in persons with nasogastric tubes, the nurse can prevent this imbalance by using only isotonic solutions for irrigation. If ice chips are used to moisten the mouth, the nurse should caution about excessive intake, which can also cause sodium to wash from the gastric mucosa and be suctioned from the stomach. For the same reason, anyone who is vomiting should be cautioned not to drink large amounts of tap water.

It is also important to monitor fluid intake carefully and observe for symptoms of hyponatremia in persons who have experienced major surgery or head injury. In these conditions, increased ADH is secreted, causing water retention in excess of sodium. Excessive water intake could therefore lead to water overload and hyponatremia.

Hypernatremia

Hypernatremia results from increased sodium intake or a decrease in body water without a corresponding decrease in sodium.

Some causes of hypernatremia include those listed below:

- Excessive salt ingestion (*e.g.*, in the treatment of diarrhea with salt in excess)
- Decreased water intake (*e.g.*, in the unconscious person because he is unable to drink)
- Prolonged diarrhea (water lost in excess of sodium)
- Excessive administration of tube feedings (these **hypertonic** solutions cause osmotic diuresis, promoting water loss in excess of sodium)

Assessment

Hypernatremia causes increased osmolarity in the extracellular fluid because of the high concentration of sodium molecules. Increased osmolarity of the extracellular fluid results in extreme thirst and dry oral mucous membranes. The relatively high sodium level disturbs neuromuscular function and, as a result, agitated behavior, restlessness, or confusion may occur. The serum sodium measurement is elevated above 147 mEq/liter. If hypernatremia developed from a water deficit, the signs of dehydration would also be present.

Nursing Interventions

Since medical treatment involves withholding salt, the physician may order a low-sodium diet. If water deficit is the cause of hypernatremia, water replacement is indicated. Water may be replaced orally, if the deficit is mild, or intravenously if it is severe.

Nursing responsibility includes evaluating the person's response to therapy by monitoring intake and output, body weight, urine specific gravity, and lab values. Mouth care is important, to prevent oral infections. The nurse is also responsible for administering intravenous or oral fluid replacement. Suggestions for increasing oral fluid intake are the same as those discussed under Extracellular Volume Deficit. If the person requires a low-sodium diet, appropriate teaching may be necessary (discussed under Extracellular Volume Excess).

Preventive Measures. The nurse can also help to prevent hypernatremia. Persons who are receiving tube feedings or hypertonic intravenous solutions should receive adequate water to replace any losses from diuresis. Supplemental water (100–200 ml per feeding) should always be given with tube feedings. Intake and output, serum sodium values, urine specific gravity, and signs of sodium excess should be assessed in these patients. Unconscious and confused persons also need careful monitoring because they may not be capable of expressing thirst or responding to it.

Hypokalemia

Hypokalemia, or potassium deficiency of the extracellular fluid, is one of the most common electrolyte imbalances encountered by nursing personnel. Therefore, a thorough understanding of the mechanisms that maintain potassium balance is essential for effective nursing care.

Some basic facts about potassium will help enhance this understanding.

- Intake occurs through natural potassium content in food. Normal adult requirement is 2 g to 4 g/day.
- Potassium is absorbed in the small intestine.
- Output occurs chiefly through urine and the gastrointestinal tract. About 50 mEq or 5% of the body's supply of potassium is lost daily.
- Normal serum potassium ranges from 3.5 to 5.0 mEq/liter.
- Potassium maintains the normal function of nerve and muscle cells.
- Potassium is necessary for synthesis of proteins and metabolism of carbohydrates.
- Potassium influences fluid balance within cells.

Because potassium is concentrated in gastrointestinal secretions, losses through diarrhea, vomiting, or gastric suctioning can result in potassium deficit. Inadequate oral intake can also lead to this imbalance. Diuretic therapy is a common cause of hypokalemia because some of these drugs promote potasssium loss along with water loss.

Assessment

Potassium is the most abundant cation in the intracellular fluid. Potassium, together with sodium and calcium, is responsible for normal nerve and muscle function. Hypokalemia stabilizes the resting membrane potential and inhibits neuromuscular excitability. Therefore, hypokalemia results in decreased neuromuscular function in every body system.

In the early stages of hypokalemia, the person may have a vague sensation of not feeling well. He may feel fatigued or appear apathetic and he may experience loss of appetite or nausea due to decreased peristalsis. In severe hypokalemia there are more serious disturbances in skeletal, muscle, cardiovascular, respiratory, and gastrointestinal function. One sign is muscle weakness and decreased muscle tone, which may be detected by noting that the muscles feel flabby (like half-filled water bottles). There may also be a weak and irregular pulse, shallow respiration, or abdominal distention due to paralytic ileus. The lab test result that confirms hypokalemia is a serum potassium level of less than 3.0 mEq/liter.

Nursing Interventions

The treatment prescribed by the physician is administration of potassium chloride by mouth or through intravenous infusion. Nurses have an essential role in recognizing and preventing hypokalemia through assessment and health teaching.

Persons at risk of developing hypokalemia, such as those taking potassium supplements, digitalis, or potent diuretics, should be carefully assessed for signs of low potassium. In each of these instances, teaching is an important intervention that assists the person in maintaining control over his health. If the person's condition permits, he should be encouraged to eat a diet that is high in potassium (bananas, oranges, and cranberry juice). Those who are taking potent diuretics should know the signs of hypokalemia and food sources of potassium. Persons taking potassium supplements should be instructed to take them with meals to decrease gastric irritation.

Nurses should be especially alert for hypokalemia in persons who are taking digitalis preparations. Anyone who is taking digitalis and has low potassium is very susceptible to digitalis toxicity, which can lead to heart block. It is important to keep this fact in mind because many persons who take digitalis are also receiving diuretics that can result in potassium loss. A knowledgeable nurse looks for potassium loss in any person receiving a potent diuretic and is alert for signs of digitalis toxicity.

Hyperkalemia

Hyperkalamia, or potassium excess, is a very dangerous imbalance, which can be life-threatening if it is severe. Renal failure is often a cause of hyperkalemia, because the failing kidneys are unable to excrete a sufficient amount of potassium. Excessive administration of potassium by intravenous infusion may cause hyperkalemia. Trauma, such as burns or crush injuries may also result in elevated serum potassium, because damaged cells release their high concentration of potassium into the extracellular fluid. Any person with these problems should be assessed carefully for possible hyperkalemia.

Assessment

Toxic levels of potassium result in abnormal neuromuscular function in every body system, causing possible numbness or tingling in the mouth or extremities (paresthesias) and muscle cramps. In addition to these sensations, the person may seem anxious, restless, or confused. Laboratory values reveal a serum potassium level that is greater than 5.0 mEq/liter. The most dangerous sign is an irregular pulse, which indicates that the person is experiencing cardiac arrhythmias. Because cardiac arrest can occur with hyperkalemia, this possibility should be anticipated in any person who has high serum potassium levels.

Nursing Interventions

The physician may prescribe a low-potassium diet along with ion exchange resins such as sodium polystyrene sulfonate (Kayexalate). This medication, which is high in sodium, is usually given as an enema. In the gastrointestinal tract sodium ions are exchanged for potassium ions. Potassium is excreted along with the resin as the enema is expelled. Peritoneal dialysis or hemodialysis may also be employed.

The nurse should recognize those who are at risk for developing hyperkalemia and assess carefully symptoms and laboratory values which may indicate this imbalance. This particularly applies to persons receiving intravenous solutions containing potassium. In these instances, the drip rate should be monitored closely to avoid excessively rapid infusion, which could lead to hyperkalemia. An adult should receive no more than 20 mEq/hr of potassium through the intravenous route. For those persons on a potassium restricted diet, nutrition teaching can help maintain potassium balance. These persons should be cautioned to avoid salt substitutes available on the market since many of these products are high in potassium.

Hypocalcemia

Hypocalcemia is a deficiency in ionized serum calcium. Calcium is the most abundant electrolyte in the body, with about 99% concentrated in bones

and teeth. The remaining 1% is very important because only ionized calcium has an effect on the neuromuscular system. Reduction in the amount of ionized calcium results in hypocalcemia (even though the actual amount of body calcium is unchanged). Other basic information about calcium includes the following:

- Intake occurs through dairy products and greens. Adult daily requirement is 800 mg/day.
- Output occurs through urine and stool. Calcium balance is associated with phosphorus levels; as phosphorus increases, calcium decreases.
- Calcium balance is regulated by parathyroid hormone, which releases calcium from bone, increases calcium reabsorption by the kidney, and increases absorption from the GI tract.
- Vitamin D is essential for calcium absorption from the GI tract.
- Normal serum calcium is 4.5 to 5.5 mEq/liter or 9 to 11 mg/100ml.
- Calcium enhances the strength and rigidity of bones and is necessary for healing fractures.
- Calcium contributes to the process of blood coagulation.
- Calcium stabilizes nerve and muscle cell membranes against changes in electrical potential; it decreases neuromuscular irritability.

Causes. Hypocalcemia can result from a diet that is very low in calcium sources such as dairy products, although this is rare in the United States. Poor intake of vitamin D can also cause this imbalance, because vitamin D is necessary for absorption of calcium from the gastrointestinal tract. Renal failure contributes to hypocalcemia since the kidneys normally activate vitamin D. Hypoparathyroidism, diarrhea, and pancreatitis can all cause excessive calcium losses. Alkalosis also results in decreased ionized calcium even though total body calcium is not altered. Because the parathyroids affect calcium levels, it is important to be alert for calcium imbalance in patients who have undergone a thyroidectomy, since the parathyroid glands may have been removed accidentally during surgery.

Assessment

What symptoms should alert the nurse to possible hypocalcemia? Loss of calcium's stabilizing effect on neuromuscular function causes muscle cramps or paresthesias (tingling sensations in fingertips or around the lips). If hypocalcemia is very severe or develops rapidly, **tetany** and convulsions may occur. A flexion spasm of the wrists and ankles, called *carpopedal spasm*, may be noted. Spasm of the larynx may also occur and can cause suffocation and death.

Laboratory values may show serum calcium to be less than 4.5 mEq/liter. However, laboratory values for calcium can be deceiving because only ionized calcium has an effect on neuromuscular function. As noted earlier, total body calcium may be unchanged even though there is a decrease in ionized calcium. This means that lab tests would show normal calcium values, even though the person exhibits signs of hypocalcemia. Remember that this phenomenon can occur in alkalosis.

Bone Disorders. When calcium deficiency develops over a long period, such as with inadequate dietary intake of calcium or with vitamin D deficiency, other dysfunctions such as bone disorders may occur. Decreased serum calcium leads to increased parathyroid activity, which in turn causes calcium and phosphorus to leave the bone. This maintains normal calcium blood levels but bones become thinner, lighter, or reduced in quantity. Two conditions may result: *osteomalacia* (loss of calcium and phosphorous from the bone matrix) or *osteoporosis* (loss of both calcium and bone matrix).

Osteomalacia occurs in renal failure due to the kidneys' inability to activate vitamin D. Loss of calcium and phosphorus from bone causes skeletal deformities and chronic bone pain.

Osteoporosis is a common problem for older persons. It is felt that poor dietary intake of calcium, along with a decrease in sex hormones and possibly an inability to activate vitamin D, all contribute to calcium deficiency in the elderly. Because osteoporosis makes older persons susceptible to fractures, even a slight fall may result in a broken bone. In addition, compression fractures of the vertebrae may occur resulting in stooped posture and back pain.

Nursing Interventions

When convulsions or tetany occur, emergency treatment is required, including the administration of calcium gluconate intravenously. For chronic or milder hypocalcemia, calcium is replaced orally. Vitamin-D supplements and a high-calcium diet may also be prescribed by the physician.

Ongoing Assessment. Nursing care for the person with acute deficits includes assessing susceptible persons for symptoms and checking lab value changes that may indicate hypocalcemia. One means of identifying a potentially severe imbalance is observing for the Chvostek sign, which may be elicited by tapping the facial nerve in front of the ear with a pen. If a spasm of facial muscles occurs, this response is considered to be a positive Chovstek's sign that may indicate impending tetany. In such an instance, immediate calcium replacement is required. At the same time, the nurse should be alert for a possible convulsion and should institute seizure precautions.

Dietary and Supplemental Intake. In chronic deficits, dietary habits should be assessed, along with any reason for low dietary intake of calcium. For example, it may be that the client cannot afford dairy products or may simply dislike their taste. As part of health teaching, plan with the person to include at least an 800-mg intake of calcium each day. For elderly persons 1 g of calcium daily may be needed to prevent bone loss due to osteoporosis. Dairy foods and cheese are the best calcium sources; others include greens, nuts, and dried beans. If oral calcium supplements are necessary, additional instructions concerning intake should be offered. These tablets are often very large and should be crushed and administered with juice, which provides an acid medium most conducive to the absorption of calcium.

Hypercalcemia

Hypercalcemia is the term applied to extracellular calcium excess. This condition may occur with hyperparathyroidism or from ingesting large quantities of milk and antacids to treat a peptic ulcer. Hypercalcemia may also occur in bone cancer and in prolonged immobility. In bone cancer and bed rest, large amounts of calcium leave the bones and enter the extracellular fluid.

Assessment

Signs and symptoms of hypercalcemia include poor skeletal muscle tone, weakness, nausea, anorexia, or constipation. Hypercalcemia may cause kidney stones manifested by flank pain. If hypercalcemia is a result of calcium loss from bones, bone pain due to pathological fractures may be present. Severe hypercalcemia may cause cardiac arrhythmias or cardiac arrest.

Nursing Interventions

Hypercalcemia is treated medically by removing the underlying cause. For example, if hyperparathyroidism is the cause, then a parathyroidectomy may be performed. Large amounts of fluids are also used to promote calcium loss through diuresis and to prevent kidney stones.

Nursing interventions include assisting the person to maintain a fluid intake of 3 to 4 liters/day. In addition, 250 ml of cranberry juice twice daily may be advocated as a means of promoting acid urine and deterring the formation of kidney stones, because calcium is more completely ionized in an acid medium (Tripp, 1976). A basic nursing responsibility is to assess for signs and symptoms of possible hypercalcemia and to monitor laboratory values related to this imbalance. At the same time it is important to be particularly alert for irregular pulse, confusion, or severe vomiting, which may indicate dangerously high calcium levels.

Acid–Base Imbalances

As indicated earlier, normal serum pH ranges from 7.35 to 7.45. When serum pH rises above 7.45, a state of alkalosis (H^+ deficit or base excess) exists. When serum pH falls below 7.35, a state of acidosis (H^+ excess) results. There are two major categories of acid–base imbalances—metabolic and respiratory. Metabolic imbalances are caused by a deficit or excess in bicarbonate concentration associated with problems of metabolism or renal function. Respiratory imbalances result from changes in carbonic acid concentration associated with pulmonary problems that cause an excess or a loss of carbon dioxide.

Acid-base balance depends on the concentration of bicarbonate (base) or carbonic acid. Carbonic acid levels are associated with CO_2 levels because carbon dioxide combines with water to form carbonic acid. The ratio is usually 20:1, bicarbonate to carbonic acid. As long as this ratio is maintained, the serum, pH is normal (Fig. 22-4). Carbonic acid concentration is maintained by the lungs; bicarbonate, by the kidneys. This mechanism is important in adaptation to acid–base imbalances, as we shall see in the following discussion.

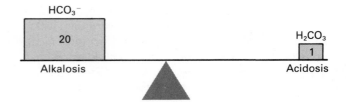

Figure 22-4
Acid–base balance in health.

Now let us discuss how nurses recognize and intervene in specific acid–base imbalances.

Metabolic Acidosis

Metabolic acidosis is caused by a deficit in bicarbonate, which leads to excess acid in relation to base (Fig. 22-5).

Causes of metabolic acidosis include hydrogen ion excess or bicarbonate loss. Bicarbonate loss occurs in diarrhea since this ion is highly concentrated in the lower bowel. Hydrogen ion excess may occur in uncontrolled diabetes (endogenous acid produced from fat metabolism), aspirin overdose (due to ingestion of acid), or renal disease (because kidneys do not excrete H^+ adequately).

Figure 22-5
Metabolic acidosis.

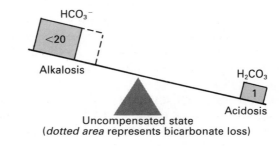

Uncompensated state
(*dotted area* represents bicarbonate loss)

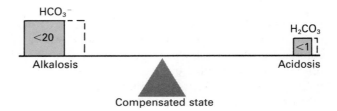

Compensated state

Assessment

Assessment is one of the most important aspects of nursing care of the person with metabolic acidosis. An alert nurse may be the first person to detect changes which indicate this imbalance. Assessment findings include the following:

- Anorexia
- Nausea and vomiting
- Lethargy, which may progress to stupor or coma
- Headache
- Warm, dry skin
- Serum $HCO_3 < 25$ mEq/liter
- Serum pH < 7.35
- Urine pH < 6.0

If metabolic acidosis develops slowly or has existed for some time, the person may adapt to this problem. Adaptation is accomplished through the lungs, which eliminate carbon dioxide, thereby lowering the carbonic acid level and returning the ratio of bicarbonate to carbonic acid to 20 to 1 (Fig. 22-2). This state, called *compensated metabolic acidosis*, is characterized by the following findings:

- Rapid, deep respirations (Kussmaul breathing)
- Decreased pCO_2
- Low normal serum pH
- Decreased serum HCO_3^-

Nursing Interventions

The physician will order replacement therapy for the bicarbonate loss by prescribing bicarbonate to be given intravenously or orally. Another form of medical therapy is intravenous lactated Ringer's solution, which corrects metabolic acidosis when lactate molecules are metabolized to form bicarbonate. The nurse is responsible for administering the IV solutions or medication carefully and for assessing the person constantly for signs and symptoms of deepening metabolic acidosis, especially respiratory rate, level of consciousness, and urine pH (Table 22-4). A return of laboratory values to near normal and a decrease in symptoms indicate a positive response to medical therapy. However, it is also important to watch for symptoms of alkalosis, which can result from overcorrection of metabolic acidosis. These symptoms are listed in the following discussion.

Metabolic Alkalosis

Metabolic alkalosis is caused by an excess of bicarbonate, that is, an overabundance of base in relation to carbonic acid (Fig. 22-6). Metabolic alkalosis may be caused by chloride ion deficit, which causes the kidneys to conserve bicarbonate ions by reabsorbing them along with sodium in the tubules. Chloride ion

---

Table 22-4
Nursing Process in Metabolic Acidosis

Assessment	Interventions
Causes: uncontrolled diabetes, chronic renal failure, aspirin overdose, diarrhea	Assess respiration, level of consciousness, urine pH, serum lab values.
Signs/symptoms: anorexia, nausea, vomiting, lethargy, headache, Kussmaul respirations,* decreased level of consciousness	Administer prescribed replacement therapy.
Laboratory values: HCO_3^- < 25 mEq/liter pCO_2 < 40 mmHg* Serum pH < 7.35 Urine pH < 6.0*	Monitor responses to replacement therapy and watch for metabolic alkalosis due to overcorrection.

* Compensatory changes

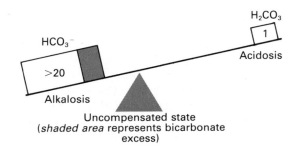

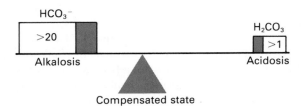

Figure 22-6
Metabolic alkalosis.

deficit is seen in vomiting, nasogastric suctioning, and diuretic therapy. Metabolic alkalosis may also be caused by an excessive ingestion of bicarbonate, taken in the form of bicarbonate of soda for gastric ulcer.

Assessment

The nurse should be watchful for signs of metabolic alkalosis in persons with the above conditions. Signs and symptoms and laboratory value changes include the following:

- Muscle twitching or tremors
- Tetany
- Convulsions (with severe imbalances)
- Serum $HCO_3^- > 29$
- Serum $pH > 7.45$
- Urine $pH > 7$

The neuromuscular changes of metabolic alkalosis are the result of low ionized calcium. In alkaline conditions, calcium ions combine with phosphate ions to form a solid, causing a calcium deficit in the extracellular fluid. The findings we see in metabolic alkalosis are actually signs of hypocalcemia.

As with metabolic acidosis, the person may adapt to metabolic alkalosis. Adaptation occurs as the lungs conserve carbon dioxide and thereby elevate the carbonic acid concentration in relation to bicarbonate (Fig. 22-3). This state, *compensated metabolic*

alkalosis, can be identified by the following signs and lab values:

- Slow, shallow respirations (often difficult to observe)
- Elevated pCO_2
- High normal serum pH
- Elevated serum HCO_3^-

Nursing Interventions

Metabolic alkalosis is usually treated by intravenous solutions of sodium chloride or potassium chloride, which supply chloride ions and reduce bicarbonate retention by the kidneys. Nursing responsibilities include administering intravenous therapy and monitoring for complications of this therapy. At the same time, laboratory values should be checked (especially bicarbonate, pCO_2, serum pH, and urine pH) and the person should be monitored for signs of improvement or worsening condition (Table 22-5). Tingling in the extremities or muscle spasms indicate worsening alkalosis. The return of laboratory values to normal levels and the disappearance of symptoms indicate improvement.

Respiratory Acidosis

Respiratory acidosis is defined as a primary gain in carbonic acid and, therefore, in carbon dioxide (Fig. 22-7). This imbalance is called respiratory acidosis because it results from disorders that cause decreased ventilation and subsequent CO_2 retention. The sequence of events that results in respiratory acidosis is as follows:

$$\text{Respiratory disorder} \rightarrow \begin{array}{c}\text{decreased}\\ \text{elimination of } CO_2 \\ \text{through the lungs}\end{array} \rightarrow$$

$$\begin{array}{c}CO_2 \\ \text{excess}\end{array} \rightarrow \begin{array}{c}\text{carbonic}\\ \text{acid excess}\end{array}$$

Respiratory acidosis may occur in such conditions as pneumonia, emphysema, and asthma or with excessive doses of narcotic analgesics or barbiturates (drugs that cause respiratory depression). Postoperative patients and elderly or obese persons are more prone to this disorder owing to decreased vital capacity (decreased ability to take a deep breath).

Table 22-5
Nursing Process in Metabolic Alkalosis

Assessment	Interventions
Causes: vomiting, gastric suction, diuretic therapy, $NaHCO_3$ ingestion	Assess neuromuscular function, urine pH, serum laboratory values.
Signs/symptoms: muscle tremors, twitching, paresthesias, tetany, convulsions, shallow respiration* (may be difficult to detect)	Administer prescribed replacement theapy (usually KCl or NaCl).
Laboratory values:	Watch for complications of intravenous therapy.
$\quad HCO_3^-\quad > 29$ mEq/liter	Monitor responses to replacement theapy.
$\quad pCO_2\quad > 40$ mmHg*	
$\quad$ Serum pH > 7.45	
$\quad$ Urine pH > 7.0*	

* Compensatory changes

Assessment

When assessing any person at risk for respiratory acidosis, the nurse should watch for the following:

- Decreased rate or depth of breathing (causes CO_2 retention)
- Dyspnea, respiratory distress (sign of ineffective respiration)
- Decreased alertness progressing to stupor or coma
- Headache
- Serum pH < 7.35
- $pCO_2 > 40$

People can adapt to respiratory acidosis. If the condition develops slowly, compensating mechanisms may be quite effective (Fig. 22-7). In the kidney, carbonic acid forms bicarbonate and hydrogen ions. Hydrogen ions are secreted into the tubules and excreted in the urine, eliminating a source of acid. Bicarbonate is reabsorbed, increasing the body's supply of base. This returns the ratio of bicarbonate to carbonic acid to nearly 20 to 1 and restores a normal serum pH. This state, *compensated respiratory acidosis*, can be identified by the following:

- Decreased urine pH (caused by H^+ excreted by kidneys)
- Increased serum HCO_3^-
- Low normal serum pH
- Increased pCO_2

Figure 22-7
Respiratory acidosis.

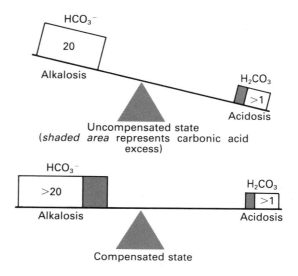

Uncompensated state
(*shaded area* represents carbonic acid excess)

Compensated state

Table 22-6
Nursing Process in Respiratory Acidosis

Assessment	Intervention
Causes: hypoventilation such as in COPD, pneumonia, drug overdose	Assess respiratory status (rate and depth of respiration, signs of distress, breath sounds), urine *pH*, serum laboratory values, level of consciousness.
Signs/symptoms: decreased level of consciousness, headache, signs of inadequate ventilation (respiratory distress, decreased respiratory rate or depth)	Support respiratory function (respiratory theapy measures, Fowler's position, frequent rest periods, oxygen therapy).
Laboratory values: pCO_2 > 40 mmHg HCO_3^-* > 29 mEq/liter Serum *pH* < 7.35 Urine *pH** < 6.0	

* Compensatory changes

Nursing Interventions

Medical therapy consists of treating the underlying respiratory disorder that caused the respiratory acidosis. The nurse can provide supportive respiratory measures such as elevating the head of the bed to allow maximum ventilation and assisting the person to rest frequently during activities in order to decrease oxygen consumption and CO_2 production. It is also important to check laboratory values and to monitor the person's level of consciousness for signs of improvement or worsening respiratory acidosis. In some instances, the nurse may also be responsible for administering prescribed respiratory therapy measures. All of these measures are intended to prevent the development of serious respiratory acidosis (Table 22-6). Further information on prevention of respiratory problems from diminished ventilation can be found in Chapter 24.

Respiratory Alkalosis

Respiratory alkalosis is defined as a primary deficit in carbonic acid. It is caused by hyperventilation, which results in loss of carbon dioxide due to overbreathing (Fig. 22-8).

Assessment

Hyperventilation can occur with anxiety, fever, or pain and may be evident by rapid, shallow breathing. Additional signs may include those below:

- Parasthesias, particularly around the mouth and in the fingers

Figure 22-8
Respiratory alkalosis.

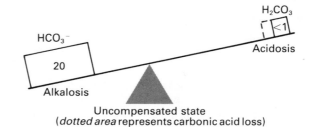

Uncompensated state
(*dotted area* represents carbonic acid loss)

Compensated state

- Dizziness or lightheadedness
- Tetany, convulsions (with severe imbalances)
- $pCO_2 < 40$
- Serum $pH > 7.45$

Often respiratory alkalosis is identified on the basis of symptoms alone, without the assistance of laboratory values.

Although the body can adapt to respiratory alkalosis, it usually takes some time to adjust to the imbalance. Therefore, signs of compensation may not be obvious. Adaptation is accomplished as the kidneys excrete bicarbonate into the urine (Fig. 22-8). This mechanism brings the ratio of base to acid closer to 20:1, which returns serum pH to near normal. This state of compensated repiratory alkalosis can be recognized by the following laboratory values:

- Increased urine pH (caused by HCO_3^-, which is excreted by the kidneys)
- Decreased serum HCO_3^-
- High normal serum pH
- Decreased serum pCO_2

Nursing Interventions

Medical therapy is directed toward the cause of hyperventilation. Treating the fever, pain, or anxiety usually decreases the symptoms of tingling or lightheadedness. When hyperventilation is caused by anxiety, the nurse may instruct the person to breathe into a paper bag so that he will rebreathe his own carbon dioxide and thereby raise the pCO_2. A person who is this anxious should be instructed to become aware of his breathing patterns and be coached to take slow, deep breaths. It is also important to allow the person to talk about his anxiety and ventilate his feelings, especially because the symptoms of hyperventilation alone can induce anxiety (Table 22-7). Providing emotional support in these instances requires a wide range of therapeutic communication skills, as discussed in Chapter 13.

Intravenous Therapy

As indicated in the preceding pages, treatment of fluid and electrolyte deficits may include intravenous (IV) therapy. IV therapy involves the administration of fluid, medications, or blood through the vein. Maintaining the safety and comfort of the person receiving intravenous solutions is an essential part of nursing care and therefore requires knowledge and understanding about the purposes and effects of this therapy.

Table 22-7
Nursing Process in Respiratory Alkalosis

Assessment	Intervention
Causes: hyperventilation related to anxiety, fever, pain	Assess neuromuscular function, labortory values.
Signs/symptoms: paresthesias, dizziness, tetany, convulsions, rapid shallow breathing	Implement prescribed therapy directed toward cause of alkalosis (*e.g.,* antipyretics).
Laboratory values: pCO_2 < 40 mmHg HCO_3^- < 25 mEq/liter* Serum pH > 7.45 Urine pH > 7.0*	Instruct to rebreathe CO_2. Give emotional support.† Increase awareness of breathing patterns.†

* Compensatory changes
† For alkalosis caused by anxiety

Table 22-8
Intravenous Solutions

Hypotonic	Solution with lower osmotic pressure than tissue fluid causes fluid shift from plasma compartment into cells and tissues; used to treat dehydration or maintain fluid balance for persons who cannot ingest fluids.	5% dextrose and water* 5% dextrose and 0.45% normal saline
Isotonic	Solution with osmotic pressure equal to tissue fluid causes no net fluid movement into or out of plasma compartment, thus expands plasma volume; used to treat blood loss or shock.	0.9% sodium chloride Ringer's solution
Hypertonic	Solution with higher osmotic pressure than tissue fluid causes fluid shift from tissues to plasma compartment; used to treat certain types of edema (such as cerebral edema) and expand plasma volume in shock. Hypertonic solutions can easily induce circulatory overload so the person should be watched carefully for symptoms.	Mannitol, dextran

* 5% Dextrose and water is isotonic when infused. However, dextrose is rapidly metabolized so the solution has a hypotonic effect.

Purposes of Intravenous Therapy

Intravenous therapy is used for a variety of purposes, including: replacing the normal daily loss of fluid and electrolytes for those who are unable to replace them orally, treating existing fluid and electrolyte problems such as dehydration, providing nutrition, and administering intravenous medications. Because IV therapy presents certain hazards, attempts should always be made to meet the person's needs with oral fluids, nutrition, or medication if at all possible. However, in certain situations, IV infusions are essential, especially for those who are unable to ingest or digest adequate water and nutrients, as might be the case in prolonged vomiting or unconsciousness or instances when an NPO order is to be in effect for more than a day. Intravenous therapy is also necessary when there is an immediate need for fluid and electrolytes, such as in shock or hemorrhage.

Types of Intravenous Solutions

There are several types of intravenous solutions to suit the purposes of therapy. The most commonly used type includes dextrose and electrolyte solutions

(Table 22-8). These solutions replace water and electrolytes but supply few calories. They are used when the person has an actual or potential fluid or electrolyte inbalance, such as in the postoperative state or in shock. Hyperalimentation solutions represent a second type of intravenous fluid and are used to meet nutritional needs, as discussed in Chapter 20. A third type of intravenous fluid is blood, which is usually given in cases of blood or plasma loss. Blood administration carries special risks and requires that all who are involved in the procedure be aware of the institutional policy for this type of therapy.

Nursing Care in Intravenous Therapy

Involving the person in his own care during intravenous therapy is essential. Often persons fear needles and view intravenous therapy as an indication of being seriously ill or as a threat of loss of independence or mobility. The following interventions may be helpful in preventing anxiety and assisting the person to participate in his care:

* Allow the person to have some choice in the site of therapy, if possible. For example, some persons may wish to avoid using the hand as the insertion site so as to have maximum mobility.

• Explain the purpose of therapy. Information helps decrease fear of the unknown and promotes feelings of control.

• Explain how the procedure will feel. Insertion produces a pinching sensation and pressure. When the needle is in place, the person will feel its presence but no discomfort.

• Explain the mobility that the person can maintain with his IV. If a joint must be immobilized during therapy, explain the reason and assist with daily activities as needed.

• Explain activities that can interfere with proper functioning of the system, such as elevating the affected arm, placing it behind the head, or pulling on the catheter or tubing.

Nurses are also responsible for maintaining the administration of IV therapy and for assessing its effects. Set and monitor the drip rate, observe intake and output, laboratory values and other pertinent observations, and watch for signs of complications of therapy. Possible complications include those below:

• *Infiltration*—The needle is dislodged from the vein and fluid enters the subcutaneous tissue. The site will be painful, edematous, hard, and cool to the touch.

• *Phlebitis*—Irritation of the vein causes local inflammation. The area will be red, edematous, hard, warm, and painful to the touch.

• *Circulatory overload*—Intravenous fluid infuses more rapidly than the pumping capacity of the heart can tolerate. Signs are discussed under ECF volume excess earlier in the chapter.

• *Infection*—Bacteria contaminate infusion solutions or equipment. Symptoms include fever, headache, malaise, and nausea.

• *Air embolism*—Air enters a vein and interferes with oxygenation of the lungs or brain. Symptoms include dyspnea, cyanosis, or loss of consciousness.

The nurse can prevent these problems by maintaining strict sterile technique during therapy, avoiding prolonged therapy at a given site, monitoring infusion rates frequently, particularly with elderly clients, children, or those with renal or cardiac problems, securing the IV site carefully with tape, and preventing air from entering an IV system. These actions can prevent client discomfort and avoid prolonged hospitalization due to complications.

Conclusion

This chapter has presented basic nursing care related to fluid and electrolyte needs. Common problems include fluid imbalances, acid–base imbalances, and deficits or excesses of electrolytes, particularly sodium, potassium, and calcium. Many of the nursing interventions for persons with fluid and electrolyte problems involve dependent functions such as administering intravenous fluids or electrolyte replacement. However, independent nursing actions are equally important and include observing susceptible persons for indications of imbalances; monitoring laboratory values, intake and output, and other signs that show response to therapy; teaching self-care; and assisting with therapeutic diets.

To exemplify how nursing care might be implemented in an actual setting, the following case study is offered.

Example □ R.W. is admitted to the hospital for removal of his gallbladder. A nasogastric tube is in place after surgery and attached to suction. R.W. is receiving IV therapy of 5% dextrose and .45% NaCl with 20 mEq of KCl/liter. Knowing that R.W. could potentially develop several fluid or electrolyte imbalances, the nurse begins preventive care. She reviews R.W.'s laboratory reports for sodium, potassium, chloride, and bicarbonate levels. She watches for lab value changes indicating potassium deficit, sodium deficit, and metabolic alkalosis due to gastrointestinal losses. In addition, she monitors R.W. for signs of these imbalances. Because R.W. is losing fluid through his nasogastric tube, she monitors him for symptoms of dehydration. She records intake and output and checks 24-hour totals for imbalances. She monitors IV infusion rate hourly to prevent fluid overload from rapid infusion. She also watches R.W. for other complications of IV therapy such as phlebitis or infiltration. The nurse communicates any adverse signs or symptoms to the physician. For instance, decreased urinary output and high specific gravity may indicate developing fluid deficit from inadequate fluid replacement. The nurse's actions, knowledge, and skill have been important in maintaining fluid and electrolyte balance for R.W. □

Fluid and electrolyte needs represent a real challenge to any health-care provider, especially for nurses, who have a major role in maintaining health and detecting early imbalances. Therefore, we must be knowledgeable about almost every aspect of a client's functional abilities and aware of those factors affecting health status. In this way, we can assist persons to adapt to stressors affecting fluid and electrolyte balance and help them to maintain health.

Study Questions

1. Mr. A. is admitted to the hospital for surgery. He experiences severe postoperative vomiting. What fluid and electrolyte imbalances should the nurse anticipate in this person? What signs, symptoms, and lab value changes would the nurse expect to see?

2. Mrs. B. has a long history of congestive heart failure. You are visiting this client in her home. Today she tells you that she feels "bloated" and that her shoes and rings feel tight. What problem is Mrs. B. most likely experiencing? What physiological mechanisms are contributing to this imbalance? How would you assess Mrs. B. further?

3. John C. is a 50-year-old client who is seen in the outpatient department for hypertension. His doctor begins therapy with furosemide (Lasix—a potent diuretic). What potassium imbalance can occur with this medication? What is the function of potassium in the body and how does this relate to the symptoms you might expect to see with an imbalance? Outline a teaching plan for Mr. C. to assist him to care for himself at home.

4. Miss D. is a 38-year-old client who underwent thyroidectomy yesterday. Why should her nurse be concerned about her calcium balance? What mechanism normally maintains calcium balance? Describe the nursing care you would plan for Miss D.

5. Mr. E. suffered a severe head injury in a motorcycle accident. His respirations are markedly depressed. Which acid–base imbalance would you anticipate in Mr. E.? What mechanisms normally maintain acid–base balance in the person? What physiological adaptive mechanisms assist Mr. E. to compensate for his acid–base imbalance?

6. Fred F. has been working full-time in addition to taking a full academic load at college for two semesters. He came to the emergency room with lightheadedness and tingling in his extremities. The doctor diagnoses his condition as hyperventilation due to anxiety. Which acid–base imbalance would you anticipate in Fred? What lab value changes may occur? What nursing care would you plan with this client?

7. Patty G., who is 1 year old, is hospitalized with dehydration associated with influenza. Patty's physician decides to begin an intravenous infusion. Why is Patty at risk for circulatory overload from intravenous therapy? What nursing actions can prevent complications from IV therapy?

Glossary

Acid: Substance that can donate a hydrogen ion or proton.

Active transport: A process that involves the movement of ions from areas of low concentration to areas of high concentration; the opposite of diffusion.

Anorexia: Loss of appetite.

Base: Substance that can accept a hydrogen ion or proton.

Buffer: Substance that can release or combine with hydrogen ions to maintain a constant *p*H.

Cation: An ion that carries a positive charge in a solution.

Diffusion: The dispersion of a dissolved substance throughout a fluid until the concentration is equal in all parts of the container.

Dyspnea: A sensation of difficulty in breathing.

Edema: Presence of abnormally large amounts of fluid in the intercellular tissue spaces.

Electrolyte: Substance capable of developing an electrical charge when dissolved in solution.

Extracellular fluid volume deficit: Isotonic fluid loss from the extracellular compartment.

Extracellular fluid volume excess: Isotonic fluid gain in the extracellular compartment.

Filtration: The movement of fluid across a membrane from an area of higher hydrostatic pressure to an area of lower hydrostatic pressure.

Hypercalcemia: Excess of ionized calcium in extracellular fluid.

Hyperkalemia: Potassium excess of extracellular fluid.

Hypernatremia: Sodium excess of extracellular fluid.

Hypertonic: Solution having a higher osmotic pressure than body fluids.

Hypocalcemia: A deficiency of ionized calcium in extracellular fluid.

Hypokalemia: Potassium deficiency of extracellular fluid.

Hyponatremia: Sodium deficiency of extracellular fluid.

Hypotonic: Solution having lower osmotic pressure than body fluids.

Isotonic: Solution having osmotic pressure equal to extracellular fluid.

Metabolic acidosis: A condition caused by a deficit in bicarbonate leading to excess acid in relation to base.

Metabolic alkalosis: A condition caused by an excess of bicarbonate or overabundance of base in relation to carbonic acid.

Oliguria: Scanty elimination of urine.

Osmosis: The passage of water through a membrane from an area of lower concentration of solute to an area of higher concentration of solute.

Osmotic pressure: The attraction for water exerted by solute particles. Solutions that have higher osmotic pressure have higher concentrations of dissolved particles and a higher attraction for water.

***p*H:** Expression of hydrogen ion concentration.

Rales: Abnormal breath sounds due to fluid or mucus in respiratory passages (trachea, bronchi, or alveoli).

Respiratory acidosis: A primary gain in carbonic acid and, therefore, carbon dioxide; caused by hypoventilation.

Respiratory alkalosis: A primary deficit in carbonic acid. It is caused by hyperventilation, which causes carbon dioxide loss.

Specific gravity: The ratio of the weight of urine to an equal volume of distilled water.

Tetany: Prolonged, painful muscle spasms, usually in hands and feet; related to hyperirritability of the neuromuscular system.

Turgor: Elasticity or resilience of the skin.

Bibliography

Adlard JM, George JM: Hyponatremia. Heart Lung 7:587–593, July–August, 1978

Felver L: Understanding the electrolyte maze. Am J Nurs 80:1591–1594, September, 1980

Fournet K: Patients discharged on diuretics: Prime candidates for individualized teaching by the nurse. Heart Lung 3:108–116, January–February, 1974

Grant M, Kubo W: Assessing a patient's hydration status. Am J Nurs 75:1306–1311, August, 1975

Guyton A: Textbook of Medical Physiology, 5th ed. Philadelphia, WB Saunders, 1976

Kee J: Fluid imbalance in elderly patients. Nurs '73 3:40–43, April, 1973

Kubo W et al: Fluid and electrolyte problems of tube-fed patients. Am J Nurs 76:912–916, June, 1976

Kubo W, Grant M, Walike B et al: The syndrome of inappropriate secretion of antidiuretic hormone. Heart Lung 7:469–476, May–June, 1978

Lancour J: ADH and aldosterone: How to recognize their effect. Nurs '78 8:36–41, September, 1978

Menzel L: Clinical problems of electrolyte balance. Nurs Clin North Am 15:559–576, September, 1980a

Menzel L: Clinical problems of fluid balance. Nurs Clin North Am 15:549–558, September, 1980b

Metheny NA: Water and electrolyte balance in the postoperative patient. Nurs Clin North Am 10:49–57, March, 1975

Metheny NA, Snively WD: Nurse's Handbook of Fluid Balance, 3rd ed. Philadelphia, JB Lippincott, 1979

Metheny NA, Snively WD: Perioperative fluids and electrolytes. Am J Nurs 78:840–845, May, 1978

O'Dorisio TM: Hypercalcemic crisis. Heart Lung 7:425–433, May–June, 1978

Sharer JE: Reviewing acid-base balance. Am J Nurs 75:980–983, June, 1975

Shrake K: The ABC's of ABG's. Nurs '79 9:26–33, September, 1979

Tripp A: Hyper and hypocalcemia. Am J Nurs 76:1142–1145, July, 1976

Urrows ST: Physiology of body fluids. Nurs Clin North Am 15:537–547, September, 1980

Circulatory and Temperature Statuses

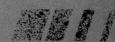

Ann Z. Kruszewski

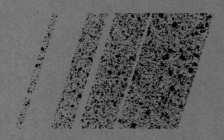

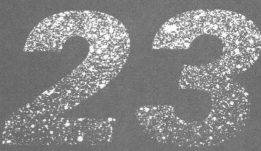

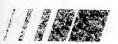

After completing this chapter, students will be able to:

● Apply principles of normal circulation to the care of the person.

● Identify stressors that can affect circulatory function.

● Apply concepts related to assessment of circulatory function.

● Identify signs and symptoms of altered circulatory function.

● List nursing actions to maintain normal circulatory function or to prevent common circulatory problems.

Because our bodies are organized into tissues and organs that perform specialized functions, a system is needed to transport materials between these areas. This function is performed by the circulatory system, which brings oxygen and nutrients to the cells and carries away wastes and other cell products.

Because every cell in our bodies is dependent on oxygen, circulatory disorders affect the function of each of our systems. Persons with circulatory dysfunction may experience problems with skin integrity, mobility, nutrition, respiration, mental and emotional well-being, and many other areas. Whereas chronic circulatory problems affect our ability to perform normal daily activities associated with jobs, school, and recreation, acute circulatory problems may threaten life itself.

This chapter explores some acute and chronic circulatory problems and the nursing actions needed to prevent dysfunction, provide support, and restore health. It also discusses the problems of temperature regulation and related nursing assessment and intervention. The close association between temperature and circulatory function stems from the fact that the cardiovascular mechanisms are the means by which heat is conserved or given off, thereby influencing our ability to regulate body temperature.

Components of the Circulatory System

The circulatory system has three components: a pump (the heart), pipes (the blood vessels), and fluid (blood). Each of these components must function adequately for the circulatory system to provide sufficient cell nourishment and oxygen. Let us look at these components individually.

Pump (Heart)

The heart pumps blood into the arterial system in order to transport oxygen and nutrients to the cells. It also pumps deoxygenated blood to the lungs. The heart must pump with sufficient force to overcome the resistance of the arterial system to blood flow. When increased arterial resistance exists, such as in hypertension and arteriosclerosis, heart problems develop. If the heart is not able to pump effectively enough to overcome arterial resistance, it eventually may fail.

In order to function as an effective pump, the heart must be structurally intact; it must receive adequate oxygen as supplied by the coronary arteries, and it must have a conduction system that works properly. For more details on the mechanisms of cardiac function, the reader is referred to an anatomy and physiology textbook.

Pipes (Blood Vessels)

The "pipes" of the cardiovascular system consist of blood vessels including arteries, veins, arterioles, venules, and capillaries. The peripheral arterial system carries oxygen and nutrients to the cells, while peripheral veins carry unoxygenated blood and cell wastes to the heart. In the pulmonary system the arteries carry deoxygenated blood to the lungs, while the veins transport oxygenated blood back to the heart. The major function of the circulatory system is accomplished in the capillaries, where oxygen and nutrients diffuse into the cells and waste substances diffuse back into the blood vessels.

One important feature of blood vessels is their ability to change diameter to accomodate the needs of the cells and the body as a whole. The caliber of arterioles and precapillary sphincters changes to maintain blood flow through tissues at exactly the level needed to meet their nutritional needs. Should blood volume fall dangerously low, blood vessels constrict thereby increasing cardiac output and maintaining blood pressure. This phenomenon is referred to again in the discussion of shock.

Fluid (Blood)

Blood is responsible for transporting oxygen and nutrients to tissues and for carrying carbon dioxide and other cell wastes away. In order to transport these substances adequately, there must be sufficient blood volume. In addition, oxygen and carbon dioxide transport depends on red blood cells that are of normal size, composition, and function.

The System as a Whole

The cardiovascular system shares the characteristic of systems in general as described in Chapter 2. The effectiveness of the cardiovascular system depends not only on the status of its subsystems (pump, pipes, and fluid) but also on how well these components work together. As with other systems, one subsystem can compensate for the inadequate function of another. For instance, if blood volume falls, the heart rate increases to maintain adequate tissue perfusion. These compensating mechanisms are important to the person's ability to adapt to internal and external stressors. Specific mechanisms are discussed in the section on circulatory problems. The important point to remember is that any problem that interferes with circulatory function ultimately affects cell nutrition and oxygenation. This in turn can lead to cell death and a significant alteration in the person's functional abilities.

General Assessment of Circulatory Status

Persons with circulatory problems are often faced with conditions that, at the least, can cause tissue damage and, at the most, may threaten life itself. The nurse's observation skills are essential to the care of these individuals. Although this section describes a complete circulatory assessment, not all the information presented here is pertinent to every situation. Thus, each assessment should be adapted to the needs of the individual client, with emphasis placed on those areas that have the most relevance for the person.

At the same time, the effects that the other statuses have on cardiovascular function should be considered as part of the general assessment. For instance, imagine that you have counted Mrs. R's pulse rate and found it to be 108. Now you must ask yourself, "What other factors might be related to this rapid rate? Is Mrs. R having pain? Is she feeling anxious? Did she just finish a strenuous activity? Is she experiencing hypoxia due to a respiratory problem?" Any of these factors could increase a person's pulse rate, yet they are all related to functional areas other than circulation. The astute nurse looks beyond the functioning of the heart, blood vessels, and blood when assessing changes in cardiovascular status.

General Observations

A great deal of information about cardiovascular function can be obtained by observing a person and knowing what to look for. Even initial observations can give clues about circulatory function. For instance, does the skin have a glowing color or is it pale or dusky (cyanosis)? Skin color may give indications of **hypoxia,** anemia, or inadequate perfusion of tissues in the area observed. Are there signs of distress such as difficulty in breathing and restlessness, or does the client appear comfortable? Any of these signs may relate to circulatory function because they can indicate inadequate oxygenation due to heart failure, inadequate perfusion of the brain, or poor local circulation. Is there evidence of edema? Generalized edema is another sign of inadequate cardiovascular function which might be noticed when first observing a client.

Interview

Fatigue, Dyspnea, and Chest Pain

The person's own descriptions are an eessential part of assessment. He may describe weakness and fatigue, which can have a circulatory origin due to hypoxia, or he may state that he has difficulty breathing during the night or when lying down (a possible sign of heart failure).

Chest pain is another symptom that may have relevance for cardiac status. In general, people tend to associate chest pain with heart trouble. However, chest pain may be due to a variety of causes, including a gastrointestinal disturbance or muscle strain, as well as angina (ischemic myocardial pain) or myocardial infarction (heart attack). Nurses in both the hospital and the community may need at times to determine whether the person experiencing chest pain needs immediate medical attention. Table 23-1 will help you distinguish the type of chest pain that may indicate an emergency cardiac condition from the types that represent less serious situations. Remember that one of the most common reactions of a person having a heart attack is to deny that something is seriously wrong. Thus, it is never safe to rely on the person's assurances that he is "ok."

Leg Pain

Leg pain may be another indication of a circulatory problem. **Claudication** is the term used to describe muscle pain due to **ischemia.** It is caused by inadequate arterial circulation to the affected extremity. Because leg pain may indicate arterial insufficiency, the nurse should assess for signs that are often associated with this problem, as will be described under assessment of extremities.

Edema

The nurse should be alert for statements that may indicate the presence of edema. The person might say, "My shoes don't seem to fit me," or "My rings feel too tight." Even a statement such as, "I seem to

Table 23-1
Interpretation of Chest Pain

Heart Attack	Other Causes
Chest pain is located beneath sternum; radiates to arms, back, or neck.	Chest pain is localized away from sternum or occurs throughout chest.
Pain is "crushing," "squeezing," or "suffocating."	Pain is sharp, burning, worsens with deep respiration.
Person is restless, pacing, expresses feeling of impending loss.	Person shows less motor activity than with heart attack.
Pain is unrelieved by rest, nitroglycerin, antacids.	Rest, nitroglycerin, or antacids relieve pain within 5 to 10 minutes.
Skin color changes, sweating, nausea, vital sign changes are present.	Skin, vital signs, gastrointestinal findings are absent or minimal.

be gaining weight so rapidly," might indicate fluid gain. A weight gain of 2 pounds indicates approximately 1 liter of fluid.

Behavioral Signs

Family sometimes can provide data about behavioral changes in the person which may represent inadequate perfusion of brain cells. For example, irritability, confusion, and forgetfulness can indicate changes in cardiovascular function.

Physical Assessment

The interview is usually conducted before the physical examination, because the client's statements can serve as clues about the physical findings that should be observed. As mentioned above, if the client states that his rings feel tight, it would be wise to look for signs of edema during the examination.

Vital Signs

The vital signs are the most basic part of the circulatory assessment. Even a rapid appraisal of the cardiovascular system should include measurement of vital signs because they can give valuable information about the heart, vascular system, and blood. The vital signs include blood pressure, pulse, respiration, and temperature. Only blood pressure and pulse are discussed here. A complete discussion of body temperature and respiration can be found later

in this chapter and in Chapter 24 (Respiratory Status), respectively.

Blood Pressure

Blood pressure is the measurement of the force of blood against the walls of the arteries. Blood pressure is one of the major determinants of tissue perfusion. If blood pressure falls, tissue nutrition diminishes and may eventually cause cellular death. Elevated blood pressure leads to pathological changes in the arteries and makes the person susceptible to heart failure. Thus, alterations in blood pressure can be a major threat to health.

Blood pressure is usually measured by an instrument called a *sphygmomanometer*. It measures blood pressure in millimeters of mercury (mm Hg); this unit represents the height to which a column of mercury would rise were it exposed to the force of blood flowing through the arteries. Blood pressure is the product of two forces: cardiac output (amount of blood ejected by the heart per minute) and peripheral resistance (resistance to blood flow through the blood vessels).

Systolic versus *Diastolic Pressure.*   There are two components of blood pressure: systolic pressure and diastolic pressure. The **systolic pressure** represents pressure during cardiac contraction and is normally within the range of 90 mm Hg to 130 mm Hg. Systolic blood pressure chiefly reflects changes in the cardiac output. For example, during strenuous exercise, when cardiac output increases to meet tissue needs for oxygen, a person's systolic pressure may rise from an average value of 120 mm Hg to 160 mm Hg or more (McBride, 1970, p. 274).

Diastolic pressure reflects the arterial pressure during cardiac filling. A normal range is 70 mm Hg to 90 mm Hg. Diastolic pressure chiefly reflects peripheral resistance. An illustration is found in persons with primary hypertension (commonly called *high blood pressure*). These individuals have increased peripheral resistance due to narrowed diameter of the arterioles. They show increased diastolic pressure (sometimes as high as 120 mm Hg) if their hypertension remains untreated.

Factors That Affect Blood Pressure. There are five physiological factors that affect blood pressure: blood volume, contractility of the heart, blood viscosity, elasticity of the arteries, and the diameter of blood vessels. As noted in Table 23-2, the contractility of the heart and the diameter of the blood vessels have the major effect on blood pressure. Only large fluctuations in the other factors cause blood pressure changes. For example, a person may lose 500 ml of blood before the blood pressure falls.

Other factors, both environmental and internal, can affect blood pressure readings. Anxiety, fear, food ingestion, exercise, and age—all are associated with increased blood pressure.

On the other hand, blood pressure decreases during sleep and in the supine position. It is important to know what factors can cause an alteration in blood pressure readings from the person's normal level. For example, a blood pressure taken when the person is first admitted to the hospital may be affected by feelings of anxiety and fear. Therefore, such a reading will most likely be much higher than normal. Yet this reading is often considered to be the baseline for comparison of future measurements. Unless the nurse recognizes this, errors can be made in interpreting blood pressure readings.

Pulse Pressures. **Pulse pressure** is another value that is used to assess circulatory function. It is obtained by subtracting the diastolic value from the systolic value. Pulse pressure ranges from 30 mm Hg to 50 mm Hg and represents the range of pressure within the arteries from the high point during ventricular contraction to the low point during filling. Pulse pressure reflects changes in stroke volume. Decreased pulse pressure is seen in early shock. Increased pulse pressure may be found in hypertension, fever, and increased intracranial pressure.

Pulse

Pulse is caused by a wave of pressure against the walls of the arteries, initiated by contraction of the left ventricle. Pulse reflects two aspects of circulatory function: the pumping activity of the left ventricle and the condition of the artery at the point at which the pulse is measured. Pulse is assessed in areas where the arteries are most superficial (Fig. 23-1). It is detected by pressing the index and middle fingers gently over the artery until the pulse wave is detected.

Table 23-2
Physiological Factors Affecting Blood Pressure

Factor	Effect
Blood volume	Influences cardiac output: ↑ volume → ↑ B.P.; ↓ volume → ↓ B.P.
Contractility of heart	Influences cardiac output: ↑ force of contraction → ↑ B.P.; ↓ force → ↓ B.P.
Blood viscosity	Influences peripheral resistance: ↑ viscosity → ↑ resistance → ↑ B.P.
Elasticity of arteries	↑ rigidity → ↓ expansion of vessels during systole → ↑ B.P.
Diameter of blood vessels	Exerts major effect on peripheral resistance: ↑ diameter → ↓ peripheral resistance → ↓ B.P.; ↓ diameter → ↑ B.P.

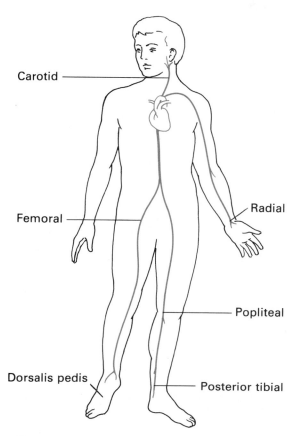

Carotid

Femoral

Radial

Popliteal

Dorsalis pedis

Posterior tibial

Figure 23-1
Peripheral pulse sites

Three characteristics of the pulse should be noted: rate, rhythm, and quality.

Rate. Rate is assessed by counting beats per minute. In the adult, normal pulse rate ranges from 60 to 100. In the infant, it is 120/minute; this rate gradually decreases with age.

Pulse rate is usually counted for 15 seconds and multiplied by four. However, there is controversy about the length of time one should count the rate to get the most accurate determination (Jones, 1970). This text recommends that slow rates (less than 60) should be counted for 60 seconds. If slow rates are counted for only 15 seconds, then errors will be multiplied by four, resulting in large miscalculations. At a slower rate, such miscalculations assume greater significance.

Rate is usually assessed at the radial artery because it is most accessible. However, it is important to remember that peripheral pulse sites reflect only pressure waves initiated by the left ventricle. Should the ventricle contract but eject no blood, a pulse wave will not be detectable at peripheral sites and rate determination will be inaccurate. The most accurate site to assess rate is over the apex of the heart. Here each ventricular contraction produces a heart sound which can be counted to obtain the apical pulse rate. The sounds are produced by the heart valves closing. Apical pulse should be assessed whenever a rapid or slow rate or an irregular pulse is present. Assessment of apical pulse is described with assessment of the precordium.

The person's resting pulse rate should be taken in order to get the truest picture of cardiac activity. Because factors such as anxiety, pain, exercise, smoking, and eating a heavy meal can elevate the pulse rate, it is important to consider the possible effects of these factors when interpreting changes in the person's pulse rate.

Pulse Deficit. **Pulse deficit** is the term for an apical rate that is greater than the radial rate. The pulse deficit is found by subtracting the radial from the apical rate. If the person's apical rate is 120 and the radial rate is 90, the pulse deficit is 30. A pulse deficit reflects inefficient ventricular contraction, one in which the ventricle contracts but no blood is ejected. This produces a heart sound but no palpable pulse wave at the peripheral artery. The nurse may note a pulse deficit in persons experiencing atrial fibrillation or premature ventricular contractions. Always check for pulse deficit if an irregular rhythm is detected, because one often accompanies the other.

Rhythm. Rhythm refers to the regularity of pulse beats. Normally there should be an equal interval between each beat. An irregular rhythm may indicate that the person has a serious deficiency in the conduction system of the heart. For this reason, irregular rhythm is often a significant finding, particularly if it represents a change from the person's previous status.

Pulse Quality. Pulse quality is often used to assess stroke volume or the amount of blood ejected with each ventricular contraction. In this case, quality of the pulse is best assessed at the carotid artery because it is the closest site to the heart. When stroke volume falls, the pulse feels weaker; when stroke volume increases, a stronger pulse is produced. Pulse quality also indicates the condition of the underlying artery. A client who has weak pedal pulses may have obstruction of the arteries supplying the leg. Assessment of pulse quality, rate, and rhythm is summarized in Table 23-3.

Table 23-3
Assessment of Pulse

	Finding	**Possible Interpretation**
Rate	Rate between 60 and 100/minute	Normal
	Tachycardia (rate above 100/min)	Sympathetic activity (fever, anxiety, pain, shock, exercise), cardiac origin (arrhythmias), medications, hypoxia
	Bradycardia (rate below 60/min)	Vagal stimulation (nausea, bowel movement), medication (digitalis), cardiac origin (heart block), increased intercranial pressure, exercise training (may be normal in athletes)
Rhythm	Regular	Normal
	Irregular	Arrhythmia
Quality	Easily palpated	Normal
	Full (bounding)	Fever, hypertension
	Weak	Arterial occlusion
	Thready	Shock

Interpretation of Vital Signs

Beginning nurses make several common mistakes when assessing a client's vital signs. Some useful points are listed here to help you analyze the person's vital signs and identify his needs:

1. Changes in One Vital Sign Are Usually Reflected by Changes in Others. For this reason, vital signs should be taken and interpreted together, along with other significant findings. For instance, an elevated pulse rate can have many causes. But if it is accompanied by an elevated temperature and respiratory rate, you can determine that these are all related to fever. Simply noting an elevated pulse rate would give little information about the person's needs.

2. Vital Signs Are Influenced by Many External Factors. Many of the factors mentioned in the previous discussion need to be considered when variances from the person's normal vital sign values are noted. For instance, if you note that your client has an abnormally rapid pulse rate and elevated blood pressure, you might ask yourself, "Did my client just perform strenuous activity?" "Is he anxious or in pain?" If so, you should try to remove the factor and recheck vital signs later (Fig. 23-2). Always consider variables that might alter vital signs any time

you obtain a reading which is not within the person's normal range.

3. Individuals Vary in Their Normal Range of Vital Signs. The nurse should not only know the normal ranges for the four vital signs but also the client's own range. The person's usual values may fall outside of normal thereby affecting the way the changes are interpreted.

Example☐ Mrs. R. is a 78-year-old woman who underwent a hysterectomy the previous day. The student nurse takes her blood pressure and finds that it is 110/88. Is Mrs. R's blood pressure normal? It does fall within the normal adult range; however, the student noted that before surgery Mrs. R. had blood pressures ranging from 160/80 to 170/90 and that she lost considerable blood during surgery. Mrs. R. is actually hypotensive due to low blood volume. If the student had not known Mrs. R's normal blood pressure range, she would have missed data that show a serious problem. ☐

4. Trends Are More Important than Single Readings when Interpreting Vital Signs. Take the following example. Mr. M. experienced a myocardial infarction today. He seems to be doing well after his admission to the hospital. But when comparing Mr. M.'s vital signs the nurse notes the following:

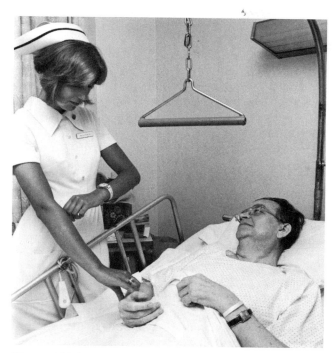

Figure 23-2
Vital signs may be affected by emotional stress.

Time	Blood Pressure	Pulse
2 P.M.	130/80	72
3 P.M.	126/86	90
4 P.M.	110/78	100

Should the nurse notify Mr. R's physician? Definitely! Although the vital signs are still within normal range, the trend is toward rising pulse rate and falling blood pressure. This may indicate shock. Whenever you note abnormal vital signs, check them again a short time later to detect trends as early as possible.

5. Vital Signs Should be Checked Whenever the Client's Condition Warrants It. To use another example: Mrs. B. experienced an incident of severe respiratory distress earlier in the morning. Although vital signs are ordered to be taken once every 8 hours, Mrs. B.'s nurse checks blood pressure, pulse, and respiratory rate as often as her condition requires. The nurse knows that vital signs will be elevated with inadequate tissue oxygenation and wants to identify changes before serious problems develop.

Assessment of Extremities

Observation of the person's extremities can yield valuable information about circulation to the body part being inspected. The nurse will wish to assess the legs of the elderly and persons with diabetes, arteriosclerosis, and chronic venous insufficiency, because many of these individuals are at risk for circulatory problems of the lower extremities. Persons with arm or leg casts should be assessed to ensure that adequate arterial circulation is being delivered to the affected extremity. The following considerations should be noted when assessing the extremities.

Skin Color

Skin color in an extremity affected by venous or arterial insufficiency may be pale, **cyanotic,** or a dusky red color. These changes are difficult to detect in darkly pigmented individuals. Refer to Chapter 18 for more information on assessing skin color.

Skin Temperature

Skin temperature may be cool if arterial blood supply to an extremity is impaired, because skin temperature reflects tissue perfusion. Skin temperature should be assessed in individuals who wear elastic bandages or have casts on an arm or leg. Cool skin temperature in the affected part may mean that the cast or bandage is so tightly applied that it is obstructing blood flow. The skin temperature of one extremity should be compared to the other in order to detect any differences between the two. This may help confirm that a temperature change is present and is not the result of other factors such as cool room temperature.

Skin Integrity

A disruption in skin integrity may indicate potential venous or arterial insufficiency of a chronic nature. If the person has inadequate arterial circulation to the legs, oxygen and nutrient supply will not be sufficient to meet cellular requirements. Tissue death and skin ulcers will occur, especially on the toes or areas where injury has occurred. In venous insufficiency, veins do not empty efficiently causing edema, which interferes with cell nutrition. Here, too, tissue death occurs resulting in skin ulcers. Lesions are usually found over the ankles in persons with chronic venous problems.

Hair and Nail Growth

The appearance of hair and nails may undergo a change in chronic arterial insufficiency. Occluded arteries are unable to deliver sufficient oxygen and nutrients to the tissues, which alters the growth of hair and nails. As a result, hair loss on the legs and thick, ridged toenails may be noted in persons with chronic arterial problems.

Capillary Filling

Capillary filling is a test to determine local circulation and vasomotor tone. It can be performed on the fingers or toes as appropriate. Pressure is applied on the very edge of the nail until the nail bed blanches (Fig. 23-3). The pressure is then released and the return of color noted: color should return in 1 second or less. Slow return indicates decreased vasomotor tone, which can occur in shock, arterial insufficiency, or with a tight cast.

Quality of Peripheral Pulses

As indicated earlier, quality of pulse can indicate patency of the artery being palpated. The quality of peripheral pulses might be assessed following an arteriogram in which an artery is injected with dye and then x-rayed. Hematomas sometimes develop in the artery following this diagnostic test. The nurse would check the strength of the pulse distal to the injection site to determine patency of the artery. Persons with diabetes, arterial insufficiency, or any condition that can occlude an artery also need this assessment. It is important to note that edema can

Figure 23-3
Assessing capillary filling

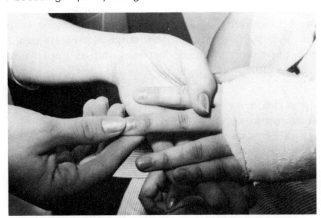

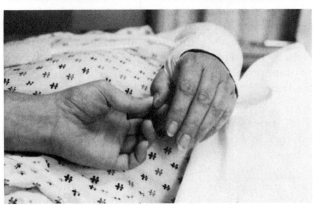

make pulse detection difficult even in the presence of patent arteries.

Venous Pattern

Dilated veins when the person assumes a standing position can indicate inadequancy of the venous system. This observation is important in persons with a history of venous problems. The nurse does not make this observation to establish a medical diagnosis; rather, this evaluation can assist in identifying future changes in the client's status. Such observations may determine a need for changes in nursing care or the need to refer the client for medical intervention.

Edema

Edema is the collection of fluid in the interstitial compartment. It is the result of an imbalance between fluid that leaves the capillary bed and that which enters. There are many causes of edema, such as tissue injury and endocrine or renal disturbances; only circulatory causes will be discussed here.

Local edema is common in persons who have chronic venous problems. In these individuals, the veins do not return blood to the heart efficiently. The result is an increase in hydrostatic pressure in the venous system and the capillaries behind it. Because venous problems most frequently affect the legs, fluid accumulates in the tissues of the lower extremities. Many of us have noticed a similar effect when our feet swell after prolonged standing. This is due to inactivity of the leg muscles whose contractions normally promote venous return by massaging the blood vessels. Interference with lymphatic drainage can also cause local edema because of increased hydrostatic pressure in this system.

Generalized edema is common in persons who have congestive heart failure. Heart failure increases hydrostatic pressure in the venous system because blood is congested behind the failing pump. (Chap. 22 contains more information about fluid retention in heart failure.) Heart failure also initiates endocrine changes that promote sodium retention; this also contributes to edema.

When assessing edema be sure to note the amount, extent, and type. *Pitting edema* feels soft and will show an imprint when a fingertip is pressed against the skin (Fig. 23-4). *Brawny edema* feels hard or gelatinous. Brawny edema is most common in impaired lymphatic drainage. Edema may be generalized or confined to a specific body part. Generalized edema is detectable in dependent body parts such as the ankles and feet; if the person is in bed

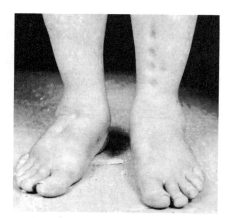

Figure 23-4
Pitting edema of lower extremities

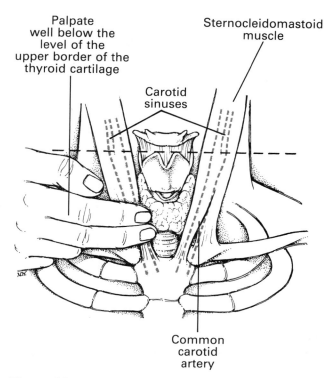

Figure 23-5
Palpating the carotid pulse

edema may be noted in the sacral area. Generalized edema may sometimes be detected by swelling in the eyelids and hands. If possible, the amount of edema should be assessed by measuring the affected body part with a tape measure. Always measure an edematous extremity along with its pair for comparison. Edema can also be evaluated by weighing the person, as described earlier.

Assessment of the Neck

Useful information about the arterial and venous systems and the pumping activity of the left ventricle can be obtained by examining the carotid pulse or the jugular veins in the neck.

Carotid Pulse

The carotid pulse may be assessed to determine rate, rhythm, and quality. Although pulse assessment is usually performed at the radial artery site, the carotid is the most easily detected pulse and is closest to the heart. If the nurse is unsure of findings obtained from the radial pulse assessment, the carotid pulse may be examined to confirm them. When palpating the carotid pulse, avoid the carotid sinus found just to the side of the thyroid cartilage (Fig. 23-5). Pressure on this area can cause a sudden drop in blood pressure or pulse rate. Palpating one side of the neck at a time also helps avoid this complication.

Jugular Veins

The appearance of the jugular vein can indicate the pumping effectiveness of the left ventricle. Jugular veins are normally distended when we are in a supine position and collapsed when we raise the trunk to a 30- or 45-degree angle. Veins which remain distended beyond this point indicate increased venous pressure. This finding is common in congestive heart failure, indicating venous congestion behind the failing left ventricle. Neck vein distention is an early sign of this problem and appears even before edema becomes apparent.

Assessment of the Precordium

The *precordium* is the area of the chest that overlies the heart. Experienced nursing practitioners can obtain much useful information from physical assessment of this area; however, these nurses also have advanced knowledge to analyze the data they obtain. For this reason, an in-depth description of the precordial assessment is not presented in this introductory text. Findings that the beginning nurse can identify and analyze are discussed.

The apical impulse is produced by the left ventricle and indicates the location of the left border of the heart. It can be palpated at the fifth intercostal space on the left side of the thorax at the midclavicular line. This point is usually located just below the left nipple (Fig. 23-6). It can also be detected in some individuals as visible chest wall movement. In conditions where the heart is enlarged, such as in long-term cardiac failure, the apical impulse is lo-

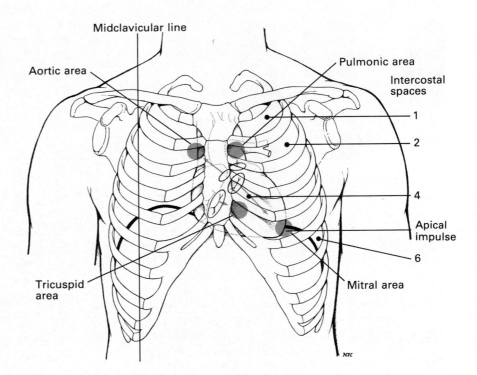

Figure 23-6
Assessment of the precordium

cated lower and further to the left and feels more forceful.

The precordial area is auscultated for the characteristics of the heart sounds. Normally, only two heart sounds are present in the adult. The first sound (S_1) is produced by the closing of the mitral and tricuspid valves at the beginning of systole; the second sound (S_2) is produced by the closure of the aortic and pulmonic valves at the end of systole. The two sounds represent one cardiac cycle and are counted as one beat when auscultating for pulse rate.

There are four areas where heart sounds are auscultated, corresponding to the four heart valves (see Fig. 23-6). The mitral area is the one most commonly auscultated. However, listening at the other areas may give information such as murmurs or extra heart sounds. Such observations should be reported to the physician if they represent a change from the person's previous status.

Nursing Process
Applied to Specific Circulatory Problems

Altered Venous Function

Nurses care for many people who have a potential for developing altered venous function. Persons confined to bed, pregnant women, and anyone undergoing surgery represent just a few who may benefit from preventive nursing care. Persons who already have chronic insufficiency of venous circulation, such as varicose veins, have a health problem they must manage the rest of their lives. Nurses have the skills to assist these individuals with their self-care activ- ities and to support them during any acute phases of dysfunction.

Venous Insufficiency

One purpose of the venous system is to return blood to the heart. Two mechanisms assist venous return from the legs: the skeletal muscle pump and valves within the veins. The skeletal muscle pump is activated by contractions that occur during walking or exercise. This action compresses veins in the legs and milks blood toward the heart. The ankle swelling which often occurs with prolonged standing is evidence of the importance of skeletal muscles in emptying leg veins. Venous valves as illustrated in Figure 23-7, maintain the flow of blood toward the heart by closing when backflow occurs. If the skeletal muscle pump or valve system is ineffective, blood pools within the venous system and leg veins dilate. This condition, called *venous stasis*, is the major physiological disruption in individuals with venous insufficiency.

One of the chief dangers of venous stasis is that it increases susceptibility to thrombus formation. A **thrombus** is a blood clot within the lumen of a blood vessel. Although the diagnosis and treatment of a thrombus is the responsibility of the physician, the nurse is also concerned with attending to and preventing this problem. Thrombi are often preventable with appropriate therapeutic nursing intervention and client teaching.

Assessment

The kind of persons who are at risk for venous insufficiency or who may already be experiencing this problem are listed in Table 23-4. Persons who

Figure 23-7

Competent valves in the veins permit the blood to flow toward the heart and prevent the flow of the blood in the opposite direction. Incompetent valves, by failing to close tightly, permit the blood to flow in both directions.

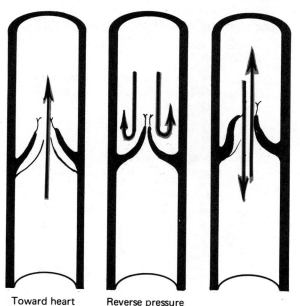

| Toward heart | Reverse pressure |

| Competent valve | Incompetent valve |

Table 23-4 Persons at Risk for Venous Insufficiency	
Mechanism	**Persons at Risk**
Venous stasis	History of venous problems
	Prolonged sitting or standing
	Pregnancy
	Advanced age
	Congestive heart failure
	Immobility (bed rest, surgery)
	Overweight
Increased blood coagulability	Birth control pills
	Dehydration
Injury to veins	IV therapy
	Leg trauma
	Fracture

have longstanding venous insufficiency may be recognized by ankle edema, distended leg veins, skin discoloration around the ankles, or ulceration at the ankles. The nurse should begin teaching and preventive care for any individual at risk for venous problems, not just those who have signs of active or chronic problems. Such early action assists clients to maintain health and avoid the short- and long-term consequences of venous dysfunction.

Should a thrombus occur, signs and symptoms depend on its extent and location, and whether inflammation is present. If the thrombus is located in a deep vein, there may be few symptoms. Findings in venous thrombosis are the result of obstructed venous flow. If inflammation is present, the following characteristic signs of this process will be apparent:

- Pain—may have various qualities such as cramping, a feeling of heaviness, aching calves, or local tenderness. Pain is related to inflammation. Discomfort that occurs with dorsiflexion of the foot is called a positive *Homan's sign*, an indication of venous thrombosis.

- Erythema—is due to inflammation.

- Local warmth—is another consequence of inflammation.

- Induration—may occur as a palpable knot in the calf.
- Edema—may be present in the entire lower extremity or only below the knee. Venous obstruction increases capillary hydrostatic pressure. This causes a net movement of fluid into the tissues.

The physician makes the actual diagnosis of venous thrombosis. However, the nurse should be able to identify the symptoms for two reasons. First, the nurse may be the first to note indications of developing thrombosis and can direct the person to medical attention. Second, the increase or decrease in symptoms may provide a basis for evaluating the effectiveness of nursing interventions.

Nursing Interventions

Nursing actions are directed toward promoting venous return from the lower extremities and preventing injury to the veins. By assisting the person to participate in the management of his health problem, the nurse can help prevent the development of acute problems such as thrombosis. Once thrombosis has occurred, the person has increased susceptibility to future venous problems including varicose veins and recurrent thrombus formation. This consequence occurs because venous valves are often damaged while the blood clot is being resolved by the body's defense mechanisms. Thus, by helping to prevent the recurrence of thrombosis, the nurse can have a significant effect on the person's future health status.

Teaching Self-Care

Teaching the person to incorporate into his daily routine those measures which promote venous return and prevent injury to the veins is an important nursing action to maintain health. Such teaching is appropriate for any person who has developed or is susceptible to venous insufficiency. Possible points to include in a teaching plan are listed in Table 23-5. Assessing the person's knowledge level and readiness to learn before beginning teaching will aid in planning appropriate methods and content for the individual learner.

Preventing Thrombosis

In the hospital, measures for prevention and health promotion should be instituted for anyone susceptible to thrombosis. Nursing interventions aim to reduce coagulability of blood, prevent injury to veins, and improve venous return. Some specific actions which will achieve these goals include:

- Leg exercises—Because movement activates the skeletal muscle pump, an excellent exercise is dorsiflexion and plantar flexion of the foot. The contraction of the calf muscles (gastrocnemius and soleus) massages blood toward the heart. These exercises can be performed by most individuals, including the elderly, pregnant women, and persons recovering from surgery. They can be performed while sitting or standing. If the person is unable to move his legs, the nurse can assist him with passive exercises. Consult with the physician before recommending exercise to persons recovering from cardiac disease, lower extremity surgery, or previous history of venous thrombosis.
- Early ambulation—This also promotes venous return by means of the skeletal muscle pump. It is an important action for persons following surgery or childbirth.
- Leg elevation—Elevating the legs promotes the return of blood to the heart by means of gravity. Persons who are ambulatory should elevate their legs whenever they sit.

Table 23-5
Teaching Plan
for Venous Insufficiency

Instruct clients as follows

- Understand how veins work and those factors which promote and prevent venous return
- Elevate legs for 10 minutes every one to 2 hours
- Exercise legs whenever possible
- Avoid prolonged sitting or standing
- Avoid sitting with legs crossed
- Avoid constrictive devices around the legs (tight garters or girdles, or stockings)
- Avoid smoking
- Maintain ideal body weight for body height and build
- Beware of the symptoms of thrombosis

- Avoidance of pressure against the popliteal space—There are four specific positions which should be avoided, to prevent pressure from being applied against the popliteal space. These four, along with correct positions, are depicted in Figure 23-8.

- Hydration—Dehydration increases the coagulability of blood. Those who are susceptible to dehydration and venous stasis such as the unconscious, the elderly, or persons who have undergone surgery should be assisted to maintain adequate fluid intake.

- Proper application of elastic wraps or stockings—Improper application of elastic stockings or ace bandages can obstruct venous circulation. Always wrap ace bandages toward the heart and never allow elastic stockings to roll up and constrict the leg. If elastic wraps are properly applied they prevent venous stasis by exerting pressure on superficial veins and encouraging blood return through deep veins.

Managing Thrombosis

If the person develops a thrombus, goals are focused on relief of discomfort, resolution of inflammation, and prevention of an **embolus.** The nurse works closely with the physician who prescribes medical therapy. Often the physician will prescribe bed rest to prevent embolization, anticoagulant medication to prevent extension of the thrombus, and moist heat to relieve inflammation. Independent nursing actions include the following:

- Elevate the affected extremity to relieve edema and increase venous return.

- Avoid pressure on the popliteal space to prevent venous occlusion.

- Do not massage the lower extremities because this can cause embolization. It is a good practice to avoid massaging the legs of any person susceptible to thrombi because a clot may be present in the absence of symptoms.

- Apply elastic wraps or ace bandages correctly.

- Observe for bleeding tendencies associated with anticoagulant medication

- When the person is sitting, always elevate legs above heart level.

When the thrombus has resolved, the person will need health teaching to prevent future incidents of thrombosis. Remember that these individuals are more susceptible to blood clots, because venous valves may have been damaged during the episode of thrombosis. The teaching plan outlined in Table 23-5 will assist the person to manage his self-care activities after hospitalization.

Altered Arterial Function

There are many health problems in which arterial blood flow is diminished. Some of these are long term, such as a chronic occlusive process in the arteries. Others occur suddenly, such as when a cast is too tight and blocks arterial flow. Whatever the cause or the nature of the problem, the result is the same: decreased tissue perfusion, inadequate cell nutrition, accumulation of wastes, and cellular death. The nurse has a responsibility to maintain or improve tissue perfusion and prevent further health problems.

Assessment

Chronic arterial problems are more common than those which occur suddenly. Persons with diabetes, those who smoke heavily, and the elderly are frequently affected by such problems. Chronic arterial obstruction occurs most often in the legs, although arteries throughout the body may be affected.

The physician will diagnose and treat chronic arterial obstruction. However, there is much that the nurse can do to assess the status of the health problem and to teach the client to do self-care. Often the nurse is the first person to recognize changes which indicate the person's condition is improving or worsening.

Changes that occur in chronic arterial obstruction include the following:

- Cool skin temperature—Skin temperature reflects perfusion of a body part, although a cool room temperature and anxiety should be considered as possible causes if the extremities feel cool. Also, temperatures in the right and left leg should be compared to one another and then to other body parts. Changes felt in just one extremity are more significant than bilateral changes.

- Weak or absent pulses—This sign indicates arterial narrowing or obstruction which interferes with transmission of pulse waves. Again both right and left sides should be compared as a way of determining whether a change is a normal pattern for the person. Frequent assessment helps the nurse detect improvement or worsening of the person's condition.

Wrong **Right**

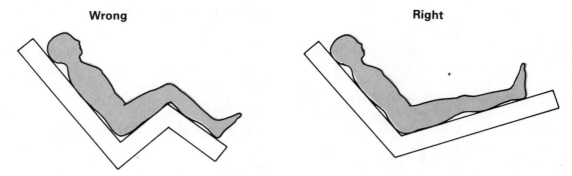

Adjust bed position so that mattress does not put pressure on the popliteal space.

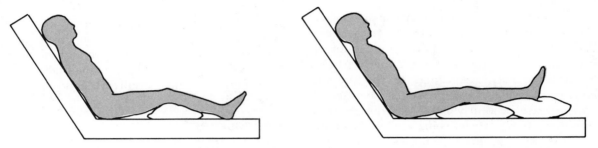

Position pillows underneath the entire leg to prevent pressure at the popliteal space.

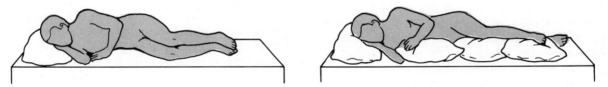

Avoid resting legs on top of each other when the person is in the lateral position to avoid pressure points at the knees.

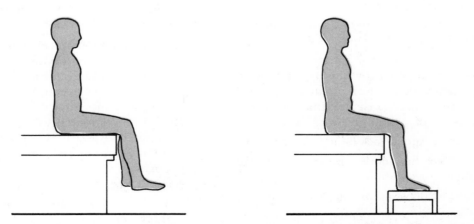

Avoid dangling legs unsupported when sitting. Rest feet on a stool to prevent pressure points at popliteal space.

Figure 23-8
Positioning to prevent venous stasis

- Leg pain—The characteristics of pain may vary depending on the cause and location of arterial obstruction. Pain may be constant or intermittent; it may be present at rest or begin with exercise. (Exercise pain, called **claudication,** was described in the assessment section of this chapter.) The cause of pain is not certain. It may be due to the build-up of wastes, such as lactic acid, or to arterial spasm. If the person experiences claudication, the nurse can assess his progress by noting how far the person can walk before pain begins and comparing future exercise tolerance to this baseline. This information is useful when evaluating the effectiveness of an exercise program in decreasing claudication.
- Alterations in skin appearance—The skin may appear shiny, dry, and tight, hair growth is sparse, and nails are thick and ridged in the affected extremity. These signs are sometimes called *trophic changes* because they are caused by poor tissue perfusion which diminishes cell nutrition. (The term *trophic* refers to nutrition.) Nail and skin changes create grooming problems as will be discussed in the section on nursing care. Skin color may be pale, cyanotic, or dusky red, indicating diminished perfusion. Skin lesions may appear and become a serious problem for the person. Because cell nutrition is inadequate, these areas heal poorly. Chronic ulcers may become gangrenous and may necessitate amputation of a toe, foot, or leg. Prevention of skin lesions is a critical part of nursing care.

Acute arterial obstruction can occur if the vessel is injured due to development of a hematoma, if an embolus lodges in an artery, or if a cast becomes too tight. In any of these situations the nurse might observe the following in the affected extremity:

- Absent pulse(s)
- Cool skin temperature
- Pale or cyanotic skin color
- Numbness or tingling
- Loss of motor function

Acute arterial obstruction is an emergency situation requiring immediate nursing intervention. It is important to recognize these signs as early as possible because tissue necrosis occurs rapidly.

Nursing Interventions

Nursing interventions for persons with chronic arterial insufficiency include care that supports the client's current level of function and health education that will enable him to manage his own health problem. Client education is presented first because supportive care involves performing parts of the teaching plan that the person is unable to do for himself.

A teaching plan with rationale is shown in Table 23-6. The nurse should identify teaching methods and content that are appropriate for the client's individual needs.

Supportive nursing care has three objectives: to maintain or improve tissue perfusion, to prevent infection or injury, and to improve exercise tolerance.

Maintaining Tissue Perfusion

Maintaining or improving tissue **perfusion** is accomplished by avoiding vasoconstrictors and keeping metabolic needs of the tissues to a minimum. The nurse should never apply heat or cold directly to affected limbs because heat increases metabolic activity and cold causes vasoconstriction. In addition, room temperature should be at a level that is comfortable for the person. Proper positioning is also very important. Usually the legs are maintained at heart level. Pressure should not be applied against the popliteal space, as can occur when the legs are dangled over the side of the bed or when the knee gatch on the bed is elevated.

Preventing Infection or Injury

Preventing infection or injury is an important objective because ischemic tissues heal poorly. To avoid injury to the toes or feet, the client should wear slippers or shoes at all times. If the client is not capable of performing the daily foot care routine shown in Table 23-6, the nurse should assume this for him. Any heat therapy should be closely monitored; such applications can cause injury because of the fact that many of these persons have decreased pain perception in the affected extremity.

Improving Exercise Tolerance

Leg pain can limit the person's mobility considerably and alter his entire life-style. Some individuals can only walk three or four blocks before pain forces them to stop. If the person has difficulty with claudication and does not have foot problems such as open lesions or blisters, he may benefit from a mutually planned exercise program. Such a plan would incorporate walking into the daily routine. A typical goal involves walking two or three times daily and continuing just beyond the point of pain (Ream, 1977). It is felt that exercise is useful in developing collateral circulation, although recent evidence shows that it may reduce claudication by improving met-

Table 23-6
Teaching Plan for Arterial Insufficiency

	Content	Rationale
Each Day:	Wash feet with mild soap and water, dry carefully, especially between toes.	Washing decreases potential pathogens; drying prevents maceration, reduces tendency to skin breakdown.
	Examine feet for cuts, blisters, fungus infection.	Allows early detection of problems.
	Wear a clean pair of white cotton socks.	Cotton's absorbency prevents skin maceration. White socks prevent possible skin irritation from dyes.
	Wear well-fitting shoes.	Decreases potential skin trauma (e.g., blisters, pressure lesions).
Special Care:	If feet are injured, cover the area with a gauze dressing; report to physician immediately; stay off feet.	Decreases risk of further injury or infection.
	Trim nails straight across; be careful not to cut skin. If nails are thick, consult podiatrist for foot care.	Prevents ingrown nails or trauma to skin that heals poorly.
	In cold weather dress warmly and wear warm footwear.	Cold induces vasoconstriction, which reduces circulation.
Avoid:	Smoking	Nicotine is a vasoconstrictor.
	Crossing legs	Obstructs arterial blood flow.
	Tight clothing on legs	Obstructs arterial blood flow.
	Tight boots	Obstructs arterial blood flow.
	Direct heat such as heating pads, hot water bottles, hot bath water	Heat increases metabolic rate and increases tissue needs of O_2; also there is risk of injury from burns related to decreased pain perception in extremity.
	Going barefoot	Potential injury to feet from cuts, abrasions.
	Cold exposure	Cold induces vasoconstriction.
	Treating own corns, calluses, or other foot lesions.	Potential for infection from improper treatment.

abolic capacity of muscles (Ekroth *et al*, 1978). After several weeks of exercise, the person should notice that he can walk greater distances without pain, thereby reinforcing his desire to continue with his exercise plan.

Dealing with Acute Arterial Obstruction

Acute arterial obstruction is treated according to the cause. In the case of obstruction from a cast, the cast is split to relieve pressure against the arteries. If arterial obstruction is the result of a hematoma or embolus, emergency surgical intervention may be necessary. While the person is awaiting surgery, the nurse provides supportive care as described in the care of chronic obstruction. In particular, it is important to avoid heat, cold, and pressure to the affected limb.

Shock

Many persons think of shock as an emotional state; however, health professionals also define shock as a distinct physiological syndrome with specific signs and symptoms. **Shock** occurs when there is a decrease in circulating blood volume leading to inadequate tissue perfusion. Decreased circulating blood volume is caused by a fall in cardiac output. Cardiac output is determined by two factors: stroke volume (the amount of blood ejected by each ventricular contraction) and heart rate.

Cardiac output = stroke volume × heart rate

Let us examine more closely some of the factors that affect cardiac output.

Stroke Volume.   Stroke volume is affected by the contractile force of the heart and venous return. Should the heart be unable to pump effectively, such as following myocardial infarction, cardiac output may fall so low that the tissues do not receive adequate oxygen. Likewise, with a fall in venous return (the amount of blood returning to the heart), there will be insufficient blood volume for the ventricles to deliver to the tissues. Decreased venous return occurs in hemorrhage or severe dehydration. Venous return may also drop if the size of the vascular system increases through vasodilatation, because this allows blood to pool in the capillaries and venous system.

Heart Rate.   Heart rate is influenced by the autonomic nervous system, whereby parasympathetic stimulation slows the heart and sympathetic stimulation increases it. Because cardiac output is affected both by heart rate and stroke volume, an increased rate can usually compensate for decreased stroke volume and maintain adequate blood supply to the tissues. In this situation, increased heart rate is an adaptive mechanism that maintains cardiac output.

From this discussion, we can identify the potential causes of shock—decreased blood volume, massive vasodilatation, and decreased pumping effectiveness of the heart. Each of these problems is related to a variety of types of shock, including cardiogenic shock, neurogenic shock, anaphylactic shock, septic shock, hemorrhagic shock, and hypovolemic shock. Some examples of these problems and the different types of shock they produce are shown in Table 23-7.

Assessment

With so many types of shock, it is obvious that nurses need to be alert to the possibility of this problem occurring in any susceptible person. This includes those who have undergone surgery or childbirth, or those who have suffered trauma, burns, severe dehydration, head injuries, myocardial infarction, allergic reactions, severe infections, or any situation in which circulating blood volume may be diminished.

Table 23-7
Types of Shock

Type	Possible Cause	Mechanism
Cardiogenic shock	Myocardial infarction	Failure of cardiac pumping activity
Neurogenic shock	Spinal cord injury	Massive vasodilatation
Anaphylactic shock	Allergic reaction	Venous pooling
Septic shock	Massive infection	Decreased venous return
Hemorrhagic shock	Hemorrhage	Decreased blood volume
Hypovolemic shock	Severe dehydration	Decreased venous return

Shock occurs in stages, each of which is accompanied by specific signs and symptoms. Because shock can often be treated successfully if it is recognized early, nurses need to be able to recognize the indications of shock in its early stages to give the person the best chance for recovery. The findings may vary depending on the type of shock and the stage at which it is noted. The following discussion presents the events that occur in early, intermediate, and late hypovolemic or hemorrhagic shock, the most common types.

Early Shock

Early shock occurs when an event such as bleeding causes a loss in circulating blood volume greater than 10% of the total blood volume. Cardiac output falls and there is a transient drop in arterial blood pressure. This initiates two adaptive mechanisms that maintain blood flow to vital organs and return blood pressure to nearly normal. First, the decreased cardiac output and low arterial pressure cause capillary pressure to fall below that in the tissues. Fluid from the tissues moves into the capillaries and a much-needed boost in blood volume results. Loss of tissue fluid causes thirst, one of the early signs of shock.

The other adaptive mechanism is a release of norepinephrine and epinephrine in response to the drop in arterial pressure. These hormones cause vasoconstriction in the vessels supplying the skin, kidneys, liver, intestines, and lungs. This shunts blood away from these organs toward the brain and heart and also reduces the size of the vascular compartment. As a result, venous return and cardiac output increase and the systolic blood pressure is maintained at normal levels. However, vasoconstriction may cause the diastolic pressure to rise. This results in a narrowed pulse pressure. Also, urine output decreases to less than 30 ml/hr and the skin becomes cool and moist as a result of vasoconstriction. Release of epinephrine causes increased pulse rate, a mechanism that maintains cardiac output. The pulse often feels weak or thready, which reflects decreased stroke volume.

Intermediate Shock

If shock remains undetected and untreated, the signs of intermediate shock develop. Intermediate shock is characterized by continued vasconstriction. Although vasoconstriction maintains blood pressure, it also causes hypoxia of tissues in the affected areas. When deprived of oxygen, tissues must rely on anaerobic metabolism, and products of the process, such as lactic acid, accumulate. These products cause the sphincters at the entrance of capillaries to dilate, but those at the venous end remain constricted. Blood pools in the capillaries and venous return falls. The result is a decrease in cardiac output. At this point the blood pressure drops. A vicious cycle is initiated of further constriction of the arterioles and veins, further tissue hypoxia, and capillary dilatation. If inadequate oxygen is supplied to the brain, restlessness and then confusion result. Hypoxia is also indicated by rapid, shallow breathing. Accumulation of acid end products of anaerobic metabolism results in metabolic acidosis, which also causes rapid breathing. (See Chap. 22 for further explanation of metabolic acidosis.) All of these signs indicate worsening shock. However, the condition is still treatable if detected at this stage.

Late Shock

If shock is allowed to progress it will reach the late stage. At this point, stasis of blood in the capillaries and acidosis favor coagulation of blood. These tiny clots in the capillaries prevent tissue perfusion. When deprived of nutrients and oxygen, tissues die; the vital organs such as the kidneys, lungs, heart, and brain fail; and death occurs. Even vigorous treatment will not save the person's life.

Nursing Interventions

Nursing care of the person in shock involves working interdependently with the physician as well as functioning independently. One of the first actions the nurse takes after identifying that the person is developing shock is to notify the physician, who determines treatment of shock. Therapy involves intravenous fluid replacement, drugs, oxygen, and other modalities. Fluid replacement is essential to the treatment of most types of shock because it increases circulating blood volume and improves cardiac output. The nurse is responsible for carrying out medical orders. However, there are three other independent nursing functions that are equally important. These are assessing the person for response to therapy, reducing oxygen demands, and giving psychological support.

Assessing Response to Therapy

Assessment involves evaluating cardiac, respiratory, renal, and neurological function. Important parameters such as vital signs and urine output are assessed hourly, or more often if the client's condition warrants. However, the nurse is continually observing the person for other signs, such as restlessness and pale skin color, to determine his status. Since the condition of persons in shock can worsen suddenly, the nurse must be constantly alert to changes. Cardiac function is reflected in vital sign changes described earlier, as well as in the condition of the skin. Return of vital signs to the client's normal range indicates a positive response to therapy. Irregular pulse indicates the development of cardiac arrhythmias due to myocardial hypoxia, a serious sign. The nurse must be aware of the client's normal vital signs in order to evaluate changes correctly.

Respiratory function is indicated by rate, rhythm, and depth of breathing. Onset of rapid, shallow respiration is often a sign of hypoxia. Additional signs of hypoxia as described in Chapter 24 may also be noted (see Table 24-7). Any of these may indicate that the client's condition is worsening. Renal function is evaluated by monitoring the person's intake and output. Urine output should be maintained at a rate of 30 cc/hr or more. An indwelling catheter is inserted into the bladder to permit frequent monitoring. Recording fluid intake is important as a comparison for urine output. The nurse watches not only for signs of hypovolemia but also for indications of circulatory overload from too rapid fluid replacement or cardiac failure. Neurological function is reflected in the person's behavior. Restlessness and anxiety are early signs of cerebral hypoxia. If hypoxia worsens, the person may become confused or difficult to arouse.

Reducing Oxygen Demands

There are several independent nursing actions that can reduce the client's oxygen requirements and improve perfusion of vital organs. One such consideration is to avoid overheating the person, which can happen if the room temperature is too warm or if heavy bedcovers are used. Just enough covering should be placed over the person to prevent shivering. If the person becomes overheated, blood vessels in the skin dilate to promote heat loss. This diverts blood away from the vital organs and is obviously undesirable.

Positioning is also important in maintaining blood flow. Depending on the type of shock, the person may be positioned flat in bed or with the legs slightly elevated. Trendelenberg postion (head dependent and legs elevated) is no longer recommended. This position reduces ventilation and contributes to hypoxia because the abdominal organs rest against the diaphragm. It is also important to turn the person at least every 2 hours. Turning promotes ventilation of all areas of the lung; this is important in shock, in which lung perfusion is uneven. By improving ventilation, the nurse is improving oxygenation.

Assisting the person to decrease energy demands and reduce anxiety is also important. Often the person is anxious and unable to rest because of the constant activity and monitoring that is taking place. By providing rest and emotional support, the nurse reduces the person's oxygen needs.

Giving Psychological Support

Psychological support is also important in improving the person's comfort. Persons in shock are often anxious because of the effects of cerebral hypoxia. In addition, they are the center of a great deal of unfamiliar activity and equipment. This can threaten the person's safety and security needs and sense of control. It is important to explain treatments and equipment to the person, even if he is unconscious. Carry out procedures in a calm and confident manner and, if possible, help the person verbalize his fears. Sleep is often disrupted because of frequent treatments and monitoring. Organizing activities to provide uninterrupted periods can help the person to meet sleep needs.

The problem of shock is the subject of much current research and new information is continuously being published. There is much more to medical and nursing intervention than can be discussed here. This section provides only basic information to help the beginning nurse identify when a person is developing shock and how basic care should be provided. The readings listed at the end of this section provide more information about the assessment, treatment, and mechanisms of shock.

Body Temperature Status

Body temperature problems occur frequently in people who are sick. Fever is a common manifestation of many illnesses. This section reviews the mechanisms that control body temperature, discusses fever as a health problem, and presents nursing care of the person with a fever.

In order to assess body temperature and care for persons with dysfunctions, the student first needs to know how temperature is normally controlled. Two different processes are going on continuously in the body: those that promote heat loss and those that promote heat retention. The temperature reading which we obtain with a thermometer represents the net effect of these processes. Factors that promote heat loss and gain are shown in Table 23-8.

The task of balancing heat production and heat loss belongs to the hypothalamus. This portion of the brain contains receptors that are sensitive to temperature. Should body temperature begin to fall below normal range, the hypothalamus initiates processes which increase heat production and retention. If body temperature rises, processes that promote heat loss begin. In this way, body temperature is maintained between 36°C and 37.2°C (97°F and 99°F).

General Assessment

Body temperature reflects the metabolic activity of cells, since heat is a by-product of cellular activity. Elevated body temperature is accompanied by increased pulse and respiratory rates so these vital signs are assessed together. Normal oral body temperature ranges from 36° to 37.2° Celsius or 97° to 99° Fahrenheit. Oral temperature readings can be altered by drinking or eating. In addition, body temperature can be influenced by factors such as exercise, sleep, the menstrual cycle, circadian rhythms, and metabolic rate (Sims–Williams, 1976; Guyton,

1976). In most people, peak temperature occurs in the afternoon or early evening (Conroy and Mills, 1970, p. 19).

Body temperature is commonly measured at three sites: oral, rectal, and axillary. Oral temperature recordings are felt to be most accurate (Molnar and Read, 1974), followed by rectal and then axillary determination.

When assessing temperature, the nurse should consider the person's normal range and correlate findings with other observations such as the person's skin temperature, his subjective feelings of warmth or coolness, and presence of perspiration.

Nursing Process Applied to the Problem of Fever

Fever is defined as an elevation in body temperature greater than 37.2°C (99°F). It is often precipitated by an infection or inflammation that may result from trauma, burns, surgery, allergic reactions, or microorganisms. These processes release substances called *pyrogens*, which cause the hypothalamus to adjust the body temperature 1 to 4 degrees higher. For example, if the person's previous temperature averaged 37°C (98.6°F), the inflammation process would cause the temperature to rise to anywhere between 38°C (100.4°F) and 41°C (105.8°F).

Table 23-8
Factors that Promote Heat Loss and Gain

	Mechanism	Rationale
Heat Gain	Increased metabolic rate	Increases heat production by cells
	Sympathetic nervous system activity	Increases metabolic rate; induces vasoconstriction which reduces heat loss from skin
	Shivering	Muscle activity and increased muscle cell metabolism produces heat
	Thyroid hormone activity	Increases metabolic rate
Heat Loss	Sweating	Promotes evaporation
	Vasodilatation	Increased blood supply to skin brings heat to body surface
	Radiation	Heat lost to atmosphere in form of rays
	Conduction	Heat lost to another object through direct contact
	Convection	Heat lost through air currents
	Evaporation	Heat lost through process of converting water to vapor

Assessment

The fever process is often described in three phases: onset, course, and termination.

Onset

During the onset stage, which usually lasts 10 to 40 minutes, body temperature rises in response to heat-producing mechanisms initiated by the hypothalamus. These mechanisms were described in Table 23-8. The person will shiver, feel chilly, and appear pale, and piloerection will occur. Increased metabolic rate from thyroid stimulation and shivering increases the cellular oxygen consumption and carbon dioxide production. Heart rate increases to supply the cells with oxygen, and respiratory rate increases in response to elevated carbon dioxide tension in the blood. Since the temperature is rising during this phase, the nurse should check the person's temperature often.

Course

Now the temperature has stabilized at a higher level. Metabolic rate remains high, which increases oxygen needs and carbon dioxide production. Pulse and respiratory rates remain elevated. The person loses a large amount of water in the form of vapor in exhaled air. This may lead to dehydration and complaints of thirst and dry mouth, along with a decrease in urine output, dry skin, and a loss of weight. Children sometimes experience convulsions with high fevers of rapid onset. Adults more commonly experience delirium with temperatures greater then 40°C (104°F), although convulsions may also occur at very high levels. Symptoms that occur in prolonged fever are fatigue and muscle weakness, possibly due to tissue breakdown. Anorexia is also common in prolonged fever.

Termination

In the termination stage, the hypothalamus readjusts body temperature back to its lower, normal level. To achieve this end, mechanisms which promote heat loss are initiated by the hypothalamus (see Table 23-8). As a result, the person's skin appears flushed and is warm to the touch. Sweating may be moderate if the temperature falls slowly, profuse if it falls rapidly. The nurse will note that the person's temperature readings fall during this stage.

Each person's response to fever is highly individual. The severity of symptoms depends on factors such as the cause of fever, the person's age, and the degree of temperature elevation. Low-grade fevers (less than 38°C or 100.4°F) produce less severe symptoms. The elderly are prone to delirium, and children are more likely to convulse during a high fever. The nurse should be aware that signs of fever are varied and should assess susceptible persons carefully for this problem.

Nursing Interventions

Nursing interventions vary according to the characteristics of the fever. For low-grade fevers which usually cause fewer comfort and safety problems, nursing responsibilities include assessing temperature frequently, keeping the individual comfortable, and working with the physician to treat the cause of the fever. High fevers, however, cause problems in themselves and are dealt with by maintaining comfort and safety, providing hydration and nutrition, reducing heat production, and promoting heat elimination.

Maintaining Comfort and Safety

Persons experiencing the stress of fever often feel uncomfortable and fatigued. To offset these problems, the nurse should try to decrease stimuli in the environment and help the person to conserve energy. Establishing frequent rest periods and quiet and minimizing interruptions can increase comfort. Comfort is also promoted by changing damp bed linens and clothing frequently if the person perspires heavily. If the person is restless or confused, he should be observed closely to prevent injury. Raise the side rails to prevent a fall from bed.

Maintaining Hydration

High fevers frequently cause increased water loss, which can lead to dehydration. As much as 3 liters of fluid per day can be lost. Because most of this loss occurs through perspiration and water vapor in exhaled air, it is not detectable directly. Remember that persons with decreased level of consciousness or young children will not be able to express thirst, which is a sign of dehydration. The nurse needs to monitor the person's fluid balance frequently and watch for signs of dehydration as described in Chapter 22. To improve hydration, liberal fluid intake of at least 3 liters per day should be encouraged. If the person is unable to replace fluids orally, the physician may order intravenous therapy.

Maintaining Nutrition

High fevers are usually accompanied by increased metabolic rates. This means that calorie intake must also increase to meet cellular energy needs. If these are not supplied, fat and protein will be metabolized into energy, resulting in tissue breakdown and accumulation of acid end-products. Compounding the problem of increased calorie needs is the anorexia which is frequently experienced. It can be a challenge to determine what foods appeal to these clients and how to provide concentrated calories. Assessing each client for his preferences and offering liquids, such as milkshakes or eggnog, may achieve these ends. If there is concern about adequacy of caloric intake, the nurse may weigh the person. Weight loss can occur with dehydration as well as with inadequate nutrition, so it may be difficult to evaluate nutritional status. Chapter 20 contains more information about nutrition assessment and caring for persons with appetite loss.

Reducing Heat Production and Increasing Heat Elimination

Independent and interdependent nursing functions are used to achieve this goal. Independently, the nurse can assist the person to decrease activity in order to reduce heat production from muscular work. Other measures include keeping the room temperature cool (68°F–70°F) to promote heat loss by radiation from the skin to room air and by avoiding heavy covers, which insulate the body and prevent heat loss from the skin.

If the person's temperature exceeds 38.4°C (101°F), the physician usually begins therapy to reduce the temperature; frequently, antipyretic drugs are ordered. The nurse should recheck the person's temperature after administering these medications to evaluate their effectiveness. Cooling baths, which promote heat loss through evaporation, are another measure that the physician may order to lower body temperature. This measure is used more often with young children whose small body area makes it more effective and practical. The water should be tepid to start to prevent shivering, which raises body temperature. Gradually, cooler water is added. Prior to

therapy and during the bath, the person's temperature is checked periodically to evaluate the effectiveness of treatment. A more common method of cooling in adults is the hypothermia mattress or cooling blanket, which consists of a large rubber pad, through which a cooling liquid is pumped. It is positioned underneath or over the person, promoting heat loss both by conduction and by convection. A temperature probe may be inserted into the rectum to allow continuous temperature monitoring.

Conclusion

Some of the common problems that persons experience with circulatory dysfunction include altered venous and arterial function and shock. Nurses who care for these individuals assist them to achieve oxygenation in all body cells. Nursing interventions are directed toward maintaining tissue perfusion and reducing oxygen demands. The circulatory and temperature statuses are closely related, because vasoconstriction and vasodilatation are means of regulating body temperature. Fever is a common phenomenon that accompanies illness and may become a problem in itself if it is prolonged or very high. Nursing care involves preventing the consequences of fever on nutrition, fluid and electrolyte, balance, skin, and comfort, as well as implementing measures to lower body temperature.

Because nurses have the privilege not only of affecting the quality of the person's life but also of maintaining life itself, we need to be aware of how the person adapts biologically and psychologically to altered functions brought about by circulatory impairment. Knowledge of adaptive mechanisms enables nurses to assist the person through preventive health measures such as health teaching, supportive care during acute dysfunction, and restorative care to promote maximum health.

Study Questions

1. Mr. Young's pulse rate is 124/minute when you check it at 6 P.M. What other information would you need to interpret this finding?

2. Mrs. Green tells you that her feet seem swollen at the end of the day. How would you assess her further?

3. What indications suggest that the nurse should assess the client's apical pulse?

4. What persons are most at risk of developing altered venous function? What preventive measures should be included in a nursing care plan? Why are preventive measures important for these individuals?

5. Mr. Jones has chronic arterial insufficiency in both lower extremities. What findings would you expect on assessment? Outline a teaching plan to assist Mr. Jones to care for himself.

6. Steve Smith has just had a cast applied to his right arm. What signs would you teach him to look for that indicate inadequate circulation from a tight cast?

7. What are the early signs of shock? Why is low blood pressure considered a later sign of shock? What are the nursing responsibilities for a person in shock?

8. What are the physiological effects of an elevated temperature?

9. What are the major problems a person with a prolonged high fever can develop? What nursing care will prevent these problems?

Glossary

Claudication: Ischemic calf muscle pain brought on by exercise.

Cyanosis: A bluish or grayish skin color due to increased amounts of reduced hemoglobin in the blood.

Diastolic pressure: Arterial blood pressure during ventricular filling.

Edema: Presence of abnormally large amounts of fluid in the intercellular tissue spaces.

Embolus: A clot or other substance brought by the blood from one vessel into another.

Hypoxia: Inadequate oxygenation of body tissues.

Ischemia: Inadequate circulation to a body part.

Perfusion: Flow of blood through a tissue or organ.

Pulse Deficit: A condition in which a difference exists between the number of ventricular contractions (as determined by the apical pulse rate) and the pulse rate measured at a peripheral site.

Pulse pressure: The mathematical difference between the systolic and diastolic blood pressures, reflects changes in stroke volume.

Shock: Condition of inadequate tissue perfusion caused by a decrease in circulating blood volume.

Systolic pressure: Arterial blood pressure during ventricular contraction.

Thrombus: Clot formation within the lumen of a blood vessel.

Bibliography

Argondizzo N: Patient assessment: Pulses. Am J Nurs 79:115–132, January 1979

Bates F: A Guide to Physical Examination. Philadelphia, JB Lippincott, 1979

Conroy RT, Mills JN: Human Circadian Rhythms. London, J&A Churchill, 1970

Davis-Sharts J: Mechanisms and manifestations of fever. Am J Nurs 78:1874–1877, November, 1978

Eddy ME: Teaching patients with peripheral vascular disease. Nurs Clin North Am 12:151–159, March, 1977

Ekroth R, Dahllöf A-G, Gundevall B et al: Physical training of patients with intermittent claudication: Indications, methods, and results. Surgery 84:640–643, November, 1978

Fitzmaurice J: Venous thromboembolic disease: Current thoughts. Cardiovasc Nurs 14:1–4, January–February, 1978

Guyton A: Textbook of Medical Physiology, 5th ed. Philadelphia, WB Saunders, 1976

Hauser D: What to do first when a patient complains of chest pain. Nurs '76 6:54–56, November, 1976

Jackson B: Chronic peripheral arterial disease. Am J Nurs 72:928–934, May, 1972

Jones M: Accuracy of pulse rates counted for fifteen, thirty, and sixty seconds. Milit Med 135:1127–1136, December, 1970

Jones D, Dunbar CF, Jirovec MM: Medical Surgical Nursing: A Conceptual Approach. New York, McGraw-Hill, 1978

Manzi C: Edema; How to tell if it's a danger signal. Nurs '77 7:66–70, April, 1977

McBride C, Blacklow R: Signs and Symptoms, 5th ed. Philadelphia, JB Lippincott, 1970

Molnar G, Read R: Studies during open heart surgery on the special characteristics of rectal temperature. J Appl Physiol 36:333–336, March, 1974

Nichols G, Ruskin MM, Glor AK et al: Oral, axillary, and rectal temperature determinations and their relationships. Nurs Res 15:307–310, Fall, 1966

Nichols G, Kucha D: Taking adult temperatures: Oral measurement. Am J Nurs 72:1091–1092, June, 1972

Ream I: Counseling patients with leg pain. Nurs '77 7:54–57, October, 1977

Roberts B: The acutely ischemic limb. Heart Lung 5:273–276, April, 1976

Ryan R: Thrombophlebitis: Assessment and prevention. Am J Nurs 76:1634–1637, October, 1976

Secton D: The patient with peripheral arterial occlusive disease. Nurs Clin North Am 12:89–99, March, 1977

Simpson MM: Prevention of deep vein thrombosis. Am Heart J 91:400–401, March, 1976

Sims-Williams A: Temperature taking with glass thermometers: A review. J Adv Nurs 1:481–493, November, 1976

Tharp G: Shock: The overall mechanisms. Am J Nurs 74:2208–2211, December, 1974

Wiley L: Staying ahead of shock. Nurs '74 4:19–27, April, 1974

Respiratory Status

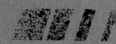

Ann Z. Kruszewski

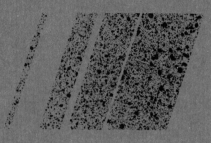

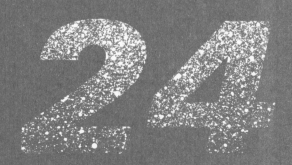

After completing this chapter, students will be able to:

● *Apply principles of normal respiratory function to the care of the person.*

● *Identify stressors that can alter respiratory function.*

● *Assess the person's respiratory status using interview and physical examination skills.*

● *Identify persons who are susceptible to disruptions of respiratory function.*

● *Identify common signs and symptoms of altered respiratory function.*

● *Describe nursing actions to maintain and restore normal respiratory function.*

● *Describe interventions to assist persons with respiratory dysfunction to cope with life style changes.*

Respiration is the process of supplying oxygen to body tissues and removing carbon dioxide. Because oxygen is essential to normal cell function and life, alterations in respiration affect every body system. This means that nurses who assist persons with respiratory dysfunction must consider the effects of these disorders on the whole person, not merely on the respiratory status.

Acute respiratory problems may be life-threatening and call for emergency measures. Chronic problems, while not so critical, may have a profound effect on a person's life-style, by limiting daily activities, mobility, social contacts, and even finances, or by necessitating changes in employment and housing. Nursing care of people with these problems involves helping them not only to cope with their oxygenation needs but also to deal with the life-style changes that chronic respiratory disorders bring. Of equal importance are preventive measures which nurses can assist persons to utilize in order to avoid respiratory illness.

This chapter discusses the assessment of individuals who are at risk for respiratory difficulties and describes the common problems related to oxygenation. Nursing approaches are presented with the focus on assisting the whole person to adapt to stressors affecting respiratory function. In order to understand these effects, nurses need to be knowledgeable about normal respiratory anatomy and physiology. Let us begin with a brief review of the major concepts.

Process of Respiration

The respiratory tract consists of a series of tubes or passageways that begin at the nares and end at the alveoli. Figure 24-1 shows a portion of the lower respiratory tract. These structures play a vital role in the process of respiration. This process consists of three phases: ventilation, gas exchange and transportation, and cellular respiration.

Ventilation

Ventilation is the process of moving air into and out of the lungs. Effective ventilation requires that air reach the alveoli; this means that the airway must

Figure 24-1
The respiratory tract

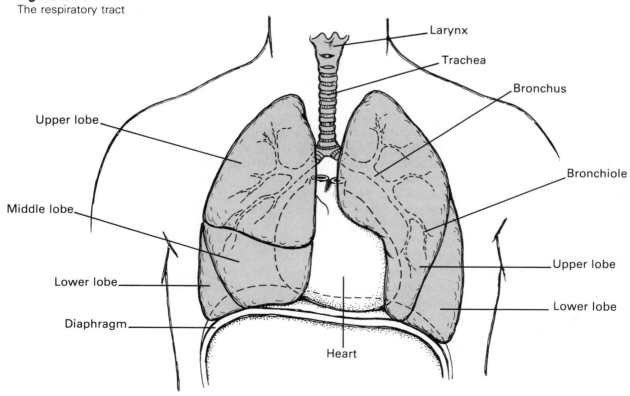

be patent and the thoracic cage, lungs, and muscles of respiration must be intact and functioning properly.

Ventilation consists of two phases: inspiration and expiration. During the inspiratory phase the thorax expands longitudinally, as well as outwardly and laterally. The lungs move outward along with the chest wall, drawing air into the lungs. The movement of the chest wall during inspiration is created by contraction of the diaphragm and external intercostal muscles. Whereas inspiration is an active process, expiration is usually passive. As the thorax and lungs return to their normal resting position during expiration, the size of the thorax decreases and air moves out of the lungs. In the presence of respiratory distress, expiration often becomes an active process in which the abdominal muscles are used to push the diaphragm upward, thereby forcing air out of the lungs.

Ventilation is controlled by several mechanisms, the most important of which is the central nervous system. The respiratory center is located mainly in the medulla and is sensitive to carbon dioxide and hydrogen ion concentration in the surrounding tissue fluid. Even very slight increases in concentrations of either substance stimulate ventilation, resulting in an increase in the rate and depth of breathing.

Ventilation is also affected by oxygen deficiency, though to a much lesser extent. Chemoreceptors, which are located mostly in the carotid and aortic bodies, are stimulated when the partial pressure of oxygen in the arterial blood (pO_2) falls below 70 mm Hg. Normally the pO_2 is 90 to 100 mm Hg, so low oxygen tension ordinarily is not a very important factor in controlling ventilation.

There are several conditions in which oxygen does act as a powerful stimulus for respiration. One such condition is emphysema in which there are chronically high levels of carbon dioxide in the tissues. Instead of stimulating the central nervous system to increase ventilation, the high CO_2 levels gradually have a toxic effect and depress respiration. Fortunately, low oxygen tension in the arterial blood still stimulates respiration through the chemoreceptors in the carotid arteries and aorta. We call this condition *respiration by hypoxic drive*. Nurses who work with people who have emphysema must never administer oxygen in high concentrations. If this happened, arterial oxygen tension would rise, removing the only stimulus for breathing. Ventilation would decrease markedly and the person would lapse rapidly into a coma.

Ventilation is also controlled by respiratory movements. As the lung inflates, stretch receptors located in the lungs are stimulated. This signal is relayed to the respiratory center in the brain which inhibits further inspiration. This process, known as the *Hering-Breuer reflex*, partially controls ventilation by limiting the volume of air that enters the lung.

Movements of muscles and joints also stimulate ventilation. Most of us notice an increase in the rate and depth of breathing during exercise. Because exercise has these effects on respiratory rate and depth, assessing respirations after a person has been active may yield data that are elevated above normal values.

Ventilation can be altered voluntarily, such as when we talk or are conscious of our breathing pattern. Thus, it is best to avoid counting respirations when a person is conscious of the fact that he is being observed for this purpose, because he may inadvertently alter his breathing pattern. However, it is also important to check respiratory rates serially to document major changes. The factors controlling ventilation are summarized in Figure 24-2.

Stressors such as an obstructed airway and a depressed respiratory center interfere with ventilation. When ventilation is ineffective, oxygen supply to the tissues is limited, resulting in **hypoxia.**

Diffusion and Transportation

Diffusion is the transfer of a substance from an area of high concentration to one of low concentration. Diffusion of gases occurs both in the alveoli and at the cellular level. In the alveoli the partial pressure of oxygen is high, while that of carbon dioxide is low as compared to pressures in the pulmonary capillaries. Therefore oxygen moves into the pulmonary capillaries and carbon dioxide enters the alveoli by the process of diffusion. At the cell level the diffusion gradient causes oxygen to move into cells and carbon dioxide to move into the capillaries. Diffusion at the alveolar level depends on the partial pressure of oxygen in the alveoli and the thickness of the alveolar–capillary membrane.

Many factors can affect the process of gas exchange. For instance, in pulmonary edema, fluid interferes with diffusion between the alveoli and capillaries. When ventilation is inadequate, as in depressed breathing, less oxygen is available for diffusion into pulmonary capillaries.

Adequate diffusion is also dependent on matching the distribution of air in the lungs with blood flow in the capillaries. If alveoli are ventilated but the capillaries supplying them are not perfused,

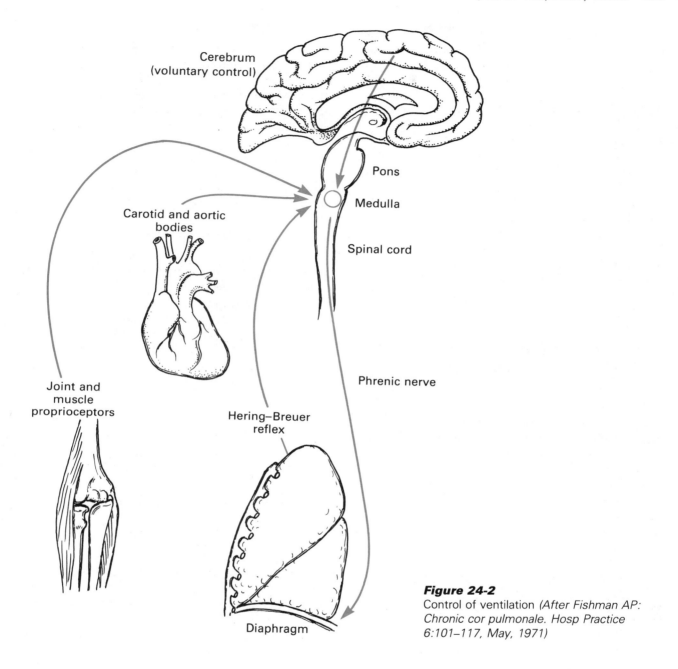

Cerebrum
(voluntary control)

Pons

Medulla

Carotid and aortic
bodies

Spinal cord

Joint and
muscle
proprioceptors

Phrenic nerve

Hering–Breuer
reflex

Diaphragm

Figure 24-2
Control of ventilation *(After Fishman AP:
Chronic cor pulmonale. Hosp Practice
6:101–117, May, 1971)*

diffusion cannot take place. Likewise, if capillaries are perfused but alveoli are not ventilated gas exchange cannot take place. These conditions are termed *shunts.*

Oxygen is transported in the blood in two ways: in the plasma or in combination with hemoglobin. Approximately 3% of oxygen is transported to tissues dissolved in the plasma; the remaining 97% is combined with hemoglobin (Guyton, 1976, p. 552). Because oxygen is transported mostly by hemoglobin, it is easy to see how persons with anemia often experience hypoxia and resulting fatigue. Carbon

dioxide is transported away from cells by the same mechanisms.

Another important factor for transportation of gases is cardiac output. In heart failure, oxygen cannot be delivered in adequate amounts to meet tissue demands. The result is hypoxia, fatigue, and inability to perform normal daily activities.

This discussion of diffusion and transportation demonstrates how closely the respiratory and circulatory systems work to supply cells with adequate oxygen. Because of this interrelationship individuals with circulatory problems often have accompanying respiratory difficulties. In the presence of a circulatory or a respiratory problem it is important to assess the abilities of both systems together to supply oxygen.

Cell Respiration

The process of utilization of oxygen and production of carbon dioxide as a waste product takes place in the cells. In order for effective respiration to take place, the lungs and circulatory system must supply enough oxygen to meet the demands of the cells, and they must eliminate the carbon dioxide produced during cell metabolism. In certain conditions, such as fever, cell metabolism is increased. The increased pulse and respiratory rates which nurses often observe in febrile persons reflect the attempt to increase oxygen supply and eliminate carbon dioxide.

Protective Mechanisms of the Respiratory Tract

There are several mechanisms that protect the lungs from foreign bodies and microorganisms. In health these mechanisms function so effectively that the lower respiratory tract is normally sterile. However, under certain conditions, protective mechanisms may not function adequately, resulting in respiratory infection or airway obstruction. For this reason, it is important to understand these protective mechanisms as well as factors that may interfere with their function.

Upper Respiratory Tract

In the upper respiratory tract, inspired air is cleansed, warmed, and humidified. The stiff hair or vibrissae in the nares trap inhaled particles. In addition, the nasal septum and turbinates, by directing airflow into narrow streams, force many particles to come in contact with the mucous secretions of the nasal walls where they are trapped. The cilia which line the epithelium of the nose transport foreign particles continuously toward the pharynx. Here they are expectorated or swallowed. Other irritants are expelled by the sneeze reflex, which cleanses the nasal passages through a rapid expulsion of air.

The swallowing reflex is another important protective mechanism, which prevents food from entering the lower respiratory passages. It is controlled in the central nervous system by the fifth, ninth, and tenth cranial nerves. Persons with impaired swallowing function, such as may occur following a stroke

or during decreased consciousness, are in danger of aspirating food, oral secretions, or vomitus into the lower respiratory tract. A *tracheostomy* (an opening into the trachea) presents a different problem. In this instance, inspired air bypasses the upper respiratory tract defense mechanisms and passes directly into the trachea. Because of this diversion, respiratory secretions are often more viscous and difficult to cough out since air is not humidified by the upper airway. Some tracheostomized individuals have difficulty performing a normal swallowing maneuver, which increases their potential for aspiration.

Lower Respiratory Tract

The lower respiratory passages also rely on certain protective mechanisms, including the cough reflex, ciliary activity, alveolar macrophages, and lymphocytes. The cough mechanism clears the trachea and bronchi of foreign bodies and secretions. Irritation of the respiratory passages by substances such as mucus, smoke, or foreign bodies sends impulses to the central nervous system, which initiates a cough. Five actions comprise a cough:

- Deep inspiration
- Closing of the epiglottis and vocal cords trapping air in the lungs
- Contraction of the abdominal muscles that push against the diaphragm and increase pressure in the lungs
- Sudden opening of the vocal cords and epiglottis
- Rapid expulsion of air from respiratory passages carrying foreign bodies and mucus into the pharynx

The cough reflex may be compromised in numerous situations, such as in people who are not fully conscious or those who are receiving drugs that depress the central nervous system. Similarly, persons with weakened chest wall muscles or a painful abdominal incision may not be able to generate an effective cough, owing to their inability to take a deep inspiration. In all these instances, there is a risk that pulmonary secretions will be retained or that the airway will be obstructed by mucus or foreign bodies.

Another protective mechanism of the lower respiratory tract is the ciliated epithelium, which lines the respiratory passages. Cilia continuously move in an upward waving motion toward the pharynx, propelling the mucus that covers the respiratory tract and transporting small particles and bacteria to the pharynx where they are expectorated or swallowed. The effectiveness of this mucociliary transport mechanism is compromised by cigarette smoke, anesthesia, dehydration, or any condition that thickens or increases the amount of mucus. Nurses should be aware that persons with these risk factors are susceptible to respiratory infection and retained secretions.

Alveolar macrophages and lymphocytes serve as other protective mechanisms. Alveolar macrophages are cells which are capable of phagocytosis. They engulf and destroy bacteria and small foreign particles that have made their way into the terminal bronchi and alveoli. Cigarette smoking and heavy ingestion of alcohol interfere with the action of alveolar macrophages. Lymphocytes produce antibodies against microorganisms in the lung. The action of lymphocytes is severely restricted in immune deficiencies, which occur in persons who have leukemia or those receiving anticancer drugs. As a result, their risk of respiratory infection is increased (Dowell and Freeman, 1977).

Factors that Affect Oxygenation

From the previous discussion we can identify a list of factors that are essential in maintaining an adequate supply of oxygen and removing carbon dioxide. These factors are presented in Table 24-1, along with examples of health alterations that may result in

respiratory problems. Being aware of these factors can help identify those individuals who are at risk for developing respiratory problems and who may therefore need special nursing attention to maintain respiratory function. Detecting these problems early and preventing oxygen deficiencies in these individuals depends to a large degree on a careful and thorough assessment of respiratory function.

General Assessment of Respiratory Status

The amount of detail covered in the initial assessment of respiratory function depends on the circumstances. Not all persons need a complete respiratory assessment. For instance, a 19-year-old woman attending a clinic for a routine physical examination might need only a basic assessment. A 54-year-old man who smokes heavily and is awaiting surgery would need a detailed observation of respiratory status.

At the same time, it is important to remember that assessment is an ongoing process and is not limited to the initial interview. Assessment of respiratory status is continual, particularly if there is a potential danger that oxygenation problems will develop.

Table 24-1
Factors that Affect Oxygenation

	Factors	Examples of Health Disruptions
Ventilation	Neurological control	Decreased level of consciousness, drug overdose
	Patent airway	Increased respiratory secretions, aspirated foreign bodies
	Intact thorax	Chest wall trauma
	Muscle control	Muscle disease, aging, prolonged illness
Diffusion	Matching ventilation and perfusion	Chronic obstructive lung disease
	Adequate O_2 in alveoli	Airway obstruction
	Functional alveolar–capillary membrane	Pulmonary edema
Transportation	Adequate cardiac output	Hemorrhage, cardiac failure
	Adequate hemoglobin level	Anemia
Cell Uptake of Oxygen		Fever

Initially, though, respiratory assessment is carried out during the interview and physical examination. Physical assessment relies on the skills of inspection, palpation, percussion, and auscultation, as described below.

Interview

The interview is the means by which we determine the person's perceptions, his experiences with respiratory symptoms, and his health practices. Thus important subjective data concerning respiratory function can be obtained by inquiring about a wide range of possible symptoms and signs, including dyspnea, fatigue, cough and sputum production, pain with respiration, and a possible history of smoking.

Dyspnea

One of the first signs to check is the presence of **dyspnea**—a sensation of difficult or labored breathing. Clues to the existence of this problem may be revealed by subjective statements the client makes such as, "I feel short of breath," "It's as if I'm suffocating," "I can't seem to catch my breath," "I feel weak," or "I get tired quickly." Because persons with normal respiratory function experience dyspnea with strenuous activity such as running up stairs, it is important to determine what level of activity brings on this sensation. For instance, a person who experiences dyspnea after walking one block or doing light housework probably has some respiratory dysfunction. This information can be used in planning nursing care, for these individuals will need frequent rest periods between activity.

Fatigue

Because respiratory problems interfere with oxygenation, fatigue may accompany respiratory dysfunction as an indication of hypoxia. As with dyspnea, it is important to correlate fatigue with the degree of activity involved. Fatigue after mild activity such as bathing or preparing a meal may indicate hypoxia. Again, nurses can use this information for planning and prioritizing activity because persons who are easily fatigued need frequent rest periods.

Cough and Sputum Production

As indicated earlier, a cough is a protective mechanism for clearing the lower respiratory tract. However, the presence of a cough, especially if it is persistent, may indicate a respiratory problem. Thus, it is important to determine how long the cough has persisted. Coughs lasting longer than 2 to 3 weeks may indicate a serious respiratory condition. It is also important to note the character of the cough (dry, moist, croupy, hacking), its frequency, and when it is most evident.

Sputum production is related to irritation of the lower respiratory tract. The irritation stimulates the mucous glands to produce increased amounts of mucus, which is then coughed up as sputum. Normally the respiratory tract produces 100 ml of mucus per day. However, when the respiratory passages are irritated, ten times this amount may be produced (Wade, 1977, p. 11).

If a cough produces sputum, the amount, color, consistency, and odor should be noted. Normally sputum is clear. Green or yellow sputum which has a foul odor may indicate the presence of infection. Thick sputum indicates a need for hydration because respiratory mucus is normally 95% water. Frothy sputum may result from pulmonary edema. **Hemoptysis** (blood in the sputum) is a serious finding that may be seen in tuberculosis or carcinoma of the bronchi. Persons with this symptom should be referred immediately to a physician.

Smoking History

Smoking has many implications for respiratory function, including its effect on ciliary activity as described earlier. Smoking has also been correlated with certain pulmonary and cardiac conditions such as emphysema, chronic bronchitis, lung cancer, and diseases of the arteries. It may also pose a risk for pulmonary complications in heavy smokers who undergo surgery.

Because of these effects, it is important to identify whether the person smokes, how long he or she has smoked, and the number of packs smoked per day. In view of the fact that people are beginning to smoke at an earlier age and that more women are now using tobacco, it is useful to obtain information about the person's attitudes and beliefs toward smoking and whether or not any attempts have been made to stop. Nurses can play an important part in preventive health care by teaching about the effects of smoking and by helping people to change their smoking habits.

Pain with Respiration

Painful respiration can result from inflammation of pulmonary structures such as the pleura (pleurisy) or from trauma to the thorax (surgical incisions, rib fracture). Painful breathing is often accompanied by shallow respiration in an attempt to limit movement of the thorax. The nurse might look for this finding when assessing respiratory rate and depth in persons experiencing painful breathing.

Inspection

A good deal of useful information about the person's respiratory status can be obtained just by looking at him. Included in this aspect of assessment is the inspection of respiratory rate, rhythm and depth, skin color, breathing posture, chest contour, the muscles used in breathing, and possibly clubbing of the fingers.

Respiratory Rate, Depth, and Rhythm

Respiratory Rate

Respiration in many ways is the most inaccurately assessed of all the vital signs; often respiratory rate is ignored altogether or estimated rather than counted. Yet much can be learned by assessing respiration. Therefore, establishing a baseline respiratory rate by counting the rate for 1 minute is essential to a good respiratory assessment.

Respiratory rate is affected by age and other factors. A normal rate in infants is 26 to 34 breaths per minute; in adults it is 14 to 20 per minute. Increased respiratory rate (**tachypnea**) may indicate hypoxia. **Bradypnea** (decreased rate) is seen when the respiratory center in the medulla is depressed, such as in drug overdose or head injury.

Depth of Respiration

Assessing the depth of respirations provides important information concerning *alveolar ventilation*, the amount of fresh air reaching the alveoli (Fig. 24-3). If respiratory depth is very shallow, air only moves into and out of the trachea and bronchi (dead space breathing). Because air does not reach the alveoli, carbon dioxide is not removed from the lungs, nor is oxygen supplied. Nurses should be aware that the consequences of this breathing pattern are **hypercapnea, hypoxemia,** and eventual hypoxia. This

Normal Adult
Alveolar ventilation = (tidal volume − dead space) × rate
7000 ml/min = (500 ml − 150 ml) × 20/min

Shallow Breathing
3000 ml/min = (300 ml − 150 ml) × 20/min

Figure 24-3
Determinants of alveolar ventilation

shallow breathing pattern is often seen in persons experiencing chest wall pain.

Considered together, the rate and depth of breathing can also yield useful information. Rapid, shallow breathing may be a sign of pain, anxiety, or hypoxia. Rapid, deep breathing, known as *Kussmaul breathing*, is seen in metabolic acidosis.

Respiratory Rhythm

Respiratory rhythm indicates the status of the neurological controls of breathing. Normally, respirations are regular, with an equal interval between each breath. Irregular respiration due to short periods of **apnea** is not unusual in newborns or elderly persons, particularly during sleep. This is probably caused by changes in respiratory center excitability. **Biot's breathing,** in which respirations vary in depth with irregular periods of apnea, is seen in brain damage and may be a prelude to death. **Cheyne–Stokes respirations,** in which periods of hyperpnea alternate with periods of apnea, may be seen in cardiac failure (Fig. 24-4).

While observing respirations the nurse can also note the duration of inspiration and expiration. Normally, expiration is 1½ times as long as inspiration but it may be longer in certain respiratory diseases. Prolonged expiration is often seen in emphysema due to air trapping, which makes it difficult to move air out of the lungs.

Cyanosis

People with respiratory problems sometimes have a bluish or gray color to their skin—a condition termed **cyanosis.** Cyanosis is caused by increased amount of deoxygenated hemoglobin, which is bluish in color.

There are two types of cyanosis: peripheral and central. Peripheral cyanosis is usually seen in isolated body parts such as the fingers, nose, or earlobes. It is sometimes seen in cold weather, because cold causes vasoconstriction and slower blood flow to exposed body parts. Because of the slower blood flow, cells extract more oxygen from the blood, thereby increasing the level of deoxygenated hemoglobin. Central cyanosis usually has a more serious cause because it indicates a generalized increase in deoxygenated hemoglobin throughout the tissues. It can be best detected where capillaries are numerous such as the lips, tongue, or nailbeds.

Although central cyanosis may indicate hypoxia, it is usually considered an unreliable sign. For one thing, changes in skin color are difficult to detect, especially in poor lighting or in dark-skinned individuals. Cyanosis also is affected by skin thickness.

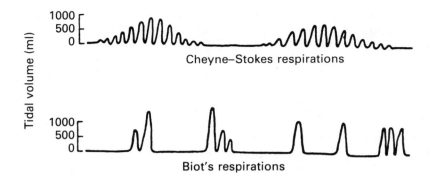

Tidal volume (ml)

1000
500
0

Cheyne–Stokes respirations

1000
500
0

Biot's respirations

Figure 24-4
Disturbances in respiratory rhythm. (*A*) With Cheyne–Stokes respirations, periods of hyperpnea alternate with periods of apnea. (*B*) With Biot's respirations, respirations vary in depth with irregular periods of apnea. (*Cherniack R* et al: *Respiration in Health and Disease, 2nd ed, p. 120. Philadelphia, W B Saunders, 1972*)

It is much easier to observe skin color changes in infants, children, and elderly persons because their skin is relatively thin. Another reason that cyanosis is an unreliable sign of hypoxia is that it only occurs when there are at least 5 g or more of unoxygenated hemoglobin per 100 ml of arterial blood. Persons with elevated hemoglobin concentrations may easily have 5 g/100 ml of unoxygenated hemoglobin and appear cyanotic even though hypoxia is mild. On the other hand, anemic individuals (who have low hemoglobin levels and use all available hemoglobin to transport oxygen) may only become cyanotic when they are severely hypoxic. Even in persons with normal hemoglobin levels, cyanosis does not appear until the arterial oxygen tension has fallen very low (pO_2 less than 50 mm Hg). Therefore cyanosis is usually a late sign of hypoxia. The nurse should be able to identify other signs of hypoxia long before cyanosis appears. These findings are covered in more detail in the discussion of respiratory distress.

Muscles Used for Breathing

When a person has difficulty breathing, accessory muscles of respiration such as the neck and shoulder muscles, the scalenes, sternocleidomastoids, and trapezius may be used to assist ventilation. Pronounced shoulder movement may be observed when these accessory muscles are used. The abdominal muscles also assist forceful expiration by moving the diaphragm up and the lower ribs down and inward, thereby decreasing the size of the thorax. **Retractions** (drawing in of the spaces between the ribs or just below the rib cage) represent another indication of accessory muscle use.

Posture

Persons with respiratory problems often assume a posture that facilitates their breathing. For instance, people experiencing dyspnea often maintain a sitting position that allows maximum chest expansion with the least effort. Persons with chest wall pain may lie on the affected side to diminish movement and discomfort.

Clubbing

Clubbing is the term used to describe a particular change in the appearance of the fingers and toes.

Figure 24-5
Clubbing. *(Left)* The angle between the nail and digit is about 20°. *(Center)* Flattened angle represents early stage of clubbing. *(Right)* In advanced clubbing, the nail is rounded over the end of the finger. Note also that the distal phalanx is bulbous and of greater depth than the proximal portion of the finger (interphalangeal depth).

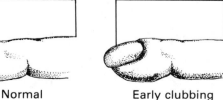

Normal   Early clubbing

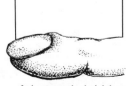

Advanced clubbing

Early clubbing is evident by a loss of the angle between the nailbed and the finger. The nailbed also feels soft and spongy. Later, the digits become enlarged and bulbous so that they look like clubs (Fig. 24-5). Clubbing may be an indication of pulmonary disease, particularly cancer or emphysema, and cardiac disease, especially congenital heart conditions. The specific mechanism which causes clubbing is not known.

Changes in Chest Contour

Normally the lateral diameter of the thorax is twice as large as the anteroposterior diameter. In emphysema, however, these diameters become equal, resulting in a condition known as *barrel chest* (Fig. 24-6). This change fixes the chest in the inspiratory position, which increases the work of breathing. In essence, the person must work harder to move air into and out of his lungs and often uses accessory muscles to aid ventilation. Barrel chest is normal in children younger than 6 years and in some older individuals; therefore, the finding is less significant in these age groups.

Other chest deformities that may interfere with respiration are *kyphosis* (outward displacement of the thoracic spine) and *scoliosis* (lateral displacement of the thoracic spine). Individuals with these deformities may be at higher risk of developing pulmonary problems. The nurse should pay special attention to the respiratory status in these people.

Palpation

Palpation can frequently confirm what the nurse has detected from inspection. It is used to determine chest expansion, fremitus, and respiratory secretions.

Chest Expansion

Chest expansion can be determined by standing behind the client and placing your hands on the sides of the chest wall with thumbs parallel to the spine. Ask the person to exhale then inhale deeply. You should observe your thumbs moving apart at the same rate and separating an equal distance from the spine (Fig. 24-7). Reduced movement of one side of the chest wall may indicate diminished air movement through the affected area, as occurs in **atelectasis.**

Fremitus

Fremitus may be assessed by placing the side of the hand on the chest wall and asking the person to say

a resonant word such as "ninety-nine." When the person speaks, vibrations pass from the larynx through open airways and are transmitted to the chest wall. The intensity of the vibrations are noted by placing the side of the hand on the chest wall and moving from side to side down the thorax while the client repeats the word "ninety-nine." Diminished fremitus is noted when there is bronchial obstruction such as in atelectasis. Increased fremitus is noted when there is a patent bronchus and increased transmission of sounds through solid tissue. This occurs in pneumonia, when the alveoli become occluded with inflammatory exudate.

Figure 24-6
Comparison between normal and barrel chests

Normal   Clinical appearance   Cross section of thorax

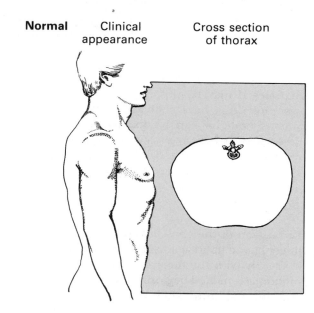

Barrel Chest   Clinical appearance   Cross section of thorax

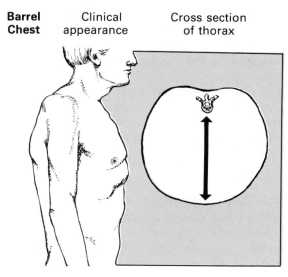

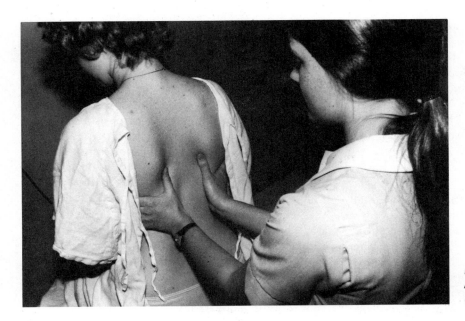

Figure 24-7
Assessing chest expansion
(Photo by Bob Kalmbach)

Respiratory Secretions

At times it may be possible to palpate respiratory secretions that have collected in the large airways. Such secretions can be felt as coarse vibrations. Persons who have excessive respiratory secretions need special nursing care to clear their airways. These measures are described later in the chapter.

Percussion

Percussion of the chest involves placing the middle finger of one hand against the chest wall and striking it sharply with the fingertip of the other hand. This motion is repeated beginning at the top of the thorax and moving from side to side down the chest. Normally percussion of the thorax produces a high pitched resonant note because lungs are filled with air. Solid tissue produces a lower pitch or dull sound. Percussing over bone, the diaphragm, or heart thus results in a low, duller sound, as does percussing over a tumor and over areas where alveoli are blocked by inflammatory products as in pneumonia. To develop the skill of percussion, students may find it helpful to practice on one another until they can distinguish among the different percussion sounds.

Auscultation

The skill of auscultation also requires practice. The chest is auscultated by placing the diaphragm of the stethoscope firmly against the chest wall, beginning at the apex of the lungs and moving down alternating sides of the thorax. Throughout the process, one side of the thorax is compared to the other as the person takes a full breath. Both the anterior and posterior thorax are auscultated in this fashion (Fig. 24-8). Breath sounds are more easily heard if the client is sitting and breathes through his mouth slightly more deeply than normal. The normal breath sounds are listed in Table 24-2.

Figure 24-8
Technique for auscultation of posterior chest

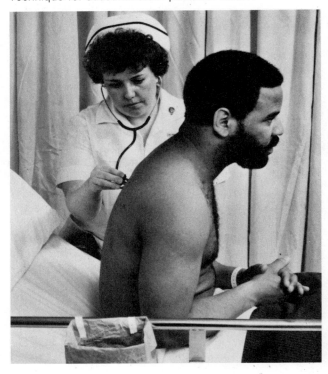

Table 24-2
Breath Sounds

Sound	Origin	Characteristics
Normal Sounds		
Vesicular	Alveoli	Low pitched, soft, swishing
		Heard over most of adult chest
Bronchial (tracheal)	Trachea	Loud, high pitched, hollow
		Expiratory phase louder and longer than inspiration
Bronchovesicular	Mainstem and larger bronchi	Louder than vesicular sounds
		Equal inspiratory and expiratory phases
		Heard at second or third intercostal space to right of sternum in adults
		Heard over most of infant chest
Adventitious Sounds		
Rales (inspiratory sounds due to mucus or edema)		
Fine rales	Alveoli	Fine, crackling sounds
Medium rales	Bronchioles	Louder, more distinct than fine rales (like carbonated beverage fizz)
Coarse rales	Trachea, bronchi	Loud, gurgling sounds
Rhonchi (inspiratory or expiratory sounds due to airway narrowing)		
Sibilant rhonchi (wheezes)	Bronchioles, bronchi	High pitched, wheezing, whistling sounds
		Caused by airway narrowing
		Common in asthma or emphysema
Sonorous rhonchi	Bronchi	Low pitched, snoring, rattling sounds caused by partial airway obstruction from mucous plugs
Pleural friction rubs (inspiratory and expiratory sounds)	Pleura	Common in pleurisy
		Grating, crackling sounds caused by inflamed pleura moving against each other

The intensity of breath sounds should also be checked. In normal persons, sounds diminish slightly in intensity as you move toward the lung bases. An area of diminished intensity other than this may indicate decreased ventilation through that portion of the lungs. Abnormally placed **bronchial** or bronchovesicular **breath sounds** are also an indication of respiratory problems. This finding indicates that the alveoli have become blocked or compressed and that sound is being transmitted from the larger airways, as can occur in pneumonia. **Adventitious sounds** represent another respiratory abnormality and are listed in Table 24-2.

Diagnostic Tests

Blood gas studies, pulmonary function tests, sputum cultures, and chest x-rays are commonly used diagnostic tests for determining the functioning of the respiratory system. Although nurses are usually not responsible for ordering diagnostic tests, the results of the reports can be used to plan nursing interventions and to identify any changes in respiratory function.

Blood gas studies are the partial pressures of oxygen (pO_2) and carbon dioxide (pCO_2), usually measured in arterial blood. Serum pH is another value, which is determined from blood gas studies. Because nurses are often the first to see the client's laboratory values, they should be familiar with normal values and the implications of changes. The arterial pO_2 reflects the oxygen delivered to the cells. The arterial pCO_2 is a good indication of the effectiveness of alveolar ventilation. Elevated pCO_2 indicates ventilation which is not eliminating carbon dioxide effectively (**hypoventilation**). Low pCO_2 indicates that the person is exhaling too much carbon dioxide (**hyperventilation**). Normal values for arterial blood gases are shown in Table 24-3.

Pulmonary function tests include measurements of lung mechanics and lung volumes. The various types of lung volumes and capacities are summarized in Table 24-4. These measurements can be used to understand the physiology of certain types of respiratory dysfunction. For instance, a person with a decreased vital capacity has impaired ability to take a deep breath. This condition exists in persons with high abdominal incisions, which limit inspiration due to pain.

Two additional diagnostic tests are the sputum examination, which may reveal useful information, such as the presence of infectious organisms, and chest x-rays, which can provide useful information for planning nursing care. For instance, if the client is developing atelectasis, the nurse can reinforce preventive measures such as deep breathing exercises.

Holistic Assessment of the Person

Persons with respiratory problems are often coping with changes in many systems aside from the respiratory system. When assessing these individuals, the nurse should consider the need to obtain information about other functional areas in addition to respiratory function. For instance, chronic respiratory problems may have a profound effect on lifestyle by limiting a person's ability to perform normal activities of daily living. Dyspnea may interfere with shopping, work, or hobbies. Sociocultural status, including family role, finances, and relationships with friends, may also be affected by limited respi-

---

Table 24-3
Arterial Blood Gas Studies

Study	Normal Range	Interpretations
pO_2	80–100 mm Hg	↓pO_2 = hypoxemia
pCO_2	35–45 mm Hg	↑pCO_2 = hypercapnea
		↓pCO_2 = hypocapnea
pH	7.35–7.45	↑pH = alkalosis
		↓pH = acidosis

Table 24-4
Lung Capacities and Volumes

Measurement	Definition
Tidal volume	Volume of gas inspired or expired during each respiratory cycle (depth of breathing)
Inspiratory reserve volume	Maximum amount of gas that can be inspired from the end-inspiratory position
Expiratory reserve volume	Maximum volume of gas that can be expired from the end-expiratory level
Residual volume	Volume of gas remaining in the lungs at the end of a maximal expiration
Total lung capacity	Amount of gas contained in the lung at the end of a maximal inspiration
Vital capacity	Maximal volume of gas that can be expelled from the lungs by forceful effort following a maximal inspiration
Inspiratory capacity	Maximal volume of gas that can be inspired from the resting expiratory level
Functional residual capacity	Volume of gas remaining in the lungs at the resting expiratory level

Definitions from Comroe JH: The Lung, 2nd ed, p. 9. Chicago, Year Book Medical Publishers, 1962

ratory capacity. Cardiovascular function is often altered by changes in the respiratory system, as indicated by an elevation in vital signs, which occurs during respiratory distress.

Nutritional alterations often occur with respiratory problems due to dyspnea, the effort required to eat, and certain medications such as bronchodilators, which cause nausea. Yet, calorie needs may be greater in these persons because of the extra energy expended in breathing. On the other hand, persons who are overweight may face an added risk of respiratory problems because their increased abdominal girth limits excursion of the diaphragm and forces them to work harder to move the chest wall while breathing.

In terms of mental status, changes that accompany oxygen deficiencies may be manifested by restlessness or impaired judgment. To verify these changes, it is important to assess the client and obtain information from family members about changes in mentation.

Since fatigue and dyspnea from long-term breathing problems can interfere with the ability to walk and move about, the person's mobility status should be assessed along with environmental factors. For example, persons living in two-story homes may find that they are unable to climb the stairs and therefore must confine their living quarters to the first floor. Rest and comfort status may also be affected by respiratory difficulties because shortness of breath and painful breathing can interfere with sleep.

It is also important to consider the interaction between psychological function and respiration. Persons who are anxious may show signs of rapid, shallow breathing indicating hyperventilation. On the other hand, respiratory problems may cause emotional changes. Very often people who have difficulty breathing are anxious. Whereas acute respiratory problems often make persons feel that their life is in danger, persons with a long-standing breathing problem may feel that they have lost control over their lives because of the life-style changes that occur. They may also show signs of grief (depression, anger, denial) or experience feelings of helplessness.

Changes in one of the person's systems are accompanied by changes in almost all other systems. Nurses should be mindful of this interrelationship when assessing the effects of breathing problems on the person's ability to function. Consider the person as a whole and look beyond the respiratory system when assessing and planning care.

Nursing Process
Applied to Specific Respiratory Problems

When caring for individuals with respiratory dysfunction, it is important to remember that the primary function of the respiratory system is to supply oxygen and remove carbon dioxide. When respiratory problems exist, these functions are not performed effectively. The result may be hypercapnea, hypoxemia, and hypoxia. This section synthesizes some of the common problems that accompany any type of respiratory dysfunction, including problems of increased respiratory secretions, ineffective ventilation, airway obstruction, respiratory arrest, and respiratory distress. Although the specific nursing interventions for each condition may vary, they all are based on two major goals:

- Assisting the person to improve oxygen delivery and carbon dioxide removal
- Helping the person to cope with the effects of respiratory problems on other functional abilities

Increased Respiratory Secretions

As indicated in an earlier portion of this chapter, mucus production and removal represents one of the protective mechanisms of the respiratory tract. When the cough, gag, and sneeze reflexes are functioning along with the other protective mechanisms, the airways can be cleared of secretions. However, if large amounts of secretions are produced or if the protective mechanisms of the respiratory tract are not functioning properly, mucus may accumulate in the airways, causing several problems, such as those listed below:

- *Obstruction* of the respiratory tract and reduced ventilation, leading to possible hypoxemia, carbon dioxide retention, and hypoxia.
- *Infection*—Microorganisms that are not removed by the mucociliary cleansing mechanism and alveolar macrophages can multiply readily in the lungs.
- *Atelectasis*—If a bronchus or bronchiole is completely obstructed by a mucous plug, air cannot enter the alveoli distal to it. Gas is absorbed from the alveoli into the pulmonary capillaries, and the airless alveoli collapse. The result is atelectasis.

Susceptible Persons

Because retention of pulmonary secretions can have serious effects, it is important that nurses identify those persons who are at risk. Generally, these individuals may have one or both of the following problems: altered lung protective mechanisms and production of copious secretions. Persons who may develop problems from retained secretions are described in Table 24-5.

Assessment

Retained respiratory secretions may be suspected on the basis of any of the following observations:

- Cough productive of sputum, or moist-sounding cough
- Dyspnea (if secretions obstruct a major airway)
- Palpable coarse vibrations on the chest wall
- **Rales** or **rhonchi**
- Temperature elevation

These findings indicate that the person needs nursing measures to promote clearance of respiratory secretions.

Nursing Interventions

There are many interventions that can assist the person to clear his airway of respiratory secretions, including an effective coughing regimen, humidification, fluids, positioning, postural drainage and percussion, and suctioning. Some of these interventions are more appropriate for certain individuals or conditions than for others. In some settings, certain interventions are considered to be dependent nursing functions, so it will be necessary to consider the policies of the agency in these instances.

Coughing
Effective coughing is one of the most important actions to maintain a clear airway. Therefore, it is an important part of the nursing care for anyone with respiratory infection or chronic respiratory disease, or those undergoing surgery. This is especially true if the person is considered to be at risk because of such factors as heavy smoking or a decreased level of consciousness.

Table 24-5
Causes of Increased Respiratory Secretions

Cause	Mechanism
Smoking	Inflammatory changes in respiratory tract epithelium
	Impaired or damaged cilia
	Increased mucus production
	Bronchospasm
	Reduced effectiveness of alveolar macrophages
	Reduced effectiveness of lung protective mechanisms allowing blanket of dirt and bacteria-laden mucus to remain in lungs
Chronic respiratory problems (emphysema, chronic bronchitis, cystic fibrosis)	Altered lung protective mechanisms (similar to smoking effects)
Aging	Decreased cough effectiveness due to weak respiratory muscles
	Decreased ciliary activity
	Altered immune responses
Decreased level of consciousness	Depressed cough, gag, and swallowing reflexes
	Inability to close glottis properly and depressed cough reflex increases likelihood of aspiration of gastric contents
Tracheostomy	Upper airway protective mechanisms are bypassed causing decreased humidification and production of thick mucus
	Decreased ciliary effectiveness due to thick mucus
	Increased potential for aspiration due to impaired swallowing mechanism
	Reduced effectiveness of cough
Painful chest conditions, muscle weakness	Decreased forcefulness of cough
Drugs	Depressed cough reflex, rate and depth of breathing due to narcotics and barbiturates
	Depressed ciliary activity, diminished swallowing reflex due to anesthetics
	Increased viscosity of secretions due to anticholinergics (e.g., atropine)
Dry environment, dehydration	Increased viscosity of secretions due to decreased humidification, reducing effectiveness of ciliary clearance

A review of the mechanisms of coughing will show that an effective cough depends on the ability to take a deep breath and to contract the respiratory muscles actively (especially the diaphragm and abdominal muscles). For most people this action is easier to carry out when they are sitting up and leaning slightly forward (Lagerson, 1973). For those who have an abdominal or thoracic incision which makes it difficult to contract the respiratory muscles, coughing can be more effective if the incision is splinted with a blanket or the hands. Place your hands on the person's abdomen and instruct him to take several slow deep breaths, using the abdominal or lower thorax, so that your hands appear to move as he inhales (Fig. 24-9). After three or four deep breaths have him inhale and then perform a series of at least three short coughs. This requires less effort than a single forced cough and prevents

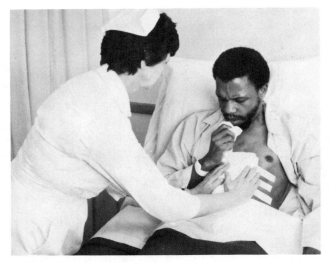

Figure 24-9
Staged coughing with wound support is designed to help produce an effective cough without excessive increases in airway pressure or pain. *(Respiratory Care: Concepts and Techniques, an audiovisual publication of JB Lippincott, 1980)*

airway collapse or spasm in persons with chronic obstructive lung disease (Moody, 1977, p. 106). The coughs should be low pitched and hollow sounding, indicating that they are produced in the thorax rather than the throat. Coughing at the end of expiration may be helpful in decreasing incision pain after surgery (Beland and Passos, 1981, p. 374). If sputum is coughed up, note the amount, color, and consistency.

The effectiveness of coughing in preventing respiratory problems in susceptible persons has been documented both in literature and by research. Yet people do not always adhere to a routine for coughing or practice effective health behavior as discussed in Chapter 9. Coughing can be considered a preventive health behavior which may or may not be adopted, depending on the person's perception of his health status. For instance, a person may not perform coughing exercises because he does not know their benefits. In this case, teaching would be an appropriate nursing action. Some individuals may not believe that coughing will have a beneficial effect on their health or they may not realize that they are at risk of developing respiratory problems. In such instances, an explanation of the cause of respiratory problems may be useful.

Other barriers to performing coughing exercises include pain or dyspnea produced by coughing. One woman who had recently undergone abdominal surgery told the student nurse, "I'm trying not to cough because it hurts so much." Yet prior to surgery

this woman had been carefully taught a coughing procedure and the rationale behind it. Such an example shows that we must not assume that individuals are performing coughing exercises simply because they have been taught to do them. We need to follow up with discussions about other problems the client may be having. At the same time we can point out the benefits of coughing and provide assistance while the exercises are being performed. Concrete evidence of improvements, such as relief of fever or improved breath sounds may help the person to continue his exercises.

It may also be necessary to assist the person in other ways to overcome problems that may interfere with the cough regimen. As mentioned earlier, splinting the abdominal incision to prevent pain postoperatively or encouraging a series of short coughs to prevent dyspnea in a person with emphysema may be in order. In such instances, the person is more likely to continue these preventive behaviors if he perceives that they are beneficial to his health.

Humidification
There are times when it may be necessary to provide some kind of humidification to enhance respiratory function, since moisture thins tracheobronchial secretions, thus facilitating ciliary transportation of mucus. This is an important consideration for anyone who is bothered by dry tenacious secretions or for those who have undergone a tracheostomy or have a respiratory infection. In such instances, humidification is supplied by means of a nebulizer. This device delivers water droplets suspended in gas, which are inhaled. For persons receiving oxygen therapy, moisture may be needed to prevent drying of the respiratory mucosa. To achieve this end, the oxygen is bubbled through the humidifier.

Fluids
Fluid intake has a direct effect on the viscosity of sputum (Dowell and Freeman, 1977). Recall that respiratory secretions are 95% water. Because dryness of the respiratory mucosa interferes with the ciliary clearance mechanism, it is important to maintain an adequate fluid intake in persons who have increased respiratory secretions. Encourage a fluid intake of 3 to 4 liters of fluid per day unless there is a danger of fluid overload, such as in cardiac or renal failure (Moody, 1977).

Positioning
Turning a person and changing his position helps promote drainage of lung segments by means of gravity. Immobilized persons often cough sponta-

neously immediately after turning, indicating that pooled secretions are draining out of the major bronchi.

Positioning is also important in persons who are in danger of aspiration, such as those who are unconscious or semiconscious (the group at greatest risk of aspiration). These patients should be positioned on their side, preferably with the head dependent. They should never lie on their back, to prevent tracheal pooling of regurgitated secretions (Fig. 24-10).

Postural Drainage and Percussion

Postural drainage is another means of using gravity to drain secretions from the airways. The person is positioned so that secretions drain from the small airways into larger ones where they may be removed by coughing. Turning the person, as described in the previous paragraph, is a form of postural drainage. Postural drainage is used for persons with increased pulmonary secretions such as in asthma, emphysema, pneumonia, cystic fibrosis, and some postoperative states. Not all positions are necessary when this technique is used, nor can all positions be tolerated by every individual. For instance, certain positions may cause dyspnea in some people and should be avoided. The same is true if a head-down position results in unstable vital signs in a person with cardiovascular problems. Postural drainage is not done within 1 hour after eating, to prevent vomiting. The amount of time in each position and the number of times per day each position is used are individualized according to the person's needs.

Percussion is a technique that is often used in

Figure 24-10
Positioning the unconscious person
(After Cameron JL, Zuidema GD: Aspiration pneumonia. JAMA 219:1195, Feb 28, 1972)

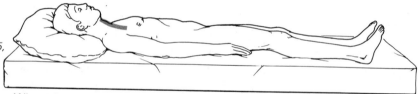

When the person is supine, tracheal position encourages aspiration of gastric contents and pooling of respiratory secretions.

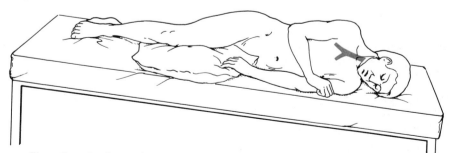

Elevating the foot of the bed and positioning the head dependent puts the trachea above the pharynx. Placing the person on the left side positions the right bronchus, which is straighter than the left, above the trachea. This position decreases the possibility of aspiration.

conjunction with postural drainage to assist in the removal of secretions. It is used for the same respiratory conditions as postural drainage, except that it is rarely performed on postoperative patients. The technique is carried out by cupping your hands (as if carrying water) and rhythmically clapping the chest alternately with each hand by flexing the wrist. This action dislodges pulmonary secretions. It is usually performed for 1 to 2 minutes in each postural drainage position, after which the person is allowed time to cough. The area over the breasts, spine, and kidneys should not be percussed. Nor should percussion be done if the person has chest wall disease, pulmonary hemorrhage, untreated tuberculosis, or painful chest conditions.

Percussion and postural drainage take 20 to 30 minutes, depending on how many different positions the person assumes. Positions for postural drainage may be determined on the basis of chest auscultation, chest x-rays, or prior knowledge of which positions produce the most sputum. The effectiveness of therapy can be evaluated by auscultating the lungs before and after this procedure. The specific techniques of percussion and postural drainage are described in the skills manual that accompanies this text.

Suctioning

At times it may not be possible to cough up excessive respiratory secretions, either because of weakness or a decreased level of consciousness which depresses the cough reflex, or possibly because of conditions that produce copious secretions, such as pneumonia. If the person cannot cough up secretions effectively, mechanical suction of the tracheobronchial tree may be necessary. This procedure involves inserting a catheter into the trachea to withdraw the secretions. It is an unpleasant experience for the person and presents several hazards, including hypoxia, infection, and trauma to the tracheal mucosa.

- *Hypoxia*—Suctioning removes oxygen as well as secretions and may thus cause hypoxia. In some persons this can lead to cardiac arrhythmias. Because of this potential hazard, oxygen administration should never be discontinued during suctioning. Administering oxygen prior to, during, and after suctioning is recommended.
- *Infections*—Pathogens may be introduced into the tracheobronchial tree if careful clean or sterile technique is not maintained.
- *Trauma to the tracheal mucosa*—Even careful suctioning causes some damage to the airway. Repeated suctioning can cause erosion of the tracheal mucosa and bleeding.

Because of these hazards, suctioning is performed only when necessary. Signs that the person needs suctioning include moist breathing or moist coughing that does not clear secretions, elevated temperature, changes in pulse and respiratory rates, or increasing adventitious breath sounds (Amborn, 1976). As with postural drainage the lungs should be auscultated before and after suctioning to evaluate the effectiveness of therapy. Additional nursing interventions include providing emotional support throughout the procedure to reduce anxiety and fear and administering mouth care after suctioning.

Ineffective Ventilation

Diminished ventilation is often a problem during prolonged bed rest or after surgery. In both situations vital capacity and functional residual capacity are diminished, indicating decreased ability to take a deep breath. Several factors cause these changes, as indicated in Table 24-6. Following surgery, the major problem is a decrease in the sigh mechanism (the deep breaths we automatically take very 5 or 10 minutes). During bed rest, the major problem is often decreased chest wall movement, which limits the ability to take a deep breath. These two conditions can lead to reduction in surfactant production and subsequent respiratory problems such as atelectasis. Pulmonary surfactant, which is produced by the alveoli, lowers the surface tension within these air sacs and keeps them inflated. Surfactant activity appears to depend on adequate ventilation and the sigh mechanism. Without this, alveoli tend to collapse, causing atelectasis.

There are several risk factors that increase ventilation problems in persons who are confined to bed or undergoing surgery. They include the following:

- *Age*—Decreased muscle strength and diminished elasticity of the chest wall diminish the ability to breathe deeply and ventilate the alveoli (Burnside, 1976, p. 290).
- *Overweight*—A large abdomen and increased weight of the chest wall limit movement of the diaphragm and thorax. This decreases ventilation in overweight individuals, especially when they are in a supine position.
- *Narcotic analgesics*—Morphine sulfate and other narcotics act on the respiratory center. Persons receiving these medications experience diminished respiratory rate as well as a depressed sigh mechanism.

Table 24-6
Ventilation Changes in Postoperative States and Bed Rest

Following Surgery	*During Immobility*

Pain—leads to
  ↓ ability to deep breathe
  ↓ sigh
	Supine position—leads to
	  ↓ diaphragm and chest wall movement, leading to
	  ↓ vital capacity

Anesthesia—leads to ↓ sigh (longer surgical procedures increase this effect)	

Abdominal distention—leads to
  ↓ thoracic cage expansion, leading to
  ↓ vital capacity
	Abdominal distention—leads to
	  ↓ thoracic cage expansion, leading to
	  ↓ vital capacity

- *Preexisting pulmonary disease*—Such conditions limit ventilation, which is further compromised by bed rest and surgery.
- *Location of the surgical incision*—Persons who have undergone upper abdominal or thoracic surgery are at higher risk for developing respiratory problems. Pain limits the ability of these individuals to take a deep breath.

Assessment

The following observations may indicate diminished ventilation in persons who have undergone surgery or are confined to bed:

- Decreased chest excursion
- Rapid breathing (more than 30/min)
- Absent or diminished breath sounds in one or more areas of the lung fields (Johnson, 1975, p. 1474)

If ventilation problems continue, carbon dioxide will not be eliminated effectively, nor will oxygen be supplied to tissues in adequate amounts. The result is hypoxia and hypercapnea, as evidenced by the following signs:

- Headache
- Inability to concentrate
- Restlessness progressing to lethargy and stupor
- Elevated pulse and blood pressure.

Elevated temperature is often an indication of atelectasis in susceptible individuals (Johnson, 1975, p. 1475).

The early signs of diminished ventilation are often subtle and difficult to detect. It is best to begin preventive measures immediately after surgery or at the onset of bed rest, whether obvious respiratory changes are present or not.

Nursing Interventions

The most effective means of preventing atelectasis in susceptible individuals is periodic deep breathing (Fig. 24-11). This exercise has the effect of a sigh. It promotes surfactant activity and decreases the tendency of alveoli to collapse. Recent evidence indicates that deep breathing should be carried out hourly in order to achieve maximum effectiveness (Risser, 1980). One method of encouraging deep breathing is to place your hands on the person's abdomen or lower thorax and instruct him as follows:

- Take a slow, deep breath through your nose and expand your abdomen so that my hand appears to move out as you inhale.
- At the end of inspiration hold your breath for 3 seconds. (This sustains inflation of the alveoli.)

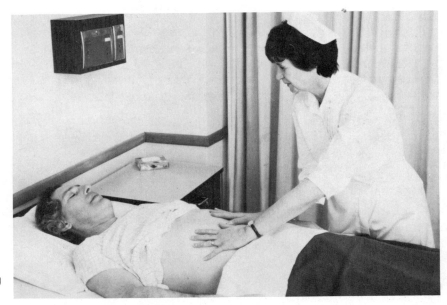

Figure 24-11
Technique for teaching deep-breathing exercises

- Exhale slowly.
- Perform this maneuver yourself several times each hour.

Another means of achieving the same end is to use an incentive spirometer. While there are many types of spirometers, one common type consists of a clear, plastic, vertical chamber that contains a small ball. The person takes a deep breath through a mouthpiece connected to the chamber and tries to raise the ball to a preset level. Fig. 24-12 shows another common type of spirometer. The procedure outlined for deep breathing must be followed in order to achieve the best effect from this device.

Deep breathing and incentive spirometry, like coughing, are only effective if the person believes that they have value and uses them. The general nursing approaches used to encourage client participation in coughing exercises are also helpful for encouraging deep breathing. Education and support of clients are important actions that may increase their sense of control and encourage their participation in deep breathing exercises.

Respiratory Distress

The term respiratory distress is used here to describe any condition in which the work of breathing is increased or in which ventilatory demands exceed ventilatory capacity.

Respiratory distress often creates a vicious cycle. As the person struggles to take in air, the work of breathing increases. This work increases the oxygen requirements, which contributes to the person's struggle. Often accessory muscles are used inefficiently, which further increases oxygen needs. This increases ventilation demands, which worsens respiratory distress. Because of the endless struggle to get air, anxiety is often acute in these persons. Such individuals need nursing assistance to break the chain that contributes to respiratory distress. In some instances, this will require that they alter their lifestyle to cope with their breathing limitations. Nursing assistance can often substantially improve the quality of life for such people.

Assessment

Respiratory distress may be seen in any condition that increases the work of breathing such as emphysema, asthma, or pulmonary edema. It is also seen in conditions that limit ventilation ability such as pneumonia or pulmonary embolism. Hypoxemia and hypoxia are often components of respiratory distress. Therefore, many of the signs the nurse sees are related to oxygen deficiency in the tissues.

It is easy to identify the person who is struggling to breathe. It is more of a challenge to recognize respiratory distress in its early stages before hypoxia becomes severe. It is important that the nurse be able to recognize respiratory distress early and take appropriate actions to prevent worsening hypoxia. The early and late signs of respiratory distress are listed in Table 24-7. The early signs include an elevation in blood pressure, pulse, and respiratory rate that occur because decreased pO_2 stimulates the peripheral chemoreceptors and the vasomotor center. Low pO_2 also alters cerebral function causing restlessness, anxiety, and impaired judgment.

The later signs as indicated in Table 24-7 are more extensive. Included in this list is telegraphic speech, in which the person must pause after every few words to take a breath. Obviously, the nurse should avoid prolonged interviews with these individuals. Accessory muscles are often used ineffec-

Figure 24-12
Incentive spirometry

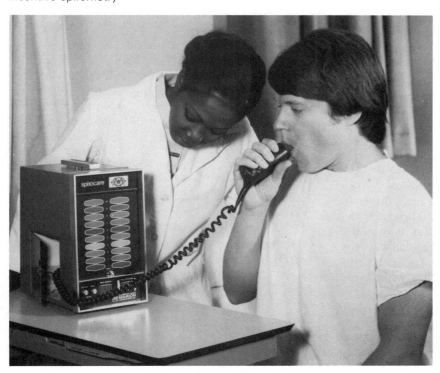

Table 24-7
Manifestations of Respiratory Distress

Early Signs and Symptoms	Later Signs and Symptoms
↑ blood pressure	Dyspnea
↑ pulse rate	Accessory muscle use
↑ respiratory rate	Licking lips
Restlessness	Flared nostrils
Anxiety	Telegraphic speech
Impaired judgment	Cyanosis
	Confusion (with slow onset of hypoxia)
Headache	Frantic behavior (with rapid onset of hypoxia)
	Stupor, coma ⎫
	↓ pulse rate ⎬ Very late signs
	↓ blood pressure ⎭

tively in respiratory distress. The vital sign changes indicated in Table 24-7 are very late signs and indicate that the heart and brain are seriously deprived of oxygen.

Not everyone suffering from respiratory distress will show exactly this pattern of symptoms. The manifestations of hypoxia depend on how rapidly this problem has developed and how long it has existed. For example, in pulmonary embolism the person is severely anxious and has elevated vital signs. In chronic lung disease such as emphysema, the person may be dyspneic and using accessory muscles.

Nursing Interventions

During acute phases of respiratory distress, nursing interventions are directed at decreasing the work of breathing and reducing demands on ventilation. Staying with the person, talking slowly and calmly, and asking him to breathe with you are important steps in relieving anxiety and reducing oxygen demands. It is often helpful to elevate the head of the bed and place pillows under both arms so that the upper arm rests 60 to 90 degrees from the body. This position reduces the work of breathing by making expansion of the thorax easier and decreasing the use of the shoulder girdle. At the same time the person should be encouraged to move the diaphragm to assist breathing. Reducing activity and providing frequent rest periods helps conserve oxygen during acute respiratory distress. Because oxygen therapy is often a part of the medical plan for persons suffering from respiratory distress, nursing care is planned accordingly. Details of this care are summarized in Table 24-8. Mouth care is also an important nursing consideration since many individuals breathe through their mouths during periods of acute respiratory distress, thereby drying the oral mucosa and causing discomfort or infection.

When episodes of respiratory distress are frequent, such as in chronic respiratory or cardiac conditions, the nurse can assist the person to maintain optimal function by helping him to adjust his life-style as much as possible. This might include such measures as mutually planning the arrangement of his living quarters to avoid wasted steps and incorporating frequent rest periods into his daily activities. The loss of normal function may lead to feelings of anger and depression, and the person may need nursing support to move through the grieving process. Interventions for individuals experiencing a loss are described in Chapter 29.

Persons with obstructive lung disease such as emphysema or asthma may benefit from breathing exercises, which can prevent or alleviate incidents of respiratory distress due to increased resistance to airflow during expiration. Edema, spasm, or collapse of the airways interferes with the movement of air out of the lungs because the airways normally narrow during expiration. Often accessory muscles are used ineffectively in an attempt to move air out of the chest. This increases oxygen needs and contributes to respiratory distress.

The nurse can assist the person to improve his breathing patterns by teaching new breathing techniques. The best time for such instruction is during periods of comfort, not during an episode of respiratory distress when anxiety over the struggle to breathe would interfere with the ability to learn. The following steps will help in teaching a new breathing technique:

- Assist the person to a sitting position and provide support for his arms (pillows or a small table).

- Encourage the person to inhale through his nose and slowly exhale through pursed lips. Pursed-lip breathing keeps airways open by creating positive pressure during expiration.

- Ask the person to prolong expiration twice as long as inspiration.

- Have the person lean forward during exhalation and contract the abdominal muscles which thereby assist the movement of the thorax.

- Place your hands on the abdomen and press gently upward.

As the person practices this technique it will become automatic and can be used to prevent episodes of respiratory distress during exertion.

Acute Airway Obstruction

Although the respiratory passages can become blocked at any point, obstruction of the upper airway is most serious because it leads rapidly to severe hypoxia and death. The trachea can become blocked for many reasons, including edema and tumors, or the tongue may occlude the pharynx of unconscious individuals if they are positioned on their back.

One of the most common causes of airway obstruction is the aspiration of foreign bodies. Foreign body obstruction ranks sixth as a cause of accidental death in the United States (American National Red Cross, 1976, p. 2). Frequently the cause is poorly chewed food that lodges in the throat. In

Table 24-8
Nursing Care of the Person Receiving Oxygen

Intervention	Rationale
Avoid fire hazards: 　Static electricity 　Electrical equipment 　Smoking	Oxygen supports combustion.
Provide humidification.	Oxygen is a dry gas, can decrease effectiveness of respiratory protective mechanisms by drying mucosa.
Explain equipment, purpose of therapy.	Information promotes sense of control. Anxiety can increase oxygen demands.
Change tubing, masks, *etc.* frequently (daily is recommended).	Microorganisms can breed in equipment.
Provide skin care (when mask is in use), nares care (when cannula is in use).	Oxygen flow is irritating to skin.
Assess respiratory status.	Status indicates response to therapy.
Watch for signs of oxygen toxicity: 　Pain below sternum 　Dyspnea 　Cough 　Rales	Oxygen is a drug with potentially toxic effects; in high concentrations over extended time it can cause decreased lung compliance and airway irritation.
Avoid high oxygen concentrations for persons with chronic lung disease.	Oxygen can cause respiratory depression in persons breathing by hypoxic drive.

children, small candies, toys, popcorn, or nuts are common culprits. The American Red Cross recommends the following precautions to avoid airway obstruction by foreign bodies:

- Cut food into small pieces and chew thoroughly, especially if dentures are worn.
- Avoid laughing and talking during chewing and swallowing.
- Avoid excessive alcohol intake before and during meals.
- Do not allow children to walk, run, or play while they have food in their mouths.
- Keep small foreign bodies out of the reach of infants and small children. (American National Red Cross, 1976, pp. 2–3)

Unconscious people are especially vulnerable to upper airway obstructions caused by the tongue's occluding the pharynx. To avoid this danger, an unconscious person should not be positioned on his back. For those who are susceptible to copious respiratory secretions, coughing and other airway clearance techniques should be instituted. Through proper health teaching and preventive care, nurses play a major role in assisting persons to maintain a patent airway.

Assessment

Airway obstruction may be partial or complete. In either instance hypoxia may develop quickly. A person with a partial airway obstruction requiring immediate intervention can be identified by the following:

- Weak, ineffective cough
- **Stertor**
- **Stridor**
- Dyspnea
- Cyanosis
- Use of accessory muscles, intercostal retractions

Persons who have aspirated a foreign body that completely obstructs the trachea will show these signs:

- Inability to cough or speak
- Clutching the throat with the hand
- Cyanosis

In unconscious individuals, a possible airway obstruction may be evident by the signs just listed for partial airway obstruction. If a foreign body has completely blocked the airway, the signs will be apnea and an inability to ventilate the person through artificial respiration.

Nursing Interventions

A recently developed technique for relieving airway obstruction is the *abdominal thrust* or *Heimlich maneuver*, introduced by Dr. Henry Heimlich. The abdominal thrust maneuver involves placing the hands against the victim's abdomen just below the diaphragm and sharply pushing inward and upward. This technique forces air from the lungs, thereby moving the foreign body out of the airway. The student should consult the American Red Cross or the American Heart Association for the standard procedure for relieving airway obstruction. Methods are continuously reviewed and revised by the Red Cross and Heart Association and yearly updating is recommended for all health professionals.

Respiratory Arrest

Complete cessation of breathing is called *respiratory arrest* and may be due to many causes. The nurse should anticipate possible respiratory arrest in anyone who has neurological, respiratory, or cardiac problems or is seriously ill. Drowning is one common accidental cause of respiratory arrest. Respiratory arrest leads quickly to cardiac arrest and death if the person does not receive immediate assistance. Hypoxia results in irreversible brain damage in 4 to 6 minutes.

Assessment

Respiratory arrest should be checked in any individual who suddenly loses consciousness. One way to assist the person is to support the neck with one hand, place the other on the forehead, and tilt the head backward. If a neck injury is suspected, alternate methods for opening the airway, as described by the American Red Cross, must be used. Tilt the head back to open the airway, which is often blocked by the tongue in unconscious persons. Next, place your ear near the person's mouth and look toward his chest. Listen, feel, and watch for breathing. If breathing cannot be detected, assume a respiratory arrest. The person's carotid artery is also palpated; if he is pulseless, assume a cardiac arrest has occurred.

Nursing Interventions

The technique for artificial respiration is not described here because methods are continuously being revised. The American Red Cross and the American Heart Association develop standards for this procedure and conduct classes to teach them. The student should consult either of these organizations for the most recent procedures for treating respiratory and cardiac arrest.

As a student nurse in the hospital, your major responsibility is to get immediate assistance for the client. If you discover a respiratory arrest, call for another nurse and begin artificial respiration if you have been instructed in this procedure. Know how to summon the emergency team in your hospital. Even if you do not actively assist the client by performing resuscitation measures, these actions provide assistance to those who can best help the client.

Conclusion

This chapter has presented an overview of nursing care of the person with respiratory dysfunction. No matter what the specific disorder, anyone with this type of dysfunction is at risk for inadequate oxygenation and carbon dioxide removal. Because all cells depend on oxygen, respiratory problems potentially affect the function of all other body systems, as well as quality of life.

Problems that may be experienced by persons with respiratory dysfunction include increased respiratory secretions, ineffective ventilation, respiratory distress, and acute airway obstruction. Nurses use assessment skills to determine which of these problems their clients are experiencing and intervene appropriately. Some of the most important nursing interventions for respiratory dysfunction are directed toward maintaining a patent airway through effective coughing, humidification, fluids, positioning, postural drainage and percussion, or suctioning. In emergency situations nurses may take actions to clear an obstructed airway or institute artificial respiration. Other nursing interventions for persons with respiratory problems include establishing effective breathing patterns, positioning for maximum ventilation, reducing activity demands, and administering oxygen. Nursing interventions may also involve assisting persons to make or to adapt to lifestyle changes based on their current abilities.

The nurse who is providing person-centered care not only deals with clients' oxygenation needs but also considers the effects of their needs on other functional abilities. By preventive, supportive, and restorative interventions, nurses can assist these individuals to regain control over any abilities that have been lost and to maintain abilities they still have. In this way, nurses assist persons to achieve the broad goal of functioning at their highest level.

Study Questions

1. Why should respiratory rate be checked without the person's awareness? Why would you avoid checking respiratory rate after the person has exercised?

2. What is the effect of narcotic drugs on respiratory function?

3. What is the effect of smoking on the respiratory tract?

4. Why does shallow breathing contribute to ineffective ventilation? What relationship does this have to anatomical dead space?

5. What information can be obtained by auscultation of the chest? When might the nurse use this skill?

6. Name two respiratory alterations that commonly occur in persons following surgery. Why are persons with high abdominal incisions most likely to develop respiratory complications? List nursing actions that can prevent these.

7. How would you position an unconscious person? Why?

8. Why are persons who are immobilized prone to respiratory complications? What nursing interventions can prevent these problems?

9. Mr. S. has chronic obstructive lung disease. He is coughing up a moderate amount of thick, yellow sputum. He has numerous rales and rhonchi in all lung fields. What nursing care is appropriate for this person?

10. What signs and symptoms indicate early respiratory distress to the nurse? Is cyanosis a reliable indicator of respiratory distress? Why?

11. Describe the nursing care of a person who is experiencing respiratory distress. How would you position this person? Why?

12. What is the nursing care for a person receiving oxygen therapy? Why would you avoid giving high concentrations of oxygen to persons with chronic obstructive lung disease?

Glossary

Adventitious sounds: Abnormal breath sounds.

Apnea: Cessation of respiration in the resting expiratory position.

Atelectasis: Lack of air and collapse of alveoli in all or part of a lung.

Biot's breathing: Respiratory pattern characterized by uneven tidal volumes and irregularly occurring periods of apnea.

Bradypnea: Slow rate of breathing (fewer than 10/min) with no appreciable change in depth.

Bronchial breath sound: Loud, "hollow" breath sound caused by air rushing through the trachea and being deflected by the larynx and carina; heard normally over the trachea and cervical vertebrae.

Cheyne–Stokes respirations: Waxing and waning of depth of respirations alternating with regularly occurring periods of apnea; indicates cerebral anoxia and is often a prelude to death.

Cyanosis: Bluish or grayish skin discoloration due to presence of increased amounts of reduced hemoglobin in the blood.

Dyspnea: Difficult breathing; refers to a person's subjective sensation of breathlessness.

Fremitus: Vibrations transmitted through the bronchi and lungs to the chest wall when the person speaks; can be palpated (tactile fremitus) or auscultated (vocal fremitus).

Hemoptysis: Presence of blood in the sputum.

Hypercapnea: High carbon dioxide tension (pCO_2) in the blood.

Hyperventilation: Increased rate and depth of breathing greater than required to maintain normal pCO_2 (results in decreased pCO_2).

Hypoventilation: Occurs when volume of fresh air entering alveoli is not sufficient to meet metabolic demands; results in increased pCO_2.

Hypoxemia: Low oxygen tension (pO_2) in the blood.

Hypoxia: Inadequate oxygenation of body tissues.

Rales: Abnormal breath sound due to fluid or mucus in respiratory passages (trachea, bronchi, or alveoli).

Retractions: Drawing inward of intercostal or suprasternal areas during inspiration; indicates increased respiratory effort.

Rhonchi: Abnormal breath sound due to mucus, edema, or airway narrowing in bronchioles or larger airways; may be high pitched and musical (sibilant) or low pitched and snoring (sonorous).

Stertor: "Snoring" or labored, noisy breathing due to obstruction of large airways (*e.g.*, tongue falling back).

Stridor: "Crowing" or high-pitched sound on inspiration caused by partial obstruction of large airways (*e.g.*, foreign body, laryngeal edema or spasm, croup).

Tachypnea: Rapid breathing (more than 24/min), with no appreciable change in depth.

Ventilation: The process of moving air into and out of the lungs.

Vesicular breath sounds: Soft, swishing sounds caused by air moving through alveoli; normal breath sound that is heard over entire lung except large airways or over scapulae.

Bibliography

Amborn S: Clinical signs associated with the amount of tracheobronchial secretions. Nurs Res 25:121–126, March-April, 1976

American National Red Cross: First Aid for Foreign Body Obstruction of the Airway. Washington, DC, American Red Cross, 1976

Bakow E: Sustained maximal inspiration—a rationale for its use. Resp Care 22:379–382, April, 1977

Bartlett R, Gazzaniga AB, Geraghty TR et al: Respiratory maneuvers to prevent postoperative pulmonary complications. JAMA 224:1017–1021, 1973

Beland I, Passos J: Clinical Nursing, Pathophysiological and Psychosocial Approaches, 4th ed. New York, Macmillan, 1981

Bendixen H, Egbert LD, Hedley-White J: Respiratory Care. St. Louis, CV Mosby, 1965

Bode F: Axioms on smoking and the respiratory tract. Hosp Med 14:35–55, September, 1978

Burnside I: Nursing and the Aged. New York, McGraw-Hill, 1976

Cameron J, Zuidema G: Aspiration pneumonia. JAMA 219:1194–1196, February 28, 1972

Cherniack R, Cherniack L, Naimark A et al: Respiration in Health and Disease, 2nd ed. Philadelphia, WB Saunders, 1972

Comroe J: Physiology of Respiration, 2nd ed. Chicago, Yearbook, 1974

Demers R, Saklad M: The Etiology, Pathophysiology, and Treatment of Atelectasis. Resp Care 21:234–239, March, 1976

Dowell A, Freeman E: Lung defense mechanisms. Resp Care 22:50–59, January, 1977

Foss G: Postural drainage. Am J Nurs 73:666–669, April, 1973

Morrison M: Respiratory Intensive Care Nursing, 2nd ed. Boston, Little, Brown, 1979

Guyton A: Textbook of Medical Physiology, 5th ed. Philadelphia, WB Saunders, 1976

Johnson M: Outcome criteria to evaluate postoperative respiratory status. Am J Nurs 75:1474–1475, September, 1975

Lagerson J: The cough—its effectiveness depends on you. Resp Care 18:434–448, July-August, 1973

Moody L: Primer for pulmonary hygiene. Am J Nurs 77:104–106, January, 1977

Price S, Wilson L: Pathophysiology, Clinical Concepts of Disease Processes. New York, McGraw-Hill, 1978

Prior J: Analysis of breath sounds. Consultant 18:112–117, April, 1978

Rifas E: How you and your patient can manage dyspnea. Nurs '80 10:34–41, June, 1980

Risser N: Preoperative and postoperative care to prevent pulmonary complications. Heart Lung 9:57–66, January-February, 1980

Sladen A: Maintenance of a patent airway. Hosp Med 13:56–67, August, 1977

Tecklin J: Positioning, percussing, and vibrating patients for effective bronchial drainage. Nurs '79 9:64–71, March, 1979

Wade J: Respiratory Nursing Care, 2nd ed. St Louis, CV Mosby, 1977

Zavela D: The threat of aspiration pneumonia in the aged. Geriatrics 32:46–51, March, 1977

Rest and Comfort

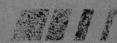

Mary L. Hunter

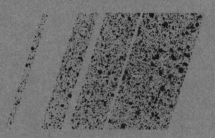

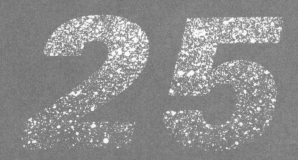

After completing this chapter, students will be able to:

- Describe the phenomenon of pain.

- Describe how the gate control theory suggests an approach to pain intervention.

- Discuss the role of endorphins in the pain experience.

- Describe the experience of pain from the holistic perspective, considering the physiological, psychological, and sociocultural facets of the pain response.

- Write a plan for the assessment of pain.

- Describe interventions for both acute and chronic pain.

- Describe the phenomenon and phases of sleep.

- Describe how sleep is affected by the physiological, psychological, and sociocultural factors in our lives.

- Plan interventions around the clock to facilitate sleep.

- Describe how energy conservation is affected by pain and sleep.

Throughout this text we have discussed the movement of energy among subsystems and the importance of conserving energy. Because physical dysfunction and psychological stress can have a draining effect on stamina and vitality, one of the most important nursing interventions for promoting health and well-being is to help our clients conserve and replenish their own internal energy. Scheduling daily activities to avoid fatigue and exhaustion, planning nutritious meals to restore energy reserves, and assisting in problem solving to overcome emotionally draining situations are just a few of the measures that can be incorporated into the plan of care when called for.

Because we are holistic beings, there is an interrelationship between our physical status and our emotions. As a result, fatigue and inactivity are frequently accompanied by feelings of sadness and depression. On the other hand, people who are active generally feel happy and motivated, and those who are happy are generally active.

When energy is drained by severe pain and minor discomforts, physical exhaustion and depression can result. Assisting an individual to conserve energy during periods of prolonged pain can be a real nursing challenge. The purpose of this chapter is to help nurses understand how rest and comfort affect each other and how we can help others achieve both. When we are relaxed, rested, and free from pain and discomfort we can maintain and replenish our energy stores and maximize our functional abilities. Therefore, the single concept of rest and comfort can perhaps best be explained by focusing on the phenomena of pain and sleep.

Part One: Pain

Phenomenon of Pain

Throughout civilization, man has sought to understand the phenomenon of pain. Yet the answers still elude us. As we seek to understand, we must view pain as more than just the response to a noxious stimulus. Instead we must examine it from a broader perspective that not only identifies pain as a form of discomfort but also envisions it as a great protector and a phenomenon that binds us together in a common understanding of the sufferings and joys of others, as well as ourselves.

Definition of Comfort

Comfort is defined as "the feeling of consolation or relief; the sense of being soothed; a state of ease with freedom from pain and anxiety, and a satisfaction of bodily wants; hopeful in time of grief or pain." These ideas all imply a link between the physical and the psychological responses to stress. The reference to hope in the last definition underscores the importance of providing a hopeful atmosphere in helping others face the future, regardless of their particular affliction. As such, hope serves as an underlying principle in carrying out the nursing process.

Definition of Pain

Pain can be defined as a sensation that creates mild or severe discomfort. The onset of pain may be spontaneous and intense or slow and dull, sometimes increasing in severity. Pain, as a subjective phenomenon, arises from within and cannot be observed by an outsider. Only the response to pain, such as wincing or crying, can be seen. How intense the pain is depends on the perception of the person experiencing it and how he describes it.

Sternbach defines pain as "an abstract concept which refers to (1) a personal, private sensation of hurt; (2) a harmful stimulus which signals current or impending tissue damage; (3) a pattern of responses which operate to protect the organism from harm" (1968, p. 12).

Pain as a Protective Mechanism

Pain also has a positive side. Pelletier states, "Sages of all civilizations have noted that pain is a great teacher, since it informs the person that he must change his life and grow" (1977, p. 320). As a protective mechanism, pain forewarns us of danger. Consider how someone with an impaired neurological system that does not transmit pain impulses can suffer severe injury because of an inability to perceive the danger involved.

Pain is also protective in that it motivates us to seek treatment or medical assistance. We may delay treatment of illnesses that are not associated with pain. Yet many serious diseases initially do not cause pain. Cancer, for example, may not cause pain until the disease has reached advanced stages. We must rely on other symptoms to know that we need medical attention.

Acute Pain

Acute pain may vary in onset. It may begin spontaneously as a fairly severe feeling or it may begin as a mild discomfort and reach a more severe level after minutes or hours. Acute pain usually is of short duration but it is probably the most common symptom that causes persons to seek help. Thus acute pain is often described as serving a useful purpose. C.S. Lewis has written, "Pain is unmasked, unmistakable evil; every man knows that something is wrong when he is being hurt" (1955, p. 80).

Acute pain does not necessarily indicate whether the problem is minor or serious. Pain from flatus or cystitis, for example, is often acute and severe even though each of these conditions is readily treatable. Likewise, severe, acute chest pain may indicate a life-threatening heart attack or benign indigestion. Acute pain is also associated with surgical incisional pain.

Chronic Pain

Chronic or prolonged pain is usually described as lasting beyond 6 months. Although chronic pain may also be severe, it is generally characterized as occurring in periods of intense discomfort followed by a certain amount of, or even complete, relief. Because chronic pain, such as that associated with back ailments, headaches, and arthritis, is so widespread and incapacitates millions of people, it is often called a disease in itself.

Chronic pain is sometimes described as having no useful purpose. However, Miller states, "By enforcing rest, pain assists recovery" (1978, p. 128). Chronic pain helps us to avoid further stress to an injured part of the body; it may also help us avoid situations that add to our psychological suffering. Nevertheless, chronic pain can be devastating and is regarded as a nightmare by many who experience it. Chronic pain invades the person's whole life, often affecting his family and social relationships as well as his job and recreational interests. Nonetheless, many persons in pain report that they have gained a tremendous amount of self-awareness and an understanding of life and the needs of others as a result of their experiences with chronic pain.

Pain Threshold and Pain Tolerance

The term **pain threshold** refers to the point at which a person becomes aware of the pain sensation—the beginning of pain perception. Sometimes a person is described as having a high or low pain threshold. Actually studies on pain indicate that pain threshold is generally the same for most people. However, it is **pain tolerance** that may vary. Armstrong describes pain tolerance as "the point at which an individual

feels that the pain can no longer be tolerated. The severity and duration of the pain necessary to reach tolerance vary ... Tolerance may be decreased by such factors as anxiety, fatigue, anger, stress, and boredom" (1980, p. 385). Trying to define pain in terms of tolerance and threshold is not always useful, because each person perceives and experiences pain in his own unique way.

Physiology of Pain

The complex neurological mechanisms involved in the pain experience are not entirely understood. There are many accepted facts and many speculative theories, some of which will be described below.

An Early Theory

One early theory describes the physiology of pain as a relatively simple mechanism in which the pain response begins when a pain stimulus activates the pain receptors. Sternbach states, "A pain stimulus is one which produces or threatens to cause some tissue damage and which elicits an escape or avoidance response" (1968, p. 28). The stimulus may arise from chemical, electrical, thermal, mechanical, and bacteriological agents and may originate from internal or external sources. The pain stimulus then activates the pain receptors, which are believed to be specialized nerve cells distributed throughout the body.

Information from the pain receptors reaches the central nervous system through ascending nerve pathways. As this information reaches the thalamus, we become aware of the pain sensation and learn something about the location and strength of the stimulus. When the information reaches the cerebral cortex, we become more involved with the pain sensation, trying to interpret its meaning and seeking ways to avoid further stimulation. Our response to the pain sensation incorporates all our subsystems, as will be described later in the chapter.

This early theory, although accurate as far as it goes, does not provide an adequate explanation of why people respond so differently to the pain experience, nor does it really address the neurological system in all its complexity. A less simple theory—the **gate control theory**—offers a more comprehensive view of pain transmission and perception. This theory was first proposed by Melzack and Wall in 1965 and is still widely accepted. However, some scientists speculate that the processes involved in the pain response are even more complex than that described in the gate control theory. In addition, there is little physiological proof of the gate control theory. The theory, however, does provide an excellent understanding of the pain experience, which nurses can use when developing interventions to help persons find relief.

Gate Control Theory*

The **gate control theory** proposes that the substantia gelatinosa (SG), an area of specialized cells in the dorsal horn of the spinal cord, acts as a gating mechanism. This gating mechanism alters and modifies the arriving pain sensations before they reach the cerebral cortex and evoke the perception of pain (Fig. 25-1). In order to understand the theory, let us consider three major factors that interact at the gate. The first factor is the pain receptors and pain fibers and their interaction at the gate. The second is the effect on the gate of cognitive and emotional elements, which are also called higher central nervous

*This section was prepared by Terry M. VandenBosch, clinical nurse specialist, University of Michigan Hospitals.

Figure 25-1
The gate theory depends on the concept of two "parallel" fibers, both with cell bodies in the dorsal root ganglia. The large fiber has basically an inhibitory effect on pain perception, the small fiber basically a facilitative effect. The large fiber acts upon the substantia gelatinosa (SG) and stimulates it. Such stimulation prevents firing of the T cell, which is necessary for pain perception. The small fiber can overcome or modify the large fiber's influence on the SG or it can directly stimulate the T cell to fire. The large fiber may also act directly on the brain's central processing mechanisms, although the pathways of this action have not been defined. Impulses may be either inhibitory or facilitative. If the latter, the result will be firing of the T cell, producing pain perception and endocrine and muscle responses. *(Hospital Practice, Special Report: Recent Studies on the Nature and Management of Acute Pain, January 1976. Reprinted with permission.)*

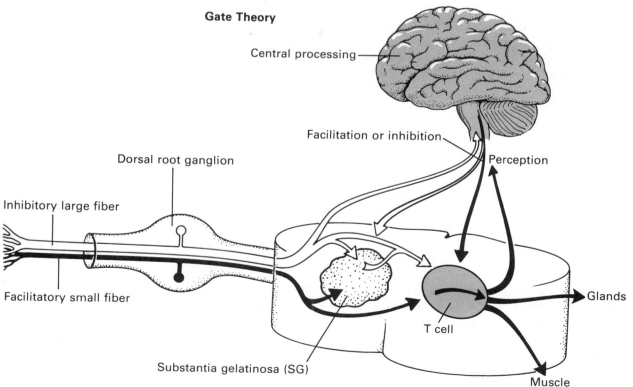

Gate Theory

system functions. The third is the descending neural input from the brainstem.

Pain Fibers

Two major types of pain fibers, important in the study of pain, are small-diameter and large-diameter pain receptor fibers. Small-diameter fibers transmit high-threshold or more intense pain sensations. Certain small-diameter fibers rapidly transmit intense, highly localized pain sensations, while others slowly transmit a vague, dull, or crushing pain that is more generalized, making it difficult to locate the exact area of pain. Receptors for the small-diameter fibers are free nerve endings located in the skin and deeper body structures such as tendons, muscles, and internal organs. These receptors send out pain impulses when they are stimulated by chemical, thermal, or mechanical agents.

There are many chemical agents in our body that can cause pain. Bradykinin and potassium, which are released when a cell is destroyed, can stimulate a pain sensation. Lactic acid in muscles is another chemical whose build up can cause pain. Thermal agents include causes such as fire or hot water. Examples of mechanical agents are strong blows to the body or changing the dressing on an open wound.

Large-diameter fibers transmit the sensations of touch, vibration, warmth, and light pressure. Receptors for the large-diameter fibers are located mainly in superficial structures. Large-diameter fibers are myelinated and conduct impulses rapidly. However, they adapt to stimuli, whereas small-diameter fibers do not. Adaptation means that the large-diameter fibers do not continue sending impulses to the gate with long-term, continuous stimulation. An example of adaptation of these fibers is diminished sensation and awareness, which occurs as we wear wristwatches or rings over a long period of time.

Impulses that are created by stimulation of the receptors of large- and small-diameter fibers are conducted along the fibers to the cell bodies in the dorsal root ganglia. The cell fibers then synapse at the substantia gelatinosa (SG). The interaction of the large- and small-diameter fibers at the gate is one cause of the alteration or modulation in the pain sensation. Stimulation of the large-diameter fibers that synapse at the SG inhibits and modifies the pain sensations arriving on the small-diameter fibers (Melzack and Wall, 1970). For example, a pregnant woman is taught to modify the pain sensation by using a method of rubbing her abdomen during labor contractions.

Cognitive and Emotional Factors

Within the central nervous system is a pathway for a constant input from the brain down to the gate in the spinal cord. Normally this input is inhibitory and keeps the gate or SG partially closed to painful small-diameter fiber sensations. A high anxiety level decreases the inhibitory input and allows the pain sensation to pass through the gate unchecked.

The Gate

The pain sensations arriving at the gate can be modulated by the large-diameter fibers and one's emotional state before one has actually perceived the pain. Three features help determine how much pain a person perceives. The first is the ongoing cognitive and emotional input that precedes and coincides with the pain stimulus. The second is the intensity of the pain stimulus in terms of numbers of fibers stimulated and the frequency of impulses. For example, a small burn to the finger would not stimulate as many receptors as a burn to the hand. The third is the relative balance of activity in large *versus* small fibers (Melzack and Wall, 1970).

Some neurophysiologists maintain that the gate (SG) is also a storehouse for pain memory. They state that pain impulses are recorded in the SG in a way similar to photographic film registering visual events. If the original injury is not reactivated, the pain images gradually fade. However, the memory traces of the pain can be revived by a different irritant focus and the same pain can be reestablished (Mehta, 1973). This, in part, could account for some chronic pains that have no obvious physical causes. A common example of this phenomenon is low back pain. The cause of the pain may be removed by surgery, yet the pain often returns for no apparent reason.

Areas of the brain stem receive input about somatic, visceral, and autonomic activity. The brain stem also has a pathway for constant inhibitory input to the gate. Changes in somatic, visceral, and autonomic activity can affect the amount of inhibition of pain impulses that occurs at the gate. An example of this might be the person who finds that pain is minimized by increasing his activity level.

Neuro Transmission After the Gate

After being altered at the gate, the pain impulses go to the transmission cells (T cells) which, like the SG, are located in the dorsal horn of the spinal cord. The T cells transmit the impulses along spinal cord pathways to the thalamus, reticular formation, limbic system, and the cerebral cortex. The reticular formation and limbic system are in part responsible for emotions and sympathetic responses to the pain sensation. The cerebral cortex helps us interpret and evaluate the pain. Thus the pain sensation evokes emotions and thoughts, as well as physical reactions.

Consider the following points concerning the gate control theory and the pain experience:

- Because modulation of the pain sensation occurs at the gate, there is no direct relationship between the amount of tissue damage and the amount of pain a person experiences.

- Emotions and thoughts about pain affect the amount and quality of pain a person perceives.

- A person can perceive physical pain from emotional causes.

- Because there are many factors that interact to modulate the pain sensation, multiple interventions are appropriate for pain relief.

- The gate control theory can help predict what kinds of interventions would be appropriate.

Responses to Pain

Physiological Responses

The early investigations of prominent scientists such as Walter Cannon (1929) have helped us understand the effects of pain on the body. The physiological changes resemble the effects that result when the sympathetic nervous system is activated due to fear, rage, or fight or flight. Such effects include a faster heart rate, higher blood pressure, greater secretion of epinephrine into the bloodstream, increased blood sugar, less gastric secretion and motility, decreased blood flow to the viscera and skin, dilated pupils, and sweating. In some instances, nausea and vomiting accompany the pain.

When a person experiences severe pain the above responses may occur. Theoretically, these responses prepare the body for the activity that is necessary to avoid further pain. However, the person cannot sustain this sympathetic response in its initial fervor and continue to survive. Therefore the parasympathetic nervous system responds with its compensatory mechanism, and the body begins to adapt to the painful sensation. The vital signs and other responses revert to the individual's usual levels. In some instances of severe prolonged pain, the blood pressure, pulse, and respiratory rates may decrease below their own normal levels, and fatigue and exhaustion can occur. If intervention does not take place, a state of shock can result.

More recent research has indicated that endogenous (within the body) substances called **endor-phins** with morphinelike characteristics are released in response to the pain sensation. Endorphins are peptides found in different areas of the body, such as the central nervous system, the adrenal glands, and certain cells of the intestine. These peptides provide our own natural supply of a pain-relieving substance.

Our natural endorphin response is apparently quite effective in acute pain but less so in chronic pain. Some investigators have suggested that our endogenous pain-relieving system is dulled or depleted by chronic pain. It may be that endorphins are released to help us cope with severe acute pain with its potential for shock but become less active as pain continues. However, the cognitive and emotional factors discussed in the gate control theory may stimulate or even inhibit the release of endorphins.

Psychological Responses

Although the psychological response to pain varies greatly among people, there are certain general responses that we can explain. When pain first occurs, it dominates the person's thought processes. The severity of the pain stimulus and the amount of fear evoked determine how long this pain-centered state lasts. Often, within a few moments, the person recognizes danger and attempts to avoid further pain. He may try to remove himself from the cause if possible, he may cry out for help, or he may even deny the danger and attempt to continue his usual activities. This last response is sometimes noted in those who are experiencing a heart attack or a sudden severe injury.

Prolonged pain may elicit a grief response, causing feelings of guilt, anger, depression, and abandonment. Some people may question why the pain has happened to them and they may view it as punishment for some wrong deed. Others may attempt to bargain with God or with their care giver for relief from pain. Still others may respond to pain by denying its existence and assuming a stoical manner, refusing to acknowledge the pain and determined to bear it without complaint.

Eventually those who experience continued severe pain become exhausted. They may moan or cry occasionally, but often they say very little because having severe pain is a very lonely experience. Others may want to talk a great deal about their sufferings. The observable response to pain does not necessarily indicate the amount of pain being experienced.

Behavioral responses to pain, although they may actually be physiological in nature, are really a reflection of the person's psychological state. Often there are facial grimaces and a clenching of the fists or an attempt to protect the body part by assuming a certain position or by twisting and turning in bed or pacing the floor.

Whatever the manifested response, pain usually involves the whole person. Even a small localized area of pain, such as a cut or burn on the finger, can cause severe discomfort, forcing us to alter our activities to avoid further pain to the injured area. Headache pain is a good example of how our entire being can be affected by discomfort. Saper and Magee state, "A headache occurs at the center of the mind; it affects the captain of the ship and disrupts the control center of the body; ... They [headaches] attack the very essence of you" (1978, p. 16).

Factors that Affect the Painful Experience

Physiological Factors

Adequate nutrition and rest during a painful experience contribute to a person's sense of well-being and a possible lessening of the pain. In certain instances, exercise and range of motion to affected joints also increase comfort. The amount of exercise advisable depends on the particular disease or injury involved. Deep breathing exercises contribute to a sense of well-being and may reduce the muscle tension so often implicated in severe pain.

If more than one pain exists, the response is different than if only one type of pain occurs. For example, if an individual who experiences chronic pain from arthritis also has a headache, both the joint pain and the headache together may seem worse than if each pain occurred by itself. On the other hand, some persons are not even aware of a second painful stimulus if the dominant stimulus is severe enough. A clinical example illustrates this point.

☐ Mrs. Barnes had a great deal of pain in her left foot as a result of compromised circulation to her extremities. When the doctor drew an arterial blood sample from her arm, usually a painful procedure, Mrs. Barnes did not wince or even seem aware of the sensation. When asked later if she had felt pain during the procedure, she responded that she had not really noticed; all she could think about was her foot. ☐

Psychological Factors

It is well accepted that states of anxiety, anger, and fear compound pain, possibly because these emotions inhibit high levels of endorphin release to cope with pain.

It is difficult to separate physiological and psychological components of the pain experience. Familiar examples of the mind–body–pain relationship include the tension headache, or stomach cramps in a child who is anxious about school. Although in these situations the original stressor is psychological, the body has responded physiologically and the pain is very real.

When the original stressor is physiological, such as a surgical incision, people who are able to meet their basic needs of safety, love, and self-esteem usually cope well with this pain. Those who are not able to meet these basic needs may describe their pain as very severe. As described in Chapter 2, an exchange of energy between systems helps in coping with stress. If the stressor is great enough, the discomfort and pain will be experienced in both the original system and the one that is mobilized to help cope.

Anxiety about the meaning of pain may also intensify the response. For example, a person who believes that the pain means cancer, or a recurrence of cancer, may feel severe pain. However, the pain may diminish or become more tolerable if he learns that it is not due to cancer. Generally, if we understand the meaning of pain, even when it is related to a serious cause, we are better able to cope with it.

Sociocultural Factors

Our response to pain is unique because it represents a culmination of our past experiences with pain, the way we learned to respond to pain by watching significant people in our lives, and cultural patterns and mores.

People from certain cultures respond in certain ways to pain. Some respond in a stoical manner, often refusing pain medications and preferring not to give vent to their sufferings. Others respond with great verbal anguish. It is important to recognize that, although these responses may serve as assessment guidelines, they are not always accurate and must be considered within the context of many other observations to reflect a more precise picture of how a person responds to pain.

Example 1 □ Mrs. G, who spoke only Spanish, was having a dressing changed by a student nurse in the presence of another student and an instructor. She wept and cried out frequently, calling upon God for help. Finally, one of the students, Barbara, who spoke a little Spanish, tried talking to her. As soon as Mrs. G. heard someone speaking her own language, she stopped crying and burst into a flood of Spanish. She and Barbara chatted during the rest of the dressing change. Mrs. G. didn't say much about the pain except that it was not too severe. She was more interested in the student. Later when Mrs. G.'s son was informed of the episode, he explained that his mother had not really been in severe pain, but she had used crying as a way of communicating because crying out in pain is a common and acceptable practice in her culture. As soon as she realized that she could communicate in another way, she no longer needed to cry. □

Our response to pain is shaped by other social factors that developed from childhood experiences and the response of others we have observed. In addition, as we experience pain we are affected by family members, friends, and care givers who observe us and respond in particular ways.

Example 2 □ Kathy, a 28-year-old woman who had injured her back in a fall, had experienced incapacitating pain for 2 years since the accident. The physicians had done everything they could to help her and were now telling her she would "just have to live with the pain as nothing more could be done." She was very conscious that pain had become the center of her life, disrupting her entire life-style and affecting her relationships with family and friends. But aside from these concerns, Kathy had become aware that her 4-year-old daughter was suffering from migraine headaches and had begun to emulate her pain behavior. She believed that the child was not only imitating her mother's pain response but the pain experience itself. □

People at times are rewarded by secondary gain if others who observe their pain provide them with a way of meeting basic needs which the pain represents. This does not mean that the pain is less severe or even due to less serious causes. However, an understanding of secondary gain provides guidelines to help us plan nursing interventions.

Spiritual Factors

Some people tend to ascribe religious meaning to their pain, believing perhaps that the pain is a punishment for sins or that it will help to make them strong. Take, for example, the following quote from the Bible:

> For it became Him . . . in bringing many sons unto glory, to make the captain of their salvation perfect through their sufferings. (Hebrews 2:10)

Even people without strong religious beliefs often beseech God to help them during severe pain and suffering. Nurses frequently hear comments such as, "Oh God, make it stop hurting." Other spiritual resources or a particular philosophical approach can be of help in coping with pain.

Environmental Factors

Most of us are aware, when we have a headache, that light and noise aggravate our pain. Other common environmental factors, such as changes in weather, temperature, and exposure to heat or cold, can affect pain. Damp or rainy weather often causes an increase in the level of muscle and joint discomfort. Even sunlight, which most of us welcome, can be painful to skin that is sunburned or otherwise damaged.

Pain may also be affected by changes in one's home environment. The removal of familiar objects, for example, may cause anxiety and stress, thereby accentuating the pain. The need to enter a hospital changes one's environment drastically, and in addition, provides little satisfying sensory stimulation. Decreased environmental stimuli, like increased stimuli such as light and noise, can increase the pain sensation.

(Nursing Process follows)

Nursing Process
Applied to the Problem of Pain

Assessment

"Pain is whatever the experiencing person says it is, existing whenever he says it does" (McCaffery, 1968, p. 95).

Because pain is subjective, we are often tempted to place our own value judgments on another person's pain. This is especially true if we have intervened in every way we know and still have not relieved the pain. Frustration, exasperation, and feelings of failure interfere with our ability to be objective, and we begin to assume that the client is lying, manipulating, or just plain crazy. McCaffery's words have helped many nurses maintain their proper perspective during these frustrating experiences.

Trying to help another person cope with pain can indeed be an exhausting experience, not only to care givers, but to family and friends as well. All of these people, in addition to the person in pain, need help and support from others. In order to maintain objectivity during the pain assessment, nurses may want to consider the following ideas:

- Pain can be experienced whether or not there is a known physiological reason for it.

- The person in pain may not exhibit certain expected behavior, such as crying out, holding the painful area, or avoiding certain activities.

- Only the person experiencing the pain knows how it feels and knows what best relieves the pain.

- Care givers can assist, but the person in pain also holds a major responsibility for its management.

- Some persons may use their pain to achieve certain results, such as attention, tangible gifts, or another's discomfort. The use of pain may be conscious or unconscious, but the pain is still experienced, and the underlying problem must be identified and managed.

- Persons with the same pain stimulus, such as cancer or a surgical incision, may experience very different levels of pain.

- Psychosocial, cultural, environmental and religious factors are all a part of the pain experience.

Hopefully these suggestions will help nurses maintain a balanced view of the pain experienced by their clients and will assist them in making their assessments and planning nursing interventions.

Pain assessment is based on both subjective data, the person's verbal description of his pain, and objective data, the nurse's observations. Moreover, the nurse must be aware that a synthesis of several different data is necessary before an accurate pain diagnosis can be made. This is especially important because a number of the following assessment guidelines, if taken in isolation, may suggest a very different picture of pain than the person is actually experiencing (Table 25-1).

Characteristics of Pain

- *Description*—Ask the person to describe the pain using words that indicate the kind of pain he is feeling, such as: jabbing, throbbing, dull, stinging, and so forth. Be aware, however, that sometimes language can be deceiving. For example, the person who describes his pain as stabbing may never have been stabbed. Ask for several descriptive words.

- *Intensity*—The severity of the pain can be described with words such as mild, uncomfortable, distressing, horrible, or excruciating.

- *Location*—Try to determine the location or site as specifically as possible. Pain may be localized and easily pinpointed or diffuse and difficult to locate. Use palpation in some instances to help the person determine location. This assessment is important in distinguishing between pain that is expected, such as that from the operative site, and pain that occurs independently of a known problem.

- *Rhythm*—Determine whether the pain is continuous or intermittent and whether it varies in intensity. Assess the patterns of any variation.

- *Duration*—Assess whether the pain is acute or chronic and how long the person has had the pain.

- *Factors that precipitate or affect pain*—Assess possible factors that may be associated with the pain, such as the time of day when it occurs, the amount of exercise the person engages in, whether certain foods, coughing, bright lights, or noise trigger the pain, or whether there is any worry or conflict in the person's life. The person's

**Table 25-1
Pain Self-Assessment Guide**

1 How long have you had your pain?

2 What started or caused your pain?

3 Describe your pain; choose from the following list or add your own words:

Pulsating	Gnawing	Aching	Punishing	Penetrating
Throbbing	Cramping	Heavy	Cruel	Tight
Flashing	Wrenching	Tender	Blinding	Numb
Pricking	Hot	Splitting	Annoying	Cold
Boring (like a drill)	Itchy	Tiring	Intense	Nagging
Sharp	Dull	Fearful	Unbearable	Nauseating
Pinching	Sore	Terrifying	Spreading	Your own word(s)

4 Where is the pain located in your body? Can it be described as occurring at a certain place or places? Is it more diffuse (extending over a wide area)?

5 What is the pattern of your pain?

Constant, steady
Rhythmic, periodic, intermittent
Brief, momentary, transient

Describe the intensity of your pain.

Mild

Horrible

Uncomfortable

Excruciating

Distressing

How long have you had pain?

6 What factors make it worse?

Time of day

Inadequate ventilation

Exercise

Sleep

Lack of exercise

Worry

Certain foods

Arguments or conflict

Coughing

Other

Bright lights

7 What other physical signs do you notice when your pain is at its most intense or distressing level?

Pulse rate—speeding or slowing

Dry mouth

Respiratory rate—speeding or slowing

Jerking or spasmodic muscle movement

Perspiration

Nausea and vomiting

Diarrhea

Other

8 How do you cope with your pain?

Medication

Talking with others (about pain or other things)

Changes in position

Rest

Anger

Exercise

Imagery

Applications of heat or cold

Meditation

Relaxation techniques

Prayer

Pacing activities

9 How does your pain affect the following:

Your family relationships

Your sexual functioning

Your daily living activities such as bathing, dressing, preparing and eating food, rest or sleep, exercise, elimination, driving, doing hobbies, housework, gardening, etc.

Your social relationships

Your recreational activities

Your job

10 What is your emotional response to your pain?

Grin and bear it

Will cope somehow

Sad or depressed

Sense of being strong

Helpless or hopeless

Sense of feeling superior to others who do not have pain

individual patterns of behavior are especially important in this regard, because what affects one person's pain does not necessarily affect another's, even though the stimulus for pain may be the same.

Physiological Signs of Pain

Although physiological signs vary among individuals and even within the same person throughout the episode of pain, assessing each client and determining his particular pattern will help reveal important signs such as changes in blood pressure, pulse, or respiratory rate; dry mouth; muscle tension; nausea and vomiting; diarrhea or constipation; and diaphoresis.

Psychological and Behavioral Signs of Pain

Body Movements. Changing position, protecting a body part, twisting, turning, pacing the floor, making faces, clenching the fists, contracting other muscles, and engaging in purposeless or inaccurate movements are all musculoskeletal signs involved in the response to pain.

Voice Patterns. Alterations in tone of voice, pitch, and speed of speech, as well as unusual sounds such as grunts and groans, may reflect pain. Higher pitch and fast speech sometimes accompany acute pain, whereas slow, low-pitched speech, often with a sobbing quality, may be present with chronic pain.

Response to the Environment. Assessing how the person seeks help from others during a painful experience and whether or not he can respond to the help offered are important points to note. Does he reach out to the care giver or passively accept touch? Does he barely allow touch or even actively reject it?

What is the person's response to the physical aspects of the environment such as light, noise, and temperature?

How easily the person is distracted from the pain may also need to be considered. Distraction can be a useful approach under certain circumstances. Some people can be distracted and helped to substitute a pleasurable experience for the pain, such as having visitors, verbalizing about the pain, or even reading. Others cannot make these substitutions. The degree to which a person can be distracted, however, does not necessarily indicate the amount of pain felt.

Distractability is a useful criterion for assessing episodes of severe, acute pain. If the person is completely centered on his pain and cannot be distracted, it may indicate that the pain is very severe. Knowing the person's typical patterns of pain response is necessary to analyze the significance of his ability to be distracted.

Coping Mechanisms. It is important to determine what coping mechanisms are used, on both a conscious and a subconscious level. Observe for the use of physiological mechanisms such as position changes, exercise, immobilization of a body part, abdominal breathing, muscle relaxation exercises, massage, patterns of rest and sleep, or eating certain foods.

If medications are used, check the names of the drugs, the amount, and the frequency with which they are taken. When a person enters a hospital or other health-care agency with the problem of pain, ask for the most recent type and dose of medication he has taken. This will ensure the lapse of time necessary before the next dose is given.

Determine which psychological mechanisms are used for coping. Does the person verbalize his suffering readily or need encouragement to do so? Does he cry or show anger? Has he attempted to use such mechanisms as imagery, meditation, or prayer? How does he ask family and friends for help?

The Meaning of Pain. Some people can ascribe meaning to their pain through psychological, philosophical, or spiritual means. This ability may depend on prior illness, the length of the pain experience, and the person's internal strengths and external resources.

Some of the most common concerns associated with pain are the fear of cancer or its recurrence, impending death, inability to have children, potential loss of a body part, and punishment for wrongdoings.

Social Functions and Life-Style

Chronic pain can have a marked effect on the person's ability to function and follow his normal life-style. Pain often alters interactions with family and friends, affects sexual functioning, impairs the ability to carry out recreational and hobby interests, and results in less effective job performance.

These kinds of changes can be very debilitating, can disrupt long-term relationships, and may result in job loss with added financial concerns. No matter how devoted family members and friends may be, living with a person who suffers from chronic pain can become exhausting. The nurse will want to collect data in all these areas in order to identify possible difficulties and allow problem solving to begin.

Other Functional Areas

Maintaining comfortable patterns of nutrition, rest, sleep, mobility, and elimination are essential for anyone experiencing pain. Each of these areas is affected by discomfort because of the difficulty involved in trying to eat a healthy diet, sleep well, exercise, and follow typical elimination patterns when pain is severe. In fact, if such disturbances are not attended to, the pain can be accentuated. The nurse will want to assess the client carefully and suggest some problem solving approach, in order to intervene in the total pain experience. For more detail on the assessment guidelines associated with the various functional statuses, see the relevant chapters in this unit.

In addition to physiological assessment, it is important to consider the person's emotional response to pain. Does he feel sad, depressed, or hopeless? Does he try to be strong and bear it? Is he determined to cope or has he given up? Refer again to Table 25-1 which provides a guide to pain assessment that may assist the nurse and the client to understand the pain patterns experienced.

Nursing Interventions

Nurses who deal extensively with people in pain often conclude that acute pain is undertreated, whereas chronic pain is overtreated. Some physicians and nurses frequenty worry that prescribing narcotics for acute pain will lead to drug dependency. On the other hand, medication is often prescribed for those in chronic pain because it is so difficult to meet their constant need for pain relief. It is unfortunate that medications are used so readily instead of relying on natural methods for relieving pain or encouraging the individual to assume more responsibility for his pain management.

Acute Pain Interventions

Severe acute pain is a crisis situation, and must be treated as such. Pain from such problems as heart attack, renal calculi, gallbladder disease, cerebral disorders, and severe injury require immediate attention to prevent shock. When these illnesses occur, the body mobilizes all its resources in an attempt to cope with the problem. The result is an elevation of blood pressure and of pulse and respiratory rates, in addition to other physiological changes. Because the body cannot sustain this level of activity for long, physicians prescribe narcotic and sedative medications on a fairly liberal basis at the beginning of an emergency situation. It is the tendency to cut down on these drugs after the immediate crisis has passed that can result in the undertreatment of acute pain.

In addition to administering drugs, nursing interventions include proper positioning and relieving anxiety. Acute pain can be a frightening experience resulting in muscle tension, vasoconstriction, and additional pain. To promote relaxation and the release of endorphins that reduce the pain, the nurse should speak in a soothing, quiet voice to provide reassurance, use back rubs and other relaxation techniques when appropriate, and control the physical surroundings to create as peaceful an environment as possible. The nurse assesses the person's understanding of his condition and provides information which is needed to reduce anxiety and pain.

In the instance of pain related to surgical incisions, although the extent of the incision varies greatly depending on the surgery, acute discomfort can be expected to occur for at least 2 to 3 days postoperatively. Anxiety related to the outcome of surgery is often present but is less acute than in a life-threatening situation such as during a heart attack.

To manage postoperative pain, physicians often order a narcotic. The order may be specific about time and dosage or it may be less exact, such as "morphine 8–10 mg, q 3–4 hr." This kind of order requires that the nurse assess the pain and provide the dosage best suited to the particular person.

Because of the fear of drug addiction, nurses and clients sometimes are hesitant to use the full amount of medication ordered, even when it is needed. Although the need for medication depends on the extent of the surgery and the person's individual situation, the full prescribed amount of narcotics is often necessary for 2 days postoperatively. Nurses who follow this plan after carefully assessing individual needs often find that their clients are able to ambulate more frequently, cough and deep breathe more effectively, and achieve a more restful sleep, all of which contribute to a smoother postoperative course.

It is important to remember, however, that although narcotics can be therapeutic, they also can cause side-effects such as nausea, dizziness, and respiratory depression, which diminish both ambulation and efforts at coughing and deep breathing. When side-effects are anticipated, one solution is to carry out these activities prior to the narcotic injection. This allows a period of rest until it is time again for ambulation and respiratory exercises. With this plan, it is the rest time, rather than the drug, that makes it easier to carry out the necessary postoperative activities.

Overall, the primary intervention when helping a person in acute pain is to consider all his basic needs. Moreover, use of the holistic approach recognizes that pain affects all the person's systems and aids in planning effective care.

Chronic Pain Interventions

Chronic pain stems from a wide range of causes including headaches, back disorders, arthritis, former injuries, and cancer. In some instances there is a definite pathology, in others none is observable. To some degree, the pain response occurs independently of the stimulus. Even in instances in which the stimuli are similar, such as with whiplash injuries common in car accidents, the pain is felt in very different degrees. Some people suffer for a lifetime from what might appear to be a simple injury; others are uncomfortable for several days and then recover completely.

People who suffer from chronic pain are subjected to a variety of unsympathetic views from society in general and from some health-care professionals in particular. Some are told that they must live with pain because nothing can be done to correct the cause. Others are made to feel that they are lying or neurotic. Men are sometimes admonished for being unmasculine if they complain about pain, and adults in general are supposed to have higher pain thresholds than children. Thus, it is obvious why people in pain feel abandoned, beyond help, and often hopeless.

In recent years, however, there has been a growing willingness to address the issue of chronic pain and develop ways to help people manage the pain. One outgrowth from this change in philosophy is the emergence of pain centers.

Pain Centers

A pain center is a place where a person can go to seek help with chronic pain. A multidisciplinary pain center should include the following: "(1) an initial outpatient pain clinic, (2) an inpatient pain service for diagnosis of pain problems and treatment of patients with intractable pain, including pain from cancer, (3) a psychotherapeutically oriented chronic benign Pain Unit, (4) facilities for clinical and basic pain research, and (5) affiliations for an adequate teaching program" (Crue *et al*, 1979, p. 3).

The first holistic approach to managing chronic pain was begun in 1971 at the Pain and Health Rehabilitation Center in LaCrosse, Wisconsin. Here Dr. C. N. Shealy and his associates have treated thousands of persons by means of a comprehensive program of diagnostic studies and physical and psychological interventions. Many other pain centers have emerged, verifying that chronic pain is a valid and credible concern and providing hope that help is available.

One young woman described her experience at a center for the treatment of headaches.

Example □ "My headaches interfered with my ability to sleep and then to eat properly, and finally they affected all my family relationships. I went everywhere for help but was given only prescriptions for pain and informed that since there was apparently nothing physically wrong with me, nothing could be done. Finally, I learned about the headache clinic and called to make an appointment only to be told that it would be months before they could see me. However, after I told the person on the phone that I was desperate, she found a spot for me on their emergency schedule. My first visit lasted the entire day. I was seen by a doctor, a nurse, and a psychologist and was given a series of tests to determine that no other problems were present. A schedule was started to taper my medications, and I was told how I could be involved in a total program of pain relief. However, the most important thing I learned that day was that there was hope. I have fewer headaches now, but even those I have are more bearable just knowing that I am being helped." □

Medications

As previously suggested, chronic pain is frequently overtreated through a combination of many different pain-relieving agents including analgesics (often combined with narcotics), tranquilizers, muscle relaxants, and sedatives for sleeping. Although the tendency in acute pain is to withhold the drugs after the initial crisis because "the person will get over the pain in a few days," the tendency in treating chronic pain is to pour in the drugs for lack of knowing what else to do.

There is one time when large amounts of narcotic medication may be appropriate; that is when a person has pain from cancer and is dying. Large amounts of morphine sulfate are often used because this drug seems to be more effective and has fewer side-effects than other narcotics.

Another drug combination first used in 19th-century England and eventually introduced in the United States is an oral preparation called the *Brompton's cocktail*, named after the hospital where it was apparently first used. This mixture contains a variable amount of morphine (from 10–80 mg), 10 mg of cocaine, 2.5 ml of 98% ethyl alcohol, 5 ml of a flavoring agent, and a variable amount of water to equal a dose of 20 ml. In England, heroin is sometimes substituted for morphine. An antinauseant medication, often thorazine, is usually administered along with the mixture. Brompton's cocktail, when administered on a regular 3- to 4-hour schedule, not only relieves pain but does so without causing the mental clouding and grogginess that is so common with a variety of other medications. It also diminishes the fear that pain will return.

Nursing Interventions. When administering medication to anyone in severe pain from cancer, the nurse should consider the following interventions:

- Provide the smallest amount of the least potent medication that will give comfort. However, as the disease and the pain progress, do not hesitate to administer the unusually high dosages that may be prescribed at that point.
- Give enough pain medication to prevent pain or give adequate relief.
- Offer appropriate amounts of medication to give comfort but not so much as to cloud the person's thought processes.
- Administer medication on a regular and not a p.r.n. basis as the pain increases in severity.
- Consult with the physician to plan for a higher dosage of medication if assessment indicates the need.

Use of Placebos

The term *placebo* is derived from the Latin word meaning "I shall please." **Placebos** are generally thought of as substances that have no pharmacological effect but are given to satisfy a particular need. Sterile water or saline may be injected as placebos, or gelatin capsules containing sugar may be administered orally. Some authorities, however, believe that placebo can be defined much more broadly, "A placebo may be defined as *any* medical treatment (medication or procedure including surgery) or nursing care that produces an effect in a patient because of its implicit or explicit therapeutic intent and not because of its specific nature (physical or chemical properties)" (McCaffery, 1979, p. 260).

According to Simonton and colleagues, "The only active ingredient in the treatment appears to be the power of the *belief—the positive expectations*—patients have that they have received a helpful treatment" (1978, p. 20). There are a great many reports in the literature about positive placebo responses. In order to keep a perspective about placebos, consider the following ideas:

- Placebos are usually used to relieve pain but can be used for other purposes such as anorexia or insomnia.
- Some persons experience relief from their problem following a placebo, and some do not.
- Positive placebo responses may occur whether the pain is physiological or psychological and cannot be used to diagnose from which system the pain has originated. In other words, one cannot say that if there is a placebo response, the pain originated from a psychological problem.
- An apparently positive placebo response may be the result of other analgesic measures, such as a backrub or relaxation technique that was employed at about the same time.
- Persons may state that their pain has diminished after receiving a placebo because they wish to please the care giver.
- Persons may experience relief from placebos. However, this relief lasts only a short time if other contributing problems are not satisfactorily resolved.
- Placebos may provide a positive response, because the positive expectation comforts the person and possibly stimulates the release of his own endorphin supply.

Establishing a Caring Relationship

Twycross (1975) has described chronic pain from cancer as being meaningless, having no predictable end and acting as a constant reminder of the disease. Furthermore, the pain is likely to get worse before it gets better, frequently expanding to occupy the person's whole attention and isolating him from the world around him.

The importance of using the concept of caring as a framework for helping the person in chronic pain is worthy of emphasis here. This is especially true because, aside from medication, there are a variety of other interventions for chronic pain and the pain of cancer, some of which can be used alone or in conjunction with drugs.

The first step is to establish a trusting relationship by helping the person understand that you are concerned about his pain and expect to provide assistance in its management. The next step is to help the person attain control over his pain by building positive expectations and hope that his future, if not free from pain, can at least contain periods of comfort. One aspect of this approach is to teach the person that he, as the one who knows the most about his pain, has control over it and is responsible for its management. This will maximize his strengths, help him to build self-esteem, and counter the depressions that so often accompany chronic pain. Once this trusting relationship has been established, the following measures can be considered.

Psychological Interventions for Chronic Pain

Relaxation Techniques. There are several relaxation techniques that can be used to diminish pain. Perhaps the simplest technique is rhythmic breathing, which can be carried out as follows:

- Position yourself in a relaxed position, knees slightly bent and back and neck well supported.
- Stare at an object straight ahead or close your eyes, as you prefer.
- Breathe in deeply using abdominal muscles.
- On exhalation, repeat a pleasant word or relaxing expression.

Suggest that this skill be practiced for 5 minutes several times a day, so that it will be easier to use under stress.

Distraction. Substituting pleasure for pain can be an effective method of distraction. Simonton and colleagues relate the story of a man who went fishing with a friend, even though he was suffering from severe pain. Although he was not sure that he could manage the expedition, even for a few hours, he discovered that he had considerably less pain while he was engaged in this pleasurable activity. Although the pain returned, he nonetheless had several hours of relative comfort (1978).

Sometimes just visiting with friends or reading a favorite book can accomplish the same objective. Other forms of distraction include listening to someone read aloud or listening to music and using pictures or paintings to add interest to the surroundings. The kinds of distraction employed must be chosen by the individual and related to his own particular interests.

Another form of distraction is mental imagery; this takes a good deal of concentration but, if practiced, can become quite useful. One form of imagery involves a conscious use of imagination to call to mind pictures of pleasant scenes or happy memories. The pleasant feelings associated with these thoughts can serve as a substitute for pain. Another form of imagery suggests that the person concentrate on a picture of himself as healthy and pain free. As McCaffery states, "If we give the patient an image of how he is sick, we should also give him an image of how he will recover" (1979, p. 156).

Spiritual Resources. The nurse can assist the person to use spiritual resources by obtaining the services of a chaplain, clergyman, or rabbi, if the person so desires, or can pray with him if so inclined. Also, the person may wish to discuss his spiritual thoughts, either with the nurse or another member of the staff.

Staying with the Person. McCaffery has written an article entitled, "Don't Just Do Something: Sit There" (1981, p. 58). After we have done all that we can do to relieve the pain, it may be enough just to sit with the person as a means of showing support. We can also encourage family or friends to be present, if the person so desires.

Social Systems Interventions for Chronic Pain

There are a variety of pain interventions associated with the social system of the person. These are most commonly related to the family and significant others.

- Include family and significant friends in the plans to help the person manage pain.
- Assist family members to understand and cope with any life-style changes that may occur as a result of living with a person in pain.
- Assist family members to incorporate the person's needs, such as nutritional practices and exercise activities, into their own daily programs of healthy living.
- Assist family members to remain independent and to carry out those life-style activities that are most important to them.
- Help family members to go through the grieving process for their own losses as well as for the losses of the person in pain.
- Spend time listening to family members as they express their frustrations and worries concerning the person in pain.

- Help all concerned to solve the problems created by pain, in order to facilitate adaptation.

Summary. It is important to recognize that all the psychological interventions listed here serve to relax, comfort, and soothe the person in pain. If we can create this therapeutic environment, we will assist people both to mobilize all their strengths and to learn to manage chronic pain in the interest of leading a more comfortable life.

Physiological Interventions

Many interventions that can be used to relieve the actual physical sensation of pain are related to cutaneous stimulation, which is the act of stimulating the skin in order to lessen pain. Included in these measures are the application of hot and cold packs, the use of pressure, and the application of ointment. When carrying out these measures, it is important to assess the skin frequently to ensure that adequate circulation and tissue integrity are maintained.

Application of Hot and Cold Packs slows the conduction velocity of pain impulses to the brain and the return flow of motor impulses to the muscles in the painful area. Blood flow, edema, and the inflammatory response are increased by heat and decreased by cold. Heat also has a soothing effect, thereby promoting a sense of well-being and reducing stiffness in sore joints. It should be noted, however, that many persons find the application of cold to be more effective than heat in relieving pain. Both measures can be tried to see which one suits the person's particular needs.

Readily accessible means of applying cold include immersing a body part in cold water or using cold wet soaks, ice, reusable commercial cold packs, and ice caps or bags. Readily accessible means of applying heat include warm showers and baths, warm moist soaks, heating pads, and hot water bottles.

Massage promotes muscle relaxation and circulation and can be used most effectively on the upper and lower back and the neck, arms, and hips (Fig. 25-2). However, do not massage the legs, to prevent dislodging a thrombus. (For more detail, see Chap. 23.)

Pressure can be applied by pressing down with the heel of the hand or the fingertips and using a circular motion in one place. This measure is useful for painful areas over the back, arms, or bony prominences.

Ointments. The application of analgesic ointments, particularly those with menthol, produces a sensation of warmth. It is not completely clear why menthol ointments relieve pain, but they are effective for back and joint pain and can be used on the neck, forehead, and scalp to relieve headaches.

Figure 25-2
Backrubs promote relaxation and sleep. *(Photo by Bob Kalmbach)*

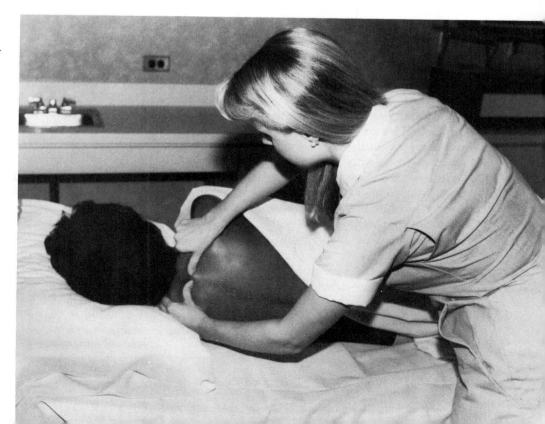

Rest and Activity.   Because pain can be exhausting, rest is essential. Activity and planned exercise can be helpful in promoting muscle tone and circulation, maintaining skin integrity, and creating a sense of well-being. Generally, planning periods of rest and activity according to the individual's needs can be very beneficial.

Nutrition.   Feelings of discomfort are frequently accompanied by poor eating patterns, especially if nausea is present. Helping the person to maintain the highest possible state of nutrition will assist him in coping with the pain. Chapter 20, The Nutritional Status, contains further discussion on this point.

Elimination.   People in pain often experience elimination problems, especially constipation. This is an additional stressor that often increases the pain. Chapter 21, the Elimination Status, provides interventions for bowel elimination problems.

Part Two: Sleep

More than 200 years ago Dr. Samuel Johnson wrote

> Sleep is a state in which a great part of every life is passed ... Yet of this change, so frequent, so great, so general and so necessary, no researcher has yet found either the efficient or final cause; or can tell by what power the mind and body are thus chained down in irresistible stupefaction; or what benefits the animal receives from this alternate suspension of its active powers.

Prior to Dr. Johnson's writing, and throughout most of history, sleep and dreams were left to the realm of the mystics and others who claimed occult powers. Dreams were often thought to be predictors of the future. The Bible speaks of angels appearing in dreams, with specific instructions or warnings of impending danger. Shakespeare provided us with a comprehensive description of disturbed sleep in the character of Lady MacBeth. Even fairy tales such as Sleeping Beauty and Rip Van Winkle have revolved around the phenomenon of sleep.

Sigmund Freud's work on dreams in the early years of this century marked the beginning of a scientific approach to the study of sleep and dreams. Nathaniel Kleitman's work entitled *Sleep and Wakefulness,* first published in 1939, was one of the early scientific treatises on sleep. Since that time many highly sophisticated studies have described the neurological and biochemical aspects of sleep.

Although scientific study of the sleep state has progressed substantially, Dr. Johnson's words remain surprisingly true today. Researchers still believe that the purposes of sleep cannot be definitively stated. Although sleep consumes about one third of each person's day and is thought to be essential to life itself, it is truly a mystery world. However, we do know now that sleep does not cause the suspension of active powers, as Dr. Johnson suggested. In fact sleep is a very active process, as will be described in the following discussion on the physiology of sleep.

Physiology of Sleep

Definition of Sleep

Sleep can be defined as a phenomenon in which there is a period of unawareness accompanied by a set of physiological and psychological behaviors that are different from the waking state. Hartmann defines sleep as "a recurrent, easily reversible condition characterized by relative quiescence and by a greatly increased threshold for response to external stimulation" (1973, p. 21).

Some authorities suggest that a reduction of mental and physical activity occurs during sleep. However, although many bodily functions are diminished, certain ones become or remain very active during sleep. For example, secretion of growth hormone is increased during sleep, especially in adolescents and children. New skin cells are created at twice the usual rate, and various proteins are synthesized. The brain does not rest during sleep but experiences an increase in cerebral blood flow and engages in greater neuronal activity during certain periods of the sleep cycle.

Central Nervous System Control of Sleep

Certain neurons in the brain-stem core release a biochemical transmitter known as 5-hydroxytryptamine (5HT) or **serotonin.** When serotonin increases to a certain level, it acts as an inhibitor to the reticular activating system (RAS), resulting in sleep. Eventually, a decrease of the serotonin level occurs, releasing the inhibition on the RAS, and wakefulness returns.

The sleep-producing system and the arousal system of the brain actually oppose each other. Thus the activity of one suppresses the activity of the other, producing the sleep–waking cycle. Other brain regions, especially those associated with the limbic system, which is concerned with emotions, also affect sleep patterns. Emotions and other factors that affect sleep are discussed later in the chapter.

Measurement of Sleep

Through the use of the **electroencephalogram (EEG)**, the **electrooculogram (EOG)**, and the **electromyogram (EMG)**, scientists have discovered two distinct phases within the sleep state: **non-rapid eye movement** (non-REM or **NREM**), and **rapid eye movement (REM).** These phases were so named because frequent bursts of rapid eye movement can be observed to occur under closed eyelids during certain periods of sleep.

The REM and NREM phases are characterized by very different tracings on the EEG, the EOG, and the EMG, as well as by different sets of behavior. During sleep REM and NREM occur in a cyclic pattern known as the *basic rest activity cycle* (BRAC). BRAC probably occurs throughout wakefulness as well as sleep. In sleep it consists of several stages, including the alert or wakefulness state, the readiness-for-sleep state, the alpha state, four stages of NREM sleep, and finally the REM phase (Fig. 25-3).

Readiness for Sleep

When we are not sleeping, we are said to be alert or in the state of wakefulness. Each night at bedtime the body readies itself for sleep. The body temperature decreases, respirations slow, the muscles relax, and we begin to yawn. Yawning is really an exaggerated respiration, an adaptive mechanism to replenish the body's oxygen supplies following the slowing of respirations.

Just before actually falling asleep, we enter the **alpha state** of consciousness. This state is characterized by increased relaxation and rambling thoughts. The EEG shows tracings of the alpha waves, which are regular in form and of a fairly low amplitude (Fig. 25-4). This is the same state that can be induced by relaxation and deep breathing techniques or by meditation. For most persons, however, it occurs

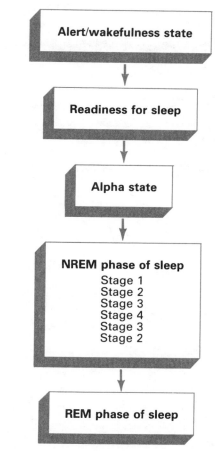

Figure 25-3
Wakefulness and sleep

normally at the onset of sleep without any conscious intervention.

NREM Phase of the Sleep Cycle

Following the alpha state, the NREM phase of the sleep cycle occurs. This phase is characterized by four stages differing primarily in depth of sleep and distinguished by changes in EEG, EMG, and EOG tracings. Figure 25-4 depicts the EEG tracings. There is more NREM during the earlier part of the night and less in the latter part. Generally, when subjects are awakened during NREM sleep, they do not report dreaming. However, some investigators suggest that a characteristic mentation may occur during this phase, one that is believed to be more definitive and closer to our waking thoughts than the dreaming we usually remember (Vander *et al.*, 1980).

Stage 1. This is the stage of sleep onset. The person is very relaxed and subjectively "feels" drowsy. He is

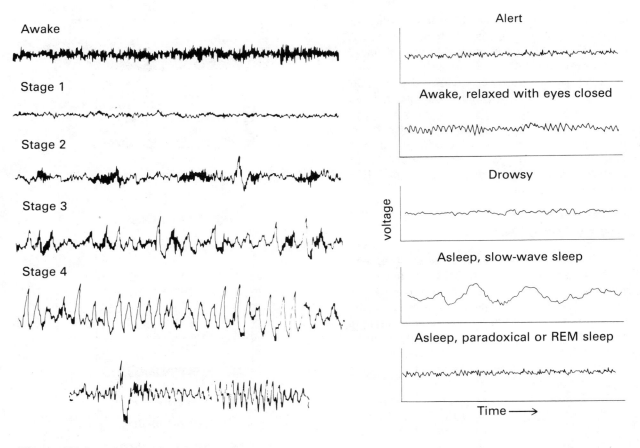

Figure 25-4
EEG tracings differentiating the phases and stages of sleep. (Left, *reproduced from Dement WC: Some Must Watch While Some Must Sleep, with permission of W W Norton & Company, Inc. Copyright © 1972, 1974, 1976 by William C. Dement; right, from Vander, Sherman, Luciano: Human Physiology, 3rd ed. Copyright © 1980 by McGraw-Hill. Used with the permission of McGraw-Hill Book Company)*

still somewhat aware of his surroundings and may jerk involuntarily and awaken. When aroused during this stage, he may deny having been asleep. Stage 1 consists of only about 5% of our total sleep and is characterized by an EEG tracing that has a fairly low frequency and low amplitude.

Stage 2. During stage 2 the person is unaware of his surroundings but awakens easily. This stage comprises 50% to 55% of our sleep. The EEG tracings consist of spindles (brief bursts of fast, low-voltage waves) and K-complexes (sharply rising and falling high-amplitude waves). Spindles and K's are interspersed amidst an irregular, low-frequency, low-amplitude EEG pattern.

Stage 3. At this point the person is more deeply asleep and more difficult to arouse. This stage constitutes about 10% of our sleep. The EEG tracings

show low-frequency, high-voltage waves called *delta* waves.

Stage 4. This is a very deep, restful sleep that makes up 10% of our sleep time. It is composed of more slow, high-amplitude delta waves than occur in stage 3. Both stages 3 and 4 are often known as **delta sleep** or **slow-wave sleep (SWS).**

After the person has progressed through the four stages of NREM, sleep gradually becomes lighter. The EEG resembles first stage 3 and then stage 2. At about this point the first episode of REM sleep occurs. This phase constitutes the last 20% of the sleep cycle.

Physiological Responses During NREM Sleep

During the stages of NREM, the pulse and respiratory rates gradually become slower, and systolic blood pressure and temperature decrease. The metabolic rate also slows, but growth hormone is secreted at higher levels. Oxygen consumption, brain temperature, and cortical blood flow are also decreased during NREM sleep.

REM Phase of the Sleep Cycle

During REM sleep the EEG tracing resembles that of the alert state. REM sleep is characterized by particular brain-wave patterns, dreaming, and physiological responses that are described later in the chapter. This phase is sometimes called *the fifth stage* of sleep, and is entered only after approximately 30 to 60 minutes of NREM sleep. REM sleep constitutes about 20% of our sleeping time. A person deprived of REM sleep for several successive nights spends more time in REM sleep on subsequent nights. This phenomenon is known as **REM rebound** and causes the total amount of REM sleep to remain fairly constant over time.

Dreaming

The dreaming that takes place during REM sleep can be happy or sad, peaceful or frightening, but it is almost always curious and often bizarre. Dement states, "The essence of dreaming is that we see, hear, smell, touch, and taste things that are not really there" (1976, p. 85). Dreams basically are an hallucinatory experience that occur during sleep. They are said to be drawn from life experiences, although at times the dream events bear little apparent resemblance to our real experiences.

The EEG tracings of infants demonstrate that they experience REM sleep. It is not known, however, if they have either visual or auditory dreams. Persons who have been blind since birth also dream, but their dreams consist of sounds rather than images. These persons display the usual EEG and EMG tracings but do not experience the rapid eye movement. Persons who become blind later in life generally experience the visual dreaming and rapid eye movements that occur in people who can see.

Because of the link between dreaming and rapid eye movements, Dement and his associates conducted studies to determine whether subjects were "watching" their dreams. They termed this notion the *scanning hypothesis.* Although they could predict the eye movements based on the subject's report of his dreaming with a fair amount of accuracy when reading the EEG tracings, other investigators were skeptical. Subsequent studies were not conclusive, and we still lack data that would provide the reason for the rapid eye movements of REM sleep.

Dreams remain an intriguing and mysterious experience in our daily lives. Frequently, upon awakening, we need to sort out the dream from reality. On the other hand, when dreaming a particularly frightening or distressing dream, we can remind ourselves while still asleep that we can awaken and be rid of the difficult circumstances.

Physiological Responses During REM Sleep

Physiological responses during REM sleep include frequent bursts of rapid eye movements, muscular twitching, and profound muscular relaxation that gives the effect of almost total paralysis. Some investigators believe that if this decrease in muscle tone did not occur, the accompanying muscle jerking would cause the person to thrash about and awaken.

Although the EEG tracings during REM sleep resemble the alert state, the person is usually very difficult to awaken. Moreover, although REM sleep may be thought of as light on the basis of the EEG, it is often considered deep because of the patterns of muscle contraction found on the EMG. Because of these contradictions within REM, this phase is commonly known as **paradoxical sleep.**

During REM sleep pulse rate, systolic blood pressure, cerebral blood flow, metabolic rates, and temperature all increase as compared to NREM sleep. Oxygen consumption, brain temperature, and cortical blood flow are all elevated in REM. Penile erections and increased vaginal blood flow also occur during REM. At times, the respiratory rate is very irregular and may fluctuate, along with the pulse rate, to levels above that of the waking state.

Basic Rest Activity Cycle (BRAC)

A typical night's sleep begins at the alert state, after which the person enters the alpha state and then NREM, stages 1, 2, 3, and 4. After at least 30 to 60 minutes or longer, the patterns on the EEG begin to shift upward to about stage 2, at which time the first period of REM occurs. Following 15 to 20 minutes of REM, the EEG pattern again indicates progression through the stages of NREM. There are generally four to six of these cycles during a typical night's sleep, averaging about 90 minutes each. The amount of time spent in each of the phases varies, with more stage-3 and stage-4 sleep occurring in the earlier part of the night, and more REM in the latter portion (Fig. 25-5).

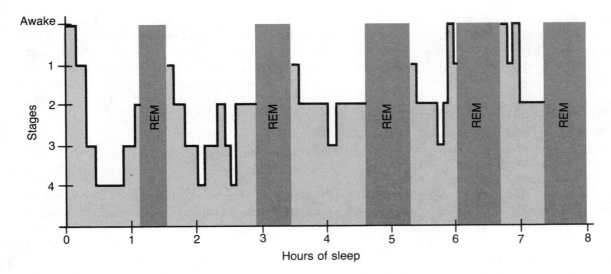

Figure 25-5
Sequences of phases and stages in a typical night's sleep *(Reproduced from Dement WC: Some Must Watch While Some Must Sleep, with permission of W W Norton & Company, Inc. Copyright © 1972, 1974, 1976 by William C. Dement)*

This periodicity of phases in the sleep cycle has been called the *basic rest activity cycle* (BRAC) by Nathaniel Kleitman and others who have studied the phenomenon. There is also speculation that a similar kind of cycling exists during wakefulness. Although factors that occur during the day disrupt the cycle, our functioning in everyday life clearly demonstrates the phenomenon. For example, some persons note a fairly regular need for a break from work every hour and a half or so. They may also function more effectively at certain times of the day. Perhaps for a while after lunch they feel sleepy and find it difficult to function at a high level. Others work better in the evening than the morning. Such observations suggest that activity and rest patterns are unique for each person.

Functions and Purposes of Sleep

The functions and purposes of sleep have been studied long and arduously. After hundreds of studies by as many investigators, the results are inconclusive and often conflicting. Many theories have been proposed, but the reasons why we sleep and dream remain elusive. However, because sleepless-ness is one of the most common functional complaints and 30 million Americans suffer from insomnia, it is clear that sleep is essential, whether or not we understand why.

Sleep deprivation studies have been one popular way of trying to determine the purposes of sleep. In such studies, subjects are prevented from sleeping or are awakened frequently. Investigators have placed volunteer subjects in sleep laboratories and system-atically awakened them during various portions of the sleep cycle. Several studies have even totally deprived subjects of sleep. The results have been inconclusive. In some instances, the subjects contin-ued their usual functioning, although in a somewhat lethargic and ineffective manner, and exhibited a flattened affect.

At least one clinical experience suggests that certain problems may occur following a period of sleep deprivation. In this instance, persons receiving treatment for an eye disorder were given eyedrops every 15 minutes throughout the 24-hour day for approximately 2 weeks. They slept at intervals but were constantly awakened for the drops. The nurses reported that confusion was the greatest problem these people experienced. Confusion was especially marked in older persons, who may have been slightly confused at the start of the treatment, and in those who had another sensory deficit such as decreased vision or hearing.

Purpose of REM Sleep

As mentioned earlier, REM deprivation usually causes a REM rebound effect in subsequent nights (Dement, 1960). Dement's REM deprivation study has been replicated many times with similar results, indicating that REM sleep is essential. Dement also noted that, during waking hours, subjects deprived of REM sleep were anxious and irritable and experienced an increased appetite. They were also aware of difficulty in concentrating. Various studies suggest that the importance of REM may be associated with helping us adapt to anxiety-provoking stimulation and improving our memory of material that is of personal significance. Apparently REM sleep also may be involved in retention of learned material and the learning of new or difficult tasks. For example, one study demonstrated that persons who were relearning speech after having a stroke had a much higher incidence of REM sleep (Greenberg and Dewan, 1969).

The idea that REM sleep is involved with tasks requiring higher mental capacities is also supported by the fact that persons who are severely mentally deficient experience considerably less REM sleep than do persons whose mental capacities are within the norm. Other studies have noted that persons experience more REM after days when they have had stressful experiences or difficult tasks to perform. Wolman states, "These findings suggest that REM sleep does have a role to play in the consolidation of such ego functions as learning, coping, memory, and problem solving" (1979, p. 37).

Purpose of NREM Sleep

REM sleep has been studied more extensively than NREM sleep. Perhaps this is because REM sleep is more interesting and mysterious and raises more questions than NREM. Whatever the reason, there are fewer studies confirming the purposes of NREM sleep.

Agnew, Webb, and Williams (1964, 1967) were able to design a study similar to Dement's 1960 study to determine whether there would be a NREM rebound. They discovered that depriving a person of stage-4 sleep for several nights did indeed result in a stage-4 rebound on subsequent nights, thus indicating the need for the deep sleep that characterizes this stage. Again, as in the REM studies, it was noted that subjects did not experience serious consequences from stage-4 deprivation, although they were physically lethargic and depressed. Investigators have also demonstrated that physical exercise and, in some cases, sexual activity and severe hunger have caused more NREM sleep to occur.

Hartmann's Purpose-of-Sleep Theory

Many theories about the purpose and function of sleep have resulted from extensive investigation into the nature of sleep. Perhaps the most comprehensive view of the purpose of sleep has been postulated by Hartmann (1973), who believes that REM sleep restores our mental functioning after the wear and tear of everyday existence. REM accomplishes this by allowing the catecholamine-dependent neuronal systems in the brain to recuperate. In developing his theory, Hartmann used the accepted fact that catecholamines play a critical role in adaptive function, such as psychomotor coordination, learning, memory, vigilance, attention, and so forth. He also believes that NREM is essentially related to the synthesis of proteins, which are biologically essential and related to the growth or regeneration of body tissues. Thus, NREM helps restore us physically.

Theories are likely to change as more investigation is done.

Factors that Affect Sleep

Many factors affect individual sleep patterns. Only as we understand ourselves and our unique psychological and physiological make-ups can we take steps to cope with our own sleep alterations. Sleep patterns are as individual as are the approaches people use to help them sleep.

Our Biological Clocks

The term **circadian rhythms** was coined to describe the fluctuations of biopsychological activities throughout the 24-hour day. Circadian is derived from two Latin words that mean "about a day." Temperature, respiration, mood, alertness, and hormonal secretion, as well as sleep-cycle patterns, fluctuate at regular intervals throughout the 24-hour day.

Evidence indicates that a circadian biological rhythm occurs in relation to the secretion of serotonin, norepinephrine, and melatonin and is closely associated with the sleep–waking cycle. The release of such hormones as adrenal cortisol, antidiuretic hormone, and prolactin also apparently occurs on a circadian cycle and affects our patterns of daily living.

Consider the circumstances of people who are morning or night persons. Morning people prefer to arise early, and function well before noon, but fade toward evening. Usually they prepare for bed by 10 P.M. Others have difficulty getting started in the morning, flounder around until lunchtime, and do their best work in the afternoon and evening. These people may not be ready for bed until well after midnight. Investigators have discovered that morning and night persons who marry each other often participate in fewer activities together, generally have more conflict, and experience a greater threat of divorce.

Although individual biological clocks can sometimes be altered to fit the demands of society, people often have difficulty adapting to these changes in their normal rhythm. For example, persons entering the hospital setting must try to adapt to a different environment as well as to altered health. These factors of altered environment and health, together with the person's unique circadian rhythms, have implications for sleeping patterns in the hospital setting. Nurses can use their knowledge of sleep cycles and biological rhythms to help people plan their daily rest and activity patterns.

Changes in the Physiological State

General Considerations

Sleep patterns are affected in various ways by illness. Some persons sleep heavily during an illness, whereas others find that sleep comes with difficulty. Pain and other discomforts are often incorporated into one's dreams and may play a part in their plots. At times during illness, and frequently following surgery, there is an increased need for sleep that causes some people to nap at intervals throughout the 24-hour day. This is partly associated with anesthesia and medication and partly with the energy required to stabilize bodily functions.

Chronic Disease States

Many chronic diseases affect patterns of sleep. Some disturb sleep; others seem to be exacerbated during sleep time. For example, persons with asthma tend to lose sleep because they awaken frequently during the night and early morning. Although they do not seem to lose REM sleep, they experience less stage-4 sleep. Depressed persons also experience a decrease in total sleep time, have less slow-wave sleep (stages 3 and 4 NREM), and awaken more frequently during the night than nondepressed persons.

On the other hand, sleep may have an effect on some dysfunctions. For example, persons with diabetes mellitus have abnormally wide variations of blood glucose levels noted during their sleep.

Nutrition

Because sleeping and eating are two essential functions that govern daily activities, they undoubtedly affect each other. Exactly how this occurs is difficult to say, because research data on the subject are often inconclusive and conflicting. However, we can consider typical patterns with which we are familiar. The newborn infant sleeps a great portion of each day but awakens most often when hungry. After he is fed and comforted, he becomes quiet and often returns to sleep. For many people, the ability to sleep is often linked to feelings of hunger or fullness. Some persons awaken during the night with severe hunger pangs and must get a snack before they return to sleep. On the other hand, rich or spicy foods sometimes cause indigestion and disturb sleep during the night. Many of us can recall feeling sleepy after eating a large meal. Some persons complain that certain foods cause them to have nightmares. Consider the following whimsical verse:

> If ever I ate a good supper at night,
> I dream'd of the devil
> and wak'd in a fright.
>
> Christopher Anstey

A definitive study of the links between sleep and nutrition has been done by Crisp and Stonehill, who investigated changes in sleep associated with changes in weight. They conclude, "Weight loss is associated with a reduction of total sleep, compounded of more broken sleep and earlier waking. Weight gain is associated with an increase in total sleep compounded of less broken sleep and later waking" (1976, p. 166). They also indicate that there is evidence to suggest that persons with anorexia nervosa and obese persons on a low-calorie diet experience reduced amounts of sleep during the second half of the night.

L-Tryptophan

The essential amino acid L-tryptophan and its effect on sleep has been the subject of much recent investigation. Hartmann states, "Brain serotonin levels may be directly dependent on circulating plasma L-tryptophan levels, and these levels are influenced rapidly by dietary protein and L-tryptophan" (1974, p. 394). Since L-tryptophan occurs naturally in food and especially protein, investigators have speculated that drowsiness following a large meal may be due to the intake of L-tryptophan. This substance is also the reason why warm milk is so effective as a bedtime drink. The usual diet of the adult contains from ½ to 2 g of L-tryptophan daily. Doses as low as 1 grain have been found to be effective in producing sleep-

iness. Table 25-2 indicates common foods and their levels of L-tryptophan.

At the present time, L-tryptophan is sold in tablet form in health food stores. Although some sleep authorities have suggested that the substance could become the "perfect sleeping pill," others are more cautious, as is the FDA (Food and Drug Administration), preferring to await documentation on the effects after long-term use.

Stress

Consider the following words of Hans Selye (1978) from his classic work, *The Stress of Life:*

> The stress of a day of hard work can make you sleep like a log or it can keep you awake all night. This sounds contradictory, but if you come to analyze the work that helps you to sleep and work that keeps you awake, there is a difference. Muscular activity or mental work which leads to a definite solution prepares you for rest and sleep; but intellectual efforts which set up self-maintaining tensions keep you awake (p. 423).

Selye further reminds us that "hormones produced during acute stress are meant to alarm you and key you up for peak accomplishments . . ." (p. 424). High levels of these hormones within the circulation definitely affect our ability to sleep.

Most of us know that we need to unwind after the wear and tear of a typical day. At periods of high stress in our lives, many of us notice changes in sleep patterns.

Work that leads to problem solving is the key to a restful sleep. When we are upset, angry, fearful, behind in our work, involved in conflicts with others, or experiencing periods of grief and loss, we often find ourselves unable to fall asleep. We may be troubled by disturbing dreams and wake up frequently during the night. On the other hand, some persons describe the opposite problem. They are drowsy and sleepy all the time; they frequently sleep for extended periods, presumably to avoid having to cope with their problems.

Insomnia itself is a stressor. If we do not sleep well we must try to get through the next day with inadequate rest. Our work then overtires us, contributing to more insomnia. The cycle becomes vicious and too often we turn to sleeping pills for relief.

Sometimes the seemingly needless mental activity that goes on during periods of heavy stress and that causes periods of insomnia is a part of our necessary "work" to face and then cope with problems and conflicts. One final word from Selye offers

Table 25-2 L-Tryptophan Content of Common Foods

Food	Portion	L-Tryptophan (mg)
Bread, whole wheat	1 slice	29
Cheese, cheddar	1 oz	98
Cheese, swiss	1 oz	100
Chicken	1⅓ oz	115
Cottage cheese	1 cup	336
Egg	1	112
Ham	1 slice	49
Hamburger	¼ lb.	259
Ice cream	1 pint	158
Macaroni	½ cup	60
Milk, nonfat	½ pint	137
Milk, whole	½ pint	119
Noodles, dry	1 cup	102
Oatmeal, dry	1 cup	146
Peas	½ cup	34
Peanut butter	1 oz	109
Peanuts, unsalted	20 nuts	67
Pork chop	1 oz	96
Rice, dry	½ cup	157
Spinach	½ cup	47
Steak	1 lb	297
Tuna, canned	¾ cup	914

Adapted from Trubo R: How to Get a Good Night's Sleep. Boston, Little, Brown & Co, 1978

a hopeful view, "Stress keeps you awake while it lasts (even when it outlasts its cause) but prepares you for sleep later when your reaction to it is finished" (p. 425).

Age

Sleep patterns are age-linked. Sleep changes in both quantity and quality from birth to old age, with babies sleeping as many as 20 hours a day and elderly persons as little as 5 hours. Moreover, there is considerably less of stages 3 and 4 sleep in the older person, whereas a baby spends much of his time in those stages. Feinberg believes that age-related changes in sleep patterns primarily reflect alterations in the physical status activities of the central nervous system (1969). He indicates that total sleep time is high in childhood, shows a major decline during adolescence, and then reaches a plateau until old age when it declines sharply again.

Some investigators believe that this alteration in total sleep time occurs because of the need of the baby and small child to develop nervous system maturity. There is also a hypothesis called the *sleep–cognition hypothesis* related to the development of cognition, which purports that certain brain activities that go on during childhood are somehow related to sleep.

One study of age-linked sleep patterns indicated that children awaken more slowly than older persons, suggesting that the intensity of sleep decreases with age. It has also been noted in many studies that REM sleep is present in unusually high levels in infancy and childhood. It is not known whether REM sleep in babies is accompanied by dreaming; the main reason we do not know about their dreams is that they cannot report them to us!

Elderly persons can often go to sleep readily enough but find they awaken many times during the night and may be unable to return to sleep. This is not surprising because the major portion of the older person's sleep is spent in stage 2 of NREM, from which one is easily awakened. It is partially because of this light sleeping that many elderly persons feel they sleep poorly and frequently worry about becoming ill because of this. Currently there are no data to support the idea that lack of sleep is likely to cause illness, but it can affect one's sense of well-being.

Exercise

It is generally accepted that exercise during the day causes a deeper sleep and that exercise immediately before bedtime causes a more restless sleep. How-ever, a review of the literature on the subject of exercise and sleep patterns indicates that the evidence is far from conclusive. Shapiro and co-workers, from one of their studies, state, "The results show a specific and graded increase in Slow Wave Sleep with increasing physical fatigue" (1975, p. 189). The method used to create increased fatigue was to cause a progressive increase in daily exercise.

A study done by Walker and associates (1978) on runners and nonrunners demonstrated that the runners had a greater proportion as well as a larger absolute amount of NREM sleep than nonrunners. Although these studies focus on the difference between athletes and nonathletes, and between those who exercise and those who do not, they primarily emphasize the uniqueness of each individual. Nurses will need to assist their clients to assess their own exercise and sleep patterns and determine what changes will promote a healthy life-style.

Environment

Environmental conditions that relate to the sleep experience include noise, light, temperature, ventilation, type of bed, and the presence of other sleepers in the same bed or room. Alterations in the person's typical sleep environment may cause a less effective or less restful sleep.

Generally when we change environments, we notice a change in our sleep patterns until we adjust. Persons traveling, for example, may sleep in different beds and experience different environmental conditions each night. Moreover, if one travels through several time zones, a phenomenon known as "jet lag" may exist. The change in time requires that we adjust our bed and arousal times to be in concert with each place we visit. Certain persons find this adjustment difficult and may feel chronically tired while traveling.

The hospital environment is often implicated in the alterations of usual sleep patterns. Changes occur in the sleep environment but, more importantly, changes in nutrition, exercise, and family and social relationships contribute to alterations in sleep patterns. The hospitalized person is at a high risk for experiencing insomnia and sleep deprivation. Interventions to assist these persons are discussed later in the chapter.

Drugs and Alcohol

General Considerations

Whenever a person takes a new medication, he should be advised to observe its effects on his patterns of sleep and wakefulness. Although some drugs purportedly have no side-effects, each person will react on an individual basis. Classes of drugs often noted to cause daytime sleepiness include tranquilizers, antihistamines, analgesics, and anti-hypertensive agents. Surprisingly, antibiotics may cause daytime sleepiness in certain persons.

Many drugs may also alter the amounts of REM or NREM sleep. Information from drug companies or other pharmacology references do not always explain the particular effect that a given drug may have on patterns of sleep and wakefulness.

Stimulants

One particular group of drugs, the stimulants, such as dextroamphetamine (Dexedrine), amphetamine (Benzedrine), phenmetrazine (Preludin), and methylphenidate (Ritalin), delay sleep onset, decrease the total amount of sleep, and change the patterns of REM and NREM sleep. Caffeine is the most commonly used stimulant that causes these effects. Most of us know that coffee is a major source of caffeine. However, caffeine also occurs naturally in tea, cocoa and chocolate. Colas, certain other soft drinks, and a host of nonprescription remedies such as pain relievers, diuretics, cold remedies, and weight control agents have caffeine added by the manufacturer (Consumer Reports, October, 1981).

Agents Used to Induce Sleep

Hypno-Sedatives. The hypno-sedatives represent a large group of drugs that induce sleep by imposing a general depressant effect on the total brain, including a severe respiratory depression that can cause death. They provide sleep, but it is an unnatural sleep that some authorities have likened to being hit over the head with a hammer. All hypno-sedatives disturb sleep to one degree or another. Some disturb REM and others disturb NREM sleep. Although they do produce sleep instantly when first used and are a great relief to those who are unable to sleep, within a short time they actually decrease sleep. Sleep therapists differ in how they use these drugs. Some never use them; others use small amounts with caution and under certain circumstances.

Until recently the hypno-sedative barbiturates such as pentobarbital (Nembutal) and secobarbital (Seconal) were commonly prescribed drugs. However, because these drugs have an addictive potential in addition to causing severe disturbances in REM sleep, they are now used to a lesser degree and with greater caution. Initially these drugs provide several nights of excellent sleep. After about a week, however, REM sleep, which is severely depressed by the drug,

breaks through the effects of the drug and causes excessive and disturbing dreams. This is the REM rebound phenomenon described earlier. In order to regain a peaceful sleep, the person often increases the drug dosage. Some may also begin to take an alcoholic beverage, which is known to depress REM. The combination of pill and alcohol only compounds the problem.

Dr. Jerrold Maxmen (1981), in his book *A Good Night's Sleep*, describes how innocently the pattern of taking a sleeping pill and drinking alcohol can begin. Eventually, it develops into a ritual and establishes a cycle that is difficult to reverse without help. Maxmen points out that as recently as 1976 an estimated 9,000,000 Americans took barbiturates for sleep. These drugs were also implicated in an alarming number of accidental and intentional drug overdoses. We need to be aware of who actually takes these drugs. The typical sleeping pill abuser is not the heroin user, the cocaine sniffer, or any one else who fits the classic picture of an addict or criminal. In fact, those most likely to take sleeping pills are from the mainstream of society and have one or more of the following concerns: boredom, overwork, anxiety, loneliness, anger, or grief.

The dangers of taking the hypno-sedative barbiturates are exceeded only by the dangers of withdrawing from them suddenly and without careful supervision. Table 25-3 lists a typical progression of

---

Table 25-3
Typical Progression of Withdrawal Symptoms from Barbiturates

Weakness

Restlessness

Tremulousness

Insomnia

Lightheadedness or dizziness on standing up due to postural hypotension

Increased pulse and heart rates

Anxiety

Fever

Convulsions

Psychosis—visual and auditory hallucinations, confusion, feelings of persecution, delirium

Continued seizures

Death

withdrawal symptoms that are likely to occur if long-term barbiturate use is stopped without a specific plan. Nurses should be on the lookout for such symptoms, because people who are habitual users of barbiturates do not or cannot always reveal their dependency when admitted to the hospital for other health problems. Withdrawal symptoms can be obscured or complicated by disease processes and may reach the danger point before an accurate diagnosis is made.

In an attempt to cope with the disastrous effects of the barbiturates, physicians began prescribing another hypno-sedative, a benzodiazepine called Dalmane. For a while, this drug was thought to be the answer to sleep problems because it had a minimum effect on REM sleep patterns and therefore did not cause the disturbing REM rebound phenomenon. However, Dalmane was found to disturb slow-wave sleep (stages 3 and 4) and also to remain and accumulate in the body long after it was taken. These effects often result in daytime grogginess, sleepiness, and clumsiness. Persons on Dalmane sometimes find themselves in need of amphetamines or "uppers" in order to stay awake during the day, thus creating the problem of greater insomnia the next night.

One of the safer hypno-sedative drugs for sleep is a somewhat old-fashioned generic product, chloral hydrate. This drug has a minimal effect on the phases and stages of sleep and generally does not cause daytime drowsiness. However, its effectiveness may not last more than a week, and taking increased doses of this drug is not only habit forming but dangerous, since an increased dose can become lethal much more quickly than is the case with barbiturates. Thus chloral hydrate is primarily useful for short-term problems.

An interesting fact about chloral hydrate is that, in combination with alcohol, it can cause an almost immediate and uncontrollable sleep. The combination of the two substances has been popularly termed a *Mickey Finn*.

Sedatives. These drugs used for sleep are generally the common mild tranquilizers such as chlordiazepoxide (Librium), diazepam (Valium), and meprobamate. They actually create relaxation rather than sleepiness, an effect that helps to induce sleep. They have been considered an answer to the sleeping pill dilemma but in actuality, though milder than the barbiturates and flurazepam (Dalmane), they cause most of the same problems. They also are increasingly implicated in physical and psychological dependence.

Over-the-Counter (OTC) Sleep Products. Popular drugs in this category, which can be obtained without a prescription, include Sominex, Nytol, and Sleep-Eze. These are heavily advertised on television and are touted to be safe, effective, and not habit forming. They generally produce sleepiness because of their antihistamine component. Antihistamines, however, are normally used to reduce allergic symptoms. Drowsiness is actually a side-effect; therefore it is the side-effect, rather than the true action of the drug, that enables it to be used as a sleeping medication. Nevertheless, the action of the drug, particularly dryness of oral and nasal passages, will also be experienced.

Persons should be cautioned about the presence of scopolamine, an anticholinergic agent, in many OTC sleep products. Although the FDA has made serious attempts to have scopolamine eliminated from OTC sleep products, the drug may still be present in certain products. Maxmen (1981) cautions us that, although OTC sleep aids really do not contain enough scopolamine to produce sleep, they do contain enough to cause dryness of mucous membranes, blurred vision, constipation, irregular heart beats, and stomach distress. Scopolamine is also contraindicated in persons with glaucoma and heart conditions. Elderly persons are especially sensitive to scopolamine and often experience memory impairment, confusion, and disorientation with its use.

The placebo effect produced by OTC products is probably the best reason for their use. Many persons find that these agents work because they *expect* them to work. Unfortunately, these products also have the potential for harm.

Drug Combinations. Sleeping pills alone provide a potentially harmful effect, but they are even more dangerous when taken in combination with drugs that are used for other problems such as pain, anxiety, grief, endocrine disturbances, hypertension, respiratory distress, or severe depression. If several such drugs are taken together they can have an addictive, synergistic, or antagonistic effect. Sometimes they produce other side-effects that create new health problems. We must be aware of the deleterious and often disastrous effects that steroids, antihypertension agents, bronchodilators, and the like can have when taken in combination with hypno-sedatives, tranquilizers, and stimulants.

Nursing Implications

Why, if sleeping agents are so dangerous, are they prescribed by the millions? The answer, of course, is very complex. Physicians who prescribe sleeping agents may do so from a genuine desire to help. Others prescribe these products because they provide an easy answer to the demands of certain patients. Treating a person from the holistic perspective may take more time and energy than some health-care providers are willing to give.

The drug companies also play a major role in the overuse of sleeping medication—a problem that is of major national health concern. They are reluctant to give up or even cut back on their multimillion dollar industry. Moreover, local pharmacists assist these companies by encouraging their customers to buy OTC sleeping agents.

A consideration of these powerful groups may cause us to wonder how we can combat such forces. Nurses must avoid falling into the trap of handing out sleep medication in the hospital setting without first inquiring whether a sleeping pill is needed or wanted. However, the truth is that the ultimate responsibility for healthy living rests with the individual person. Healthy sleep patterns are within the control of each person. Yet many people need assistance in exercising that control.

The answer to the major health dilemma of the sleeping pill lies only partly in continued health education programs and perhaps in more effective legislation that places controls on the manufacture and the prescribing of the drugs. There are two other more important interventions. First, as health-care providers, we must become committed to providing support for the use of natural means to deal with sleep problems and to helping persons realize that they can control their own patterns of sleep and wakefulness. Second, it is our opinion that the major portion of the answer lies in assisting persons to cope effectively with life and to take responsibility for healthy living.

Nursing Process
Applied to the Rest and Sleep States

Assessment of Rest and Sleep Patterns

Remembering that sleep patterns vary according to the individual will assist the nurse to make a comprehensive rest and sleep assessment. Assessment may begin by determining whether the client is comfortable with his particular mode of rest and sleep and if he feels refreshed after a nap or a night's sleep. Generally consider whether he feels rested enough to carry out the activities of his daily life and if he is able to conserve energy for the large tasks that often occur.

Sleep Patterns. Assess the number of hours slept in each 24-hour period, usual sleep and arousal times, number of naps, and time of day naps are usually taken. If the person has difficulty sleeping, determine whether the problem is with falling asleep, awakening frequently, or awakening several hours before the usual arousal time. Assess also whether the person has unpleasant, frustrating, or nightmarish dreams and the effect of anxiety, stress, and environmental changes on usual sleep patterns.

Sleep Environment. Assessing the usual sleep surroundings can help the nurse plan interventions with those persons who encounter a different environment when they enter a hospital or travel. Assess for type of bed, number of pillows and blankets used, ventilation and room temperature preferred, and amount of light and noise tolerated.

Bedtime Routine. Most of us carry out a number of activities before going to bed. These activities are a part of our bedtime routine, although we are hardly conscious of them. If asked to identify our routine, most of us would mention brushing our teeth, bathing or showering, attending to skin care and perhaps saying goodnight to other members of the family. How many of us would be aware that a snack or a glass of warm milk or reading for a while are a part of the bedtime routine? Even putting out the dog and locking the door are important activities that we do, not only at the end of the day, but as part of our bedtime routine. Persons coming into the hospital expect to alter their routines. However, they may need to identify their bedtime activities and feel assured that others will take care of things while they are away. This will help promote relaxation and sleep. Recognizing typical activities that can be carried out in the hospital will also assist in bringing about sleep.

Sleep Aids. Certain sleep aids, such as warm milk, a bath or shower, and reading were suggested as a part of bedtime routine. Other aids include alcoholic beverages and sleeping medications. Although persons often find that these aids assist them in falling asleep, they may also discover that alcohol and drugs cause other problems. Determine the amounts used and how helpful or problematic these aids are. Be alert for symptoms of withdrawal from these drugs.

Alterations in Sleep Patterns. Assess how a person's particular health concerns have affected his sleep patterns. Additional data that help in determining alterations in sleep patterns and in planning interventions include all areas that have an affect on sleeping, namely, exercise, nutrition, stress, and so forth.

Personal Beliefs about Sleep. Some persons believe that they need a certain amount of sleep in order to function. They worry that they will become ill if they do not sleep as long as they expect. Others believe that their dreams provide information from a higher authority. Children especially hold unusual beliefs about sleep. Some children, particularly those who are ill, may equate sleep with death and worry that they may die if they fall asleep. These beliefs are difficult to assess because they may be subconscious, or the person may not want to discuss them. The alert nurse can uncover fears about the sleep state when assessing other areas of stress and anxiety.

Interventions to Enhance Normal Sleep

There are five basic nursing interventions that might be considered first in assisting others to attain restful sleep.

General Interventions

- Assist the person to recognize that he has control over his sleep patterns and can achieve a restful sleep by natural means.
- Help the person identify his own sleep patterns, preferred sleep environment, and bedtime routine.
- Assist the person to maintain or establish a sleep pattern that is comfortable and restful for him.
- Help the person identify factors that affect his sleep patterns.
- Consider patterns of rest and activity throughout the day, evening, and night when helping the person plan for nighttime sleep.

The following words of Hans Selye can be considered when assisting ourselves and others to attain a comfortable night's sleep, "Whatever you do during the day, your next night's sleep depends largely on how you have spent your previous day" (1976, p. 423). This is why it is so important to remember that not just the night nurse or the care provider who is with the person at night is responsible for helping to achieve a restful sleep.

Daytime Interventions

- Assist the person to engage in activity that is appropriate for his condition. Plan periods of rest and activity throughout the waking time.
- Help the person to identify nap times. Naps are revitalizing if taken at the same time each day and for a planned amount of time.
- Help the person avoid the habit of constantly dozing off and on throughout the day. Certain critically ill persons and those who have just had surgery will do more napping during the day. Even these people, however, will benefit from a more regular sleep pattern, and the nurse should try to help with establishing that pattern.

Evening Interventions

- Assist the person to plan to slow down his activities in the evening, a "winding down" before bedtime.
- Help the person identify and carry out his usual bedtime routine; help him adapt that routine when hospitalized.
- Provide a gentle backrub.
- Suggest reading or quiet music.
- Help the person devise a plan for decreasing alcoholic intake before bed and avoiding the use of sleeping medications. Suggest medical intervention to assist him with withdrawal from drugs if he takes large amounts.
- Be aware that anxieties are often greater at night. Provide opportunities for verbalizing or exploring concerns and fears; suggest that these concerns be discussed with another member of the family or a trusted friend.
- Suggest that your client plan to take certain medications for pain or respiratory distress before trying to fall asleep. Although these medications may also affect sleep patterns, they often do so less than the uncomfortable symptoms they are designed to relieve.

- Plan ahead so that all treatments, vital signs, or other procedures can be carried out before the person tries to go to sleep.

After-Midnight Interventions

- If the person is having difficulty sleeping, try to assess the problem. Determine whether there is a specific concern or an uncomfortable physical symptom.

- Choose the appropriate evening interventions and try again.

- When the person is asleep, group all necessary activities together so as to disturb him as little as possible.

- Try to provide a minimum of 3 hours of undisturbed sleep before awakening the person to do a treatment or take vital signs. This generally provides about two full sleep cycles.

- Be very cautious about waking any person during the night. Frequently the nurse can check respirations and take a pulse gently without disturbing a person who is sleeping. Temperature alterations can often be assessed by placing a hand close to or gently on the skin. Nurses need to make individual clinical judgments, depending on needs and acuity, about how often the person must be disturbed for special treatments or observations.

- Reassure the person that if he sleeps poorly for several nights, he can make up his sleep in far less time than the amount missed. For example, after 3 to 4 days of sleep deprivation, the healthy subject can make up sleep in 12 to 14 hours on the recovery night and an extra hour or so on the following night (Kleitman, 1963). Several recovery nights might be required for the ill person. Kleitman's original work on this subject has continued to be substantiated by more recent studies.

- Suggest use of the self-assessment of sleep patterns (Table 25-4).

Insomnia

O sleep, O gentle sleep,
Nature's soft nurse, how have I frighted thee,
That thou no more wilt weigh my eyelids down,
And steep my senses in forgetfulness?

Shakespeare's *Henry IV*, Part II

Insomnia is a distressing functional problem suffered by some 30,000,000 Americans. It can be defined as the inability to attain the amount of sleep that one believes is necessary for healthy functioning. The person who cannot sleep understands very well the emotion contained in the words of Henry IV.

The wide variations in sleep patterns among people make it imperative to consider the individual person's concern. One person's insomnia may not be another's. Insomnia can take many forms: difficulty falling asleep, waking many times during the night, or waking early before the usual time to arise. The causes of insomnia are many, and not all are known. According to Dement (1976) scientists believe that a disturbance in the basic mechanism of circadian rhythm may be at the root of certain insomnia problems. In other instances, factors such as stress, age, exercise, and pain affect sleep, as mentioned earlier in the chapter.

Diagnosing insomnia can be difficult. Dement describes persons seen in his sleep laboratory who believed they had not slept more than 3 hours a night for some time. He and his researchers discovered through the EEG and the EMG that about half of the persons who believed they slept little actually slept much more than they realized. They were simply unaware of the amount of time they slept. Dement does not know why this happens, but he emphasizes that an accurate diagnosis of insomnia cannot be made without the use of the EEG and EMG.

Assessment

When assessing the person who experiences insomnia, consider all the areas suggested in the general sleep assessment. Try to help the person identify stressors that may be causing the sleeping difficulty and determine whether these problems are likely to be temporary or long term.

Nursing Interventions

Since insomnia can be a very perplexing problem, its severity and the circumstances surrounding the insomnia should be considered for each individual person. When insomnia is associated with a current hospitalization or other known stressors, nursing interventions will revolve around solving the specific problem. If the insomnia is a long-standing and major health concern, a different approach may be needed. While using the interventions described in

Table 25-4
Self-Assessment Guide for Sleep Patterns

1 Examine your own sleep patterns; consider making a chart about your sleep experience.

  What time do you usually go to bed at night?

  What time do you usually get up in the morning?

  How long does it take you to fall asleep?

  How long do you stay asleep?

  How many times do you awaken during the night?

  Can you return to sleep after you awaken?

  Are your sleep patterns different from what they used to be?

  Does this worry you?

  Do you take naps? Are they at the same time each day and for about the same length of time?

2 What factors affect your sleep patterns?

  Exercise?

  Certain foods?

  Exciting events?

  Stressful events?

  Anxiety or anger?

3 What is your bedtime routine?

  What sorts of things do you do to settle your house: put out the dog, put out the lights, lock up, last-minute chores to get a start on the next day?

  Do you take a shower, brush your teeth, do special hair or skin care?

  Do you read or listen to music?

4 What kind of environment do you need for sleep?

  Special kind of bed?

  Blankets and pillows?

  Light and noise?

  Window open or closed?

5 What do you do when you can't sleep?

  Do you stay in bed?

  Do you get up and do something?

  Can you lie quietly and think about your life?

  Do you pray?

  Do you begin to feel more worried, anxious, or angry?

  Can you let your imagination roam? Can you replace unpleasant or anxious thoughts with happy memories, beautiful scenes, poetry, or thoughts that give you good feelings?

6 Describe your dreaming patterns.

  Do you dream?

  Can you tell how much?

  Are your dreams affected by anything you do during the day?

  Are your dreams pleasant or upsetting?

this section, the nurse may also want to refer the person to a sleep disorder clinic.*

Interventions for insomnia should encompass all those mentioned earlier in this section. When a person experiences severe insomnia, the nurse will want to intensify the effort, particularly in helping the person carry out a personal sleep assessment and in considering all factors that may affect the sleep state. The following are other interventions which sleep experts often suggest:

- Do relaxation exercises.—Although these will not be described here, the work of Dr. Herbert Benson, whose book appears in the bibliography at the end of this chapter, suggests a useful technique.

- Exercise.—Assess your exercise habits and plan a moderate amount of exercise during the day. This often promotes relaxation and sleep.

- Avoid smoking.—It is a fact that heavy smokers take longer to fall asleep, awaken more frequently, and have less REM and stage-4 sleep. This pattern may be associated with nicotine withdrawal, which can occur within 3 hours of the last cigarette and which causes a more restless sleep. It may also cause awakening when the need for a cigarette arises.

- Follow a regular sleep schedule.—It is especially important to awaken and arise at the same time each day, even if you have not gone to bed at the usual time. Staying in bed longer than usual confuses our biological clocks. People often notice a disruption in their sleep cycle when they stay up late on Saturday night, sleep longer Sunday morning, and then find it difficult to fall asleep Sunday night. Some authorities even suggest that the idea of "Blue Monday" comes not so much because Monday is the first day of a long week but because we disrupt our sleep cycle over the weekend so much that we feel lethargic and irritable on Monday.

    Part of establishing a sleep schedule is to go to bed only when sleepy. Most sleep researchers advise the person with insomnia to get out of bed if he cannot sleep and spend the time in another room. It is suggested that the time be used to read books or newspapers that one normally has no time to read or to listen to music.

* To learn about the closest clinic, write to:

The Association of Sleep Disorders Centers
c/o Sleep Disorders Center
SUNY at Stony Brook
Stony Brook, NY 11794

- Avoid naps.—It is very tempting to take a nap if one has not slept well the night before. However, often the ability to fall asleep at night is based on the length of time since one has slept. Therefore, taking naps simply compounds the problem of nighttime wakefulness.

- Control the environment. Establish the ideal sleep environment, namely, eliminate as much noise as possible, control temperature and ventilation, and obtain a comfortable bed.

- Eliminate caffeine in the evening and try a snack containing L-tryptophan.

- Avoid alcohol after dinner.

- Immediately before retiring, set aside some time for relaxation.

- Be aware that being on a diet can result in lighter sleep.

- Look for opportunities to verbalize fears, anxieties, or concerns prior to bedtime. Find a reliable person in the family, a friend, or health-care provider in whom you can confide as needed.

- If you awaken in the middle of the night, remain calm, quiet, and if necessary do relaxation techniques. If you become distressed or get out of bed, you will awaken completely.

Table 25-5
Interventions to Overcome Insomnia

- Use relaxation techniques.
- Exercise moderately throughout the day.
- Avoid smoking.
- Follow a regular sleep schedule.
- Avoid naps.
- Establish a quiet and comfortable environment.
- Avoid caffeine in the evening.
- Take a snack containing L-tryptophan (warm milk).
- Avoid alcohol after dinner.
- Relax prior to going to bed.
- Do not oversleep.
- Learn all you can about sleep medications.

- Do not oversleep.—If one has been awake half the night, it is very tempting to stay asleep into the next morning. This will completely confuse one's natural circadian rhythm and compound the problem for the next night.

- Learn what you can about sleeping medications. Persons who are taking sleeping medications need to have full information about these drugs. If they have been taking the drug for a long time, a program for withdrawal with medical interventions should probably be instituted.

Sleep Deprivation

Sleep deprivation may occur in one of three ways: REM deprivation, NREM deprivation, or total sleep deprivation. Insomnia can create symptoms of sleep deprivation, but unless the problem is very severe, most persons who have difficulty sleeping do attain some sleep and generally some rest.

Assessment

REM deprivation, or the absence of dreaming, may be caused by the ingestion of certain drugs, commonly the barbiturates and alcoholic beverages. General disruptions in usual sleep patterns, such as those experienced while traveling or trying to sleep in a hospital (particularly the intensive care unit where one's sleep is constantly interrupted), may also cause REM deprivation. Persons with this problem have been noted to be anxious and irritable and to have an increased appetite and difficulty concentrating during the waking hours.

NREM deprivation or slow-wave sleep deprivation can occur in the same situations as those mentioned for REM deprivation. One of the more popular sleeping pills, Dalmane, disrupts NREM sleep. Elderly persons spend the largest part of their sleep time in stage 2 and often feel the lack of NREM or restful sleep. Persons with conditions such as sleep apnea, hypothyroidism, and diseases causing respiratory distress often do not attain slow-wave sleep and may feel chronically tired.

Persons experiencing NREM deprivation and particularly those missing stage 3 and 4 (Slow Wave sleep) generally act physically lethargic and depressed. Often they have difficulty carrying out the repetitive and sustained tasks of the next day.

Total sleep deprivation rarely occurs except in the laboratory setting. Persons hospitalized in intensive care units frequently experience partial sleep deprivation. After 3 to 5 days in this setting some persons respond with symptoms commonly called **intensive care delirium.** Symptoms usually include increasing fatigue and exhaustion, difficulty concentrating, feelings of persecution and sometimes paranoia, occasionally hallucinations, and usually an overwhelming desire to sleep. Persons respond by dozing at intervals throughout the day but have difficulty attaining a restful sleep because of the frequent interruptions so common in the intensive care unit.

Nursing Interventions

Many interventions to assist the person to attain rest and sleep and to deal with insomnia have already been described. In addition to those mentioned, the nurse needs to orient the person to the date and time of day frequently, because awareness of time is often disrupted when the day is not divided by regular activities. Providing explanations of all treatments and procedures done and giving emotional support is necessary to help the person regain control over his sleeping patterns and his life.

Somnambulism and Related Disorders

Somnambulism or sleep walking and related disorders such as enuresis (bedwetting) and night terrors occur primarily in children and during NREM stage-4 sleep. Generally these disorders called **parasomnias,** are outgrown before adolescence and exert their primary effects on worried parents, the children often being blissfully unaware of the experience.

Assessment

Although psychic trauma or conflict is often viewed as one of the causes of sleepwalking, William Dement, renowned sleep researcher, states, "Laboratory studies have shown that these episodes [from all parasomnias] arise in the oblivion of the first deep stage-4 sleep of the night and are generally associated with body movements and intense autonomic activation" (1976, p. 79).

Certainly it is appropriate when assessing children with a parasomnia disorder to determine whether emotional conflicts or stressful events have occurred recently. In addition, it is wise to assess actual behavior, especially in somnambulism, in order to help parents provide a safe environment for the child.

The few adults who sleepwalk are usually well aware of how they behave during these episodes, having had others describe it to them over the years. If these persons are hospitalized for other reasons, they can usually describe their behavior and needs during an episode. Nurses will want to be alert for those who seem to sleepwalk in the hospital setting. Often they are persons who have awakened feeling confused and walk about in an attempt to reorient themselves. They will have different needs than the person who really sleepwalks.

Nursing Interventions

Dement (1976) is adamant that parasomnias should not be treated in children. He believes that treatment is generally ineffective and only causes unnecessary anxiety. If parents and health-care providers remain patient, the child will outgrow the problem.

Somnambulism. Providing a safe environment is the primary concern of those caring for anyone who sleepwalks. Furniture should not be moved out of place, and any other features of the usual environment should not be changed. Doors leading to stairways should be kept closed and open stairways, guarded. When a child is found sleepwalking, guide him back to bed but do not awaken him. "Because sleepwalking occurs during the deep stage-4 sleep, awakening the person can result in confusion and fear" (Usdin, 1973, p. 39).

Enuresis. Interventions for enuresis generally include making the bed in a such a way that it can be changed easily and reassuring the child that this disturbing problem will disappear before adolescence. It is advisable, however, for the child to have periodic medical attention while the problem lasts to assess for renal or urinary tract disorders. One common practice that is considered inadvisable is to limit the child's fluid intake, especially prior to sleep. Often the child does this himself in an attempt to stop the bedwetting. Limiting fluid intake prior to sleep may reassure parents and children but is of questionable value.

Night Terrors. Interventions for night terrors primarily include calming and reassuring the person or child. The nurse can help the parents plan methods for supporting the child psychologically and then allay the parents' concerns, helping them to remain patient until the child outgrows the problem.

Other Sleep Disorders

Other sleep disorders include narcolepsy, sleep apnea and its possible relationship to sudden infant death syndrome (SIDS), hypersomnia, and nocturnal myoclonus (kicking legs). Several of the nursing interventions mentioned throughout this chapter may assist with certain aspects of these disorders. However, their mechanisms are often unclear, and medical intervention is usually necessary.

Conclusion

Assisting others to attain and maintain rest and comfort is an exciting challenge for nursing. The physiological, psychological, and social responses demonstrated by persons experiencing pain or altered sleep patterns suggest the importance of holistic nursing care. We are aware that those who perceive themselves as rested and free from pain more often feel active, relaxed, and happy, whereas those who cannot attain comfort may feel sad, anxious, and fatigued.

The physiology of both pain and sleep remains unclear to scientists. There is a great deal of research being done in both areas, and theories have changed considerably over the last 30 to 40 years. As we learn more about the physiology of pain and sleep, we can identify ways in which this knowledge can assist us in planning appropriate nursing interventions. More nursing research in both areas would be useful and would provide needed answers to questions about energy conservation, rest, and the alleviation of pain.

Our knowledge of stress and basic human needs helps us to understand how these concepts affect the total human experience and cause such a variation of response in pain and sleep. We can also note, however, that health-oriented activities such as exercise, as well as nutritional and elimination patterns, affect our total being and especially our abilities to feel rested and comfortable.

There are many natural means for achieving necessary rest and comfort. However, until recently interventions that included medications and surgical procedures were relied upon heavily. Nurses will want to become aware of natural interventions that can be used for the relief of pain and fatigue. Foremost among those interventions is helping persons un-derstand that they are responsible for their own rest and comfort. Although health-care providers are able to assist with these problems, the primary respon-sibility for solutions rests with each individual per-son.

Study Questions

1. Mrs. Jones comes to the ambulatory care clinic describing an unrelenting, debilitating headache. Although she has had the headache for 3 days without relief, after an hour in the clinic with a caring nurse and doctor she begins to experience relief. Considering the concepts of pain as a protective mechanism, acute pain, and the gate control theory, how would you describe Mrs. Jones's pain and her response to the pain?

2. Mr. Thompson has been in and out of health-care clinics and hospitals for many years with the complaint of back pain. He states the pain has prevented him from working and necessitated his reliance on welfare.
   a. Indicate several reasons why nurses might judge Mr. Thomp-son before assessing his pain.
   b. Indicate the data that should be elicited in order to make an accurate assessment of the pain he is experiencing.
   c. Identify a plan of care for this man, suggesting nursing inter-ventions that will help him cope with chronic pain.

3. Suggest several reasons why persons should be encouraged to participate in the assessment and intervention of their own pain.

4. Identify what factors might cause a person to have a positive placebo response.

5. Assess yourself in relation to pain. How do you respond with mild or severe pain? How important do you believe medications are for relieving pain? How do you relieve your own pain? How do you express pain? Is there anything in your cultural back-ground that causes you to respond in a particular way to pain?

6. Place the correct designation from the left in the blank at the right.
   a. Sleep state   ____ Relaxation and rambling thoughts
   b. NREM sleep   ____ Vivid, elaborate dreams
   c. REM sleep   ____ Interruption of the waking state
   d. Alpha state   ____ Paradoxical sleep
   e. Wakefulness   ____ Slow-wave sleep
   f. BRAC   ____ Studied through use of EEG, EMG, and EOG
                         ____ Increased during morning naps
                         ____ Decreased by hypnotics
                         ____ Delta sleep
                         ____ Alert

_____ Decreases during the latter half of the night

_____ Stage 3

_____ Decrease in pulse and respiratory rates

_____ Periodicity of phases

7. Indicate the factor affecting sleep patterns that may be involved in each of the following situations:
   a. Night person or morning person _____
   b. Restless sleep _____
   c. Flying across country _____
   d. Asthma _____
   e. Weight loss _____
   f. L-tryptophan _____
   g. Frequent awakening during stage-3 NREM _____
   h. Anger and fear _____
   i. A restful sleep _____
   j. Hospitalization _____

8. You are caring for an elderly lady in her home. She states that she sleeps poorly at night and feels tired and irritable the next morning. Indicate factors that may be affecting her sleep. Suggest which areas you would assess and ideas for a plan of care.

9. The hospitalized person often has difficulty sleeping. Indicate the factors in hospitalization that may disrupt usual sleep patterns. Consider data the nurse would want to collect and suggest interventions to help this person adapt to the hospital setting.

10. Define somnambulism and indicate what interventions you would suggest to parents whose child has this problem.

Glossary

Alpha state of sleep: a state of consciousness occurring just prior to falling asleep, characterized by increased relaxation and rambling thoughts.

Basic rest–activity cycle: the cyclic pattern, or periodicity of phases of REM and NREM, that is present during sleep. There may be a similar cycling of rest and activity during wakefulness.

Circadian rhythms: the fluctuations of biopsychological activities throughout the 24-hour day.

Comfort: the feeling of consolation or relief; the sense of being soothed; a state of ease with freedom from pain and anxiety, and a satisfaction of bodily wants; hopeful in time of grief or pain.

Delta sleep: the deep restful sleep of stages 3 and 4 NREM; also known as slow-wave sleep.

Electroencephalogram (EEG): a tracing of the electrical activity of the brain.

Electromyogram (EMG): a tracing of muscle contraction resulting from electrical stimulation.

Electrooculogram (EOG): the tracing of eye movements.

Endorphins: endogenous substances with morphinelike characteristics that are released in response to the pain sensation.

Enuresis: incontinence of urine during sleep.

Gate control theory: a theory which proposes that specialized cells in the dorsal horn of the spinal cord act as a gating mechanism that alters and modifies the arriving pain sensations before they reach the cerebral cortex and evoke the perception of pain.

Hypnosedative: a drug that produces sleep.

Insomnia: the person's inability to attain the amount of sleep or the reenergizing from sleep that he believes necessary for healthy functioning.

L-Tryptophan: an essential amino acid present in dietary protein, which may influence the level of brain serotonin and thereby cause sleepiness.

Non-rapid eye movement sleep (NREM): the phase of sleep characterized by four stages of varying depth of sleep.

Pain: a sensation that creates discomfort ranging from mild to agonizing.

Pain threshold: the point at which the person becomes aware of the pain sensation.

Pain tolerance: the point at which pain can no longer be tolerated by the person.

Paradoxical sleep: a synonym for REM sleep referring to the antithetical circumstances within this phase of sleep.

Parasomnias: disorders that occur during sleep, such as somnambulism, enuresis, night terrors.

Placebo: from the Latin meaning, "I shall please"; an intervention that produces a desired effect because of its therapeutic intent, not because of specific properties.

Rapid eye movement sleep (REM): the phase of sleep characterized by rapid eye movements and dreaming.

REM rebound: a phenomenon that causes the total amount of REM sleep to remain fairly constant. It occurs when a person is deprived of REM sleep for several successive nights, and then spends more time in REM sleep on subsequent nights.

Sedative: a drug that produces a calming, quieting effect and enhances sleep when taken at bedtime.

Serotonin: a biochemical transmitter, also known as 5-hydroxytryptamine or 5HT, that acts as an inhibitor to the reticular activating system, thereby allowing the person to fall asleep.

Sleep—a phenomenon in which there is a period of unawareness accompanied by a set of physiological and psychological behaviors that are different from the waking state.

Slow-wave sleep (SWS): the deep restful stages of 3 and 4 NREM; also known as delta sleep.

Bibliography

Pain

Armstrong M: Current concepts in pain. AORN J 32, No. 3:383–390, 1980

———: A short simple tool for assessing your patient's pain. Nurs '81 11, No. 3:48–49, 1981

————: Anxiety and the aching back. Emergency Med 12, No. 3:125–128, 1980

Benson H: The Relaxation Response. New York, Avon Books, 1976

Beyerman K: Flawed perceptions about pain. Am J Nurs 82, No. 2:302–304, 1982

Bond M: Pain: Its Nature, Analysis and Treatment. Edinburgh, London and New York, Churchill Livingstone, 1979

Bonica JJ, Liebeskind JC, Albe-Fessard, DG: Advances in Pain Research and Therapy, Proceedings of the Second World Congress on Pain, Vol. 3. New York, Raven Press, 1979

Brena SF: Chronic Pain: America's Hidden Epidemic. New York, Atheneum/SMI, 1978

Brena SF: Pain and Religion: A Psychophysiological Study. Springfield, Ill, Charles C Thomas, 1972

Cannon WB: Bodily Changes in Pain, Hunger, Fear, and Rage, 2nd ed. New York and London, Appleton & Co., 1929

Conway–Rutkowski, B: Getting to the cause of tension headache. Am J Nurs 81, No. 10:1946–1949, 1981

Cousins N: Anatomy of an Illness. New York, WW Norton, 1979

Crue BL: Chronic Pain: Further Observation. New York, from City of Hope National Medical Center, SP Medical and Scientific Books (a division of Spectrum Publications), 1979

Cummings D: Stopping chronic pain before it starts. Nurs '81 11, No. 1:60–62, 1981

Davis AJ: Brompton's cocktail: Making goodbyes possible. Am J Nurs 78, No. 4:611–612, 1978

DiBlasi M, Washburn CS: Using analgesics effectively. Am J Nurs 79, No. 1:74, 78, 1979

Ersek RA: Pain Control with T.E.N.S.: Principles and Practice. St. Louis, Warren H. Green, 1981

Fagerhaugh SY, Strauss A: How to manage your patient's pain and how not to. Nurs '80 10, No. 2:44–47, 1980

Fagerhaugh SY, Strauss A: Politics of Pain Management: Staff–Patient Interaction. Menlo Park, CA, Addison-Wesley, 1977

Feuerstein M, Skjei E: Mastering Pain. New York, Bantam Books, 1979

Jacox AK: Assessing pain. Am J Nurs 79, No. 5:895–900, 1979

Jacox AK (ed): Pain: A Source Book for Nurses and Other Health Professionals, Boston, Little, Brown & Co, 1977

Krieger D, Pepper E, Aucoli S: Therapeutic touch: Searching for evidence of physiological change. Am J Nurs 79, No. 4:660–662, 1979

Larkins FR: The influence of one patient's culture on pain response. Nurs Clin North Am 12, No. 4:663–668, 1977

Lewis CS: The Problem of Pain. New York, MacMillan, 1955

McCaffery M: Cognition, bodily pain, and man–environment interactions. In McCaffery M: Nursing Management of the Patient with Pain, 2nd ed. Philadelphia, JB Lippincott, 1979

McCaffery M: How to relieve your patient's pain fast and effectively with oral analgesics. Nurs '80 10, No. 11:58–63, 1980

McCaffery M: Nursing Management of the Patient With Pain, 2nd ed. Philadelphia, JB Lippincott, 1979

McCaffery M: Relieving pain with noninvasive techniques. Nurs '80 10, No. 12:55–57, 1980

McCaffery M: Understanding your patient's pain. Nurs '80 10, No. 9:26–31, 1980

McCaffery M: When your patient is still in pain, don't just do something: Sit there. Nurs '81, 11, No. 6:58–61, 1981

McDonnell DE: TENS in treating chronic pain. AORN J 32, No. 3:401–410, 1980

Mahoney EA: Some implications for nursing diagnoses of pain. Nurs Clin North Am 12, No. 4:613–620, 1977

Maxwell M: How to use methadone for the cancer patient's pain. Am J Nurs 80, No. 9:1606–1608, 1980

Mehta M: Intractable Pain. London, WB Saunders, Ltd, 1973

Melzack R: The Puzzle of Pain. New York, Basic Books, 1973

Melzack R, Wall P: Pain mechanisms: A new theory. Science 150:971–979, 1965

Melzack R, Wall P: Psychophysiology of Pain. Anesthesiol Clin 8, No. 1:3–34, 1970

Miaskowski C: The Brompton cocktail. Cancer Nursing 1, No. 6:451–455, 1978

Miller J: The Body in Question. New York, Random House, 1978

Olshan NH: Power Over Your Pain Without Drugs. New York, Rawson, Wade, 1980

Owen BD: How to avoid that aching back. Am J Nurs 80, No. 5:894–897, 1980

Pelletier KR: Mind as Healer, Mind as Slayer. New York, Dell Publishing, 1977

Perry SW, Heidrich G: Placebo response: Myth and matter. Am J Nurs 81, No. 4:720–721, 1980

Saper J, Magee K: Freedom From Headaches. New York, Simon & Schuster, 1978

Schmitt M: The nature of pain with some personal notes. Nurs Clin North Am 12, No. 4:621–630, 1977

Shealy CN: Holistic Management of Chronic Pain. Top Clin Nurs 2:1–8, 1980

Siegele DS: The gate control theory. Am J Nurs 74, No. 3:498–502, 1974

Silman J: Reference guide to analgesics. Am J Nurs 79, No. 1:74–77, 1979

Simonton C, Simonton S: Getting Well Again. Los Angeles, Tarcher, 1978

Sternbach RA: Pain: A Psychophysiological Analysis. New York and London, Academic Press, 1968

Sternbach RA (ed): The Psychology of Pain. New York, Raven Press, 1980

Twycross RG: Diseases of the central nervous system: Relief of terminal pain. Brit Med J 4:212–214, 1975

Vander A, Sherman J, Luciano DS: Human Physiology: The Mechanisms of Body Function, 3rd ed. New York, McGraw-Hill, 1980

Weisenberg M: Pain: Clinical and Experimental Perspectives. Saint Louis, C V Mosby, 1975

West AB: Understanding endorphins: Our natural pain relief system. Nurs '81 11, No. 2:50–53, 1981

Willey TJ: The brain makes its own morphine. Life and Health 95, No. 4:19–20, 1980

Wilson RW: Endorphins. Am J Nurs 81, No. 4:722–725, 1981

Wolf ZR: Pain theories: An overview. Top Clin Nurs 2, No. 1:9–17, 1980

Yancey P: Where Is God When It Hurts. Grand Rapids, MI, Zondervan, 1977

Young JL: The pain of a terminally ill patient in the home. Nurs Clin North Am 12, No. 4:653–662, 1977

Sleep

Agnew H, Webb W, Williams R: Sleep patterns in late middle age males: An EEG study. Electroencephalography & Clinical Neurophys 23:168–171, 1967

Agnew H, Webb W, and Williams R: The Effect of Stage Four Sleep Deprivation. Electroencephalogr Clin Neurophysiol 17:68–70, 1964

Bassler SF: The origins and development of biological rhythms. Nurs Clin North Am 11, No. 4:575–582, 1976

Benson H: The Relaxation Response. New York, Avon Books, 1976

———: Caffeine: What it Does. Consumer Reports 46, No. 10:595–599, 1981

Clark M, Gasnell R, Shapiro D, Hager M: The mystery of sleep. Newsweek 48–55, July 1981

Crisp AN, Stonehill E: Sleep, Nutrition and Mood. New York and London, John Wiley & Sons, 1976

Dement WC: Some Must Watch While Some Must Sleep. San Francisco, San Francisco Book Co, 1976

Dement WC: The effect of dream deprivation. Science 131:1705–1707, 1960

Feinberg I: Changes in sleep cycle patterns with age. J Psych Res 10:283, 1974

Feinberg I, Braun M, Shulman E et al: EEG sleep patterns in mental retardation. Electroencephalogr Clin Neurophysiol 27:128–141, August 1969

Foulkes D: The Psychology of Sleep. New York, Charles Scribner's Sons, 1966

Ganong WF: Review of Medical Physiology. Los Altos, CA, Lange Medical Publications, 1979

Greenberg R, Dewan EM: Aphasia and Rapid Eye Movement Sleep. Nature (London) 223:183–184, July 12, 1969

Harris E: Sedative–hypnotic drugs. Am J Nurs 81, No. 7:1329–1334, 1981

Hartmann El: The Functions of Sleep. New Haven and London, Yale University Press, 1973

Hartmann E: The Sleeping Pill. New Haven and London, Yale University Press, 1978

Hartmann E, Cravens J, List S: Hypnotic effects of L-tryptophan. Arch Gen Psychiatry 31:394–397, 1974

Hayter J: The rhythm of sleep. Am J Nurs 80, No. 3:457–461, 1980

Kales A (ed): Sleep, Physiology and Pathology. Philadelphia, JB Lippincott, 1969

Kleitman N: Sleep and Wakefulness. Chicago, The University of Chicago Press, 1963

Lairy, GC, Salzarulo P (eds): The Experimental Study of Human Sleep: Methodological Problems. Amsterdam, Elsevier, 1975

Lanuza DM: Circadian rhythms of mental efficiency and performance. Nurs Clin North Am 11, No. 4:583–594, 1976

Linde SM, Savary LM: The Sleep Book. New York, Harper & Row, 1974

Luce GG, Segal J: Insomnia. Garden City, NJ, Doubleday, 1966

Luce GG, Segal J: Sleep, New York, Coward-McCann, 1966

Lugaresi E, Coccagna G, Mantovani M: Hypersomnia with Periodic Apneas. New York, SP Medical and Scientific Books, 1978

Maxmen JS: A Good Night's Sleep. New York, WW Norton, 1981

Orem J, Barnes CD (eds): Physiology in Sleep. New York, Academic Press, 1980

Oswald I: Sleep, 3rd ed. Harmondsworth, Middlesex, England, Penguin Books, 1974

Pasnaw RO, Naithoh P, Stier S et al: The psychological effects of 205 hours of sleep deprivation. Arch Gen Psychiatry, 18:496–505, Apr 1968

Paupst JC: The Sleep Book. Toronto, Macmillan of Canada, 1975

Priest RG, Pletscher A, Ward J (eds): Sleep Research. Lancaster, England, Falcon House, MTP Press Limited, International Medical Publishers, 1979

Prinz P: Sleep patterns in the healthy aged: Relationship with intellectual function. J Gerontol 32, No. 2:179–186, 1977

Rubenstein H: The Complete Insomniac. London, Jonathan Cape, 1974

Selye H: The Stress of Life. New York, McGraw-Hill, 1978

Shapiro CM, Griesel RD, Bartel PR et al: Sleep patterns after graded exercise. J Appl Physiol 39:187–190, 1975

Tom CK: Nursing assessment of biological rhythms. Nurs Clin North Am 11, No. 4:621–630, 1976

Trubo R: How to Get a Good Night's Sleep. Boston, Little, Brown & Co, 1978

Usdin GL (ed): Sleep Research and Clinical Practice. New York, Brunner/ Mazel, 1973

Vander A, Sherman JH, Luciano DP: Human Physiology: The Mechanisms of Body Function, 3rd ed. New York, McGraw-Hill, 1980

Walker JM, Floyd TC, Fein G et al: Effects of exercise on sleep. J Appl Physiol 44:945–951, 1978

Webb WB (ed): Sleep: An Active Process. Glenview, IL, Scott, Foresman and Co, 1973

Williams RL, Karacan I: Sleep Disorders: Diagnosis and Treatment. New York, John Wiley & Sons, 1978

Wolman BB (ed): Handbook of Dreams. New York, Van Nostrand Reinhold Co, 1979

Culture and Person-Centered Care

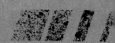

Bobbie Bloch

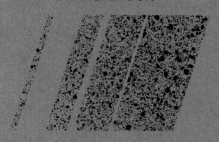

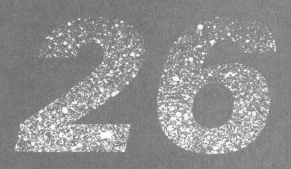

In the last two decades, American ethnic minority groups, such as Blacks, Hispanics, and Native Americans, have undergone tremendous consciousness-raising about racial and cultural identity. There is a trend away from the "melting pot" syndrome toward a cultural identity and recognition of individuals as members of the "whole" American society.

Social and political issues have caused a recent influx to America of new immigrants such as Vietnamese, Cubans, and Haitians. Like established ethnic-minority groups, new immigrants tend to adhere to familiar cultural beliefs and practices as they adjust to their new environment.

Oftentimes persons of these various racial or cultural groups have great difficulty adapting to the changes that their new environment proposes. Such changes relate to family and peer roles, language and communication process, economic and social class values, religious beliefs and practices, nutrition, and resulting physical alterations. For example, a Vietnamese peasant arriving in America experiences great confusion and anxiety related to his inability to speak English and his lack of appropriate skills to obtain a job. Sutterley and Donnelly (1973), identify such **cultural shock** as profound disorientation experienced by a person who has been thrust into an alien culture without sufficient preparation. If the rate of environmental change is too rapid, it can cause great difficulty both physiologically and psychologically during attempts to adapt.

In recent years, the nursing profession has become acutely aware of cultural variations and their impact on providing person-centered care. Official statements have been published, recognizing nursing's contribution toward meeting the "health needs of a diverse and multicultural society" (National League for Nursing, 1977, p. 13) and toward considering "individual value systems and lifestyles" (American Nurses Association, 1976, p. 4).

In response to issues raised by both new and established ethnic-minority groups, the following questions arise: What influence does a client's or a nurse's culture have on providing effective nursing care? For instance, how could the nurse provide holistic care for an Asian person who adheres to the "yin–yang" Eastern philosophy of cultural healing in contrast to the scientific healing principles and practices followed by the nurse's Western culture? What knowledge and nursing skills would be appropriate in assessing and intervening in the care of persons from different racial and cultural backgrounds? To answer these important questions, it is necessary to gain some insight into culture as a component of the concept of person and its influence on adaptation through the health-and-illness continuum.

This chapter provides a cultural approach to nursing process and considers culture as a subsystem of the person. Many cultural variables of the person are identified and explained. The relationship of cultural variables to other individual variables is considered. Bloch's Cultural Assessment Guide is presented and used to demonstrate both assessment and intervention phases of the nursing process. The chapter concludes with a case study illustration of the ideas presented.

After completing this chapter, students will be able to:

● *Recognize culture as a component of the person concept and as an adaptive mechanism in a person's environment.*

● *Describe several cultural variables of the person.*

● *Identify how cultural variables may influence health behavior.*

● *Use biopsychosocial variables to synthesize cultural data into the nursing process.*

● *Use cultural data to bring about change in the health behavior of a person who is racially or culturally different from the student.*

● *Recognize the effects of nurses' values, beliefs, and practices on persons who are racially or culturally different from themselves.*

● *Communicate acceptance of persons who are racially and culturally different from themselves.*

Culture as a Subsystem of the Person

Definition of Culture

There are numerous theories and definitions of the anthropological concept of **culture.** Downs defines culture as "a system of symbols shared by a group of humans and transmitted by them to upcoming generations" (1975, p. 45). Murray and Zentner define culture as "a group's design for living . . . [including shared] assumptions about the nature of the physical and social world, goals in life, attitudes, roles and values" (1979, p. 384). How persons resolve problems related to basic human needs is strongly influenced by their cultural backgrounds.

Characteristics of Culture

Three major characteristics of culture have been identified by Murray and Zentner (1979):

- Culture is learned.
- Culture is capable of change, but remains stable.
- There are components or patterns present in every culture.

As a small child, a person learns behaviors, values, attitudes, and beliefs within his cultural family system, a major teaching and supportive unit. This learning is largely influenced by the person's social status within a society and how he adapts to experiences in his environment. These values are learned and accepted for a time but then are modified or rejected as one is exposed to subgroups within a culture (Frances and Munjas, 1976).

The second cultural characteristic relates to language, traditions, and norms or customs that may act as stabilizers for a culture. But time, events, and location can have a great impact on these stabilizing factors of culture. For instance, Hirabayashi (1975) discusses the variations between three generations of Japanese migrants and their style of adaptation to America. The deferent behavioral traits of the first generation were detrimental to the second generation when negative stereotypes of Japanese-Americans prevailed during World War II. Thus there evolved a third, more radical, generation in the 1960s.

The third characteristic of culture is the cultural components or cultural patterns that are generally evident among all societies. These include communication systems, means of economic and physical survival, transportation systems, family systems, social customs and mores, and religious systems. These cultural components form the basis for cultural variables of the person.

Cultural Variables of the Person

The phrase "cultural variables of the person" refers to those characteristics that a person exhibits or identifies with from a particular cultural group. These variables may or may not be exhibited by every person from a cultural group. Any individual, depending on his personal experience, may have all, none, or any combination of these variables.

An understanding of the underlying development of the cultural variables of the person is essential for carrying out an appropriate and effective cultural assessment. Table 26-1 highlights those variables that form the basis of the cultural assessment tool to be discussed later.

Ethnic and Racial Identity

Ethnic origin and racial background have the greatest influence on how a person reacts and is reacted to by others in the health-care environment. Werner defines **ethnicity** as a group's "affiliation due to shared linguistic, racial, (religious), and/or cultural background" (1979, p. 343).

A person's ethnicity can be identified by any of the following:

* Language and communication process—*e.g.,* Spanish, Chinese, or Tagalog (Filipino)
* Racial background—*e.g.,* tribe, people, nation of same stock or human type such as Blacks, Caucasians
* Cultural background—*e.g.,* art, customs, laws, morals

Thus, if a nurse were assessing a person from a Hispanic background, a distinction between Mexican-American, Cuban, or Puerto Rican would be important. Likewise the nurse would need to distinguish between Iroquois or Navajo Native American. These individual groups would have very different ethnic backgrounds affecting their health and illness beliefs, health behaviors, value systems, and language and communication process.

Since the melting-pot concept is now less popular, the importance of accepting and appreciating culturally diverse people is receiving more attention. There has been a tremendous upsurge in trying to find one's ancestral "roots."

Value Orientations

Values are "intrinsic beliefs about the worth of an entity or concept" (Frances and Munjas, 1976, p. 59). As such, they provide the basis for each person's attitudes and behaviors and they assist in establishing hierarchies of needs and goals. Kluckholn and Strodtbeck (1961) defined value orientations as principles that assist in the solution of common human problems. Among the value orientations that may differ across cultures are those concerning human nature, man-to-nature and man-to-man relationships, and time.

Staples (1976) compares time orientations between Blacks and the white dominant American culture:

* Black value orientation—Schedules are flexible; activities happening now are important, as is adapting to ranges in time rather than fixed periods.
* White value orientation—Society dictates how a person regulates his life; punctuality is a high priority.

The white nurse who adheres to fixed schedules for baths, meals, medications, and sleep may find conflict with a Black person who is very flexible in his time orientation. Similarly, precise clinic appointments may have different meanings to white nurses and Black clients. Conflict and frustration can frequently be lessened with insight into value orientations different from the nurse's own.

Language and Intercultural Communication

Samovar and Porter describe **communication** as a "dynamic process whereby human behavior, both verbal and nonverbal, is perceived and responded to" (1976, p. 5). They further state that **intercultural communication** "occurs whenever a message producer is a member of one culture and a message receiver is a member of another" (p. 4). Persons from two different cultural groups will attempt to understand each other from their own cultural frameworks. Persons' cultural frameworks greatly influence their social perception, which involves attaching meaning to an object or event in their environment. For

---

Table 26-1
Cultural Variables

Ethnic and racial identity
Value orientations
Language and communication process
Family system
Healing beliefs and practices
Religious beliefs and practices
Nutritional behavior and cultural influences

instance, perceptions of pain, complaints of symptoms of illness, reactions to death and dying, and meanings attached to messages are all influenced by a person's cultural perception.

Cultural Differences

Samovar and Porter further emphasize that cultural differences are often responsible for communication problems. These cultural differences occur along a minimal–maximal dimension. For example, a maximal difference is shown between Asian and Western cultures that have numerous cultural variations and few commonalities, namely physical appearance, religion, philosophy, social attitudes, and language. On the other hand, Americans and Canadians would be considered on the minimal end of the scale, having separate but similar cultures. This type of minimal–maximal scale can also apply to differences between a nurse and client involved in the intercultural communication process. For example, eye contact and a friendly handshake are acceptable in the dominant American culture, indicating understanding and attentiveness, but they have very different meanings for the Native American. In many tribes, looking one in the eye is considered disrespectful and an intrusion upon a person's private soul that results in "soul loss" (Primeaux, 1977, p. 94). Nurses may think Native Americans are not listening or comprehending any conversation if there is no eye contact, but this is not necessarily true.

Word Connotations

Differences in word connotations affect our ability to communicate interculturally. For example, a nurse may associate "hospital" with health care. On the other hand, a Chinese American may associate "hospital" with uncleanliness and death because in the Chinese belief system, a patient's spirit may get lost and be unable to find its way home (Campbell and Chang, 1973).

Denotative meanings of words can also result in cultural communication problems. For instance, a Black youth may say, "I heard his house was really bad," which actually means, "I heard his house was really nice, good, or fantastic." Such a statement may confuse those who are not of this racial or cultural group. The Black youth's expression is a special linguistic code known as "Black argot." **Argot** means terms with "usage limited to a particular group or class; secrecy and usage are associated with members outside the dominant American culture" (Folb, 1972, p. 10).

Interracial Communication

Interracial communication is another factor that can influence the nurse–person communication process. Rich defines interracial communication as "communication between whites and nonwhites in American society with nonwhites occupying a marginal position in the society and (thus) introducing resentment and strain into the interaction" (1974, p. 13). For example, the social and environmental factors in our society have taught ethnic-minority persons to observe and listen carefully for any sign of racial discrimination. Anything that appears to be even slightly condescending can be interpreted as racism. One should not "talk down" or attempt to converse in the ethnic style of the cultural language, because it does not bring about a sense of identification and the nurse may appear awkward in trying to communicate this way. The patient may interpret this as ridiculing the style of communication (Bloch, 1976). Further study of the literature is suggested for a more in-depth discussion of racial–cultural communication characteristics of specific ethnic-minority groups.

Family System

Traditionally the family in American society has functioned as a group for the allocation, accumulation, and consumption of material resources. The family also plays a major role in personality development, identity formation, status assignment, and value orientation (Smith, Burlew, Mosley, and Whitney, 1978).

One might assess the family by looking at its structural patterns: Is it **matrilineal** or **patrilineal** with family descent determined through female or male? These structural patterns along with family roles, are culturally determined. For example, the strong feeling for family among Filipinos is derived from Chinese influence in which old traditional patterns are imposed by the family patriarch or a similarly authoritative matriarch. Respect and deference are shown for decisions made by elders (De-Garcia, 1979). Nurses may be concerned about families who hover over Filipino patients, but this can be an added asset in promoting family-centered nursing. The nurse may also find it helpful to seek out the Filipino elders when decisions are being made about patient care of an ill family member.

The psychological functioning of the family is crucial for ethnic-minority families since their psychological well-being depends on adaptation to the social and human environment. Because of racial attitudes toward these minority groups in America, the main function of the family is to promote survival. Many ethnic-minority families have shown tremendous adaptability and flexibility. Otto (1962) indicates that this resiliency is due to family loyalty and intrafamily cooperation, ability of family self-help, flexibility in performing family roles, and providing for physical and spiritual needs of the family.

Nursing Implications

If a nurse is assessing ethnic-minority families, it would be helpful to capitalize on these strengths in meeting the client's health-care needs. When nurses are interviewing ethnic-minority persons, it is important to consider the impact of the family on decisions related to nursing care. For example, in Mexican-American families, the "family" comes first and the "self" is second. The family is sought first in meeting health-care needs and others are sought when no other alternatives exist (White, 1977). One may conclude that the family unit among ethnic-minority groups is a major source of stability.

Cultural Healing Beliefs and Practices

Cultural healing beliefs are beliefs that reflect a specific cultural orientation towards health and illness. They include cause of illness, treatment measures, illness prevention, and health promotion. According to Moore and associates, "Beliefs reflect perceived relationships between culture and environment . . . [and] beliefs (may) pertain directly to cause–effect relationships" (1980, p. 199). In many instances, these beliefs contrast greatly with the traditional scientific medical theories about health and illness. Several authors (Spicer, 1979; Scott, 1974; and Snow, 1974) have discovered through research that these cultural health belief systems exist and indeed are prevalent among ethnic and cultural groups.

The cause and effects related to health and illness can be viewed from a variety of religious and socio-behavioral contexts. Some persons rely on cultural healers such as **spiritualists.** These are persons of either sex "called" by God to heal incurable diseases or solve emotional or personal problems. Why one society may resort to chants and rituals to expunge disease and another may visit a physician or hospital requires an understanding of the belief systems of each culture regarding health and illness. This diversity may also demonstrate the vast adaptive capabilities of human beings.

For example, Holland (1978) studied the health–illness concepts of Mexican-Americans in Arizona. He found, especially among poor peasant populations, a strong adherence to a "miracle-oriented" system of magicoreligious beliefs and rituals for controlling stressful life events. Disease concepts are based on this magicoreligious belief system: Good health and prosperity are maintained when there is a balance between good and evil forces. Ill health and life's difficulties occur when this equilibrium is disturbed, and then a person will suffer a host of consequences. Some illnesses may be viewed as heavenly punishment for not following social mores and others may be thought to be caused by devils or witches. Diagnosing and curing are done mainly by "curanderos," curers who use herbal remedies for simple illnesses and magicoreligious rituals for difficult illnesses. The religious component is very strong, with many Mexican-Americans requesting favors from Catholic saints during times of crises. An example of one of the traditional Mexican illnesses is the emotional disease called *susto*, which refers to any disturbing or unstabilizing experience such as accidents or fearful events that cause "fright sickness' in which the "spirit" is separated from the body. The person afflicted may experience diarrhea, elevated temperature, anorexia, listlessness, or withdrawal. Treatment is done by a curer who calls the spirit back to the person's body with prayers and candle burning before saints (Holland, 1978).

Prior to Holland's study, Snow (1974) did an ethnographic study in Tucson, Arizona. He studied the cultural healing systems of low-income black Americans. Themes indicated that this cultural group perceives the world as a hostile and dangerous place where people are liable to attack from external sources, including a punitive God, nature, malice of fellow men, relatives, friends, or strangers. Further, people were perceived as helpless and dependent on outside help. Again the use of magic was prevalent if persons felt helpless and had important wishes. Good health was associated with success in life and bad luck with illness. Natural illnesses were considered to be caused by exposure to nature's forces or to be punishment from God, whereas unnatural illnesses were those serious conditions caused by evil influences including demons and witchcraft. Treatment of illness was done by using home remedies and preventatives, such as turpentine and kerosene and not letting cold air enter a menstruating or pregnant woman's body. Cultural healers were used who had special powers to cure natural and unnatural illnesses. Powers to cure were thought to be healing gifts from God, inborn, or learned from others.

Nursing Implications

Holland and Snow's brief examples of cultural healing beliefs and practices demonstrate implications for nurses and other health professionals. It was not the intent of these examples to give in-depth information but to encourage awareness of these cultural belief systems. Although these beliefs and practices may seem bizarre, they are understandable in their cultural context. The nurse must be aware of how these beliefs affect a person's response to the health-care system. A person may reject the health-care environment due to vast differences in cultural belief systems.

According to Scott (1974), health professionals should, when feasible, use a treatment plan that demonstrates respect for and reflects a person's cultural healing system. For instance, upon a person's admission to the hospital, assess what healing remedies have been helpful and incorporate them into the treatment plan. If a person believes he has been "hexed," try to alleviate his fears by combining orthodox treatment of symptoms with a cultural healer to remove the spell.

Religious Beliefs and Practices

A person's religion may also influence his concept of health and illness, treatment programs, and recovery. Religion can also act as a resource in facing crises related to critical illnesses or death. However, it must not be assumed that all persons from certain ethnic or cultural backgrounds have the same or similar religious belief systems. Pumphrey (1977) describes several religious belief systems and their characteristics as related to birth, death, health crisis, diet, and special beliefs. The nurse should assess these characteristics in a person's religious belief system and determine their influence on the health state.

There may be a thin line between religious and cultural beliefs that makes it difficult to separate the two. For example, Filipinos have a strong sense of destiny related to their Asian background and a deep faith in God drawn from the Spanish influence in their culture. This may account for why some Filipinos resign themselves and suffer in silence, attributing their illness state to God's will (DeGarcia, 1979). Some religious groups may object to medical interventions as shown by the refusal of Jehovah's Witnesses to allow blood transfusions or the avoidance of drugs by Seventh Day Adventists unless they are absolutely necessary (Pumphrey, 1977).

Nursing Implications

Again the intent of this chapter is to alert nurses to the importance of understanding religious cultural belief systems and to encourage them to be supportive of beliefs which promote comfort and adaptation.

Nutritional Behavior and Cultural Influences

The kinds of foods eaten, the way they are prepared, and the manner in which they are consumed are practices that are embedded strongly in the behavioral systems of each culture. When a person enters the health-care setting, he brings all of his cultural beliefs and practices about food with him. Frequently, his food preferences and manner of consumption conflict with the way the hospital prepares food and serves meals. This may cause some distress if there is no means of meeting his cultural needs. For example, Schubin (1980) describes the incident of a Mexican-American patient who disappeared from his hospital room soon after undergoing major surgery. He had gone home to obtain specific cultural foods of tacos, tortillas, and beans. Later he returned, believing that these foods would speed his recovery.

Niehoff (1969) and Lee (1957) both describe "proper" and "improper" foods according to the food value characteristic of a cultural system. Such foods stir positive or negative feelings depending on how the culture views the food. For example, while North Americans are strongly adverse to insects in their diet (improper food), the Ifugaons of the Philippines regard dragon flies as a human (proper) food (Lee, 1957). Similarly, North Americans regard milk as a good food, but Southeast Asians do not. North Americans may consider ice water to be refreshing but a Chinese person believes that it shocks the system and is harmful to health. Historically, water was boiled in China because of inadequate sanitation (Campbell and Chang, 1973).

Religious beliefs and practices may strongly influence nutritional behavior. For example, Black Muslim doctrine prohibits intake of alcoholic beverages, pork, and foods such as cornbread and collards that are traditionally eaten by Black Americans. Orthodox Jews who observe strict kosher dietary laws will not eat pork and shellfish or combine meat and milk at the same meal (Pumphrey, 1977).

Finally, the influence of food in the cause and treatment of disease is related to one's cultural background. A good example is the Cinese philosophy of "chi" (air or wind), referring to energy present in all living organisms. When food is metabolized it is changed into chi and becomes either cold "yin" energy force or a hot "yang" energy force. Diseases resulting from yin excesses are classified as yin disorders. Those diseases classified as hot, such as ear infection, should be treated with cold foods such as wintermelon. Because this philosophy is passed down by family tradition, nurses can ask the family which foods support the yin–yang beliefs. These can be included in treating a family member if they are not contraindicated (Campbell and Chang, 1973).

A common belief among some Blacks, southern whites, and Haitians is that the amount of blood volume may increase or decrease related to dietary intake of certain foods. For example, "high blood" (confused with the term "high blood pressure") is said to be due to ingesting too much rich food, especially meat. To remedy this, astringent foods such as vinegar, lemon juice, pickles, or epsom salts, are taken to "bring down high blood by opening the pores and allowing loss through sweat." "Low blood" is allied with the term "anemia" (confused with low blood pressure). According to tradition, one must avoid astringent foods and consume red beets, wine, grape juice, red meat, liver, and fresh animal blood with imitative magic properties to bring low blood up (Snow, 1974).

These are just some of the nutritional behaviors influenced by culture that nurses must understand to know their implications for diet planning, diet teaching, and influences on a person's health.

Nursing Implications

When assessing a person's nutritional status, the nurse may gain clues to cultural patterns of food intake and the possible implications these patterns may have on diet teaching and illness. Although it would be difficult to have a vast knowledge of all existing food habits, nurses should be aware of the cultural food preferences of the people living in close proximity to the hospital or clinic. Whatever their own personal preferences, nurses must be careful not to impose their values about food consumption and preparation on those whose cultural nutrition patterns differ.

All of the cultural variables of the person discussed here give an overview of factors that are important in doing a cultural assessment of a person. These variables are used to formulate the data categories of the cultural assessment tool that follows. However, to do a complete assessment of a person, other variables of the person—sociological, psychological, and biophysical—must be discussed briefly, and their relationship to ethnic and cultural variables must be considered.

Relationship of Cultural Variables to Other Variables of the Person

Sociological Variables

Previous discussion centered on the family as the basic socializing unit that introduces a person to the values, attitudes, customs, and social habits of a particular cultural group. There are other social variables the nurse must assess among ethnic-minority persons: economic status, educational status, social network, and valued social institutions. The relationship between cultural variables and sociological variables is best seen in the consideration of socioeconomic influences on health care.

According to Kosa and Zola (1975), American Society is classified into three socioeconomic levels: middle and upper class, blue-collar working class, and the poverty population. There may be overlapping of characteristics of these distinctive life-styles and also variations within each stratum, but generally each stratum is influenced by the following factors:

- Amount and source of income available
- Type of occupation and prestige associated with each type
- Type and value of housing and neighborhood
- Level of knowledge and education
- Race or ethnic origin.

Kosa and Zola (1975) further proclaim that a large number of ethnic minorities (*i.e.*, Blacks, hispanics, Native Americans, and other poor ethnic minorities) are part of the lowest of the three strata, characterized by high unemployment, low income, poor housing and living conditions, and low educational standards.

Many literature sources (Ruffin, 1979; Bullough and Bullough, 1972; and Irvine, 1970) state that these socioeconomic problems have a profound effect on levels of health among ethnic minorities. Ruffin (1979) concludes:

- The effects of poverty as a social environment result in a higher degree and more serious kinds of morbidity.
- Poverty hampers the poor in maintaining or regaining their health; that is, they are less likely to seek preventive or diagnostic services without symptoms.

For example, the statistics reported by Irvine depict the percentage of Native American infants born on reservations who die annually (32.3/1000) as higher than that of the general United States population (23.7/1000). The mortality rate for Native American infants in the first year of life is 25/1000 *versus* 7/1000 nationally (1970, p. 453).

Kosa and Zola (1975) conclude that the poor and working class populations seek health care later because of economic penalties that have a greater consequence for this population than for middle-class workers. Again, the cultural beliefs related to health and illness among ethnic minorities also contribute to the decision of when a person seeks health-care services.

Nursing Implications

What should be the nurse's approach to incorporating into care both variables of poverty and ethnicity? The nurse is often a member of the dominant American group. This may cause some social distance from the ethnic-minority person regarding values, behavior, attitudes, or racial background. To provide effective person-centered care, the nurse must gain some insight into the characteristics and problems a person living in poverty experiences. This will help clarify why a person does not return for clinic visits, lacks funds for special diets, or feels inferior owing to poor living environment and educational level.

Watts (1967) discusses these issues in her article, "Social Class, Ethnic Background, and Patient Care." Watts states that nurses have difficulty in caring for patients from lower socioeconomic classes because their expectations of patient behavior contrast with actual behavior, and they have problems understanding these patients' attitudes and their expectations of nurses.

For instance, if a Black person who is poor and unemployed fails to return for a follow-up visit for chronic leg ulcers, this may be interpreted by the nurse as a lack of interest in his well-being. To this black person the value of "time" and of meeting economic needs may be more important than a return clinic visit.

Brinton's (1972) study of low-income mothers reinforces the idea of variation between low-income persons' health values and those perceived by nurses. The results showed a greater discrepancy between the priority of values that nurses perceived low-income mothers to have and the value priorities the mothers actually held (*i.e.*, nurses rated less value for health than mothers—48% *vs* 85% from mothers' responses). Based on these responses, nurses, with their attitude that low-income persons care little about health, may miss many important cues these clients give.

Nurses should be aware of the dynamics of poverty and available resources. They cannot always remedy the immediate factors relative to poverty, but genuine interest and understanding of behavior and attitudes of poor ethnic-minority persons will help to resolve conflicts in dealing with this dilemma.

Psychological Variables

The nurse's assessment of psychological variables of ethnic-minority persons will include all the mental or behavioral processes and characteristics that compose the psychological system and their impact on the health environment. For example, how does an ethnic-minority person's self-concept affect the nurse–patient relationship? The nurse must first understand how that self-concept is developed.

How this ethnic-minority person's family, peers, external environment, and society characterize his behavior strongly influences the development of his self-concept. The labeling of a characteristic of the ethnic-minority person as either "good" or "bad" is the evaluative component of his self-concept known as "self-esteem" or one's worth on a scale from very low to very high (Frances and Munjas, 1976).

Smith and associates (1978) define the self-concept of minorities as follows:

- The way minority persons see themselves from their viewpoint
- The way (nonminority) "others" view them and prescribe what minority persons should be
- The way they "wish" to be known to others and to themselves
- Combination of all three definitions above.

Nursing Implications

The nurse's perception of the ethnic-minority person and how the person relates to the nurse's perception (based on his self-concept) determines the outcome of the nurse–person relationship. Hein (1980) reinforces this statement, saying that if the nurse's role of helper is based on superiority due to negative feelings about a person, the person may not believe the nurse is sincerely interested in his needs and welfare.

The nurse should assess how the ethnic-minority person responds to psychological stress in the clinical setting. For example, how does this person respond to the psychological distress of physical pain? Davitz, Sameshima, and Davitz (1976) did an excellent cross-cultural study on nurses' beliefs about patient suffering. They found 554 nurses from six different cultures varied in their interpretations and attitudes about suffering associated with illnesses and injury (*i.e.*, cancer, trauma, infection, *etc.*).

For example, differences among cultures included: Japanese and Korean nurses believed that patients suffered a high degree of physical pain and psychological distress although the nurses did not express this belief through their own overt behavior; American and Puerto Rican nurses, on the other hand, believed patients experienced a low degree of pain and Americans misperceived the psychological distress of Puerto Rican patients. Similarities among the six groups were beliefs that children suffer less psychological distress with less awareness of implications of illness and also that women show greater reaction to physical pain than men.

A nurse should be aware of both differences and similarities cross-culturally as a way of developing sensitivity to persons with varied cultural backgrounds and avoiding stereotypic approaches in relieving psychological and physical distress.

Biophysical Variables

Nurses should have knowledge of how biophysical variations among ethnic-minority groups influence their own ability to carry out appropriate and accurate physical assessments. Some of the standard values of doing physical assessments may be labelled non-normal for Blacks, Orientals, or Native Americans. Overfield (1977) emphasizes that biological variations exist because of past environmental influences rather than innate biological differences. For example, light skin could synthesize vitamin D more effectively on the few sunny days; conversely black skin became a neutral trait where protection from the sun and heat in the tropics was not a factor.

Oftentimes, skin color and hair texture are the most visible physical characteristics the nurse observes and evaluates in doing a physical assessment. Skin color and hair texture are inherited independently of each other; melanin pigment is responsible for skin color. The more melanin present, the darker the skin color (Rook, 1970). Many ethnic-minority groups have characteristic variations in skin color (*i.e.*, Blacks, native Americans, Hispanics, Asians, *etc.*) which would influence skin color changes such as those that occur in cyanosis. More in-depth examples are discussed in the chapter on skin assessment.

It is also important to understand why certain diseases are more prevalent among ethnic or cultural groups. Ruffin (1979) suggests several reasons, including: increased exposure and susceptibility related to environmental differences, increased susceptibility related to genetic factors, and higher frequency of mutant genes caused by selected environmental factors or small groups breeding in isolation.

This author further concludes that exposure and susceptibility greatly influence the health status of ethnic-minority groups due to inadequate health standards in their communities, which lead to the greater incidence of health problems.

A final factor related to physical differences is growth and development patterns. For example, studies have shown Black children to be taller and heavier than white children between ages of 5 to 14. Also, Malina's study showed that Black children have thinner skin folds than white children regardless of socioeconomic level, indicating nutrition is not a factor. Malina suggests "that criteria for evaluating nutritional status via skin folds should be different for American Negro and white samples" (1971, p. 37). All of these variations would be very important for the school nurse or pediatric nurse practitioner doing physical assessments of children.

The previous discussion of the cultural and related variables established a basis for discussion of how these factors can influence the nursing process and cultural assessment. The last section of the chapter presents current methods of cultural assessment, a cultural assessment tool, and examples of cultural assessment as part of the nursing process.

Cultural Assessment and the Nursing Process

Approaches to Cultural Assessment

Recent literature (Spector, 1979; Bauwens, 1978; and Branch and Paxton, 1976) shows increasing interest in the impact of cultural data on the delivery of health care. Besides the development of cultural awareness, there is more emphasis on methods for assessing racial and cultural groups.

For example, Branch and Paxton (1976) in their book, *Providing Safe Nursing Care for Ethnic People of Color*, discussed "the holistic nursing model." This model "recognizes the importance of the environment and prior episodes of repeated and/or intense stress on one's capacity for adaptation, and hence on one's level of wellness" (p. 152). They surmise that the variations in the supply and demand of man's energy systems (*i.e.*, familial/affiliative, restorative, spiritual, chemical/fluid, *etc.*) influence the planning and implementation of patient care. Also, the patient, family, and significant others are crucial in carrying out the nursing process using the holistic nursing model. Branch and Paxton further conclude both that the major premise of the holistic model is based on the inclusion of culture as a factor in nursing assessment and intervention and that culture serves as an adaptive mechanism in a person's environment.

For instance, if a person comes into a hospital setting for a planned cardiovascular surgical procedure, the nurse might ask the following questions: In what energy system is the person deficient (*i.e.*, circulatory)? How will this surgery affect his living environment (*i.e.*, economic, employment)? Does the person have a strong affiliation with his family, religion (*i.e.*, strong support systems), and does the person's racial and cultural background influence his ability to adapt to the hospital setting, surgical procedure, or persons in the clinical setting?

Another example is shown in Spector's (1979) book, *Cultural Diversity in Health and Illness*, which looks at the traditional views of health and illness among four cultural groups: Asian American, Hispanic American, Native American, and Black American. In assessing these groups, Spector divided the information among the following categories:

- Traditional definitions of health
- Traditional forms of epidemiological beliefs
- Traditional names and symptoms of a given disease
- Traditional remedies
- Traditional sources of "medical" assistance
- Health and illness problems the group encounters in dealing with the health-care system (p. 208)

Spector emphasizes that the data is general and not specific to any one person. But, a person's health and illness behavior may be derived from his traditional belief system, and this would have implications for the health-care provider in understanding patient care problems and their resolution.

Bloch's Ethnic/Cultural Assessment Tool is yet another approach for assessing the cultural background of a person. This approach is based not only on assessment, but on using the ethnic and cultural data to meet the health-care needs of the person. Nurses have been given information about various ethnic and cultural group characteristics but not

about how to operationalize this data by using the nursing process.

Nursing Implications

It should be emphasized that a nurse may use a variety or combination of ways of assessing cultural data. Whatever method is successful in obtaining accurate and applicable cultural information should be used. One should avoid trying to use a "specific method" of assessment for every cultural group in the belief that this will resolve all difficulties in obtaining cultural data. Nurses use nursing process with culturally different people just as they do for any person. In the crucial step of establishing trust, nurses must accept a person's values as valid for him, but they do not necessarily have to take them on for themselves. One should use the interview and physical assessment skills as described in the initial nursing process chapter, considering physical differences when applicable.

Bloch's Ethnic/Cultural Assessment Guide

Bloch's Assessment Guide is shown in Table 26-2. This guide is adapted from Bloch's Assessment Tool and uses the same general format. The four data categories are cultural, sociological, psychological, and biophysical variables of the person. For each data category, specific guideline questions are given. A right-hand column to write the data collected has been omitted to save space.

The nursing process is based on data relevant to individualized client needs: in this case, the individualized need of the ethnic/cultural client who is the primary source of ethnic and cultural assessment data.

The cultural, sociological, psychological, and biophysical data categories include some of the major areas a nurse will identify in assessing a person of another culture or ethnic group. However, Bloch's Guide is not inclusive of all areas that may be generally applicable for gathering data on persons in clinical settings. This guide should be used in conjunction with or become a part of already accessible nursing data systems. Again, there is much literature available on these systems and interpretations of the nursing process (Murray and Zentner, 1979; La Monica, 1979; Marriner, 1979; and Yura and Walsh, 1978). But there is very little literature on adapting the nursing process to the care of ethnic-minority persons. Bloch's Guide emphasizes the

(*Text continues on page 583.*)

Table 26-2
Bloch's Ethnic/Cultural Assessment Guide

Data Categories	*Guideline Questions*
I. Cultural	
A. Ethnic origin	A. Does the person identify with a particular ethnic group (*i.e.*, Puerto Rican, African, *etc.*)?
B. Race	B. What is the person's racial background (*i.e.*, Black, Filipino, Native American, *etc.*)?
C. Place of birth	C. Where is the person's birthplace?
D. Relocations	D. Where has he lived (city, country)? In what year did the person live there, and for how long?
E. Habits, customs, values, and beliefs	E. Describe habits, customs, values, and beliefs the person holds or practices which affect his attitudes toward birth, life, death, health and illness, time orientation, and health-care system and health providers. What is the degree of belief and adherence by the person to overall cultural system?
F. Behaviors valued by the culture	F. How does the person value privacy, courtesy, respect for elders, behaviors related to family roles and sex roles, and work ethic?
G. Cultural sanctions and restrictions	G. *Sanctions*—What is accepted behavior by the person's cultural group regarding expression of emotions and feelings, religious expressions, and response to illness and death?
	Restrictions—Does the person have any restrictions related to sexual matters, exposure of body parts, certain types of surgery (*i.e.*, hysterectomy), discussing dead relatives, and fears related to the unknown?
H. Language and communication processes	H. What are some overall cultural characteristics of the person's language and communication process?
1. Language(s) and/or dialects spoken	1. Which language(s) and/or dialects does the person speak most frequently? Where? At home or at work?
2. Language barriers	2. Which language does the person predominantly use in thinking? Does the person have a need for bilingual interpreter in nurse–patient interactions? Is the person non-English speaking or limited English speaking person? Is the person able to read and/or write in English?
3. Communication process	3. What are the rules (linguistics) and modes (style) of communication process (*i.e.*, "honorific" concept of showing "respect or deference" to others using words only common to specific ethnic/cultural group)?
	Is there a need for variation in techniques of communicating and interviewing to accommodate this person's cultural background (*i.e.*, tempo of conversation, eye and body contact, topic restrictions, norms of confidentiality, and style of explanation)?
	Are there any conflicts in verbal and nonverbal interactions between the person and the nurse?

Data Categories	*Guideline Questions*
	How does this person's nonverbal communication process compare with other ethnic cultural groups and what is its impact on responding to nursing and medical care?
	Are there any variations between the person's interracial communication process or intracultural and intraracial communication process (*i.e.,* ethnic patient and dominant culture nurse, ethnic patient and ethnic nurse; beliefs, attitudes, values, role variations, stereotyping [perception and prejudice])?
I. Family influence on health–illness process	I. Does the person's family feel a need for continuous presence in patient's clinical setting (*i.e.,* is this an ethnic/cultural characteristic)? How is family valued during illness/death?
	How does the family participate in the person's nursing care process (*i.e.,* giving baths, feeding, use of "touch" as support [cultural meaning], just mainly supportive presence)?
	How does ethnic/cultural family structure influence the person's response to health/illness (*i.e.,* roles, beliefs, strength, weaknesses, and social class)?
	Are there any key family roles characteristic of a specific ethnic/cultural group (*i.e.,* grandmother in Black and some Native American families); and can these key persons be a resource for health personnel?
	What role does family play in health promotion or cause of illness (*i.e.,* would family be intermediary group in patient interactions with health personnel and making decisions regarding his care)?
J. Healing beliefs and practices	
1. Cultural healing system	1. What cultural healing system does person predominantly adhere to (*i.e.,* Asian healing system, Hispanic curanderismo)? Religious healing system (*i.e.,* Seventh Day Adventist, West African–voodoo, fundamentalist sect, Pentecostal)?
2. Cultural health beliefs	2. Is illness explained by the germ-theory or cause–effect relationship, presence of evil spirits, imbalance between hot and cold (yin and yang in Chinese culture), or disequilibrium between nature and man?
	Is illness viewed as a disruption of daily activities of living and are minor discomforts ignored?
	Is good health related to success, ability to work or fulfill roles, reward from God, or balance with nature?
3. Cultural health practices	3. What types of cultural healing practices does person from ethnic/cultural group adhere to (*i.e.,* using healing remedies to cure natural illnesses caused by the external environment, using "massage" to cure "empacho" [a ball of food clinging to stomach wall], wearing talismans or charms for protection against illness)?

(Continued)

**Table 26-2
Bloch's Ethnic/Cultural Assessment Guide** (Continued)

Data Categories	Guideline Questions
4. Cultural healers	4. Does the person rely on cultural healers (*i.e.*, medicine man for Native American, curandero for Hispanic, Chinese herbalist, Hougan [voodoo priest], spiritualist, or minister for black Americans)?
K. Religious beliefs and practices	K. Does the person's religion have a strong impact on how he relates to health–illness influences or outcomes (*i.e.*, death/ chronic illness, cause and effect of illness, or adherence to nursing and medical practices)?
L. Nutrition variables or factors	L. What nutritional variables or factors are influenced by the person's ethnic/cultural background?
1. Characteristics of food preparation and consumption	1. What types of food preferences and restrictions, meaning of foods, style of food preparation and consumption, frequency of eating, and time of eating and utensils are culturally determined for the person? Are there any religious influences on food preparation and consumption?
2. Influences from the external environment	2. What modifications, if any, did the ethnic group the person identifies with have to make in its food practices in the white dominant American society? Are there any adaptations of food customs and beliefs from the rural setting *versus* urban setting?
3. Patient education needs	3. What are some implications for diet planning and teaching the person who adheres to cultural practices concerning foods?
II. Sociological	
A. Economic status	A. Who is the principal wage earner in the family? What is the total annual income (approximate) for the family? What impact does the economic status have on the family's life-style, place of residence, living conditions, and ability to obtain health services?
B. Educational status	B. What is the highest educational level obtained? Does the person's educational background influence his ability to understand how to seek health services, literature on health care, patient teaching experiences, and any written material the person is exposed to in the health-care setting (*i.e.*, admission forms, patient care forms, teaching literature, and lab-test forms)?
	Does the person's educational background cause him to feel inferior or superior to health-care personnel in the health-care setting?
C. Social network	C. What is the person's social network (*i.e.*, kinship, peer, and cultural healing networks), and how does it influence his health–illness status?
D. Supportive institutions in the ethnic/cultural community	D. What influence do ethnic/cultural institutions have on the person receiving health services? Examples of institutions— Organization of Migrant Workers, NAACP, Black Political Caucus, Churches, Schools, Urban League, Community Clinics.

Data Categories	Guideline Questions
E. Institutional racism	E. How does institutional racism in health facilities influence the person's response to receiving health care?
III. Psychological	
A. Self-concept (identity)	A. Does the person show strong racial/cultural identity?
	Any comparisons with other racial/cultural groups or members of the dominant society?
	What factors in the person's development helped to shape his self-concept (*i.e.,* family, peers, society labels, external environment, institutions, racism)?
	How does the person deal with stereotypical behavior from health professionals?
	What is the impact of racism on the person from distinct ethnic/cultural group (*i.e.,* demonstrating social anxiety, non-compliance to health-care process in clinical settings, avoidance of utilizing or participating in health-care institutions)?
	Does ethnic/cultural background have impact on how the person relates to body-image change due to illness or surgery (*i.e.,* importance of appearance and roles in cultural group)?
	Any adherence or identification with ethnic/cultural "group identity" (*i.e.,* peoplehood, solidarity, "we" concept)?
B. Mental and behavioral processes and characteristics of ethnic/cultural group	B. How does the person relate to his external environment in the clinical setting (*i.e.,* fears, stress, and adaptive mechanisms characteristic for a specific ethnic/cultural group)? Any variations based on present life-span development?
	What is the person's ability to relate to persons outside of his ethnic/cultural group?
	Do religious beliefs, sacred practices, and talismans play a role in treatment of disease?
	What is the role of significant religious persons during health–illness (*i.e.,* Black ministers, Catholic, Buddhist, Islamic priests [Moslems, Muslims])?
C. Psychological/cultural response to the stress and discomfort of illness	C. Based on ethnic/cultural background, does patient exhibit any variations in psychological response to pain or physical disability of disease processes?
IV. Biophysical	
(Consideration of norms for different ethnic/cultural groups)	
A. Racial-anatomic characteristics	A. Does the person have any distinct racial characteristics (*i.e.,* skin color, hair texture and color, color of mucous membranes)?
	Note any variations in anatomical characteristics (*i.e.,* body structure [height and weight] more prevalent for ethnic cul-

(Continued)

Table 26-2
Bloch's Ethnic/Cultural Assessment Guide *(Continued)*

Data Categories	*Guideline Questions*
	tural group, skeletal formation [pelvic shape—especially for obstetrical evalution], facial shape and structure [nose, eye shape, facial contour], upper and lower extremities).
	How do the person's racial-anatomic characteristics affect his self-concept and how others relate to him?
	Does variation in racial/anatomic characteristics affect physical evaluations and physical care, skin assessment due to color, and variations in hair care and hygienic practices?
B. Growth and development patterns	B. Are there any distinct growth and development characteristics that vary with the person's ethnic/cultural background (*i.e.,* bone density, fat folds, motor ability)?
	What is the importance of nutritional assessment, neurological and motor assessment, bone deterioration in disease process or injury, evaluation of newborns, evaluation of intellectual status or capacity in relationship to motor/sensory development in children—how does this differ among ethnic/cultural groups?
C. Variations in body system	C. Any variations in body systems for the person of a distinct ethnic/cultural group (*i.e.,* GI disturbance with lactose intolerance in blacks, nutritional intake of cultural foods causing adverse effects in GI and fluid and electrolyte system, and variations in chemical and hematological systems [certain blood types prevalent in certain ethnic groups])?
D. Skin and hair physiology, mucous membranes	D. How does skin color variation influence assessment of skin color changes (*i.e.,* jaundice, cyanosis, ecchymosis, erythema, and their relationship to disease processes)?
	What are methods of assessing skin color changes—comparing variations and similarities among different ethnic groups?
	Note conditions of hypo- and hyperpigmentation (*i.e.,* vitiligo, mongolian spots, albinism, discoloration due to trauma). Why would these be more striking in some ethnic groups?
	Note any skin conditions more prevalent to a distinct ethnic group (*e.g.,* keloids in Blacks).
	Note any correlation between oral and skin pigmentation and its influences on variations in distinct racial groups (*norms* when doing assessment of oral cavity.—*i.e.,* leukoedema is normal occurrence in Blacks).
	Note hair texture, color, and variations among racially different groups (*i.e.,* ask the person about preferred hair care methods, any racial/cultural restrictions [*i.e.,* not washing "hot-combed" hair while in the clinical setting, not cutting very long hair of Hispanics]).
	Note any variations in skin care methods (*i.e.,* using Vaseline on Black skin).

Data Categories	Guideline Questions
E. Diseases more prevalent among ethnic/cultural group and diseases ethnic/cultural group has increased resistance to	E. Are there any specific diseases or conditions which are more prevalent for a specific ethnic/cultural group (*i.e.,* hypertension, sickle-cell anemia, glucose-6-phosphate dehydrogenase alteration or G-6PD, lactose intolerance)?
	Any diseases that the person has increased resistance to because of racial/cultural background (*i.e.,* skin cancer in Blacks)?
	Does the person have any socio-environmental diseases common among ethnic/cultural groups (*i.e.,* lead-paint poisoning, poor nutrition, overcrowding [prone to TB], alcoholism due to psychological despair and alienation by the dominant society, rat bites, poor sanitation)?

After Bloch B: Overview—Bloch's Assessment Tool: Ethnic-Cultural Variations. In Orque MS, Bloch B, Monrroy LA: Ethnic Nursing Care: A Multicultural Approach. St. Louis, CV Mosby, 1982

nurse's ability to use appropriate data collecting skills in assessing ethnic-minority persons.

Nursing Implications

It is important to note that the cultural assessment guide provides nurses with a systematic approach to collecting cultural data for persons in clinical settings. It does not supersede, but should become an essential part of, the numerous nursing assessment formats being used by nurses in both hospital and community health-care settings. It can be adapted to assess the cultural characteristics for any specific ethnic population. The focus is on identifying key cultural aspects influencing a person's health care. Maslow's basic human needs concept is still applicable in finding solutions to ethnic and cultural patient problems, using the nursing process. It assists the nurse to make culturally valid nursing diagnoses relevant to the person.

The cultural assessment guidelines are not static or all inclusive, but are subject to change and reflective of data sources that have proven helpful in assessing cultural groups. The guidelines must accommodate change or growth among racial and cultural groups to maintain current and accurate information.

It is important not to stereotype when assessing, thinking all persons who are members of a specific racial or cultural group adhere to characteristics prevalent among that group. For example, there is "a tendency to attribute generalized and simplified characteristics to a group of people in the form of 'verbal labels' (*i.e.,* lazy, stupid, apathetic)" (Brodwin and Jordan, 1975, p. 43). A person may be on a continuum of being less or more identifiable with their particular cultural group, exhibiting characteristics accordingly. Again time-change, location, family and generational system, and social system have a great impact on how a person exhibits cultural characteristics.

For example, Martin and Martin (1978) discuss the variations among Blacks caused by the effects of urban values *versus* rural values. These authors explain how rural migration to urban areas changed the role of the extended family by eroding extended-family values. Urban values of "individualism, materialism, and secularism" contrasted with the extended family values of a "mutual-aid system." Despite these variations Martin and Martin state that "geographic separation does not mean severing kinship ties; . . . it often strengthens the emotional bond between relatives" (p. 84).

From this discussion the nurse should ask: How can this tool be used in following through with the phases of the nursing process? How can the nurse identify and use any data obtained from an ethnic-minority person to problem solve and provide effective nursing care relative to his cultural background? To answer these questions let us discuss the use of Bloch's Assessment Guide in the nursing process.

Use of Bloch's Guide in the Nursing Process

The following case study describes how Bloch's Guide is used in the assessment phase of the nursing process and suggests potential nursing interventions. Emphasis is on biopsychosociocultural variables in data collection, nursing diagnoses relevant to a person's cultural background, cultural implications in developing patient–client goals, and utilization of cultural resources in planning nursing interventions.

Example □ Mrs. G, a 48-year-old obese Black woman (190 lbs, 5'2") has been admitted to a coronary care unit with hypertension and congestive heart failure. She has lived in a northern city for 3 years since migrating from Mississippi. She lives with her husband, who is presently an unemployed auto factory worker, and four children in the fourth floor of a housing project. She has to cook family meals on a small two-burner hot plate. Thus, most of the foods prepared are boiled or fried. She generally eats "heavy" foods (*i.e.,* pinto beans and ham hocks, fried chicken, collard greens and fried corn cakes, *etc.*) that are highly seasoned with salt, salt pork, or hot sauces. She does heavy work as a domestic cleaning lady. She packs a lunch for work that often consists of "leftovers" from the previous day.

While in the hospital, Mrs. G. does not want to eat prescribed low-fat, low-sodium meals, having her daughter and members of the Pentecostal church bring in her cultural foods. The nurses are upset by this behavior and ask her daughter not to bring foods from home. Mrs. G. becomes angry and very loud, stating, "Who do they think they are not letting me have my food?" Nurses find these outbursts difficult and begin to avoid Mrs. G.

Mrs. G.'s family and church members from their neighborhood Pentecostal church come to "sit up" with her frequently while she is in the hospital. They try to comfort her, saying, "The Lord knows best what needs to be done." "Don't you worry about anything, he'll make it all right. You been a good woman for your family with Mr. G. out of work and all." "Don't you upset yourself; we'll talk to the nurses!" Some of the nurses are apprehensive about being approached by large numbers of the church people, thinking they felt the same way Mrs. G. does about her diet. □

Assessment

Using Bloch's Ethnic/Cultural Assessment Guide, the nurse should ask the following question in assessing Mrs. G.: What data categories are applicable in this example? A review of the data set reveals the following:

*   *Cultural data*—Black racial background. Religious impact on cause–effect relationship towards health–illness. Conflicts in communication process with nurses. Has strong preference for cultural foods in consumption and preparation. Strong family and religious support system.
*   *Sociological data*—Some evidence of economic stress on family with husband unemployed, patient who is main source of income now hospitalized, living conditions seem difficult (*i.e.,* using hot plate for cooking indicates difficulty in supporting cost of obtaining cooking stove or paying for gas). Living in low-income housing.
*   *Psychological data*—Strong ethnic/cultural identity, especially the "we" concept (characteristics of Black culture) in which family and church members are heavily involved with patient's welfare. Becomes loud and belligerent when her needs as she perceives them are thwarted by the nursing staff.
*   *Biophysical data*—Obese, complains of shortness of breath and dizziness. Mrs. G. has dark pigmented black skin, and dark-pigmented oral cavity mucous membranes, and her hair is short, black, and wooly in texture. Studies show hypertension has a high prevalence among Black persons.

Nursing Diagnoses

Based on the analysis of the above data, what are some nursing diagnoses? Some examples might be as follows:

*   Cultural variance with nursing staff related to ethnic person's preferences for certain foods.
*   Difficulty in communication process between patient and nurse due to cultural style.
*   Anxiety and stress due to nursing response to patient's cultural behavior in the clinical setting.

Goals and Objectives

What are some examples of goals and objectives in the planning phase of nursing process that consider the cultural implications of this situation? Such goals and objectives might include these:

*   Mrs. G.'s anxiety level and stressful situations will decrease in the clinical setting.
*   Mrs. G. will demonstrate increased knowledge of the relationship of her physical condition to her cultural diet preference.
*   Mrs. G. will describe diet preferences and incorporate these into her diet plan.
*   Mrs. G. will utilize support systems as a therapeutic measure (*i.e.,* the family, minister, church members).

Nursing Interventions

What are some examples of nursing interventions that demonstrate use of cultural variables? The following examples demonstrate a range of possibilities:

- Ask Mrs. G. what her perception is of her physical condition and the relationship to diet (*i.e.*, consider Pentecostal religious orientation).

- Do not retreat from Mrs. G.'s expressions of anger. Spend time explaining the reasons for diet restrictions for cardiac patients.

- Consult the hospital dietitian about patient's cultural food preferences and style of preparation to develop a diet plan considering cultural foods if appropriate (*i.e.*, using lemon juice instead of salt for seasoning collard greens or salt substitutes if applicable).

- Utilize family and church members in patient care activities (*i.e.*, diet planning and teaching, follow-up diet plans for home considering economic resources).

- Make referrals to appropriate social services about the economic situation and implications for discharge home (*i.e.*, patient as main source of family income; ways to remedy this considering her cardiac status).

Evaluation

Nurses evaluate and look at their own behavior (*i.e.*, attitudes, values, perceptions, etc.) and how a person from a different ethnic/cultural background views that behavior and its effects on providing effective nursing care to ethnic persons. The evaluation process is continuous as you collect data and formulate approaches to problem solving with the ethnic person and family. Validation is received from the direct and genuine feedback from the ethnic person and his family that his needs are being met. Nurses also observe positive changes in the person's condition or behavior. Nurses will want to ask themselves, "Is the nursing approach relevant to the client considering his ethnic/cultural background, and does it contribute to a state of wellness?" The above brief example was described to explain how cultural data can be assessed and incorporated into the nursing process.

Nursing Implications

Finally, the nurse should evaluate personal concerns, fears, and attitudes about using the ethnic/cultural assessment guide. Nurses sometimes wonder why we need such a tool when we try to provide person-centered care for all clients. Many times nurses have stated, "I treat all my patients the same," or, "Why do I need a separate way for assessing these patients?" These responses may represent a means of denying or avoiding the nurse's underlying fears or negative feelings toward others who are racially and culturally different. For example, if the nurse harbors negative feelings toward the necessity of such a tool, this attitude may make it impossible to develop an awareness of the health needs of ethnic-minority persons. Smoyak states, "Tolerance of difference is the key to satisfying, effective, growth-producing nurse/client relationships" (1979, p. 48).

Furthermore, nurses must develop a broad knowledge base of ethnic and cultural data, especially for those ethnic populations in their own working communities. This can be done by obtaining first-hand information from ethnic–cultural communities. It is important that you as nursing students begin to work with this information as early as possible in your curriculum. You will be able to synthesize cultural data more readily if it is included in your patient assessment guides. This reinforces the concept that "everyone" has an ethnic–cultural background.

It should be emphasized that nurses not only collect ethnic and cultural data because they are informative and rich with cultural philosophies but because they facilitate nursing care. Some nurses are amazed at cultural health beliefs and practices but often do not follow through to provide effective nursing care from this knowledge base. Ruffin (1979) supports the development of "health profiles" by a multidisciplinary approach to ethnic and racial health issues. This would synthesize the findings from the fields of social science, medicine, and public health documents. As nurses increasingly see the importance of cultural diversity and its implications for health care, hopefully the health status of ethnic minority groups will improve. This will continue to be a critical issue that will need response by nurses and other health professionals in the coming years.

Conclusion

Both the dominant culture and American ethnic-minority groups have experienced recent and considerable consciousness raising about racial and cultural identity. The major characteristics of culture (*i.e.*, its learned nature, its relative stability, and the patterns present in every culture) were indicated and discussed. Several cultural variables of the person were identified, including ethnic and racial identity, value orientations, language and communication process, and family system. Each was illustrated with examples from within and beyond American society. Healing beliefs and practices, religious beliefs and practices, and nutritional behavior were all discussed in relation to culture. The relationship of cultural variables to sociological, psychological, and biophysical variables was made explicit. A major portion of the chapter considered cultural assessment and the nursing process. Besides citing approaches to cultural assessment found in recent nursing literature, we presented Bloch's Eth-

nic/Cultural Assessment Guide, which synthesizes cultural assessment into nursing process. By highlighting the key aspects of cultural, sociological, psychological, and biophysical data categories, the Guide provides a systematic approach to collecting cultural data. In addition to the data categories, guideline questions were provided within the tool. A case study was included to demonstrate utilization of cultural assessment in the nursing process. Throughout this chapter the effects of nurses' values, beliefs, and practices on persons who are culturally different were emphasized.

Study Questions

1. Describe several ways in which nurses might obtain first-hand information from ethnic communities in their local area.

2. Person-centered nursing recognizes the importance of cultural variables but gives emphasis to the person as an individual. Explain how this approach helps to avoid inaccurate generalizations about cultural differences.

3. How can the nurse intervene if clients's cultural beliefs about physical symptoms are different from nursing beliefs about physical illness?

4. How can the nurse intervene if cultural healing practices conflict with traditional scientific methods of curing?

5. Mr. Chin, an Oriental person, has been suffering from high blood pressure but continues to use large amounts of soy sauce (high sodium content) in his diet. What cultural factors must be considered in doing a diet assessment and diet therapy for this patient?

6. A sacred talisman was removed from Mr. Grayhorse, a Native American Indian, prior to surgery. This patient and family members became highly upset. What would be an appropriate intervention by the nurse in this situation?

Glossary

Argot: Language terms with usage limited to a particular group or class.

Communication: A dynamic process whereby human behavior, both verbal and nonverbal, is perceived and responded to.

Culture: A system of symbols shared by a group of humans and transmitted by them to upcoming generations; also a group design for living, *i.e.*, goals, attitudes, roles, and values.

Cultural healing beliefs: Beliefs that reflect a specific cultural group's orientation to health and illness.

Cultural shock: Profound disorientation experienced by a person who has been thrust into an alien culture without sufficient preparation.

Ethnicity: A group's affiliation due to shared linguistic, racial, religious, and cultural background.

Intercultural communication: Communication that occurs whenever a message producer is a member of one culture and a message receiver is a member of another.

Interracial communication: Communication between whites and nonwhites in American society with nonwhites occupying a marginal position.

Matrilineal: Cultural descent of the family determined through the female.

Patrilineal: Cultural descent of the family determined through the male.

Spiritualists: Persons of either gender "called" by God for healing incurable diseases and solving emotional or personal problems.

Values: Intrinsic beliefs about the worth of an entity or concept.

Bibliography

Allport GW: The Nature of Prejudice. New York, Doubleday Anchor, 1958

American Nurses Association: Code for Nurses with Interpretive Statements. Kansas City, MO, ANA, 1976

Bauwens EE: The Anthropology of Health. St Louis, CV Mosby, 1978

Bloch B: Nursing intervention in black patient care. In Luckraft D (ed): Black Awareness: Implications for Black Patient Care, pp 27–35. New York, American Journal of Nursing, 1976

Branch MP, Paxton PP: Providing Safe Nursing Care for Ethnic People of Color. New York, Appleton-Century-Crofts, 1976

Brinton DM: Value difference between nurses and low income families. Nurs Res 21:46–52, January–February, 1972

Brodwin MC, Jordan JE: Racial prejudice related to race labelling, language, and the tripartite classification of attitude. Psychology 12:48–59, November, 1975

Bullough B, Bullough VL: Poverty, Ethnic Identity and Health Care. New York, Appleton-Century-Crofts, 1972

Campbell T, Chang B: Health care of the Chinese in America. Nurs Outlook 21:245–249, April, 1973

Chung HJ: Understanding the Oriental maternity patient. Nurs Clin North Am 12:67–75, March, 1977

Davitz LJ, Sameshima Y, Davitz J: Suffering as viewed in six different cultures. Am J Nurs 76:1296–1297, September, 1976

DeGarcia RT: Cultural influences on Filipino patients. Am J Nurs 79:1412–1414, August, 1979

Downs JF: Cultures in Crisis, 2nd ed. Beverly Hills, Glencoe Press, 1975

Folb EA: A Comparative Study of Urban Black Argot, Occasional Papers in Linguistics, No. 1, pp 10–11. Los Angeles, University of California, 1972

Frances GM, Munjas BD: Manual of Social Psychologic Assessment. New York, Appleton-Century-Crofts, 1976

Freebairn J, Gwinup K: Cultural Diversity and Nursing Practice (Instructor's Manual). Irvine, CA, Concept Media, 1979

Garine I: The social and cultural background of food habits in developing countries (traditional societies). Nutr Newsletter 8:9, January–March, 1970

Hein EC: Communication in Nursing Practice, 2nd ed. Boston, Little, Brown & Co, 1980

Hirabayashi JN: The quiet American? A re-evaluation. Amerasia Journal 3, No. 1:114–127, 1975

Holland WR: Mexican American medical beliefs: Science or magic? In Martinez RA (ed): Hispanic Culture and Health Care (Fact, Fiction, Folklore). St Louis, CV Mosby Co, 1978

Irvine J: On not being upper-class. N Engl J Med 282:453, 1970

Jones JM: Prejudice and Racism. Reading, MA, Addison-Wesley, 1972

Kluckholn FR, Strodtbeck FL: Variations in Value Orientations. Evanston, IL, Row, Peterson & Co, 1961

Kosa J, Zola I (eds): Poverty and Health: A Sociological Analysis. Cambridge, MA, University of Harvard Press, 1975

LaMonica EL: The Nursing Process, A Humanistic Approach. Reading, MA, Addison-Wesley, 1979

Lee D: Cultural factors in dietary choice. Am J Clin Nutr 5, No. 2:166–170, March-April, 1957

Malina RM: Skinfolds in American negro and white children. J of the American Dietetic Association 59:34–40, July 1971

Marriner A: The Nursing Process (A Scientific Approach to Nursing Care). St Louis, CV Mosby Co, 1979, 2nd ed

Martin EP, Martin JM: The Black-Extended Family. Chicago, University of Chicago Press, 1978

Moore LG, Van Arsdale PW, Glittenberg JE, Aldrich RA: The Biocultural Basis of Health. St Louis, CV Mosby Co, 1980

Murray RB, Zentner JP: Nursing Concepts for Health Promotion, 2nd ed. Englewood Cliffs, NJ, Prentice-Hall, Inc, 1979

National League for Nursing, Department of Baccalaureate and Higher Degree Programs: Criteria for the Appraisal of Baccalaureate and Higher Degree Programs in Nursing. Publication No. 15-1251, 4th ed, New York, 1977

Niehoff A: Changing food habits. J Nutrition Education 1, No. 1:10–11, Summer, 1969

Otto H: What is a strong family? Marriage and Family Living 24:72–80, 1962

Overfield T: Biological variations. Nurs Clin North Am 12, No. 1:19–26, March, 1977

Piero P: Black-white crisis. Am J Nurs 74:280–281, February, 1974

Primeaux M: Caring for the American Indian patient. Am J Nurs 77, No. 1:91–96, January, 1977

Pumphrey JB: Recognizing your patient's spiritual needs. Nursing '77 7, No. 12:64–70, December 1977

Rich AL: Interracial Communication. New York, Harper & Row, 1974

Rook A: Introduction to the Biology of the Skin, Philadelphia, FA Davis Co, 1970

Ruffin JE: Changing Perspectives on Ethnicity and Health, A Strategy for Change. Kansas City, MO, American Nurses Association, 1979, pp. 1–45

Safilios-Rothschild C: Trends in the family: A cross-cultural perspective. Child Today 7:38–45, March–April, 1978

Samovar LA, Porter RE (eds): Intercultural Communication: A Reader, 2nd ed. Belmont, CA, Wadsworth Publishing Co, Inc, 1976

Saunders L: Cultural Difference and Medical Care: The Case of the Spanish Speaking People of the Southwest. New York, Russell Sage Foundation, 1954

Schubin S: Nursing patients from different cultures. Nursing '80 10, No. 6:78–81, June 1980

Scott CS: Health and healing practices among five ethnic groups in Miami, Florida. Public Health Reports 89, No. 6:524–532, 1974

Smith WD, Burlew AK, Mosley MH, Whitney WM: Minority Issues in Mental Health. Reading, MA, Addison, Wesley Publishing Co, 1978

Smoyak SA: Nurse and Client Ethnicity and its Effects Upon Interaction, A Strategy for Change. Kansas City, MO, American Nurses Association, 1979, pp. 46–71

Snow LF: Folk medical beliefs and their implications for care of patients (A review based on studies among black Americans). Annals of Internal Medicine 81, No. 1:82–96, July 1974

Snow LF: Popular medicine in a black neighborhood. In Spicer EH (ed): Ethnic Medicine in the Southwest, 2nd ed, pp 19–95. Tucson, University of Arizona Press, 1979

Spector RE: Cultural Diversity in Health and Illness. New York, Appleton-Century-Crofts, 1979

Spicer EH (ed): Ethnic Medicine in the Southwest, 2nd ed. Tucson, AZ, The University of Arizona Press, 1979

Staples R: Introduction to Black Sociology. New York, McGraw-Hill Book Co, 1976

Sutterley DC, Donnelly GF: Perspectives in Human Development- (Nursing Throughout the Life Cycle). Philadelphia, JB Lippincott Co, 1973

Unger R, Raymond B: External criteria as predictors of values: The importance of race and attire. J Soc Psychol 93:295–296, August, 1974

Watts W: Social class, ethnic background, and patient care. Nursing Forum 6, No. 2:155–162, Spring 1967

Werner EE: Cross-Cultural Child Development: A View from the Planet Earth. Monterey, CA, Brooks/Cole Publishing Co, 1979

White EH: Giving health care to minority patients. Nurs Clin North Am 12, No. 1:27–40, March 1977

Yura H, Walsh MB: The Nursing Process: Assessing, Planning, Implementing, Evaluation. New York, Appleton-Century-Crofts, 1978

Sexuality

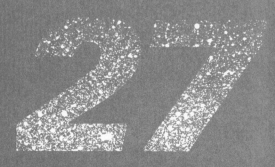

Margaret A. Banning

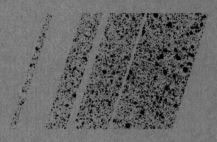

27

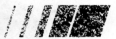

This chapter examines the intricate relationship of an individual's body image, self-concept, and self-esteem as they relate to sexuality. It explores the development of body image and sexuality throughout an individual's life span. The effect of culture on our sexual values, as well as what we feel to be normal, right, and attractive, is presented. This will assist the reader to see how disease, injury, hospitalization, or surgery can threaten one's self-concept and feelings of being a sexual person. The chapter also explores how people express these feelings. The nurse's role in assessment and counseling, including communication and teaching, is described.

After completing this chapter, students will be able to:

● *Describe the development of sexuality throughout the life span.*

● *Recognize threats to body image and feelings of sexuality.*

● *Describe acting out behavior and what it may mean.*

● *Assess sexuality during person assessment as appropriate.*

● *Recognize the need for referral regarding sexual counseling.*

● *Accept sexual values that differ from their own.*

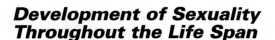

Development of Sexuality Throughout the Life Span

The subtle yet all-encompassing subject of sexuality continuously intrigues and attracts writers and researchers. Literature has been flooded with writings on every aspect of sexuality, yet the subject is still elusive. Researchers find it difficult to draw useful conclusions. What actually makes up an individual's feelings of sexuality? What critical periods or events can threaten our feelings of sexuality, and how might these emotions be expressed?

The subject of sexuality is intimately associated with feelings of self-esteem and feelings of being masculine or feminine.

Definition of Sexuality

Sexuality has been described "as a deep and pervasive aspect of the total personality, the sum total of one's feelings and behavior, not only as a sexual being but as a male or female" (SIECUS, 1970, p. 3). Individuals need to feel secure in their own sexuality because it may greatly affect their feelings of self-worth. It is also important to distinguish between sex, sex acts, and sexuality. A critical role is played by sex hormones during prenatal life. A child is born with certain sexual capacities already present, which visually affirm the child's sex for the parents. Sex acts, or behavior involving secondary erogenous zones and genitalia, are just one part of sexuality. Sexuality is being a man, being a woman, being attractive, being sensual (Griggs, 1978).

Sexuality, as one of the determinants of body image, is only part of the complete self-concept. Our self-concept or ego identity includes beliefs, values, goals, as well as the way others see us, our perception of our physical shape or appearance, what we feel about ourselves as persons, our perceptions of our functions, our moods, social status, the profession we choose or do not choose, and our ability to be mobile and independent in society (McCloskey, 1976). Let us explore the development of these feelings throughout an individual's maturation and life span.

Infancy

Hormonal Influences

Endocrine studies have confirmed the critical role played by hormones during prenatal life. These hormones are essential for the differentiation of sexual organs but may also be responsible for "programming" the brain during fetal development for a later display of either masculine or feminine behavior (Sutterley and Donnelly, 1973). These hormonal effects may facilitate adaptation to the definitions of masculine or feminine behavior taught by one's parents and society. The prenatal influence of hormones may have an organizing effect upon behavior that appears much later in the child's development.

Cultural Influences

The child's development of a sexual identity and role is influenced by many cultural factors and relationships.

The following sections describe sexual stereotyping as it has developed within this culture over the years. Pressure from society to conform to set feminine or masculine behavior can have detrimental effects on a child's optimal development. These effects are covered in greater detail under Sex Role Traits: Sexist *versus* Nonsexist Childrearing.

Cultural influences are seen even before a child is born when parents start guessing and wondering about their child's sex. When the obstetrician announces "It's a boy!" or "It's a girl!", parents immediately begin conveying this information to the child and to the world (Paluszny, 1974). First, they give a name that usually categorizes the child as male or female.

Children learn about sex roles very early in their lives, long before they enter school. They learn these roles through relatively simple patterns: We throw boy babies up in the air and rough-house with them, whereas we handle girls more delicately. We choose sex-related colors and toys for our children and encourage the energy and physical activity of the boys, just as we expect girls to be quieter and more docile. Howe (1972) suggests that although parents protest that they love children of both sexes with equal fervor, yet they are genuinely disappointed without a male heir to continue the family name.

During infancy parents send many subtle and unconscious cues that are directly related to the sex of the child. Studies have shown that mothers who breast feed their children handle boys differently from girls. Boys are given more autonomy and are allowed to assert themselves in deciding how much they want. Conformity is stressed with baby girls. The nursing mothers hover over them and encourage them to feed in a more established manner (Paluszny, 1974). Further studies also indicate that mothers touch, talk to, and handle girls more than boys. Later studies found that the girls then touched and talked to their mothers more than the boys did. The boys at 13 months were more aggressive and assertive with their toys. When confronted with a barrier, the girls would cry, but the boys would try to remove it (Goldberg and Lewis, 1969).

Childhood

Toddler

Children, by the end of their first year, discover their genitals just as they discover their fingers and toes. This wholesome curiosity causes the child to explore and handle himself. During toilet training, toddlers may explore their genitals for several seconds at a time. This will not start a masturbation habit, and children need not be distracted. Spock (1976) suggests it is better not to give children the idea that they are bad or their genitals are bad. Rather, help

children to have wholesome, natural feelings about their entire body.

Preschooler

Sex Play

The preschooler (3–6 years of age) begins to develop either a sense of initiative or a sense of guilt. There is an emergence of sexual curiosity and identification with parental models. The child consciously and unconsciously tries to pattern self after the masculine or feminine models provided by the parents. At this age many children discover that touching and manipulating the genitals releases tension and provides pleasurable sensations. The genitals may become a cause for conflict because they supply uniquely pleasant sensations but also may involve the anticipation of punishment and anxiety. This may result in body image distortion of the genital area (Blaesing and Brockhaus, 1972). In our culture curiosity about the genitals may bring punishment and hence anxiety and guilt. Nurses can be helpful in counseling parents that masturbation or sex play is normal and does not cause physical or psychological harm.

Children have learned by age 2½ or 3 which toys "belong" to each sex and which tools, appliances, and activities belong to their mommies or their daddies. In nursery school, boys who cross the sex line to play with dolls, kitchen toys, or dress-up clothes are highly criticized, and girls who choose traditionally stereotyped masculine activities such as toy trucks, blocks, or hammers may be ignored by their peers (Fagot, 1977). By age 3 to 5 years, children have already decided that certain job options will be closed to them. In one survey, when asked, "What would you like to be when you grow up?" the boys mentioned such occupations as policeman, father/husband, dentist, astronaut, truck driver, engineer, baseball player, and doctor. Girls mentioned mother/sister, nurse, ballerina, teacher, babysitter, princess, ice-skater, and baton-twirler (Papalia and Tennent, 1975).

If asked to choose occupations for the opposite sex, boys were shocked at the very idea of being a girl. "Most had never thought of it before, some refused to think about it, and one put his hands over his head and sighed, 'Oh, if I were a girl I'd have to grow up to be nothing.' " Girls were ready with their answers, saying the other sex occupations were their true ambitions . . . "But I'll never do it because I'm not a boy" (Pogrebin, 1980, p. 35).

Children attending kindergarten feel that males are more powerful, fearless, competent, and aggressive than females. Later in their development boys say that "adult men need to make decisions, protect women and children in emergencies ... fix things, support their families ... and control the money more than women do" (Pogrebin, 1980, p. 36).

Children of age 3, 4, and 5 cling to their favorite grownups, lean against them, and are physically affectionate. They like to play doctor, to see and touch each other's bodies. The nurse can help parents realize that this interest is a natural part of growing up. As long as the child has plenty of other interests there is no cause for concern. Excessive self-handling sometimes occurs in girls because they fear something has happened to make them different from boys. Simple reassurance and explanation is all that may be needed. Excessive genital handling can occur at any age as a sign of tension and worry. A nervous child worried that an ill parent is going to die may absentmindedly handle his genitals. Spock (1976) believes that if parents are uncomfortable about a child's behavior, the child recognizes this and experiences uneasiness. Parents should take a stand that is comfortable for them and may matter-of-factly tell their child to do the activity in private. Being matter-of-fact and nonjudgmental is the key.

Sex Role Traits: Sexist versus Nonsexist Childrearing

Parents who were studied by Blaesing and Brockhaus in 1972 varied somewhat in their attitudes about which traits were appropriate for one sex or the other.

> In general, muscular build, overt physical aggression, dominance, competence at athletics, competitiveness, and independence are generally regarded in our culture as desirable for boys. On the other hand, dependence, passivity, inhibition of physical aggression, competence at language skills, politeness, social poise, and neatness are some of the characteristics seen as more appropriate for girls (pp. 600–601).

Nonsexist childrearing enables each child to be all that he or she can be and communicates the message "you may" rather than "you must." With freedom of exploration and an "anyone-can-do-anything" spirit, children are free to discover their own boundaries (Pogrebin, 1980, p. 28). Nurses can be instrumental in educating parents to be flexible role models. Current literature is rich with suggestions on ways to meet this objective. Parents erroneously fear that allowing boys to do so-called feminine things or allowing girls to be aggressive or sportsminded may cause homosexual development. Yet, research demonstrates that sex roles do not decide

sexual orientation or preference. Being tough, successful, sportsminded, and a "jock" does not prevent a male from being homosexual, nor does being sportsminded and aggressive make a woman a lesbian.

Parents who practice flexible roles demonstrate a wealth of possibilities to their children. Daughters of women who work see themselves as competent and worthwhile; they have high career aspirations and see male–female roles as less distinct. An egalitarian marriage gets fathers into the home and mothers out of it. This demystifies child care as something only women have the instincts to do. It gives children "two exciting, patient, recharged parents, instead of one rarely seen stunt man and one omnipresent old shoe" (Pogrebin, 1980, p. 170).

Parents and health professionals also need to observe children while they play, because this is an area too important to be ignored. During play, children rehearse adult roles and relationships. Parents may need to intervene to promote the widest variety of play experiences. Buying nonsexist toys, encouraging sports for both sexes, and firmly challenging sexist comments are all important. Comments like, "You're a sissy," "Act like a boy," Act like a girl," and, "Who wears the pants in the family?" reinforce inappropriate sex stereotyping. Supporting flexible roles for parents and encouraging nonsexist play for children are only a few of the nursing interventions that promote optimal sexual development.

School Age

Stereotypical patterns are again reinforced for the school-age child (6–12 years of age). School textbooks describe boys making things, earning money, doing physical activities, and playing marbles while girls are cooking, sewing, buying things, and babysitting. Boys are concerned about their masculinity and avoid anything "girlish" or "sissy." Girls at this age, however, may be tomboys and play rougher games.

It is important at this point to speculate about what happens to the child who has characteristics that do not fit the norm or the child who identifies with the opposite sex? Confusion, insecurity, and conflict may arise. The stereotypical male values of being aggressive, independent, unemotional, ambitious, self-confident, and direct may conflict with stereotypical female values of being tactful, gentle, aware of the feelings of others, passive, quiet, conforming, and of having a strong need for security (Howe, 1972). Today's working woman may feel ambitious and independent yet find conflicts with her childhood upbringing that lead to feelings of insecurity, sex-role conflict, and confusion.

Adolescence

Body Image Changes

Physical growth occurs rapidly during the adolescent period, and the changes become evident to both the adolescent and those around him. The adolescent cannot easily deny growth and is thus forced to change body image. The adolescent becomes very conscious of appearance and body contour and judges his body in terms of its usefulness. "Success in using one's body is important because it contributes to the value one places upon oneself" (Dempsey, 1972, p. 610). The adolescent who feels awkward in using the physical body may be handicapped in pursuing certain chosen activities like sports. This may lead to feelings of insecurity and conflict.

A major aspect of physical maturity that occurs at this time is the growth and development of the reproductive organs and secondary sex characteristics. For girls, **menarche** marks the transition to physical maturity. The adolescent is filled with an almost sudden interest in clothes, hair, and complexion. Adolescence is a "time of peer comparison and contrast. One teenage girl's larger than average bust size becomes the envy of less endowed girls. Likewise, the deepening voice and facial hair of one boy may become the focus of attention or envy of other boys" (Roberts, 1978, pp. 273–74). The value placed by society on certain bodily traits is used by the adolescent to judge the self and whether he measures up to the ideal. The response of others contributes to feelings of high or low self-esteem.

Peer Pressure

Adolescence is a turbulent period with many peer pressures (Fig. 27-1). Peer groups set standards of acceptibility and may not accept an individual whose appearance or behavior is deviant. The literature refers to the "teenage sexual revolution" or the "new morality." Increased freedom comes with adolescence, and with it comes a sometimes unwelcome sense of peer pressure to take advantage of that freedom. Comments such as, "My virginity was such a burden to me that I just went out to get rid of it" reflect these pressures (Time, 1972). Peer pressure to have sexual relationships, as well as other social conditions, has led to an epidemic of teenage pregnancies. In the United States more than a million 15- to 19-year-olds and approximately 30,000 more who are younger than 15 become pregnant each year (Dorin, 1978, p. 50). In some instances, perhaps family deterioration leads to unsatisfied basic needs for love and safety among teenagers. This often may lead to sexual activity as much or more than peer pressure.

Psychological Needs

Some adolescents have a desperate need to feel loved and special. The state of pregnancy may help a girl feel pampered and unique. She may see pregnancy either as a way of remaining dependent on others, or, conversely, as a step toward adulthood. Depression may cause teenagers to try both sex and drugs as a temporary way of "feeling good." Others may use drugs or alcohol to avoid the pressure of a sexual

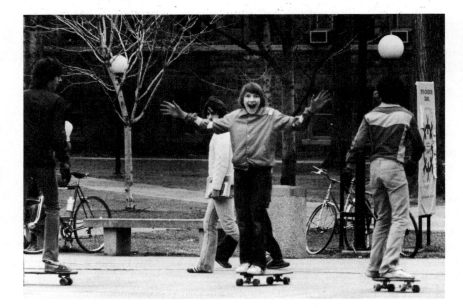

Figure 27-1
Conforming to peer behavior is an important characteristic of adolescence. *(Photo by Bob Kalmbach)*

relationship. Ignorance about birth control in spite of apparent sophistication is also an important factor.

Venereal Disease

The increase in youthful sex has been accompanied by a rising incidence of venereal disease. This is reaching epidemic proportions in high schools and colleges. Outside of the ordinary cold, syphilis and gonorrhea have become the most common infectious diseases among young people, with more cases than hepatitis, measles, tuberculosis, mumps, scarlet fever, and strep throat combined. Studies done in the 1970s show at least 3000 cases of syphilis and 150,000 cases of gonorrhea among the 27 million U.S. teenagers. During the 10 years from 1960 to 1970, the number of reported VD cases in girls from 16 to 19 increased 144%. Since three out of four cases go unreported, we must realize that these statistics do not tell the entire story (Time, 1972, p. 34).

Transitional Stress

The adolescent is faced with many decisions, such as the selection of a career, the separation from parents, and the ability to form close intimate relationships. He strives to become an adult emotionally as well as physically and to face the normal task of becoming independent and separating from parents. As a result, the adolescent is subject to feelings of loss, loneliness, and periods of confusion. His behavior may seem unusual or even irrational; he may be changeable and moody. "Flooded with new feelings and urges, the adolescent struggles painfully and uncertainly with the issue of dependence versus independence as slow steps are taken away from parents towards adulthood" (Dorin, 1978, p. 49). This move away from parents makes it necessary for the teenager to control his own behavior without dependence on parental guidance.

Support Systems

From the preceding discussion it is evident that support systems are crucial during this period. The early adolescent is physically developed yet psychologically still a child and may lack the emotional maturity necessary to manage sexual relationships. Teenagers are still very uninformed in sexual areas. Adolescents tend to overemphasize their defects and therefore undervalue themselves. Parents, peers, and health professionals can help to reinforce positive aspects of appearance and behavior to the individual. The health professional must be alert to possible depression and assess how the individual is coping with stresses. Suicide ranks as the fourth most frequent cause of death among teenagers (Dorin, 1978, p. 52). The developmental state of adolescence is a normal crisis, marked not only by increased inner conflict but also by a tremendous potential for growth. Nurses must assess the psycho-emotional status of their clients and provide support and education whenever possible.

Adulthood

Young Adult

Developmental Tasks
An adult self-image is a dynamic interrelationship among self-concept, identity, and personality. The young adult (24–45) is expected to be independent from his parents' home and care. He begins to make choices as to a life-style, the importance of work, leisure, marriage, or family. The main tasks at this age are selection of a vocation, obtaining the necessary education or training, and formulating ideas about the selection of a mate or someone with whom to have a close relationship. The following discussion centers on the last of these.

Sexual Values
Murray and Zentner (1979) have described three basic values taken by young adults towards sexuality: **absolutistic, hedonistic,** and **relativistic.** The absolutistic position views sexuality as existing for the sole purpose of reproduction. The hedonistic position considers pleasure and satisfaction to be its focus and pursues each individual's ultimate fulfillment of sexual potential. The relativistic position is the basis of the new morality, which suggests that acts should be judged in relation to their effects on other persons. Nurses need to recognize their own personal values and also that others hold different perspectives.

Sexual Patterns
During adulthood a number of sexual patterns may exist: asexual, autosexual, heterosexual, homosexual, or bisexual.

- **Asexual** is the absence of any sexual activity. Despite the media's emphasis on close intimate relationships, an individual may make a voluntary choice against sexual activity, namely masturbation or intercourse. Some marriage partners have chosen to be asexual although physiologically they are still quite capable of sexual functioning.

- **Autosexuality** is sexual gratification through one's own actions or thoughts. Masturbation and fantasies may be the choice of some individuals or may be the necessity of others, such as the single, the widowed, or prisoners isolated and confined. **Masturbation,** the erotic stimulation of one's own genital organs, commonly resulting in **orgasm,** is normal and necessary for many. It is a means of reducing sexual tension, inducing pleasure or even assessing function. Following disease or surgery it may be a means for the male to reduce fear by determining if there is still erectile function.

- **Heterosexuality** is the manifestation of sexual desire for members of the opposite sex. Although this is the choice most commonly accepted in our culture, other factors may or may not be culturally condoned. For example, whether or not the individuals are married, the number of people participating, the form of stimulation, the ages of the participants, and other factors may be points of disagreement.

- **Homosexuality,** the manifestation of sexual desire or preference towards a member of one's own sex, is accepted in some cultures and not others.

- **Bisexuality** is the anticipation and enjoyment of sexual expression with either sex.

What is "normal" is not the same for all persons or for all cultures or societies. It is important to consider normal sexual activity as an individual choice as long as it is acceptable to those adults involved and does no harm to participants or nonparticipants. There are tremendous variables within what can be seen as the normal range of sexual behavior. The degree of commitment and permanence in homosexual relationships can be equal to that in heterosexual relationships. It is a matter of choice whom one values for a warm, loving, and sexual relationship. The means of sexual gratification in any relationship is as varied as the creativity and innovation of the individuals involved. The full enjoyment and pleasure of a sexual relationship comes from the mutual growth occurring with the love and respect of the persons involved.

Sexual Abuse

Any sexual experience that involves physical or emotional abuse, such as rape, sexual abuse of a child, violence of any kind, or masochistic tendencies, is unacceptable. Sexual abuse within the family has become a growing problem, and research indicates that the father, a male relative, or boyfriend of the mother is the most common abuser. These individuals need extensive counseling and assistance in working through these tendencies. They greatly need the nurse's support but must be directed to trained and experienced professionals in the area of sexual counseling. Exploiting children by using them as subjects in pornography is big business which feeds on the "mental aberrations of buyers, viewers and producers" (Monea, 1979, p. 152). The Senate has now passed a bill to stop the sale, distribution, and production of any pornographic materials in which children are used. This type of exploitation must be reported.

Middle Adult

The developmental crisis of the middle adult (45–65) has been discussed by Erikson as generativity *versus* self-absorption and stagnation. "Generativity is a concern about providing for others that is equal to the concern of providing for the self" (Murray and Zentner, 1979, p. 341). The individual has a sense of feeling needed and important to the welfare of others.

Body Image Changes

The middle-aged adult faces a gradual aging of the physical body. Most middle-aged adults are victimized by sexual stereotypes. Western society tends to equate sexual desire and potency with bodily beauty and physique. The advertising media plays a major role in perpetuating the myth that one is sexually active only if physically attractive. "Bombarded daily with these messages, it is little wonder that the middle-aged adult with thickening midriff, partial dentures, thinning hair, and sagging breasts may discount the possibility of offering continuing sexual attractiveness to a 'significant other' " (Dresen, 1977a, p. 127).

The middle-aged adult may face illness or death of loved ones, which creates a fear about his own health and life. Divorce and widowhood may bring about feelings of isolation and abandonment. The adult realizes he looks older and feels he has less stamina and vigor. Youth and vigor are so highly valued in our society that the adult may feel depressed, irritable, and anxious about masculinity or feminity. Both men and women who suffer low self-esteem and are unable to accept a changing body may try cosmetics, new fashions and hair styles, and new young fads in the hope of attaining the physical attributes of youth. "The person tries to regain a youthful figure and face, perhaps through surgery; tints the hair to cover the signs of gray; and turns to hormone creams to restore the skin" (Murray and Zentner, 1979, p. 344). Most individuals, given time, will adjust to their changing bodies and accept these changes as part of maturity.

Menopause

Menopause, or the cessation of the menses, is a normal physiological event that occurs for women during the middle adult years. There is a permanent atrophy of the ovaries, accompanied by a decline in estrogen and progesterone production. Other physical changes may occur: the skin becomes thinner and loses its elasticity, wrinkles may begin to appear, the breasts may become turgid and tender, the nipples may lose their erectile character, and the buttocks and breasts may sag and droop. The vaginal epithelium has decreasing vascularity and eventually becomes pale and dry (Diekelmann, 1977). Consider the threats that may occur with these changes to a woman's feelings of being sensuous or attractive.

Women need to be educated that these changes are normal and that certain problems which may result from these changes can be avoided if anticipated. Nurses can help dispel the myth that menopause ends a woman's interest and participation in a regular sexual relationship. The function of the ovary has little to do with either libido or orgasm. However, a woman's view of herself as attractive, lovable, or desirable and her feelings of self-esteem can affect her feelings of sexuality and libido. The equivalent to female menopause or what may be termed "male menopause" occurs 20 years later than in the female and is covered in the following section on the older adult.

Older Adult

The older adult (65 years and older), the person in later maturity, is widely discriminated against in terms of his or her sexuality. The myth that at a certain age in life people are "over the hill" or "sexless" is widely believed despite its falseness. This myth of the sexless years may become a self-fulfilling prophecy. The person who continues to experience a strong sexual desire may feel guilty and fear being "oversexed." If, however, the individual fears a loss of sexual functioning, this stress can be so overwhelming that sexual dysfunction actually results.

Psychosocial Needs

A need for close intimate contact with another is built in at birth and does not diminish in intensity throughout maturation and into the later years. This can be the intimate exchange of the mind through thoughts and feelings or it can be the intimate exchange of physical warmth and caring demonstrated by touching, holding, hugging, or intercourse.

It is little wonder, then, that old people, frequently deprived of their mates through having outlived them, separated from family members both in terms of physical and emotional distance as a result of our mobile population with its emphasis on nuclear families, separated from meaningful employment by mandatory retirement, and experiencing increasing dependence because of chronic health problems and reduced income, should have tremendous needs for some expressions of affection and concern from another human being (Dresen, 1977b, p. 190).

Physiological Changes

Some physiological changes in sexual functioning do occur with aging, but sexual needs and interests continue into the later years. The aging process affects changes throughout the body. The sexual system is just one of the areas being affected. There is a general decrease in tone, strength, and elasticity of the tissues accompanied by a lengthening of response time. Just as it takes an older man a little longer to put his foot on the brake, it will also take him longer to have an erection. If he and his partner expect it to take longer and accept it as normal, dysfunction will not result. Unfortunately some persons question both their attractiveness and their ability to excite a partner. Erection for the male may not be as firm as during younger years, just as overall strength has decreased. The physiological changes previously mentioned for women during middle age do not reduce the capacity to achieve orgasm and enjoy sexual relations.

Male Menopause

Research has documented that men undergo a change similar to female menopause. At approximately 20 years of age testosterone levels reach their peak, then begin to drop, reaching a plateau between ages 40 and 60. After 60, testosterone levels again drop until approximately 70, when the levels become so low that they cause a serious decline in libido and sexual capacity, as well as a decline in muscular strength and aggressiveness. At this time, the man may experience hot flashes, periods of profuse sweating, anxiety, depression, and nightmares (Diekelmann, 1977, p. 146). A supportive environment is needed at this time. The man who has depended on sexual prowess to sustain a sense of masculinity may be especially distressed by a slackening ability to perform.

Summary

Body image, self-esteem, sexuality, and one's overall self-concept have now been examined from infancy to later maturity. From infancy we are taught that "being loved and wanted and being able to love and want another person are very desirable attributes and ways of validating one's gender role" (Mass and Katsuranis, 1975, p. 82). We all strive to avoid loneliness and fulfill our intimacy needs. Sexual expression often provides this fulfillment and enhances our self-esteem. Feelings of sexuality are closely related to instilled values, physical traits, interactions or relationships with those around us, and our ability to manipulate and control the environment. The effect of parental upbringing and cultural pressures clearly shapes our beliefs and values. Let us now examine potential threats, such as disease or hospitalization, which can affect an individual's self-concept and feelings of being a sexual or attractive person.

Threats to Body Image and Feelings of Sexuality

During illness, the loss of a sense of intactness, especially as related to body image, can cause great anxiety about the capacity to function sexually; feelings of self-worth and attractiveness to others are threatened at a time when need for intimacy is greatest. Loneliness and isolation add to the psychological stresses of illness. The result is sexual deprivation—loss of an important means of tension reduction at a time when it is most useful and necessary. Illness can so powerfully block normal expressions of feeling that sexual acting out occurs, sometimes in ... socially unacceptable forms, reminding us that our sexuality is a critical component of our expressive life, necessary to general well-being and devastating in its loss (Labby, 1975, p. 103).

The above quotation is an excellent introduction to an important area of emphasis for health professionals. Hospitals, institutions, illness, disease, injury, surgery, medications, and medical equipment have become accepted and expected events to the health professional. Their effect on our clients is frequently overlooked or brushed aside. Their profound effect on an individual's feelings of being normal, attractive, intact, and valued must be assessed, with the nurse playing a vital role in assisting the individual to adapt. The following sections further explain each of these areas.

Threat of Hospitalization or Institutionalization

The ability to control our environment and our appearance is crucial to our self-concept and feelings of self-esteem. Yet, the moment an individual enters a hospital or institution such as a nursing home, he is stripped of both control and privacy. The person is provided with a hospital gown, usually white and held together loosely at the back with small ties. The gown visibly conforms around body contours and leaves almost the entire back exposed. The individual may be examined by several doctors, a nurse, and possibly other health professionals. Ward beds are usually separated by curtains which, if closed completely, provide some visual privacy, but allow conversations, sounds, and odors to pass freely to the outside. The person is also subjected to many intrusive procedures that are frequently viewed and performed by several team members at once. Enemas, suppositories, catherizations, and injections may cause psychological stress and threaten the individual's feelings of being whole or attractive. Dressings and drainage tubes may be perceived as unpleasant or grotesque by the hospitalized person.

With hospitalization, the individual may lose several effective means of coping. At times of high emotional stress there is a need for family and friends as support systems to share concerns, to show support through affection and closeness, and to reaffirm that the person is still valued and special to others. Yet, our hospitalized clients are isolated from family and friends through restricted visiting hours. Even sexual activity or intimacy with one's partner, which provides a usual source of warmth, love, belonging, and security, is compromised when the ill person is hospitalized. Feelings of loneliness and abandonment are intensified. Additionally, physical activity, such as jogging, walking, or tennis, frequently a means of reducing general tension, is not available to the hospitalized person. Indeed he may be on bed rest or otherwise restricted in activity. Disease and illness themselves also threaten an individual's sense of intactness and feelings of sexuality. This is explored in the following section.

Disease and Sexual Alteration

Illness can seriously threaten sexual expression. Chronic diseases, even if stabilized with appropriate treatments and medications, can interfere with sexual activity. As in other conditions in which functional ability is compromised, it is important to focus on the person's remaining strengths. Let us remember that satisfactory expression of the sexual self can take many forms. The nurse who is comfortable with both of these ideas will be sensitive to the person's need for possible interventions. Also as Griggs suggests, "If sexual activity was not or is not a concern of the older person in his earlier or present life, then the nurse should not impose such problems or needs on the individual" (1978, p. 1352).

Illnesses are threatening partly because they interfere with the functional abilities required for activities of daily living, including sexual activity. Sexual intercourse may tax cardiac, respiratory, and mobility functions especially. During intercourse an individual with normal cardiovascular function may have an increased respiratory rate of 40/min (twice normal) and a heart rate of 160 to 180/min (sinus tachycardia). Systolic blood pressure may rise 60 to 80 mm Hg and diastolic pressure 30 to 40 mm Hg above normal resting pressures. However, in hypertensive individuals blood pressures as high as 260/150 have been reported (Labby, 1975, p. 195).

The nurse should remember that the threats of illness are real and imagined, physical and psychological, as the following examples illustrate:

Arthritis. Stiff contracted and painful hip joints may impede or complicate sexual intercourse for the arthritic person; generalized pain and fatigue, as well as steroid treatment, may decrease the person's desire for sexual activity. Progressive disfiguring may lead to feelings of unattractiveness as a sex partner.

Cardiovascular Disease. Cardiovascular disease, including coronary artery disease, hypertension, and myocardial infarctions can also interfere with sexual expression. Persons with cardiac problems often doubt their ability to resume sexual activity. If sexual activity is not discussed in the hospital, these individuals may falsely assume that the physician believes such activity is beyond their abilities (Eliot, 1975).

Sexual intercourse has been viewed as a possible life threat for those with marginally functional cardiovascular systems. However, research has now shown that sudden death during coitus is rare, approximately 1% of all sudden deaths. And, to abstain from sexual intercourse may be more stressful than to participate. Once the person has regained health after an acute episode and can tolerate modest exercise, regular sexual expression is possible. Programs are available to help increase cardiovascular performance and exercise tolerance.

The health professional can help reduce fear about sexual activity and instruct about danger signs such as angina, shortness of breath, a feeling of pressure in the chest, or irregular heart beats. Those

who experience mild angina during intercourse can sometimes take nitroglycerine beforehand. Persons who have had strokes may also fear resumption of sexual activity. Also, a stroke may result in a physical or phychological disability that may change the person's relationship or attractiveness to his or her partner.

Some persons are afraid of fumbling or failing because of changes in mobility, vision, and speech. "Anxious self-watching is not conducive to relaxed natural sexual functioning" (Renshaw, 1975, p. 68). Others feel their paralysis makes them unattractive. Suggestions such as using nonverbal cues, alternative coital positions, and emptying the bladder before sex can be helpful. Explicit communication from the nurse with both partners can greatly affect the couple's relationship.

Chronic Obstructive Pulmonary Disease. Other chronic diseases such as chronic obstructive pulmonary disease (COPD) threaten in more subtle ways. A person with COPD or an individual with bronchial asthma is prone to episodes of difficult breathing. However, when **impotence** is seen in these individuals, Labby (1975) suggests that psychological problems are more apt to be the cause.

Diabetes. Impotence in diabetic men may be as much as two to five times greater than in the general population. There is also evidence of orgasmic dysfunction in females after 5 years of diabetes (Labby, 1975). There is often a psychological component implicated in this condition, too.

Cerebral Palsy. Adults who have cerebral palsy state they received no significant sex education during their childhood development. It is an area that is either ignored or postponed to some nebulous later time (Geiger and Knight, 1975). As children they are greatly deprived in the area of touching and fail to learn ways to express closeness. They are frequently dependent on their families for care, which delays normal adolescent development and prevents socialization with children their own age. Later in life they may become partners of whoever is willing to accept them. Deprived of socialization and education, the knowledge of ways to establish relationships eludes them. Special programs, counseling, and education can teach assertiveness and appropriate social skills.

Mental Retardation. Impaired brain development has been used as an excuse to block individuals from sexual relationships. Historically, some states have prevented retarded persons from marrying and having sexual relationships. Although they may not have the cognitive abilities of an adult, these individuals do have the similar sexual desires and capabilities. However, a deficiency in social skills blocks appropriate expression of their feelings. Simple teaching, visual aids, and classes for parents are potential interventions.

Renal Disease.   Fatigue, lethargy, and listlessness may interfere with sexual desire. Dependence on dialysis machines, staff, and partner that occurs with severe disease may further threaten independence.

Although it should be natural for health professionals to discuss the implications of disease on sexual activity, this is often not so for many reasons. In addition to the fact that interactions may not be conducive to such discussions, health professionals are human beings, too, and have their own problems about sex. Furthermore, they do not always have the answers. Saying it should be natural to discuss sexual difficulties may be an oversimplification of a complex problem. Perhaps as much as anything, both partners need an opportunity to discuss feelings about altered sexual functioning in a supportive environment. Persons whose sexual functioning is altered by disease need to feel that their partners accept or at least understand the change.

Effects of Drugs

Pharmacological agents used to help persons deal with anxiety, stress, and depression can have side-effects which decrease libido or impair sexual responsiveness. Reserpine, the antihypertensive drug, also causes diminished libido and erectile failure. Oral contraceptives have been implicated in causing depression and reduced libido when taken over long periods of time (Watts, 1978). Some antidepressants contribute to impotence.

Alcoholism may decrease erectile function and vaginal blood flow resulting in sexual dysfunction. Physical abuse and alcoholism are closely related, and problems in contraception and pregnancy are more frequent. Heroin users receive other gratification and may not be interested in sexual activity. The effects of marijuana on sexual behavior are conflicting and controversial. Indeed, many pharmacological agents can affect sexual function and threaten an individual's sexual life-style.

Threat of Surgery

Surgery, even when elective and planned in advance, greatly threatens the individual's body image. The altered body part and perhaps the whole body may seem less attractive than before. Persons who expe-

rience a major alteration such as a colostomy, ileostomy, mastectomy, or radical surgery in the pelvic area are forced to alter their body concept and assimilate this change. This may cause such severe anxiety and stress that the individual is actually in crisis. The situation overcomes the person's usual coping mechanisms. There may be grief and mourning over the lost part and its meaning to the individual. The following examples suggest two surgeries that can cause alterations in the self-concept and also in sexual expression.

Stoma Creation

Stomas, such as colostomies and ileostomies, may be viewed as unsightly and odorous. The person may have difficulty looking at the area and participating in its care. He may be worried about sexual attractiveness and wonder whether the area will interfere with intimate relationships. Education and proper guidance on ways to avoid embarrassing situations are crucial.

Mastectomy

Earlier in the discussion about developmental changes, puberty was described as a time of growth and change related to secondary sex characteristics. At this time, the female's breasts become a way of validating her femininity and attractiveness. Mastectomies remove from the woman a body part valued both by her and by those around her. She may find it difficult to assimilate this change while being bombarded daily by pictures of "whole" women in revealing clothes through the media of television and magazines. The support and understanding of a partner can help to reaffirm her feelings of being valued and attractive.

Other Threats to Self-Image

Other alterations of the individual's self-concept can occur with unexpected injury, disfigurement resulting from radical excisions of the face and neck, amputation of an extremity, or hysterectomy. The adult has spent many years developing a certain self-concept and identity. Any loss threatens this identity and self-esteem. It is important to assess the meaning of the loss to the individual because certain body parts may assume more significance to one person than to another.

Psychosocial Response

As a result of changes from disease, surgery, or trauma, the person must go through a reorganization process and assimilate the change. With sexual alteration also, according to Roberts, "Adaptation to alteration in the body's function and structure depends upon the nature of the threat, its significance to the patient, previous and current coping ability, the response from significant others, and the assistance available to the patient and family as changes occur" (Roberts, 1978, p. 278).

Our culture's emphasis on a perfect or whole body may cause anger, discouragement, depression, or despair when we lose what is valued and prized. Anger and hostility may be directed towards the health team, family, and friends. Sexual acting out may occur when the individual tries to reaffirm masculinity or femininity. The role of the nurse in a support system when changes in self-concept occur is explored below.

Acting Out Behavior and What It Really Means

Acting out behavior can be defined as "the expression of certain kinds of unconscious conflicts through behavior although the unconscious impulse is not verbalized or remembered" (Wilson and Kneisel, 1979, p. 811).

- John, a nurse, answers the call-light of Mrs. Adams, a woman who has just had a radical mastectomy. As he bends over to fluff her pillow, she places her hand on his hip, strokes his thigh, and asks, "Do you find me attractive?"

- Mary, a nurse caring for Mr. Thomas who has had a prostatectomy, finds his hand on her chest while she attempts to move him up in bed.

- Peter, who is 19 years old, is being cared for by a student nurse. Peter has been severely injured in an automobile accident and is paralyzed from the waist down. He says, "I would like to sleep with you."

- Sondra, a nurse, enters the male ward to pass out medications. Three of her patients start commenting on her figure and suggest sexual activities.

- Mr. W., an 80-year-old man, hugs his student nurse visitor every time she enters and leaves his house and finally asks, "Why can't we be more than just friends?"

The behavior in all of the preceding situations seems to have a sexual connotation. When a person makes seductive gestures, masturbates in your presence, invites you to have sexual intercourse, uses sexual words, exposes sexual organs, or tries to feel parts of your body, it is difficult to be objective. The behavior seems obviously sexual and may be threatening to your feelings and role. But it is important to look beyond the obvious for the real meaning behind this behavior and assess what the person is actually seeking. This is aptly expressed in the following quote:

A number of other equally valid interpretations can be made of the patient's behavior. He may need someone to show him interest and concern. He may want a simple physical contact, to touch someone and be touched by him as an expression of friendliness and warmth. He may be asking for tenderness and acceptance in one of the few ways he can. He may be trying in some unskilled way to form some relationships with the nurse in order to reduce his isolation and loneliness. He may be trying to communicate something about himself to the nurse. He may be asking for reassurance that he is not repulsive and disliked. He may be acting out sexual fantasies which have little relation to personnel who are with him in the situation at the moment. He may be trying to find out how to manage his body in relation to someone else. He may be trying to get the nurse to notice and attend to him by engaging in behavior he knows will attract her attention and be startling or upsetting to her (Schwartz and Shockley, 1956, pp. 157–158).

Only a small amount of sexual behavior within a hospital or institution is related to a real need for physical or sexual outlets (*i.e.*, genitalia). The majority of individuals are seeking to be recognized. They may feel lonely and abandoned and need affection, intimacy, or validation that they are still attractive, or they may be asking to be loved, cared for, and soothed. We are more likely to accept our clients who seek attention by refusing to take medications or those who are angry and impatient with our care than to accept those who seek attention through sexual advances. This acting out behavior threatens our own sexuality and is seen as a threat to our role. Nurses who are comfortable with their own sexuality are better able to assess behavior and assist the client to channel his feelings and energies in a way that will be rewarding and therapeutic. Krozy (1978) developed a list of general characteristics that a sexually comfortable person might be expected to possess:

- Self-esteem and a positive body image
- Personal resolution of sexual identity and overall sexual adjustment
- Up-to-date factual knowledge

- Ability to speak openly, honestly, and confidently about any aspect of human sexuality
- Ability to accept the sexual preferences and activities of others without feeling personally threatened and without moralizing or becoming judgmental
- Skill in interviewing and using oneself therapeutically—that is, sensitivity to the client's nonverbal communication and the ability to unmask indirect cues
- Knowledge of sociocultural and religious tenets
- Ability to discuss sex with the young, middle-aged, and elderly
- Genuine concern for the individual and family
- Respect for confidentiality (p. 1036)

These characteristics require effort and practice. They are suggested as a goal. Only by being comfortable with our own sexuality can we become competent to deal with a client's concerns and help him understand the meaning of his behavior. Nurses can find ways to show warmth and concern appropriately. Touching a shoulder or hand, taking time to encourage the client to share concerns, just sitting quietly at the bedside, or helping clients with their appearance so they feel attractive and valued, all help to validate to the client his worth and importance.

Response Strategies

Let us now examine ways to handle acting out behavior appropriately as it occurs. It is important to mention that there is no one correct answer. Each of us as individuals will use our own style and personality to develop a comfortable approach. However, there are several general suggestions that might be helpful.

Judging the behavior as wrong, abnormal, immoral, unnatural, or negative is detrimental to the person and the nurse–person relationship. Responses such as, "Don't do that! How could you! You ought to be ashamed of yourself! You should know better!" are inappropriate and can be damaging to your client. The person may be unable to state his concern and might become afraid to hint at it in other ways.

A better approach is to try and look beyond the behavior to identify the underlying need and then respond appropriately. If a person makes you feel uncomfortable by touching a part of your body such as your breast or hip, you can gently remove the hand and then continue to hold it, saying, "It must

be hard for you to be separated from your family for so long." Each situation will be unique and will require a thoughtful response. Refer to the chapter on communication for suggestions of empathic responses or ways to handle anger and other emotions.

If you feel threatened by the client's behavior, your nonverbal response may convey a negative message. You need to be aware of your own emotions and express your feelings to the client. For example, "I am flattered that you want to be close to me, but it makes me feel uncomfortable when you touch me. I care about you, but touching threatens my role as your nurse." Perhaps this response may not be appropriate for you, but it is nonjudgmental and sincere. After the initial response, the nurse would then explore further the client's unmet needs and concerns.

This discussion has mentioned only the person who acts out. Many people do not act out: no jokes, no physical advances, not even questions. They may find it difficult to initiate a conversation related to their feelings of sexuality. The nurse may need to take the lead in discussions. Some persons may not want to discuss their feelings at all, and this should be respected. Many may want to deal with their feelings through discussion with close family members and friends or privately by themselves. Remember that all individuals have a right to their own values and life-style, even if it is quite different from your own. Looking at behavior for unmet needs is one of the most therapeutic interventions you can offer. Because nursing is one of the few professions involved in intimate and bodily care activities for others, clients may feel more comfortable in verbalizing their sexuality concerns.

Assessment and Counseling

The Person Assessment Guide (Appendix A) includes a section on sexuality and sexual health. The outline is meant to serve as a guide to data collection and should be individualized for each client. Not all areas or questions are appropriate for each person. Trust and confidentiality need to be established as a prerequisite to asking questions in intimate areas. Your client may have concerns about finances or urinary function and concerns of a sexual nature as well. The client may have difficulty asking questions in this area; he may be waiting for you to initiate the subject or give him permission to bring up concerns.

Assessment Strategies

After rapport and a meaningful relationship have been established, several approaches can help to ease the discussion of sexual health. At the beginning of the assessment process, clients need to know that you may be asking questions of a personal nature, in order to help plan for their needs. Tell them they need not answer these questions unless they wish to share this information. Their comments are confidential and can help you plan appropriate care.

- Start with the least sensitive topics.
- Use common terminology and avoid medical or professional terms.
- Eye contact, continuous reassurance, and a matter-of-fact approach all help to establish comfort.
- Observe for nonverbal cues.
- Only ask questions in areas in which you plan to help the client.
- Try opening leads suggested in the chapter on communication, such as, "Some women are concerned about their attractiveness to their spouse after mastectomy. What are some of your concerns?"
- Try not to suggest answers, because you may block your client's intended response. If the individual brings up concerns, help him choose alternatives that suit his religious or moral structure.
- Be sure you are not imposing your own values by the questions you ask.

Referral to Sex Counselor

There will be problems that are beyond your area of expertise and knowledge. Only a specially trained counselor is prepared to undertake intensive therapy. As a nurse, your goal is to give your client permission to air concerns and to provide factual information within your knowledge base. When they are beyond your scope, ask your client for permission to refer him or her to another health professional with sexual-counseling expertise.

It is important not to close the topic of conversation if you are uncomfortable or feel it is beyond your level of knowledge. Your nonverbal behavior may show this discomfort. A response such as, "These are important concerns, but I have limited knowledge in this area. I would like to refer you to . . .," or, if you are very uncomfortable, "I have trouble discussing topics of an intimate nature, but I know

it is very important for you to get accurate information. Please let me refer you to. . . ." Take time to consider possible responses that are nonjudgmental and positive, which will keep the topic open.

Health Teaching

Most questions and concerns are health oriented and preventive in nature. The nurse will have an active role in teaching self-breast examination for the female, testicular self-examination for the male, appropriate care of the genitals, contraception, and signs of impending infections. The nurse can also be active in counseling clients after surgery or hospitalization for illness. Detailed description of appropriate techniques for self-examination are available in most outpatient clinics. The nurse actively dispels myths and misinformation. Nursing programs promote a psychosocial approach that helps the nurse to be ready for an energetic role in the area of sexuality and sexual health.

Sexual Counseling of Parents

Nurses can also assume responsibility for counseling parents about sex education.

Sex Education for Young Children

Sex education begins early, whether parents are ready for it or not. We would all like to imagine a comfortable, private conversation while tucking a child into bed for the night. What usually occurs is a loud series of questions in the middle of a grocery store line, a crowded waiting room, or in the living room during a social evening with several guests. Children are learning about the facts of life all through childhood. They watch how parents get along and how men and women interact verbally and physically; they also see examples in books and on television.

Children start to ask "why" questions around age 3. At any age parents should try to answer a question truthfully and as simply as it is asked, clarifying exactly what the child is asking and satisfying curiosity at the appropriate level of understanding (Fig. 27-2). The first question may be embarrassing to the parent, who thinks the child is demanding answers to how intercourse and conception occur. A simple answer might be that the baby grows from a tiny egg that was in the mother all the time. Children learn a little at a time and will come back often until they are sure they have it right.

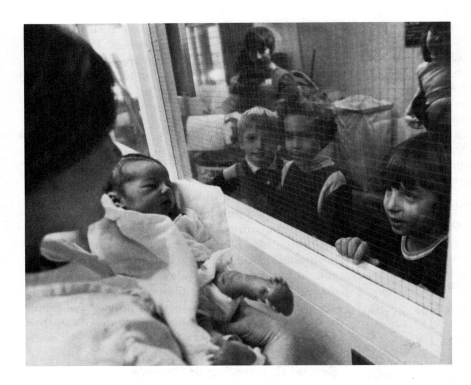

Figure 27-2
Answering preschooler's questions honestly is one means of providing early sex education. *(Photo by Bob Kalmbach)*

Answering the question on the spot is ideal, but if that is impossible, it is good to casually postpone the conversation to a private time. Children who do not receive a truthful answer may later feel uneasy when they hear the truth and also be less likely to ask the parent in the future. Nurses can help parents start answering questions early so they will begin to develop assurance for future questions that demand more exact knowledge.

Sex Education for Adolescents

Talking to an adolescent about sex is not an easy task. Parents may feel from reading articles that if they are wholesome, normal people, they should be able to discuss sex easily with their adolescent children. They may feel inadequate when they find discussions to be difficult. However, girls need to be told at the beginning of puberty what changes to expect, including physical and emotional changes and menstruation. Boys need to be told about the naturalness of erections and nocturnal emissions. One mistake parents make is to concentrate on all the dangerous aspects of sex. Some nervous mothers may make daughters so scared of becoming pregnant that boys become terrifying. Others may stress the possibility of venereal disease.

Adolescents do need to know how pregnancy takes place, what contraceptive methods are available, and how to prevent venereal diseases. Whether this information is given by the parents in the home, the teacher or nurse at school, or the nurse in the clinic, a matter-of-fact, natural, honest approach stressing all that is wholesome and beautiful is the key to counseling.

Conclusion

This chapter has examined the close relationship among one's self-concept, body image, and feelings of sexuality. Children are programmed at an early age into stereotypical feminine and masculine expectations or behavior. Children receive this programming not only at home but also at school, church, through television or anywhere they come in contact with people. The importance of nonsexist childrearing, which allows each child to be all he or she can be, has been emphasized. Stereotypical feminine qualities such as being submissive and dependent are not congruent with being a healthy, assertive, and independent adult. Stereotypical masculine qualities such as competence, control, aggressiveness, and physical prowess can lead to fear of failure, low self-esteem, and difficulty forming close and intimate relationships.

Western society builds up bodily beauty and physique to such an extent that we may never be satisfied with how we look. The media have helped to make our body expectations almost unattainable and also perpetuate sexism in our society. We must all become more active in protesting blatant sexism on the television and video screen.

Western society embraces a wide variety of sexual preferences and alternative life-styles. Some cultures are much more sexually permissive than others. In some countries parents and their children share the same bedroom, and this does not seem to interfere with the child's growth and development. In other cultures there is a variance of views on the subject of homosexuality. It is important that nurses recognize their own personal biases and preferences without imposing this value system on clients. Nurses should help clients find satisfaction within the framework of their subcultures and preferences, recognizing that each individual has a right to a partner of choice, whether of the same or the opposite sex.

It was indicated throughout this chapter that needs for intimacy, closeness, warmth, and sexual expression start early in a child's development and continue throughout the individual's life. Hospitali-zation, illness, disease, surgery, medications, trauma, and advancing age all have potential for threatening each individual's feelings of being an attractive and special person. Nurses have a vital role in education, counseling, assessment and anticipatory guidance for these individuals. Nurses who are aware of their own beliefs, values, and attitudes are better able to manipulate the environment to allow clients more opportunities to express their needs and sexuality. Using neutral terms, offering choices, and avoiding negative responses will create an atmosphere conducive to the discussion of sexual concerns.

Acting out behavior that may have a sexual connotation can be seen more realistically as a need for warmth, tenderness, friendliness, or as many other needs mentioned throughout the chapter. As nurses assess each individual client, they can respond appropriately to these needs. The understanding, concern, and simple affectionate response could make the difference for a person who is attempting to adapt to a threatening and stressful event in his life.

Study Questions

1. Describe both the blatant and subtle ways that sexual stereotyping occurs before school age.

2. How does peer pressure affect sexuality?

3. How can nurses resolve conflicts about sexual values that differ from their own?

4. How does the nurse determine what questions to ask about such a personal matter as sexual functioning?

5. Tom Jones is a 20-year-old male who has had diabetes since early childhood. Several indirect questions to you suggest that he may be concerned about impotence. How might you respond to his possible concern?

6. Mr. W., a 70-year-old widower, is recovering from a mild heart attack. He lives with his married daughter and son-in-law. He describes himself as a sexy senior citizen while his daughter describes him as a dirty old man. How would you explain this discrepancy?

Glossary

Absolutistic position: Sexuality existing for the sole purpose of reproduction.

Acting out: The expression of certain kinds of unconscious conflicts through behavior; the unconscious impulse is not verbalized or remembered.

Asexuality: The absence of any sexual activity.

Autosexuality: Deriving sexual gratification through one's own actions and thoughts.

Bisexuality: The anticipation and enjoyment of sexual expression with either sex.

Hedonistic position: A value about sexuality that has pleasure and satisfaction as its focus; advocates each individual's ultimate fulfillment of sexual potential.

Heterosexuality: Demonstrating sexual desire for members of the opposite sex.

Homosexuality: The manisfestation of sexual desire or preference towards a member of one's own sex.

Impotence: Inability of the male to perform the sexual act.

Libido: Sexual desire.

Masturbation: The erotic stimulation of one's own genital organs.

Menarche: The time when menstruation begins.

Orgasm: The climax of sexual excitement.

Relativistic position: A value about sexuality that suggests acts should be judged in relation to their effects on other persons.

Sexuality: An aspect of the total personality encompassing feelings and behavior, not only as a sexual being but as a male or female.

Bibliography

Babcock ML, Connor B: Sexism and treatment of the female alcoholic. National Association of Social Workers 26:233–238, May 1981

Blaesing S, Brockhaus J: The development of body image in the child. Nurs Clin North Am 7:597–607, December 1972

DeLora JS, Warren CAB: Understanding Sexual Interaction. Boston, Houghton Mifflin, 1977

Dempsey MO: The development of body image in the adolescent. Nurs Clin North Am 7:609–615, December 1972

Diekelmann N: Primary Health Care of the Well Adult. New York, McGraw-Hill, 1977

Dorin A: Adolescent sexuality: Adolescent depression. Ped Nurs 4:49–52, July/August 1978

Dresen SE: The sexually active middle adult. In Diekelmann N (ed): Primary Health Care of the Well Adult. New York, McGraw-Hill, 1977a

Dresen SE: Sexuality and the older adult. In Diekelmann N (ed): Primary Health Care of the Well Adult. New York, McGraw-Hill, 1977b

Ehrlich GE: Total Management of the Arthritic Patient. Philadelphia, JB Lippincott, 1973

Eliot RS, Miles RR: Advising the cardiac patient about sexual intercourse. Medical Aspects of Human Sexuality 9:49–50, June 1975

Fagot BI: Consequences of moderate cross-gender behavior in preschool children. Child Dev 48:902–907, September 1977

Finch E: Sexuality and the disabled. Can Nurse 73:19–20, January 1977

Geiger RC, Knight SE: Sexuality of people with cerebral palsy. Medical Aspects of Human Sexuality 9:70–83, March 1975

Goldberg S, Lewis M: Play behavior in the year-old infant: Early sex differences. Child Dev 40:21–31, March 1969

Gomberg ES: Women, Sex Roles and Alcohol Problems. Professional Psychology 12:146–155, February 1981

Griggs W: Sex and the elderly: Staying well while growing old. Am J Nurs 78:1352–1354, August 1978

Howe F: Sexual Stereotypes Start Early. Rockville, MD, Aspen Systems, 1972

Krisinofski MT: Human sexuality and nursing practice. Nurs Clin North Am 8:673–681, December 1973

Krozy R: Becoming comfortable with sexual assessment. Am J Nurs 78:1036–1038, June 1978

Labby DH: Sexual concomitants of disease and illness. Postgrad Med 58:103–111, July 1975

Lewis RA: Emotional Intimacy Among Men. Journal of Social Issues 34:108–121, Winter 1978

McCloskey JC: How to make the most of body image theory in nursing practice. Nurs '76 6:68–72, May 1976

Mann J, Katsuranis J: The dynamics and problems of sexual relationships. Postgrad Med 58:79–86, July 1975

Maurer TB: Health care and the gay community. Postgrad Med 58:127–130, July 1975

Monea HE: Ethnicity and sexuality: Their impact on caring. In Burnside I, Ebersole P, Monea HE (eds): Psychological Caring Throughout the Life Span, pp 142–154. New York, McGraw-Hill, 1979

Murphy WD, Coleman E, Hoon E et al: Sexual dysfunction and treatment of alcoholic women. Sexuality and Disability 3, No. 4:240–255, Winter 1980

Murray RB, Zentner JP: Nursing Assessment and Health Promotion Throughout the Life Span. Englewood Cliffs, New Jersey, Prentice-Hall, 1979

Murray RLE: Body image development in adulthood. Nurs Clin North Am 7:617–629, December 1972

Paluszny M: Sexual identity and role in children. Clin Ped 13:154–158, February 1974

Papalia DE, Tennent SS: Vocational aspirations in preschoolers—A manifestation of early sex role typing. Sex Roles 1, No. 2:197–199, 1975

Pogrebin LC: Growing Up Free—Raising Your Child in the 80's. New York, McGraw-Hill, 1980

Powell DJ: Sexual dysfunction and alcoholism. Journal of Sex Education and Therapy 6, No. 2:40–45, 1980

Renshaw DC: Sexual problems in stroke patients. Medical Aspects of Human Sexuality 9:68–74, December 1975

Roberts SL: Behavioral Concepts in Nursing Throughout the Life Span. Englewood Cliffs, New Jersey, Prentice-Hall, 1978

Schwartz MS, Schockley EL: The Nurse and the Mental Patient. New York, John Wiley & Sons, 1956

Sex Information and Education Council of the US (SIECUS): Sexuality and Man. New York, Scribner, 1970

Spock BM: Baby and Child Care, rev. ed. New York, Pocket Books, 1976

Stein PJ, Hoffman S: Sports and male role strain. Journal of Social Issues 34:136–150, Winter 1978

Sutterley DC, Donnelly GF: Perspectives in Human Development: Nursing Throughout the Life Cycle. Philadelphia, JB Lippincott, 1973

Teen-Age Sex: Letting the Pendulum Swing. Time Magazine 34–40, August 21, 1972

Valente M: Sexual advice for the mentally retarded and their families. Medical Aspects of Human Sexuality 9:91–92, October 1975

Watts RT: The physiological interrelationships between depression, drugs, and sexuality. Nurs Forum 17:168–173, 1978

Wilcox R: Counseling patients about sex problems. Nurs '73 3:44–46, November 1973

Wilson HS, Kneisel CR: Psychiatric Nursing. Menlo Park, CA, Addison-Wesley, 1979

Learning
and Teaching

VII

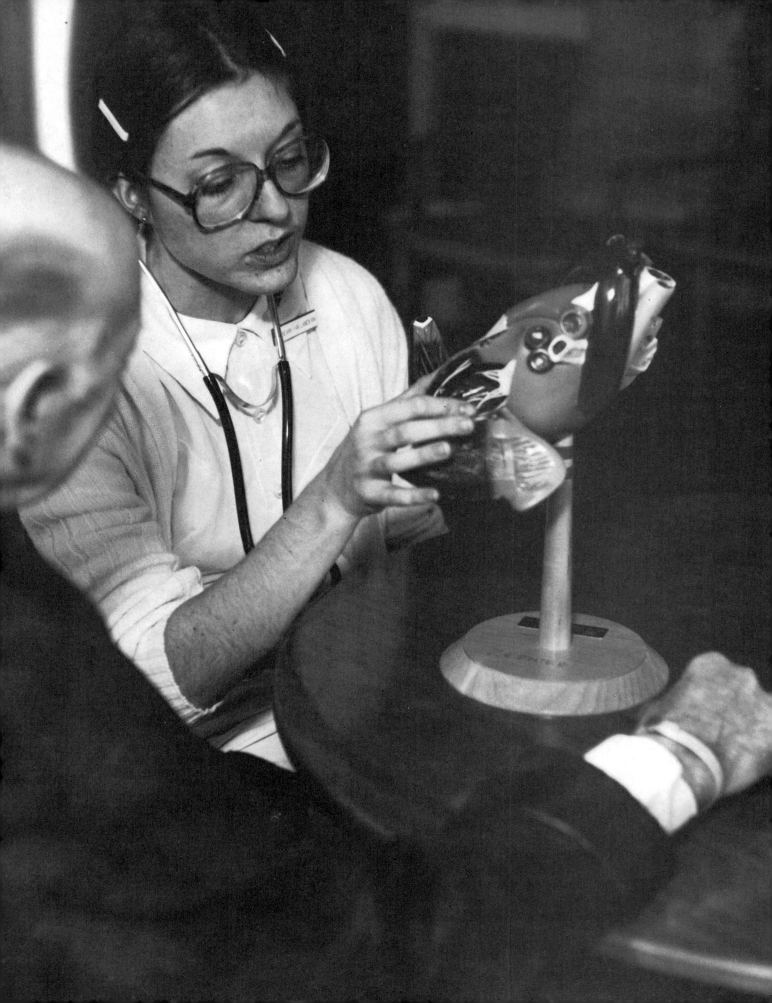

VII

Learning
and Teaching

The purpose of this single-chapter section is to emphasize the importance of the learning–teaching concept to professional nursing.

Facilitating learning is a nursing intervention that assumes greater importance as persons take more responsibility for their health. Clients need information to make informed choices, control their health situations, and mobilize their strengths. Clients may also need to learn new behaviors, new activities, and different feeling responses to internal and external stressors. Nurses individualize teaching just as they individualize other interventions. A learning need corresponds to other nursing diagnoses. It can be a problem to be solved or a strength to be augmented. To facilitate learning nurses will use all their nursing-process, interpersonal, and communication skills. Therefore, what clients learn is in part an evaluation of nurses' teaching abilities and also of their sensitivity to basic and higher-level needs.

Learning and Teaching

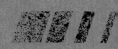

Janice B. Lindberg and Sharon Hein Jette

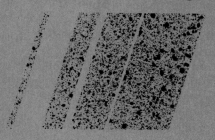

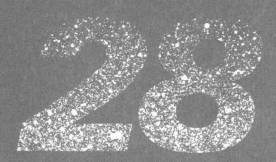

28

The purpose of this chapter is to explore the application of learning theories to nursing and to consider the process of effective teaching.

Learning involves a change in behavior and implies adaptation to an environmental situation. If nurses believe that persons grow, adapt, and develop to fulfill human potential as Maslow suggests, then learning is really the process of becoming. As such, learning is less an occasional or episodic activity and more a matter of ongoing change. At particular times, however, learning is focused to meet immediate needs. For example, within the context of nursing process, teaching is a specific nursing intervention. A particular learning is the desired outcome. As a specific nursing intervention, teaching is individualized for the person who is the object of your nursing care. To emphasize this point, we often use the phrase, "facilitating client learning" rather than "teaching" in the beginning of this chapter.

Facilitating client learning for the promotion of health is an important area of nursing practice and influence. It is an independent nursing function, the authority for which comes from the nurse's own knowledge of human health and adaptation and the skill the nurse has in promoting them. It is an independent function not bound to any particular setting or area of specialty of nursing practice. Teaching is also a nursing intervention that illustrates very well that nursing is nursing wherever it is practiced. To facilitate client learning through your teaching you need to know something about how persons are believed to learn and also how to teach your client. The knowledge we have about how persons learn comes from psychology through theories about learning.

Theories About Learning

There are many theories about learning. Theories are attempts to explain phenomena. As such, they come and go in all areas of science as people search for adequate explanations of events they do not understand. Learning is such an event. Most psychologists and educators agree that learning is a complex process. We still have much to discover about why learning occurs as it does. Psychologists who support various learning theories offer different explanations of how learning occurs. Instead of considering various theories as being in conflict with one another, it is often more useful to regard them as focusing on different aspects of learning or behaving. As Reilly suggests, numerous theories are rooted in various assumptions about man, the nature of knowledge, and the process by which persons learn (1975, p. 2).

An **eclectic** approach to learning, which the authors advocate, presumes that no one learning theory is more correct than another. An eclectic approach leads one to select from various theories, using whatever fits best from each source while being alert to the inconsistencies of different theories. For our purposes, we shall divide learning theories according to whether they emphasize behavior, cognition or thought processes, or a humanistic/holistic view of the person.

Behavioristic Learning Theories

Conditioning

Behaviorism represents learning as a process of making connections through association. Its origin is the conditioned response. This technique, developed by Ivan Pavlov (1849–1936) with his salivating dogs, was more concerned with neurology than psychology. Behaviorism itself was founded by John B. Watson (1878–1958). Using the reflex concept from neurology, Watson proposed a science of psychology that studied the individual's response to stimuli. Thus, the S–R or stimulus–response formula became the pattern or building block of behavior. Watson claimed that the process of conditioning stimulus to response was powerful enough to train or condition children for particular vocational roles. The contemporary proponent of conditioning is B.F. Skinner (1904–   ), the father of behavioral technology. Skinner concentrated on the role of reinforcement in establishing conditioned or desired responses. As Carpenter explains reinforcement in *The Skinner Primer*, it is "the central principle of learning that refers to the fact that an act becomes more frequent when it is followed by a positive consequence" (1974, p 32). Although Skinner's principles of reinforcement were developed in the animal laboratory with pigeons, they can be applied to the control of health-related behavior by means of behavior modification programs.

Behavior Modification

Behavior modification has been widely used to control smoking and also to achieve socially acceptable behavior in a variety of institutions. Behavior modification involves a carefully planned schedule of positive reinforcement when desired behavior occurs. This reinforcement may involve tokens, approval, or praise from a significant person. Positive reinforcement must be perceived as positive by the learner as well as the teacher. Punishment and negative reinforcement are also powerful and relatively easy means of controlling undesired behavior on a short-term basis. Occasionally, well-meaning authority figures such as physicians and nurses may use negative reinforcement without being aware of the ethical implications of what they are doing. As persons with health problems become aware of how behavior modification works, they may choose to provide their own meaningful reinforcement. For instance, they may use biofeedback techniques to reduce stress and promote relaxation. The consumer movement in health care has had the important effect of bringing health information and reinforcement under client or internal control. For example, expectant mothers choose natural childbirth and husbands become helpers in reinforcing healthy birthing behaviors.

Nursing Implication

The nurse possesses much information that the client could use to manage his own health behavior. Contrary to the way many people understand behavior modification, the learner's response and not the teacher's stimulus is the key to behavior change. For reinforcement to operate in any setting, the learner must believe that what is to be learned will help meet a particular need. Consider, for example, the situation of Mary W.

Example □ Mrs. W., aged 40, is approximately 50 lb overweight and was recently diagnosed as being hypertensive. She admits to being somewhat concerned about her high blood pressure. Her mother was hypertensive and died of a stroke as a young woman. Until recently, Mrs. W. did not know that decreasing her weight could possibly decrease her elevated blood pressure also. With the help of her nurse, Mrs. W. discovered that she is eating a balanced diet but that her caloric intake exceeds her energy

expenditure. Given this information, Mrs. W.'s response has been to maintain a reasonable food intake and increase her exercise. A definite weight loss and a steadily decreasing blood pressure have reinforced her to continue the diet and exercise response for several months. Note that her response brought reinforcement that influenced behavior. □

Response → Reinforcement → Future Behavior

The initial step for the nurse is to shape learning by reinforcing, hopefully in a positive manner, the adaptive behavior observed in the patient/client. This can be done without knowing either what goes on inside the person or exactly why. It is also possible and appropriate to use the natural setting and the client's response rather than worrying about contriving artificial stimuli. Any possible stimulus the nurse might contrive, such as a size-7 dress or pictures of a slim teenager, would probably be far less effective than the very real stimulus of her mother's fate, which Mrs. W. chose for herself once she had the necessary information. Because behavioral conditioning focuses on the response of the individual learner, the nurse recognizes that instruction, teaching, or facilitation, just like other nursing interventions, must be individualized to be most effective.

Mastery versus Performance

The intent of behavioral technology is to provide "mastery" of particular skills. Mastery can be contrasted with a performance approach, which attempts to assign a grade to learning. The difference between these evaluation approaches has important implications for both the learner and the teacher. The learner who has not yet mastered a particular task is not a failure and has not failed. He just has not yet "arrived" or "made it." The expectation is for everyone to pass or to learn the skill, although some will take longer than others. Someone, the teacher or nurse educator as you will see later, must facilitate learning in such a way as to increase the probability of success for the learner.

Success is maximized and the threat of failure minimized if careful assessment precedes instruction. This assessment enables the facilitator to fit both the task and conditioning to the functional abilities and strengths of the learner. In this way, the learner is also guided to accept an attainable goal. Because behaviorism is concerned with behavioral changes that are observable, it is better suited to the mastery of concrete information or well-defined motor tasks than to changing attitudes or feelings.

Cognitive Learning Theories

Cognitive learning theories focus on the complex intellectual processes of thinking, language, and problem solving. Psychologists proposing such theories included the Gestalt psychologists, Max Wertheimer and Kurt Lewin.

Gestaltists

The Gestaltists were concerned with insight, namely the "aha" experience. This insight involves a perceptual reorganization, which allows ideas to combine in such a way that 1 plus 1 = 3 rather than the usual 2. Another way to say this is that insight makes clear the relationships of puzzle pieces to each other, so that the puzzle makes sense. Consider the problem of adding together all of the numbers between 1 and 100. Some persons might laboriously begin adding 1 plus 2 plus 3 and so on. Others might see the puzzle another way, recognizing that 1 plus 100 = 101, 2 plus 99 = 101, 3 plus 98 = 101. These persons solve the problem quickly by realizing that there are 50 pairs of numbers that add to 101 and multiplying 101 by 50 to get a quick answer: 5050.

With insightful learning, the learner initially fails and later succeeds in problem solving as he develops different ways of perceiving the problem situation (Snelbecker, 1974, p. 77). Gestaltists share a philosophical view of man as a unique animal. Whereas behaviorists study learning by reducing situations to their elements, Gestaltists believe insightful learning involves discovering relationships and the larger structure of situations. Nurses often do see persons gain sudden insight into complex health situations, as the Gestaltists theorize.

Piaget/Developmental Psychologists

Some contemporary cognitive theorists like Piaget are developmental psychologists. Their important contribution to learning has been a better understanding of age-linked stages of cognitive development. This has led to teaching children at their stage of development rather than as small adults. For example, a pediatric nurse may apply Piaget's theory and use a three-dimensional model to teach a school-age child about his heart function. The nurse knows that the concept of heart as pump is insufficiently developed in the elementary school student to be understood through a verbal explanation. The cognitive development of a child at this age is at the stage of concrete operations rather than formal thought. Developmental readiness is a key factor of many cognitive approaches, as is individual readiness expressed as motivation. Cognitive theorists also believe individuals vary greatly in the amount of structure or assistance they need for learning tasks.

Humanistic Approaches to Learning

Humanistic approaches to learning are a rather recent development growing out of humanistic or "third force" psychology.

Humanistic approaches to learning emphasize the affective or feeling responses toward learning. This focus remains a prime consideration, even if what is to be learned is new knowledge or a motor skill. A humanistic approach is sometimes also called existential or phenomenological. **Existential** is a term rooted in philosophy and concerned with a person's subjective awareness of his existence. It is a self-deterministic view. Although existentialism is an idea that was popularized after World War II by such spokespersons as Jean Paul Sartre, it had origins much earlier with Kierkegaard (1813–1855). The term **phenomenological** refers to a concern for what is happening in the here and now. Behavior is dealt with in the present. There is neither the Freudian concern for the past nor the behavioristic emphasis on shaping future behavior.

The humanistic viewpoint emphasizes the importance of the person's view of self, man's unique human potential as a learner, and learning as a product of the person's perception. A hallmark of the humanistic approach is the belief that man has a basic drive toward health and self-actualization.

Humanism and Holism

The humanistic view of learning is particularly pertinent to a holistic philosophy of health care—one that focuses on the whole person. The rationale for such an approach is rooted in the belief that understanding one's health problems is essential to adapting to those health problems and moving toward health and self-actualization. This view also assumes that where no identified health problems exist, a person must still learn to manage his health care to promote continued and heightened well-being. Although each person is unique, the common basic needs shared with fellow men provide the basis for learning needs common to all persons if they are to achieve self-actualization.

Abraham Maslow and Carl Rogers represent humanistic approaches to learning. Their concepts and principles have a special relevance for nursing.

Let us look more closely at both Maslow's hierarchy of human needs and Carl Rogers' principles of learning for general applications the nurse can make to facilitate learning related to health care.

Maslow's Humanistic Approach

Maslow's humanistic approach and hierarchy of needs suggests a way to prioritize nursing interventions so that physiological needs are met first, followed by safety and security needs, love and belonging needs, esteem and self-esteem, and ultimately growth needs. In previous chapters on nursing process, we have made other applications of this hierarchy to the prioritizing of various nursing interventions. Much of traditional nursing care has involved meeting the physiological needs that an ill person was unable to meet for himself. Increasingly, nurses are also focusing their care functions toward promoting and maintaining health and assisting clients to meet growth needs that foster self-actualization. Nurses are assisting clients to use their own strengths or self-care abilities.

Facilitating learning may be an appropriate nursing intervention at all levels of the Maslow hierarchy. Imagine, for example, that a client needs to learn a new way to meet a basic physiological need: Mr. Jones needs to learn how to do intermittent self-catheterization of his bladder. If he can take care of his other physiological needs unassisted, he should be encouraged to do so. If not, the nurse would assist him as necessary before proceeding with the physiological need that has been singled out as a learning need. Even if a learning need is identified above the level of physiological needs, it is necessary to meet physiological needs before addressing higher-level needs. Think of yourself as hungry or needing to relieve a full bladder during a lecture and remember how your attention was focused on that specific need to the temporary exclusion of other needs. Thus, the Maslow hierarchy presents an approach that should assist you as a nurse to identify and prioritize meaningful learning needs.

Rogers's Humanistic Approach

Another humanistic psychologist and teacher who has been especially concerned about personalized approaches to the learner is Carl Rogers. Rogers's humanistic approach and principles of learning could easily have been written by a professional nurse. These principles, which are consistent with Maslow's hierarchy of needs, serve to highlight some of the points already made explicitly or implicitly about the humanistic philosophy of learning:

- Learning which involves a change in self-organization—in the perception of oneself—is threatening and tends to be resisted.
- Those learnings which are threatening to the self are more easily perceived and assimilated when external threats are at a minimum.
- Much significant learning is acquired through doing.
- Learning is facilitated when the student participates responsibly in the learning process.
- Self-initiated learning which involves the whole person of the learner—feelings as well as intellect—is the most lasting and pervasive.
- Independence, creativity, and self-reliance are all facilitated when self-criticism and self-evaluation are basic and evaluation by others is of secondary importance.
- The most socially useful learning in the modern world is the learning of the process of learning, a continuing openness to experience and incorporation into oneself of the process of change. (Rogers, 1969, pp. 157–164).

As is evident in the principles affirmed by Rogers, the individuality of the learner is accepted and prized. A basic trust in the human organism is taken for granted. Teaching–learning, as the humanists portray so well, is an interpersonal process. This process can be combined with and used within the context of scientific method (*i.e.*, in nursing, within the nursing process).

Common Beliefs Among Learning Theories

The nurse using an eclectic approach to learning should understand the common beliefs among various learning theories. Table 28-1 summarizes some of these common beliefs and also suggests the approaches emphasized by each theoretical perspective. Using these understandings, along with a basic knowledge of persons as unique individuals and the nursing process, the nurse is ready to consider the many learning needs of clients.

Because the human process of "becoming" is open-ended, there are always learning needs to be identified. Whether a particular learner is willing to address these is another but important consideration. A ready, active, and motivated learner is essential for any learning process to be successful. Each learner decides how much he is willing to invest in coping or mobilizing resources. What you as nurse are suggesting the learner "do" must be acceptable

Table 28-1
Comparison of Beliefs Common to Major Theories About Learning

Common Beliefs	Approaches		
	Behavioristic	*Cognitive*	*Humanistic*
Learner is the focal point of the learning process.	Rate of learning differs.	Structure needed differs.	Significance of learning differs.
Learning is a multisensory process.	Motor output activity emphasized.	Thinking process emphasized.	Feelings about learning dominate.
Readiness of the learner is important.	Reinforcement must contribute to meeting need learner is ready to address.	Developmental readiness is a key factor.	Readiness is willingness to experience the "here and now."
Learning is doing.	Action of learner starts the chain of reinforcing events that shape behavior.	Doing or activity is mental or intellectual.	The most significant doing is experiencing with the whole person, *i.e.*, feeling as well as thinking.
Learner establishes personal significance of learning.	Will determine whether reinforcement is seen as positive or negative. Whatever client learns or however he behaves is meaningful to him.	Knowledge gained is perceived by learner as helping him to adapt.	Process of learning to learn may be as important as what is learned.
The learner needs feedback.	Feedback provides information, validation, correction, reinforcement, and confirmation of self-worth as well as ability.		
	Result of action influences future action.		Person-to-person nonjudgmental feedback of great significance.
			Feedback conveys unconditional positive regard for other person as unique and valued individual.

to him at some level if it is to receive serious consideration. As you increase the acceptability to make learning more meaningful or less in conflict with the client's belief system, you will increase the likelihood of behavior change. You should consider the following questions: What is the expected outcome if the client behaves as you suggest? Can you really assure that he will feel better, be happier, or live longer? In other words, what are the alternatives and what are the probabilities? When the client seems to make a maladaptive choice, ask yourself why. Try to assume the client's frame of reference.

The nurse who strives to make learning mean-

ingful to the individual increases the chances that a nursing intervention of teaching will be effective. In order for the client to value the nurse's teaching expertise and seek it again and again, he will need to perceive the learning process and its outcome as positive. As health-care professionals, nurses have many opportunities to facilitate client learning, both in carefully planned and extemporaneous ways. Of course, other important considerations include time and resources of both the client and agencies of health-care delivery. Now that we have examined the interpersonal process of learning, we are ready to explore the process of effective teaching.

The Nurse as a Health Educator

Health Education

One of the responsibilities of the nurse as outlined in Chapter 13 (communication) is that of **health education,** facilitating another's learning to live and adapt in the healthiest possible style. All health professionals share this responsibility. Indeed, in many parts of the country, professional health educators take overall responsibility for client teaching in hospitals, schools, and commmunities. The ability of persons to learn health promotion and preventive practices, to learn to manage illness, and to learn to care for themselves and dependents underlies the health of the nation (Fig. 28-1).

Health Education Activities

Health education activities span the entire range of health care: prevention, maintenance, recovery, and rehabilitation. The nurse–educator who teaches school children basic health habits helps them to learn illness prevention. Assisting an older person to regulate and monitor several medications exemplifies health maintenance teaching. Hospital nurses teach pre- and postoperative care in order to hasten recovery from surgery. And rehabilitative nursing itself requires daily, consistent guiding and teaching of persons to implement their own self-care. Nurses working in hospice programs teach dying persons and their families how to adapt to death. Health

education, then, is a lifespan activity that includes many types of professionals, many levels of health care, and many locations. To many persons, health teaching unfortunately connotes the image of do-gooders preaching that we should avoid all the things we love best; to many others, it represents active, participative growth (Burkitt, 1977).

Health Education Categories

The scope of health education activities spans the following categories, each succeeding group representing a slightly narrower focus:

- Community health education
- Occupational health education
- School health education
- Group health education
- Family health education
- Patient–client education

In their broadest form, immunization campaigns and stop-smoking media campaigns, for example, attempt to teach large communities of persons. Health teaching done in businesses, industries, and schools attempts to maintain healthy workers and students. When focused on groups of persons, families, and friends, health teaching promotes mental and physical health of colleagues, parents, and children. Persons who are ill receive care and teaching in both formal and informal education sessions. Although nurses have focused traditionally on client and family teaching, the opportunities increase yearly for teach-

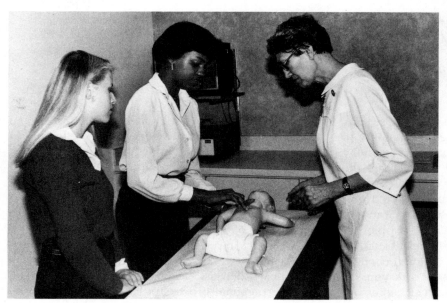

Figure 28-1
The nurse performs health education by teaching CPR skills in the community. *(Photo by Bob Kalmbach)*

ing throughout the entire scope of the categories listed above and the entire lifespan.

In 1976, President Ford signed into law the National Consumer Health Information and Health Promotion Act, defining six activities of consumer health education:

1 Inform people about health, illness, disability, and ways in which they can improve and protect their own health, including the more efficient use of the delivery system

2 Motivate people to want to change to more healthful practices

3 Help people to learn the necessary skills to adopt and maintain healthful practices

4 Foster teaching and communication skills in all those engaged in educating consumers about health

5 Advocate changes in the environment that will facilitate healthful conditions and healthful behavior

6 Add to knowledge through research and evaluation concerning the most effective ways of achieving these objectives (Somers, 1978)

Concepts of patients' rights, advocacy, consumerism, health behavior, adaptation, communication, and research pervade this law.

Credibility of the Nurse as Teacher

As a teacher, the nurse needs a certain amount of credibility. The client should perceive the nurse as competent. Frequently, ironic cartoons appear depicting obese health professionals teaching weight control or cautioning against smoking while lighting a cigarette. The saying, "Practice what you preach," applies perfectly. Clients need healthful role models as teachers. Lest you believe that you must have experienced an impairment or illness to assist another to cope with it, recall the skill of empathy as discussed in Chapter 13. An empathic understanding of illness, injury, pain, or dying makes it possible for a young, healthy nurse to teach the distressed.

Limitations on Nurses' Teaching

Most settings in which nurses practice encourage health teaching; in some, especially community health positions, nurses have total responsibility for teaching clients. When nurses practice in interdisciplinary teams, however, communication problems can arise that place limitations on the nurse's ability to teach effectively. Such limitations include those suggested by Redman (1976):

• An unclear perception of teaching as only formal sessions, omitting informal teaching

• Limited preparation in teaching within an interdisciplinary team

• Role confusion about who teaches what skills or content

• Lack of employer support for nurses to do teaching

• Lack of consumer demand for nurses to teach, showing lack of awareness of nurses' abilities

Such limitations can be minimized by careful planning and explicit understanding of which team members hold which responsibilities for teaching. With each role clarified, any team member refers for assistance to the resources of the health team to meet the total learning needs of the client.

Nursing Student as a Credible Teacher

Very early in a nursing program, the student gains a wealth of experience in health teaching: sharing knowledge of anatomy and physiology with roommates, teaching health habits and safety to family members, answering endless questions of peers on nutrition, first aid, pain relief, birth control, stress reduction, and so on. The nursing student is perceived as a resource; this perception will continue throughout your career as family, friends, and neighbors approach, saying "You're a nurse. What do you know about...?"

And yet, the anticipation of "teaching" a patient poses a very stressful challenge for many students. The idea of being responsible for someone else's learning seems overwhelming. Much of this anticipatory anxiety derives from an attitude, indeed, a cultural value that professional people should "know all the answers." The thought of not knowing the answers to a client's question appears devastating, embarrassing, disgraceful. The fact is—and it is hard to see without experience—that no professional ever can hope to have all the answers. In addition, teaching involves so much more than answering another person's questions. It is an entire process of helping another person to learn for himself. Face your mirror squarely and practice saying:

"Good question. I don't know the answer but I know how we can find out."

This is a most helpful, honest, human response, neither embarrassing nor disgraceful; such a response facilitates client involvement in learning, nursing self-confidence, and open nurse–client communication.

In fact, Redman, (1976, p. 9) defines **teaching** itself as a special type of communication that is carefully structured and sequenced to produce learning. The nurse or nursing student obviously must first communicate skillfully in order to teach skillfully. Teaching uses basic communication skills such as active listening, empathy, helping responses, and assertiveness. Other skills of supporting and crisis intervention are interwoven.

Principles of Teaching

Just as there are beliefs common to various learning theories, there are beliefs common to effective teaching or the facilitation of learning. These are sometimes called *principles of teaching.* A representative list of principles of teaching is shown in Table 28-2, enumerated by Pohl (1978).

Throughout these principles run concepts already familiar to you: nurse–client relationship, communication, client strengths, client needs, objectives or goals, environment, and evaluation. Although Pohl specifically cites the planning time necessary for

---

**Table 28-2
Principles of Teaching**

- Good nurse–learner rapport is important in teaching.
- Teaching requires effective communication.
- Learning needs of clients and co-workers must be determined.
- Objectives (goals) serve as guides in planning and evaluating teaching.
- Planning time for teaching and learning require special attention.
- Control of the environment is an aspect of teaching.
- Learning principles must be applied appropriately.
- Teaching skill can be acquired through practice and observation.
- Evaluation is an integral part of teaching.

---

teaching, informal and spontaneous teaching can occur with minimal preparation. Formal teaching requires more development time.

Nursing Process
Teaching–Learning Interaction as a Problem-Solving Process

The teaching–learning interaction is not only a communication process but also a problem-solving process. As indicated so many times in previous chapters, nursing process is the problem-solving process of professional nursing. It is logical, therefore, to approach teaching–learning within the context and organization of nursing process. This means steps of teaching–learning interaction parallel those of nursing process:

- Collecting data (assessing)
- Using the data to identify strengths and to state learning needs (identifying problems)
- Clarifying behavioral objectives (formulating goals)
- Identifying appropriate interventions
- Using teaching methods or strategies (implementing interventions)
- Evaluating both learning and teaching
- Evolving a teaching–learning philosophy and synthesizing learning theory (aggregating)

Collecting Data to Assess Learning Needs

Assessing the person's strengths and biopsychosocial needs, including growth and development needs, enables the nurse as teacher to identify problems and learning needs that are truly personalized. Data gathered for assessment do not become useful information until they are organized in a meaningful way. The nurse collecting the data may follow the format of the Person Assessment Guide (see Appendix

A) or use some other guidelines depending on the setting and circumstances. Regardless of the particular format for organizing data, assessing learner needs should include the following steps of assessment:

- Use of empathy to anticipate learning needs
- Assessing level of knowledge, skill, and attitude
- Assessing level of comprehension
- Assessing readiness to learn (motivation)

Use of Empathy

In order to project what the client may want to learn and needs to learn, use empathy. Consider the client's thoughts and feelings, as if you were in that person's situation. What questions, what uncertainties would you have? What would you be willing or able to hear? What conditions would enhance your learning? Nurses experienced in teaching soon recognize the basic information necessary to transmit to clients. Beyond the basics, however, individual learning needs are difficult to predict and demand an effective nurse–client relationship to detect. Without open, sensitive, two-way communication, a nurse never learns what the client wants and needs to learn. Indeed, the nurse will start by learning from the client.

Assessing Level of Knowledge

What does the client already know and feel about his health situation? What does the person already do? What has he already tried to do? Obviously reteaching what he already knows or suggesting what he has already tried wastes time and destroys teacher credibility. In a sense, the assessment of a client's current understanding, skill, or attitude communicates this message: "You are a competent person; you are capable of learning and adapting; I will help you build on what you already know and do." Consider what message is conveyed to a client when the nurse does not "start where he is" but reteaches what he already knows, and consider the total breakdown in the helping relationship when the nurse begins teaching far beyond the client's understanding. Solution: know what the client already knows.

Assessing Level of Comprehension

The third component of assessing a client's learning needs involves determining the person's level of comprehension. Typically, data on stage of growth and development or on level of vocabulary give a rough indication of potential comprehension. Yet far too often, the nurse stereotypes levels of comprehension based on social class, occupation, age, or years of formal education. Inbred perceptions of poor people, unskilled workers, older people, or unschooled clients label them "unable to comprehend" before they have a chance to prove otherwise; such stereotyped labels negate full life-long learning experiences acquired informally and independently through many crises and changes. Beginning with the hypothesis that all clients are capable of learning and comprehending, the effective nurse-educator sees her challenge as that of discovering how best to facilitate client comprehension.

Assessing Learner Readiness

Finally, in assessing a learner's readiness to learn, educators speak of a **"teachable moment,"** a period of time in which a learner is receptive to listen, to adapt, to learn. Ideally, then, teaching should be timed so as to take advantage of a learner's "teachable moment" so that learning more readily occurs. These moments can often be anticipated. Indeed, the entire concept of anticipatory crisis intervention derives from the fact that before a predictable crisis—childbirth, for example—a parent is open and receptive to learning and changing. Prehospitalization teaching also attempts to promote learning before a crisis.

In contrast, many other receptive movements occur spontaneously, informally, and suddenly. Palm (1971) argues that nurses tend to view teaching much too formally, missing many of the constant and unlimited opportunities for informal teaching–learning.

A crucial assessment skill is the ability to recognize the following client behaviors, which are indicative of learning receptivity:

- Direct questions—However brief or seemingly superficial, these may indicate a deeper concern for learning:
  "How am I doing?"
- Indirect questions—Often in reference to others, these may signal a need for personal information:
  "I wonder how my neighbor manages his hypertension."
- Information-seeking behavior—Often demonstrates an eagerness for new learning:
  Mr. P. listens very carefully to overhear what is being said about him, or he reads everything he can on coping with his problem.
- Withdrawal—May indicate feelings of overload,

misunderstanding, or needing to learn how to set priorities:

> Mrs. J. begins to sigh, avoids eye contact, and expresses hopelessness at any mention of caring for herself.

- Confusion, frustration, and anger—Reactions to misunderstanding or a lack of information or skills; these feelings erupt:

> Puzzled and puffing, Ms. T. tries to grasp the words used to describe the treatment she is to give her son.

Altogether, the teacher tries to assess a learner's motivation—the drives, present or future, which would facilitate learning. When a nurse-educator perceives no motivation for learning, it is possible to induce motivation by sustained psychological support. It is important to remember, however, that dealing with other perceived needs may indeed be more important. Remember also that factual information alone is a necessary but not sufficient motivator to change. Therefore, simply telling a person of the changes he must make in his diet will rarely prompt him to do so, unless he is able to express what this change in life-style means to him as a person.

Stating Learning Needs

Once the nurse identifies data indicative of a client's learning need, the question arises, "How do I work these data into a nursing process?" The answer is found in this formula:

> If the assessment demonstrates a learning need, begin a teaching–learning process *within* a nursing process.

In other words, proceed to state a learning problem or need, set mutually acceptable learning goals, enact teaching interventions, and evaluate progress.

Typically, a learning need can be stated as a problem in a variety of ways

- Limited knowledge of medications prescribed
- Distress related to inadequate information and low self-esteem
- Anxiety caused by limited ability to perform one's own personal care
- Need for continued support after discharge

Such problems, as with any problem statement,

should be validated with the client or family if at all possible:

> "I wonder if you're feeling confused about this procedure you'll have tomorrow?"

Clarifying Behavioral Objectives

At this point in the teaching–learning process, and in parallel with the nursing process, goals are formulated to direct the interventions that follow. These will clarify the expected outcomes of teaching or facilitation of learning. Specifically, learning goals are called **behavioral objectives,** or instructional objectives, in the field of education. Behavioral learning objectives are statements of what the client will do or say as evidence of learning. Such behavioral learning objectives describe the intended outcome of learning, stating the performance expected of the learner as a result of teaching (Mager, 1962). They state measurable behavior changes, such as the ones listed at the beginning of each chapter in this text. Standard format reads, "The learner will . . . ."

Because learning occurs in three domains, behavioral learning objectives are stated within each domain:

- Cognitive
- Affective
- Psychomotor

Cognitive learning objectives use verbs demonstrating results of thinking processes:

- The client will state how salt affects his blood pressure.
- J. M. will decide how to reduce the stress in his life.

Unacceptable objectives such as, "The client will (understand, learn about, accept, know) his problem." suffer from lack of specificity and impersonal, vague, and unmeasurable wording. To be sure, ask how a nurse would ever know whether this client had "understood" anything unless she saw some behavioral evidence.

Affective learning objectives reflect the client's feelings, attitudes and values:

- The client will express her reactions to her mastectomy scar.

- Ms. T. will discuss feelings of depression and loss after abortion.

The above center on the client. Unacceptable objectives (which are actually interventions) focus on the nurse, "Encourage verbalization of feelings," or "Teach compensations for visual loss post surgery."

Psychomotor learning objectives state actions and skills:

- The client will demonstrate clean technique in changing his dressing.
- Mrs. S. will decrease muscular tension as evidenced by self-message.

Again, unacceptable goals often state the nurse's psychomotor behavior, "Turn the patient every 2 hours." This is really an intervention. Writing effective learning objectives directs the nurse's choice of teaching interventions as well as evaluation of the entire process.

Identifying and Implementing Teaching Interventions

An incredible number of teaching interventions exist, some traditional, some innovative. How do you choose teaching methods and materials? Numbers of interventions—or teaching methods can be effective if chosen to match the client's learning need and behavioral learning objective. The most creative lecture will not teach psychomotor skill; clients cannot learn affective expression if they are never allowed to vent feelings.

Further consideration of the learner's ability, developmental level, cultural values, and past experiences aids the choice of teaching methods. Each client's reading ability, visual and hearing ability, and interest level differ. The nurse chooses reading materials appropriate to the reading level of the client and compensates for sensory losses when teaching. Common problems of ineffective teaching result from methods below or beyond the client's developmental stage. Children's education progresses with their levels of concentration, of abstraction, and of coordination. Growth and development knowledge must be applied when teaching children about health. In contrast, children's materials are not appropriate in teaching adults, however dependent they may be.

When teaching, nurses rely on general guidelines for matching teaching methods to client needs. Very many such guidelines have been written, most of them concentrating on the nurse. The learner–centered guide to teaching methods presented in Table 28-3 provides a contrast. This guide proposes that the nurse can facilitate learning by focusing on what the learner or client needs to learn rather than on what the teacher or nurse wants to teach.

Introspective exercises, as a method of learning, typically ask the learner to search his values and attitudes in order to answer a questionnaire or choose a hypothetical action. Values-clarification and empathy exercises, although listed as ways to facilitate learning, have been noted earlier as methods serving also to clarify ethical issues and to assess learning needs.

- Values clarification example:
  If I had only one year to live, I would:
  a. Continue my present ambitions
  b. Drop all my ambition and seek pleasure
  c. Drop all my own ambition and help others
  d. Other

Empathy simulations require that the learner "walk a mile" in another's shoes. In order to learn what it feels like to be disabled, impaired, sick, distressed, or institutionalized, the learner takes on the role of another. Such simulations range from experiencing an age-related sensory loss to mock hospitalization to "feel what it's like" in a client's role.

Roleplaying, a similar method, is based on the assumption that if a learner anticipates and acts out a conflict or situation, he will be better able to cope with it when it occurs (or recurs).

"Pretend I'm your husband," says the nurse, encouraging roleplaying. "What will you say to him when you go home?"

Roleplaying done individually, as above, assumes much problem solving. It can also be done in a support group. Reverse roleplaying asks the client to take on another's role:

"O.K. Now I'll be the wife coming home and you play your husband," says the nurse, switching roles. "React as you think he would."

Peer support is the aim of many self-help and mutual help groups. One of the original self-help groups, Alcoholics Anonymous, claims excellent success in reducing drinking problems and has generated Al-Anon for spouses and Ala-Teen for children

Table 28-3
Learner-Centered Guide to Teaching Method

Learning Need	Method
If a person needs to learn:	The nurse can facilitate learning by using:
1 Awareness of self, own attitudes, and values	1 Introspective exercises, questionnaires, values-clarification activities
2 Awareness of others' situation, attitudes, and values	2 Roleplaying, interacting with others with similar conditions or strengths or problems
3 Awareness of own behavior	3 Reverse role-playing, audio or video playback, analysis of interactions
4 Basic factual information	4 Lectures and discussion, reading, self-directed media programs
5 Concepts and relationships of ideas	5 Reading, discussion, models and graphics
6 Application of concepts to practice	6 Opportunity for guided practice
7 Manual skills	7 Skill practice, demonstration–return demonstration, programmed learning
8 Relating to others	8 Group discussion, play groups, roleplaying, counseling
9 Self-expression, self-confidence	9 Group discussion, creative arts (music, art, movement), positive reinforcement, role modeling
10 Decision making, priority setting	10 Make decisions and receive feedback
11 Adaptation to life-style change	11 Counseling, self-help and mutual help groups, contracting

of drinkers. Similar resource groups exist for persons with cancer (Living with Cancer), mastectomies (Reach for Recovery), mental distress (Recovery, Inc.), infertility (Resolve), child abuse (Parents Anonymous), and many other life crises.

Participative contracting has been demonstrated to be a teaching method of considerable success (Steckel, 1980). Using principles of positive reinforcement, nurses and clients mutually agree to set behavioral goals, set deadlines, and choose rewards for meeting goals.

Media programming now offers a wide range of sophisticated machine-assisted learning. Multimedia productions are innovative. Provocative "trigger films" of 1 to 3 minutes or less initiate discussion after viewing. Audio and video playback allow a learner to hear and see uncensored feedback on performance. Self-directed programmed instructions with tapes, video cassettes, and computers develop more flexibility and ingenuity each year (Fig. 28-2). The computer-teacher might command:

> *BEEP:* PRESS THE BUTTON INDICATING WHAT ACTION YOU WOULD TAKE TO CORRECT THIS CLIENT'S COMPLAINT. *BEEP.*

The student punches in a response.

> *BEEP:* THE CLIENT CLUTCHES HIS CHEST IN PAIN. WHAT WILL YOU DO FIRST? *BEEP.*

Ever more creative teaching methods evolve constantly. The use of artistic expression in composition, movement, music, and drama has developed particularly in mental health settings. Relaxation methods of controlled breathing, hypnosis, meditation, biofeedback, expressive exercise, and introspection prevail in learning stress reduction, self-control, and pain relief. All these methods and many others are available for nurses to employ in teaching.

Clinical Illustration

Facilitating client learning is what the nursing intervention of teaching is all about. Teaching usually involves a learning facilitation that has many dimensions. Often the more formal didactic presentation or lecture–demonstration is our initial thought about how to teach. With more attention to the matter, many of the learner-centered methods in Table 28-3 may occur to us.

Yet another approach asks the question, "What

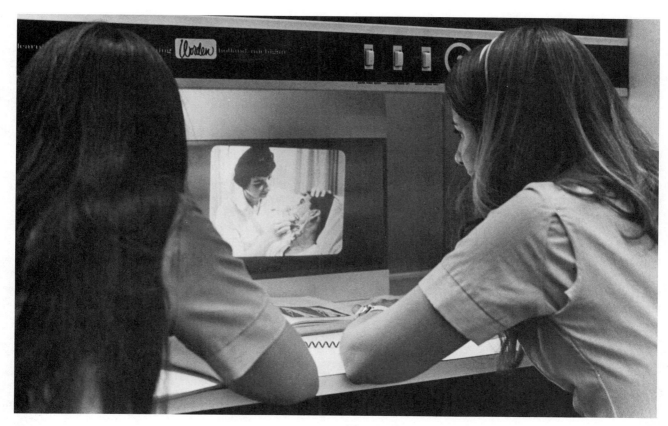

Figure 28-2
Instructional media are useful methods for learning factual knowledge or manual skills.

can I do to facilitate learning?" One of the very basic responsibilities of nursing, the creation of a supportive environment, includes the teaching—learning environment as well. For the most part, providing a setting and atmosphere conducive to communication will also enhance learning. Free from distractions, comfortable, convenient, and functional, such a learning environment provides support for the often painful process of learning. Also, an atmosphere free of psychological stress, threats, and tensions promotes learning. The ability of stress to alter perception, hearing, communication, and retention precludes the occurrence of learning (Guzzetta, 1979).

Once a supportive environment is created for the learner, two additional questions arise:

- What does the learner want to know?
- How will you as nurse/teacher know when he has learned it?

Both of these questions have a ring of familiarity and remind us that the teaching–learning interaction parallels nursing process. Utilizing the data base presented in Appendix B, we can illustrate how the teaching–learning process is used within the context of nursing process.

Example □ At the time of her present hospitalization, Mrs. R's current concern was a possible diagnosis of cancer: She underwent an emergency appendectomy while vacationing in Alabama 6 weeks ago; at that time, a questionable mass was observed on her right ovary, possible cancer. She returned home for further surgery and has been very distressed while waiting for additional surgery. (See data base in Appendix B for additional details.) □

Among Mrs. R's strengths were:

- Strong desire to recover from surgery and become independent again
- Ability to learn from and use health information
- Ability to accept help
- Strong family suppport system.

One of the identified problems in the care plan for Mrs. R. was altered respiratory status related to:

- Potential increase in bronchial secretions related to anesthesia

- Decreased mobility
- Narcotic medications

Given the general problem of altered respiratory status and the desired outcomes, one might detail specific problems or learning needs, expected outcomes or behavioral objectives, and interventions or teaching methods (Table 28-4).

Note that one of the suggested interventions is of the "lecture" or "explain" variety. Another intervention is to "demonstrate" (*i.e.*, the correct procedure for coughing and deep breathing). The other interventions are equally important to facilitating Mrs. R's learning. Not only does she have a cognitive need to know what to do and why, she also has affective or feeling needs and a need for assistance with the motor tasks. Planning for cognitive, affective, and psychomotor needs will enable persons to use strengths to their best advantage in meeting various learning needs.

Evaluating Learning

If, indeed, the nurse has developed a teaching–learning process within a nursing process, the evaluation component flows logically from the goals and interventions. Just as evaluation is an important component of nursing process, it is an equally important component of the teaching–learning process. Imagine that an evaluation of our teaching plan for Mrs. R. reveals the following: Objective 1, which was concerned with a cognitive or knowledge learning need, was met. Objective 2, which was concerned with an affective or feeling need, was also met. We conclude, however, that objective 3, the psychomotor objective, was only partially achieved. From oral and written reports, it is evident that Mrs. R. ambulates when assisted or reminded but does not take the initiative to ambulate unaided although she is phys-

Table 28-4
Specifics of a Teaching Plan for Mrs. R.

Learning Need	Behavioral Objective	Intervention
1 Cognitive—Limited knowledge of altered respiratory status	Mrs. R. will verbalize alterations in respiration and appropriate interventions for these.	Explain briefly how respiratory function is compromised by surgery, anesthesia and pain. Explain what intervention is necessary. Demonstrate procedure for coughing and deep breathing.
2 Affective—Feelings of helplessness after surgery	Mrs. R. will verbalize decreased feelings of helplessness and therefore be receptive to learning.	Spend time with her even when she does not talk. Help her vent feeling of helplessness. Listen carefully to facilitate development of trusting relationship. Acknowledge and reinforce all positive, growth-oriented behaviors. Assist her to view herself as a total person rather than focusing on limitations. Assist both person and family to express their feelings to each other.
3 Psychomotor—Decreased muscle function as a result of surgery, anesthesia, and pain medication	Mrs. R. will maintain clear lungs and will gradually increase mobility from a few steps to regular hall ambulation.	Assist with coughing and deep breathing q 1–2 hr while awake and q 3–4 hr during sleep hours. Assist with ambulation q.i.d. until able to proceed without assistance. Help her walk a bit farther each time.

ically able to do so. As a result of this evaluation, our nursing plan may be as follows:

- Continue to provide gentle reminders of the need to increase ambulation.
- Acknowledge and reinforce efforts to increase ambulation.
- Plan part of the time spent with Mrs. R. to include ambulation.
- Allow additional quiet time together when she can express other feelings or concerns.

Teaching skill develops over time and with practice. While observation of other teachers helps the novice learn methods and techniques, each teacher must employ creativity to develop his own style. With each teaching experience, a way to learn is to ask these questions:

- How would I improve this session the next time I teach it?"
- Did the client meet his goals, *i.e.*, the behavioral learning objectives?
- If so, what are the factors leading to his success?
- If not, what happened to prevent this accomplishment?
- Was a learning principle ignored or violated? Reevaluate the learner's readiness, ability, developmental stage, motivation, and the learning environment for possible clues.
- Was my teaching as effective as possible to facilitate learning? Although this is a subjective question requiring insight, peers, supervisors, and instructors may also provide valuable feedback.

- Were any teaching principles violated?
- How effectively did teaching methods match learner's needs?
- Did teaching materials compensate for any learner impairments; were they organized, creative, motivating, and accurate?

Although it is possible to measure the client's learning when using behavioral objectives, it is nearly impossible to predict what long-term influence you may have had on him or how you may have motivated his future learning, for only the learner determines what will be learned.

Conclusion

The teaching–learning interaction is described as both a communication process and a problem-solving process. Teaching is approached as the facilitation of client learning. The nurse, to be an effective teacher, must know something about how persons are thought to learn. This understanding comes from psychology through learning theories.

A person-centered approach to learning suggests providing an atmosphere in which psychological stress is purposely decreased. Using a basic knowledge of persons as unique, the nurse discharges responsibilities as a health educator by practicing nursing process. Teaching–learning interaction is viewed within the context of nursing process and therefore focused on the client as learner. In evaluating the outcome of learning, teaching is evaluated too.

Study Questions

1. Define *teaching* and *learning*. How do they differ? What is the primary focus in a nurse–client, learning–teaching interaction?

2. How can creativity enhance client learning? Give examples of creativity applied to specific situations.

3. Discuss and translate into practical examples various teaching–learning principles.

4. Discuss the significance of teaching in the home and compare with teaching in an institutional or agency setting.

5. How can teaching methods be adapted for adults? Children? Elders?

Glossary

Affective learning objectives: Learning goals concerned with feelings, attitudes, and values.

Behavioral objectives: Learning goals; statements of what a person will do or say as evidence of learning.

Behaviorism: A theoretical approach that represents learning as a process of making connections through association; developed by J.B. Watson (1878–1958) and concerned primarily with objectively observable and measurable data rather than subjective phenomena such as ideas or emotions.

Cognitive learning objectives: Learning goals that state the results of thinking processes.

Cognitive learning theories: Those theoretical approaches that focus on the intellectual processes of thinking, language, and problem solving; term includes theories of Gestaltists, Wertheimer and Lewin, and developmental psychologists like Piaget.

Eclectic: Selecting from various sources; not following any one system or theory.

Existential: Pertaining to a person's subjective awareness of his existence.

Health education: Facilitating persons' learning to live and adapt in the healthiest possible style, a shared responsibility of health professionals.

Humanistic approaches to learning: Those philosophical approaches to learning that emphasize affective or feeling responses to learning; growing out of humanistic or "third force" psychology, these approaches are also sometimes called "existential" or "phenomenological".

Phenomenological: Pertaining to a subjective perception of reality at the present time.

Psychomotor learning objectives: Learning goals concerned with actions and skills.

Teachable moment: That period of time in which a learner is receptive to listen, to adapt, and to learn.

Teaching: A special type of communication that is carefully structured and sequenced to produce learning.

Bibliography

Burkitt A: What is health education? Nurs Times (Suppl) 73, No. 25:3–7, June 1977

Carpenter F: The Skinner Primer. New York, Free Press, 1974

Guzzetta CE et al: The relationship between stress and learning. Advanced Nursing Guide 1:35–49, July, 1979

Mager R: Developing Attitude Toward Learning. Belmont, CA, Fearon, 1968

Mager R: Preparing Instructional Objectives. Palo Alto, CA, Fearon, 1962

Palm M: Recognizing opportunities for informal patient teaching. Nurs Clin North Am 6:669–678, December, 1971

Pohl M: The Teaching Function of the Nurse Practitioner. Dubuque, IA, William C Brown, 1978

Redman B: The Process of Patient Teaching. St Louis, CV Mosby, 1976

Reilly DE: Behavioral Objectives in Nursing: Evaluation of Learner Attainment. New York, Appleton-Century-Crofts, 1975

Reilly DE: Teaching and Evaluating the Affective Domain in Nursing Programs. Thorofare, NJ, CB Slack, 1978

Rogers C: Freedom to Learn. Columbus, Charles E Merrill, 1969

Smith DM: Writing objectives as a nursing practice skill. Am J Nurs 2:319–320, 1971

Snelbecker GE: Learning Theory, Instructional Theory and Psychoeducational Design. New York, McGraw-Hill, 1974

Somers A: Promoting health, consumer education and national policy. Nurs Digest 6:1–11, Spring, 1978

Steckel SB: Contracting with patient-selected reinforcers. Am J Nurs 9:1596, 1980

Synthesis
of Concepts

VIII

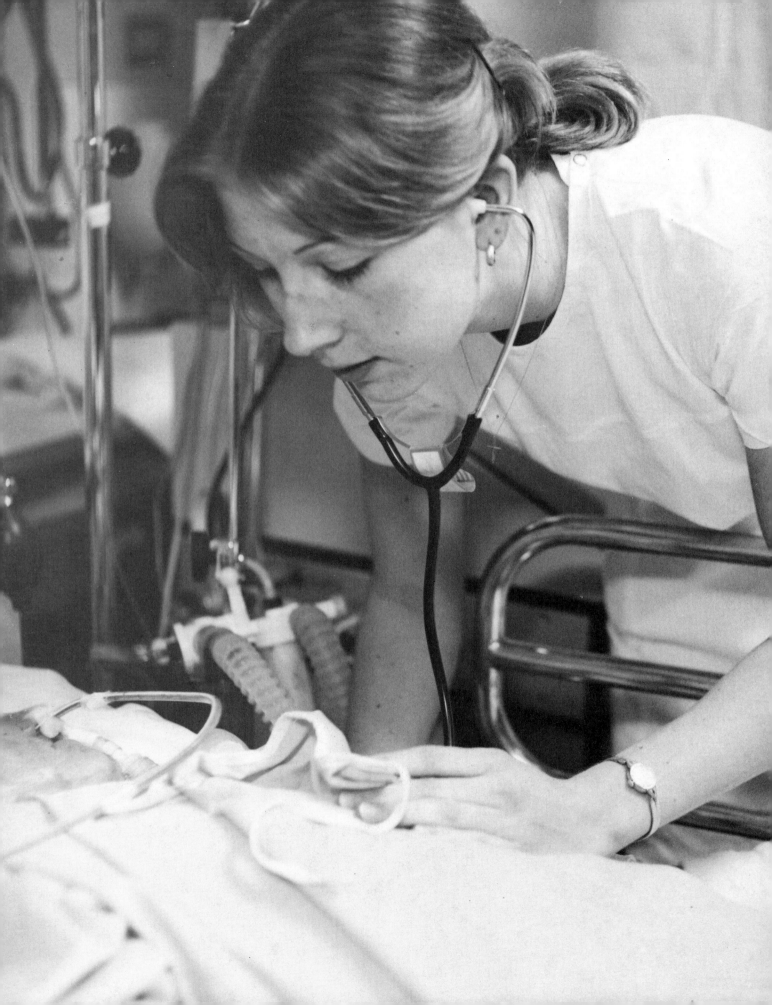

VIII

Synthesis of Concepts

Now that the discussion of basic concepts is completed, the reader may be wondering how to use them to give total person-centered nursing care. This section provides two examples of ways nurses identify and intervene for their clients' needs. The care of persons who experience loss and those who undergo surgery are described.

Each of the seven concepts presented in this book can be applied to the situation of loss. Loss is a common occurrence in the lives of all individuals. In particular, persons with health-care needs must cope with many kinds of losses, such as altered physical appearance, life-style, abilities, or the loss of life itself. Loss is a stressor and individuals adapt to losses in their own unique way. By using nursing process, nurses identify losses the person is experiencing and the strengths he has available to help him cope. Nurses' communication and teaching skills are used to intervene and assist the person to mobilize his strengths in order to adapt to losses. Professional nurses must recognize that, as persons, they are also affected by their clients' losses. For instance, nurses often grieve with their dying clients and must adapt, much as the person himself does.

The consumer movement in health-care delivery has raised issues related to the rights of dying persons. Many consumers are demanding the choice to end life-prolonging measures for themselves or family members. Such decisions have legal and moral implications for professional nurses.

The surgical experience also provides an illustration of how the seven basic concepts in this book can be used to give person-centered nursing care. Surgery is a frightening experience for most individuals and involves physical trauma to the body. For these reasons, persons experiencing surgery must adapt to many psychological and physiological stressors. Nurses use nursing process before, during, and after surgery to identify clients' unique strengths and needs. They assist clients to mobilize their strengths in order to avoid common postoperative problems. Facilitating clients' learning in the preoperative phase helps them to achieve self-care skills they need following surgery. Preoperative teaching, as well as nurses' communication skills, are essential to alleviate persons' anxiety about their surgery.

The surgical experience has been affected by recent changes in the focus of health-care delivery. Consumers are demanding more information so that they can make knowledgeable choices about the decision to have surgery, the type of anesthesia, or the type of surgical procedure. For example, more women now seek a second opinion when a hysterectomy is recommended. Women with breast cancer are requesting modified radical mastectomy or "lumpectomy" rather than the more disfiguring radical mastectomy. Such consumer behavior has implications for professional nursing practice, particularly in assisting clients to make informed choices about surgery.

We hope that after completing this section, beginning nurses will be able to use the concepts described in this book to help their clients cope with their health-care needs in their own unique way.

Nursing the Person with Loss

Sharon Hein Jette

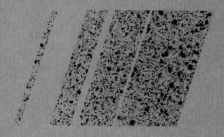

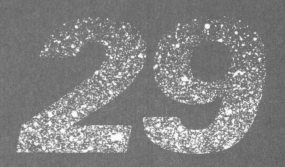

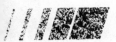

"If we did not care for others in a deep and fundamental way we would not experience grief when they are troubled or disturbed, when they face tragedy or misfortune, when they are ill or dying" (Moustakas, 1961, p. 101).

Throughout this book, the person and his strengths have been emphasized. This emphasis continues to be important in our discussion of nursing the person with loss. This chapter presents the concept of loss as a stressor and discusses the grief reaction as a means of adapting to loss, Specifically, the nurse facilitates the grief reaction by applying the nursing process in recognizing the characteristics of adaptive grief, understanding the process of grieving from various theoretical perspectives, and assisting people to grieve. In the context of loss, dying is presented as a multiple loss experience.

After completing this chapter, students will be able to:

- *Describe various losses as stressors.*

- *Describe adaptive grief.*

- *Describe factors that facilitate adaptive grief.*

- *Recognize factors that interrupt adaptive grief.*

- *Recognize dying as a multiple loss experience.*

- *Protect the rights of the dying person and his family.*

- *Apply nursing process to dying or grieving persons.*

- *Recognize personal needs related to coping with loss.*

Loss and Grief

Concept of Loss as a Stressor

All human beings cope with loss from birth to death. Indeed, birth has been described as a loss of security for both mother and children. Death, while equaled primarily with the loss of life, represents several simultaneous losses.

People's lives are filled with both losses and gains. Some losses seem rather inconsequential; others are devastating and capable of destroying a person's ability to live on. **Loss,** the absence or perceived absence of something once possessed, is a stressor acting upon the individual to produce a wide variety of adaptations. Loss threatens the individual's basic source of security in the world. Although the significance of many losses is not often apparent to the nurse as an observer, the person with loss is in need of nursing care and support.

Object Loss

Peretz (1970) described the loss of anyone or anything previously possessed as **object loss.** He categorizes four types of loss:

- Loss of significant persons
- Loss of valued possessions
- Loss of self-image
- Developmental loss

Loss can be both positive and negative; that is, not all losses are inherently negative. The loss of excess weight, for example, brings positive changes in self-image but also precipitates loss of security as

well. The security of knowing how others react to you as obese may be lost, and there may be uncertainty about the effect the new image will have. A negative loss, such as the death of a spouse, may have the positive effect of making the widow(er) more self-sufficient. Loss can also be considered either real, symbolic, or potential. For example, an amputation represents a very real loss of a limb, but it can also represent symbolic loss of beauty and potential loss of employment. In assessing the health needs of clients, the nurse must become sensitive to these characteristics of loss.

Loss of Significant Persons

This type of loss can occur not only through death but also through divorce, separations, maturation of children, relocations, and communication breakdown. An actual distance or psychological distance may separate persons once close. Single persons may perceive a loss for never having had a spouse or children; a loss of self-concept may occur when the expected roles of spouse and parent are not fulfilled. When children leave home they often leave parents with a feeling of great loss. Families are also separated when members are hospitalized. Indeed, prolonged institutionalization can lead to total separation from loved ones. But a sense of loss can occur without separation. Persons grow apart even though they may be together. Among friends or families, a communication barrier can separate people as completely as a stone wall or a thousand miles.

Valued Possessions

Perhaps you may have lost a wallet or purse and know how such a loss can disrupt normal living patterns. Losing the money, provided it did not amount to an exorbitant sum, was probably insignificant compared to the missing identification cards, appointment books, papers, keys, or personal remembrances. The significance of lost objects to the owner is difficult for anyone else to see. The value of small but irreplaceable objects and possessions may be priceless and varies within cultural groups. In America, for example, it is quite common to treat the loss of a pet as gravely as the loss of a family member. The loss of home or homeland is widely regarded as a major loss, especially when persons are displaced against their will. Children are distressed at the loss of favorite playthings that brought them security and enjoyment. For older people, the accumulation of a lifetime of valued remembrances makes moving oftentimes difficult. Indeed, moving away at any point in life usually means leaving something cherished behind. Few people exist who cannot point to something they value highly which, if lost, would hurt and leave deep feelings of loss. The significant objects with which we identify are often difficult to replace; in losing or leaving them behind, we lose a piece of our identity.

Changes in Self-Image

Throughout life each individual creates for himself and for the world a reflection of who he is. This self-image includes aspects of body image and appearance, social roles, and cultural and personal belief systems. At times a person may strive to change his image; at other times his image is changed by outside forces.

Changes in one's own perceptions of worth, competence, usefulness, prowess, or bodily function can also precipitate feelings of loss. Sometimes losing a comfortable role in life results in great insecurity. For example, upon graduation, students are often overwhelmed to find that the transition from student to professional is quite a challenge. New mothers and fathers faced with the care of an infant are commonly unsure of the expectations of parenthood. Any situation that causes altered body image, such as pregnancy, weight changes, or hair loss, can alter self-image. Enforced retirement presents one of the greatest challenges to workers to change their patterns of productivity. One's beliefs are incorporated into self-image; a change in religious beliefs, cultural practices, or health beliefs can result in feelings of loss and insecurity.

Developmental or Maturational Losses

Throughout a span of years, certain events or turning points are inevitable in the process of maturing. These maturational crises are frequently equated with losses and can challenge the individual to learn new ways of adapting. The birthing process may well be the first such crisis of an infant's life, for he must leave the ultimate security of the womb. Losses of childhood include weaning, teething, and toilet training, this last is both a loss of control over others and a gain of self-control.

At several points, losses of security are evident: going off to school, staying away from home, taking responsibility for work or possessions. These losses are mirrored in subsequent years when one becomes a young adult and moves away from parents, establishing one's own home and making career decisions. Some maturational losses are losses of innocence; learning the realities of the world is painful.

The aging process begins at birth but accelerates in midlife to add further challenges to the maturing adult. Age-related changes in physical appearance and body function produce loss of self-concept as well as developmental loss. At whatever age, the developmental task of dying presents the individual and others caring for him with several losses all at once.

Multiple Loss

Burnside (1973) describes the concept of multiple loss that is characteristic of aging and dying. The older person with multiple loss typically experiences an accumulation of losses. He may be adapting to changes of body function and body image due to the aging process, decreased productivity and income after retirement, separation from home and possessions, and the deaths of friends and family. In the case of a dying person, he may perceive that he is losing everything and everyone of value all at once. Nurses caring for persons with multiple loss need to identify and treat all of the losses and their interactions.

Positive and Negative Losses

The immediate connotation of the word "loss" is a negative one, as is the connotation of "death" in American society. However, each person and each cultural group relates in a unique way to loss, so that any loss has negative and positive attributes.

Loss of chronic pain after joint replacement surgery, for example, is a positive outcome but may represent loss of **secondary gain.** Secondary gain is, "the social and psychological uses a client may make of symptoms, for example, gaining sympathy, psychological support, financial advantages, or special treatment by virtue of being labeled 'ill' " (Wilson and Kneisel, 1979, p. 825). Divorce, separation, and death may actually be a positive relief from physical or mental suffering. To stop smoking or lose weight, although physiologically positive, may provoke emotional insecurity or cravings. In any event, the nurse cannot assume that a given loss will necessarily be negative or positive. Consider the following example:

Nurse A.: "I'll bet you were glad to be rid of those extra pounds ... you look very trim." (assumption)

Client: "Actually it's harder now because I'm unsure how to act."

Instead of assuming the client's reaction, the nurse should validate the actual feelings he has:

Nurse B.: "You were overweight for so long; now what is it like to be thin?" (validation)

Client: "Actually, it's harder. ..."

Real and Symbolic Losses

Tangible or real losses of valued people and objects indicate the absence of something once present. **Potential losses** are those perceived as likely to occur in the future; both real and potential losses cause anxiety and grief. A pregnant woman who is exposed to rubella, for example, may become extremely anxious over the potential loss of her infant.

In contrast, **symbolic losses** represent a range of intangible attributes lost: pride, status, innocence, honesty, privacy. "Loss of face" is a phrase symbolizing embarrassment and loss of pride. Cheating or stealing may be effective coping mechanisms for some persons but a moral loss of honesty, or guilt, may follow. Other persons may describe a loss of privacy felt in crowded housing, in large families, or in cases of assault or rape. Even a very positive experience such as a job promotion brings with it a symbolic loss of secure status at a lower level. As nurses teach, counsel, and provide care, we must be able to assess not only the apparent real losses but also the more subtle symbolic losses of life.

Biophysical, Psychological, Sociocultural, and Spiritual Losses

Just as man is multidimensional, so are his losses. Often a loss occurs in one sphere that eventually affects another sphere. This pattern can accelerate, producing a spiral effect in which one loss leads to another. Figure 29-1 represents a common spiral pattern, beginning with a biophysical hearing loss that often leads to feelings of social isolation and

lowered self-esteem. These feelings in turn lead to withdrawal from social interaction and eventually to psychological depression. Depression, then, manifests as biophysical disturbances of sleep and appetite ... and the cycle continues.

Adaptation to Loss: The Grief Reaction

Adaptive Grief

Thaler (1966) described **grief** as a universal, normal, and developmental adaptive process in reaction to loss. The common term, bereavement, is basically equivalent to the grieving process. This grief process allows the individual to resolve a loss over time. More than 35 years ago, psychiatrist Erich Lindemann (1944) identified acute grief as a syndrome with psychological and somatic symptoms; he differentiated "normal" grief reactions from "morbid" grief reactions that are chronic and unresolved. His pioneer work has helped to define the concept of **adaptive grief** as a resolution of loss that frees up energy previously bound to the loss.

> After an unexpected divorce, Mrs. B. found that she was unable to consider dating other men for almost a year. During this time her actions, thoughts, and feelings were focused on her ex-husband.

Adaptive grief is a healthy process, one which nurses should therefore understand and facilitate in clients.

Adaptive grief may be either anticipatory or reactive to a loss. **Anticipatory grief** begins before the loss occurs and once its inevitability is known; homesick feelings before moving, for example, are common in anticipation of future loneliness. Grief also occurs in anticipation of a maturational loss or crisis such as childbirth or retirement. **Reactive grief,** in contrast, occurs after a loss is sustained.

Characteristics of Adaptive Grief

Adaptive grief is universal but is manifested differently in each culture. Shedding tears, for example, may be very acceptable behavior in some cultures but unacceptable in others. Meditation and quiet prayer may prevail in some ethnic groups, whereas wailing or chanting is more characteristic of others.

Nurses must exercise caution not to judge the grief behavior of other people as "abnormal" in comparison with their own cultural norms; this tendency to judge one's own cultural norm as su-

PSYCHOLOGICAL   SOCIOCULTURAL

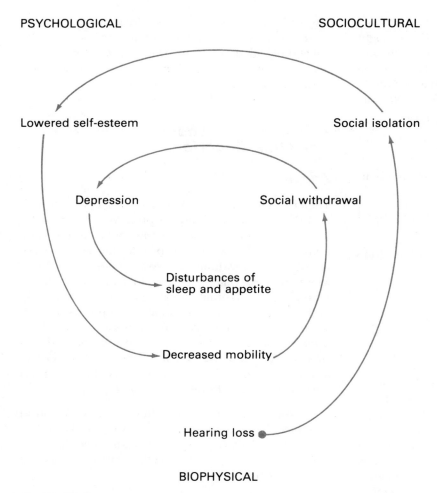

Lowered self-esteem   Social isolation

Depression   Social withdrawal

Disturbances of
sleep and appetite

Decreased mobility

Hearing loss

BIOPHYSICAL

Figure 29-1
Spiral of losses

perior is called **ethnocentricity.** For all peoples, however, grief is a period of intense psychic pain and suffering.

Level of growth and development affects an individual's grief behavior. The young child's concept of loss is limited by his abstract thinking abilities. He may react to any temporary separation with great fear and distress because he believes the loss is permanent. Older children learn to mimic the acceptable grief behaviors of adults. It is very tempting to conclude that the uncontrolled outbursts of a youngster reflect more intense suffering than the restrained grief of an adult. Such a conclusion would fail to account for cultural learning and developmental maturity.

Symptoms of adaptive grief are many and varied, including physical reactions and psychosocial effects (Peretz, 1970). The following reactions are considered adaptive and healthy grief behaviors.

Immediate Physical Reactions
Immediate physical reactions include dyspnea, deep sighing, uncontrolled crying, difficulty swallowing, muscular weakness, inertia, and physical exhaustion. Indeed, even neurogenic shock can occur in response to sudden loss.

Psychological Feelings
Common psychological feelings include anxiety and muscle tension, restlessness, loneliness, emptiness, and confusion. Feelings of distance from others evoke a detachment from life. A painful preoccupation with and yearning for the lost person or object occurs. Other psychological reactions are guilt feelings, such as, "If only I had been nicer to him; now it's too late." Since most human relationships are filled with both kind and unkind interactions, a grief-stricken person usually recalls and regrets some previous behavior.

Another related behavior is irrational anger projected at the lost person or at the closest target person. A nurse trying to comfort the bereaved will often be a target for irrational anger. The griever rejects touch, rejects offers of help, or explodes over small details. He has unpredictable mood changes, from abusive to withdrawn, and expects others to understand him and his needs.

Recently told that his son was seriously ill, Mr. T. shouted at the nurse, "Why do you always leave him alone? He's always alone!"

Another characteristic feeling is loss of time perspective. The griever may actually become confused about the time of day or date. Commonly he is unable or unwilling to look to the future; efforts to assure him that "time will heal" or that "you'll adjust" are futile because he cannot anticipate ever feeling better. It is preferable to help the grieving person to set short-term goals for the next day or the upcoming week. Long-range planning becomes extremely difficult when he is so preoccupied with the past and the present grief.

Depressive Symptoms

At times, depressive symptoms occur. These typically include decreased appetite and weight loss, although some persons do increase food intake; insomnia, especially early morning waking; lethargy and psychic immobilization.[5] The person may complain of helplessness (*i.e.*, I can't"), hopelessness (*i.e.*, "It's no use"), and worthlessness, ("I'm not worth it"). Usually decreased verbal comunication and vague somatic complaints of pain and discomfort follow.

Such signs and symptoms of depression are expected and necessary for the person to heal after a loss; generally, the more severe the loss, the more severe the depression, but this varies among individuals (Fig. 29-2), The duration of depressive behavior also varies, typically with 6 to 12 weeks of acute grief

Figure 29-2
The grieving person requires time to resolve his loss. *(Photo by Bob Kalmbach)*

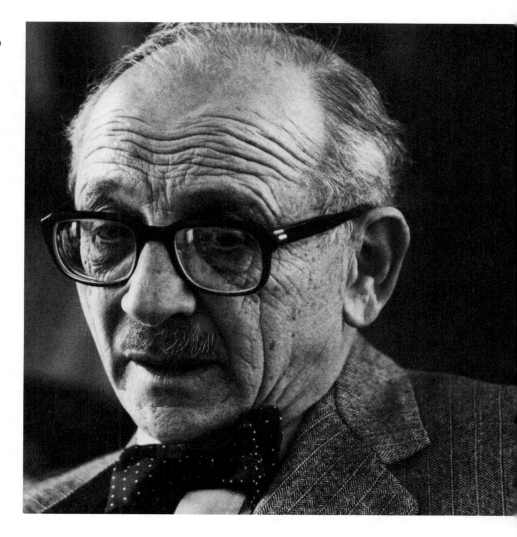

symptoms and up to 2 years of grief resolution (Hodge, 1971). Beyond 2 years, chronic unresolved grief with prolonged depression is not considered adaptive and usually demands professional intervention to resolve. Placing time limits on adaptive grief, however, is difficult because individuals may resolve the loss much more quickly or may need to suppress and delay the reactions.

If a client appears to be making no progress in moving beyond the loss, however, he may be in a state of chronic unresolved grief, also called **morbid grief.** This state represents a failure to adapt to loss. Such a failure may result from overwhelming guilt, personal identification with the lost object or person, or fear of living beyond the loss. In most cases, persons with morbid grief do not fulfill their family and work responsibilities, signaling the need for professional assistance in grief resolution. The nurse should recognize that some persons may develop multiple illness problems as a result of unresolved grief.

Process of Grieving

Several theorists and clinicians have attempted to organize the above listed reactions into a process of grieving. These processes are ordered into phases or stages of grief work through which the individual proceeds toward resolution. Much of the current knowledge about loss and stages of grief comes from observation and interview with dying people and surviving grievers. McGrory (1978) points out the hazards of using any staging theory. Although they provide an organized framework, stages also promote stereotyped expectations about what people should experience. The following examples of grief stages allow us to understand better what the client and family may experience. Any attempt to use these stages to judge what client reactions should be or to force movement through stages is unjustified and unwise. These stages are a basis for understanding, not mandates.

Engel: Stages of Grieving

George Engel, a psychotherapist, viewed grief as an emotional wound and identified three stages of grieving to heal the wound (1964).

- Shock and disbelief—These immediate reactions are accompanied by numbness, disorganization, immobility, and denial of reality.
- Developing awareness—When the pain of loss penetrates the conscious awareness of the person, feelings of emptiness, anger and hostility,

frustration, and guilt emerge. These endure as long as necessary for the person to gain full awareness of the meaning of the loss.
- Restitution—After gaining full awareness, the griever accepts that he must cope realistically. He begins to resume personal routines and seeks new pleasures without shame or guilt.

Glaser and Strauss: Stages of Awareness

Glaser and Strauss (1965) developed four stages of awareness to describe the interaction between the dying person and the family and health professionals; because dying is a situation of multiple loss, these stages resemble Engel's stages of grief.

- Closed awareness—At this first level the client has no knowledge of his dying condition and no anticipation of loss. Family and health professionals may know, however, and change their behavior accordingly so that the client's awareness increases.
- Suspicious awareness—A game of hide-the-truth may develop in which the dying person seeks information and the family or professionals choose to deceive him for his benefit or their own. This stage provokes denial and anger.
- Mutual pretense—At some point both the client and family or staff become aware that the other knows of the impending death, but no one speaks. Often this period of awkward pretense only serves to increase anger and guilt feelings.
- Open awareness—This level of awareness indicates full and open communication between the dying and survivors. At this point the individual may plan and express his preferences, hopefully with the support of family and staff. A flood of anger and depression may be released, however, if the pretense has been prolonged. With an open interaction, this can be resolved so that the dying person can make as many choices as possible in his remaining lifetime.

Kübler–Ross: Stages of Dying

Building on this earlier work, Elisabeth Kübler–Ross (1969) refined five stages of grieving during the dying process. She observes that not all dying persons move through the same sequence of all five stages. Individual variation is great even though a general pattern emerges:

- Denial and shock (No, not me!)—The immediate response of shock gives way to denial attempts. The person cannot yet believe the impending loss and so seeks to protect himself by intellectual denial and avoidance of the subject of death. Eventually such pretense collapses when the person is able or ready to feel the reality. If denial is prolonged, the client needs continued support in his struggle to face reality.

- Anger (Why me?)—In gaining some reality of his fate, the client often resents his misery compared to the health and happiness of others. Family and staff care givers receive the bitter projections of irrational anger, as decribed earlier. A key response of care givers is to tolerate this essential venting without feeling it as a personal attack, for eventually it will subside.

- Bargaining (Yes, me . . . but . . .)—The third stage of dying is one of wishing for extended time, a peaceful death, or other requests to ease the reality of losing everything. Bargaining with God or another higher power is common, but so is bargaining with professional staff. The client seeks to exchange "good" behavior for an extension of life long enough to finish some business. This ploy helps him adapt to reality, sustains his hope and minimizes his losses.

- Depression (Yes . . . me.)—Some depression is inevitable and normal during such a massive grief process as dying. Kübler–Ross found that the predominant need to withdraw into oneself was preparatory for a final separation. The dying person needs time to review his life, to seek what psychiatrist Avery Weisman (1977) terms the "significant survival"—making the remaining life most meaningful.

- Acceptance—The final stage of acceptance depends upon the client's ability and time to work through previous feelings with the support of care givers. He will have grieved for the loss of valued things and finished all meaningful business. The nature of this acceptance can involve peaceful, calm acknowledgment of the losses, discriminating positive from negative consequences, forgiving of self and others, or inner resolution, even yearning to die.

Kübler–Ross identifies hope as the element essential to growth throughout this grieving process. The hope of a peaceful death and freedom from pain sustains many persons facing death. Hope springs from cultural and religious beliefs about the meaning of this life and other future lives or states of existence. As nurses we provide hope by encouraging the dying to live as fully as possible. We never wish to deprive the dying person or his family of the hope needed to face death.

Do Stages Really Exist?

Current education and research on death seek to validate these stages and provide more data about their variations for different ages and cultures. Kowalsky (1978) suggests that "acceptance" or "adjustment" may be unrealistic expectations; a more appropriate goal would be successful "adaptation," in which the person may not be required to accept a grave loss but can still adapt to it.

Theories of universal grieving processes remain controversial. Schneidman (1976), for example, disputes the concept of predictable stages. Instead, he identifies a complex mixture of intellectual and affective states that are not universal in type or sequence. These feeling states and behaviors include disbelief, hope, anguish, terror, acquiescence and surrender, rage and envy, disinterest, pretense, daring, and even yearning for death, all amidst pain and bewilderment at the situation. Schulz and Alderman (1974) conclude that clinical research on the dying process does not clearly support five distinct stages. Kastenbaum (1975) notes that no existing theories of the grief process account fully for client's age and sex differences, ethnicity, or the effect of the social environment.

Assisting People to Grieve

All of the theories and stages of grieving and dying hold implications for nurses who assist people to grieve. Nurses very often are the care givers most in contact with grieving persons and families at home and in institutions. In order to assist people to grieve, we need an awareness of the factors facilitating and interrupting adaptive grief (Peretz, 1970).

Factors that Facilitate Adaptive Grief

The nurse can assist a person to proceed through an adaptive grief process by the following means:

- Listening to the concerns expressed by the griever(s) without defending, justifying, or explaining away any complaints. This includes effective use of silence.

- Anticipating and providing basic comfort and safety, at home or in an institution. Simple gestures such as providing a tissue or a glass of water are greatly appreciated.

- Acknowledging the reality of the loss and feeling reactions.

- Avoiding diminishing the significance of the loss. Do not, for example, make statements like, "You'll soon be pregnant again and can replace this child."

- Identifying and reinforcing the person's strengths, maintaining hope by building on his capabilities. A sincere, "I know you will never forget him but I will help you find the strength to understand his death," provides empathy, support, and hope to the bereaved.

- Maintaining an open relationship through even the most difficult phases of grief when, as a result of anger or rejection, the relationship may be strained.

- Allowing the griever to experience the pain and express feelings as he is ready and able to do so; although moderate use of sedation or distraction may be helpful, it may also allow him to suppress, ignore, or delay grieving.

- Allowing privacy and freedom from distraction when requested or needed. This demands flexible scheduling of physical care or other interruptions.

- Helping people to anticipate what will occur and when. This lowers their anticipatory anxiety so they may realistically prepare.

- Facilitating as much control and choice as possible in decisions of activities, treatments, or problem solving. This must be done without overwhelming the person's limited energy reserve.

Factors that Interrupt Adaptive Grief

In contrast to the above measures which facilitate grieving, the nurse can interrupt adaptation to loss in the following ways:

- Reinforcing denial, arguing with denial, or joining a pretense between the individual and family. By agreeing that he will soon be well or, "You're better off without him," one can delay acknowledgment or reinforce denial. Denial is an essential defense mechanism and a helpful buffer from pain, but by reinforcing denial we increase the person's dependence on it.

- Engaging in punishing reactions (on the part of the nurse) that show rejection and control. The nurse who returns projected anger to persons or family risks increasing their guilt and closing the lines of communication.

- Bargaining with the griever or family, thereby raising false hopes. Promising gifts or rewards to a grieving person only distracts him and may make him distrust you.

- Advocating a quick solution is shortsighted. Overuse of tranquilizers or alcohol during grieving, making major life change decisions, or returning too soon to daily responsibilities may temporarily help but may delay grief resolution.

- Providing secondary gain in the form of prolonged attention, increased affection, or a dependency relationship. Such reactions may remove the griever's incentive to complete adaptive grief work. It is necessary for the griever to trust the nurse at the same time he strives for self-sufficiency and recovery from loss.

Indications of Progress in Grieving

When the grieving person is showing adaptive grief resolution, he typically presents a pattern of decreased preoccupation with the loss over time, increased ability to resume future-oriented planning, and gradual return to life responsibilities. Some persons delay resolution by returning immediately to daily responsibilities and future planning.

Other measures of progress in grieving include resumption of pleasurable activity without feeling guilt and the establishment of new relationships, new possessions, or new goals.

Dying: A Multiple Loss Experience

Dying, viewed from the perspective of the dying person, can be considered a multiple loss. The family is losing one person; but the dying person is losing everything all at once. He is losing the people he loves, the possessions he values, and life as he knows it. Although it is theoretically possible to anticipate and prepare for this inevitable multiple loss, it is difficult to anticipate one's own death.

In the past two decades, educators and researchers have expanded the understanding of grieving to include the specific grief process of dying. Death is no longer the taboo subject it was even 10 years ago. Today a wealth of written materials and media illuminate several approaches to the multiple loss of dying. The need continues for controlled study of the experience in order to validate these various approaches in differing age groups, sexes, cultures, and environments.

Cross-Cultural Perspectives on Dying

Values of life and death vary throughout the world, but even in the United States a picture of evolving values and practices is seen. When nurses become care givers to a dying person of an ethnic or racial group other than their own, they will see many variations in styles of adapting. Some native American Indians, for example, express grief and honor for the dead by preparing favorite foods of the deceased and expressing a desire to bring such foods or possessions to the hospital (Joe, 1976). American Blacks rely very heavily on support of family members and the church during times of grief or death. Large groups of extended family may wish to visit the hospital or home of a dying relative. The Irish wake and the Jewish shiva are both examples of grief vigils for the dead but they vary greatly in solemnity. Christian faith provides its members with a strength, a "dying grace," in the hope of the next life.

Pain and suffering may be expressed differently based on cultural norms. Kalish and Reynolds (1976) found that Japanese-Americans valued the controlled expression of grief emotions and would attempt to sustain emotional control if bereaved. Although many nurses are inclined to stereotype this behavior as "stoic," it may express strong feelings of pain (Davitz *et al*, 1976).

Hospice versus Hospital

Care for the dying has changed within American culture during this century. Whereas earlier generations died at home among families as a norm, today the majority of deaths occur in hospitals and nursing homes. These institutions have been accepted as places appropriate to die, especially for the old and chronically ill. There is, however, a growing demand for alternatives of care for the dying person and his family. Recognizing that the needs of the dying person at home place enormous stress on the family, the **hospice** alternative has gained recent success.

Hospice is a philosophy and program of active relief of distress and personal involvement of the dying with family and care givers. It is a concept rather than a place; it need not be equated with home death, either. The model for this concept is St. Christopher's Hospice, founded in 1948 to provide "hospitality" or a place of refreshment and rest for those on the journey of dying (Saunders, 1977). The hospice program offers home care, institutional care as needed, control of chronic pain, support for family, and hope for the dying.

Rights of the Dying Person and Family

Annas (1974) contends that the dying person needs an advocate to help him assert his rights. He believes nurse-advocates should provide the opportunity for clients to enjoy the following rights:

- Right to know the truth when he is ready to hear it.
- Right to confidentiality and privacy.
- Right to informed consent to treatment.
- Right to choose a place to die.
- Right to choose the time of death.
- Right to determine the disposition of his body.

Several laws have assisted the client to achieve these rights. The Euthanasia Education Council in New York City developed a Living Will to provide a moral obligation (and a legal obligation in a few states) to help the client fight loss of control. All states recognize the Uniform Anatomical Donor card as a legal expression of the person's wishes for his body or body parts. Institutional policies and procedures should also incorporate these rights.

The nurse can protect these rights by maintaining an open relationship with client and family, observing for signs of readiness to hear reality, protecting confidentiality, and teaching what to expect in impending treatment.

Client's Adaptation to Dying

Reactions to death vary not only according to cultural patterns but also according to developmental level.

Children

Nagy (1959) developed three levels at which children comprehend death. In her view, the child under 5 equates death with separation. From approximately 5 to 9 years, he realizes the permanent and personal nature of death. After 9 to 10 years of age, death becomes understood as inevitable and universal. Subsequent work in child psychology examines more of the cultural and socioeconomic variables in the child's view of death. Bluebond–Langner (1977), for example, hypothesizes that adults and children have similar concepts of death, which are expressed differently.

Clinical observations show that children do think of death and do incorporate death play as a part of their development. Although their words fail to express what they feel when dying, children may adapt by using play, visual arts, or movement to communicate nonverbally. Creative nursing demands that we provide outlets for the child to express his dying. Nursing of the dying child should include roles of advocacy and information-sharing on this difficult journey.

Adolescents

To the adolescent, the chance of death is usually so remote that it is easy to deny the risks of street violence, dangerous driving habits, or taking drugs. Usually the teenager has adopted a concept of time, life, and death that shields him from considering his own death. But at a stage of life when self-concept is so dependent on his physical appearance and ability, the adolescent with any disability or disfigurement may find it difficult to adapt. The dying adolescent typically rebels against any disfiguring or dependent aspect of terminal illness because it threatens his self-concept. Typically he expresses feelings of frustration at not experiencing adulthood fully, anger at the energy of his peers, and loss of control over his own body (Kastenbaum, 1977).

Adults

Williams (1976) described three common fears of death as described by adults:

- Fear of a painful death
- Fear of loneliness or of dying alone
- Fear that life (or his life) is meaningless

Nurses are very likely to hear and see these fears expressed, and they very much need to be able to respond by listening, using empathy, and problem solving. Adult clients will show certain expectations; most expect the oldest in their families or the most frail with chronic illness to die first. When these expectations are violated, when an apparently healthy adult dies in the prime of life, adaptation is often more difficult because of less mental and economic preparation.

Older Adults

In old age, death may be not only expected and anticipated but also welcomed; just as often, however, death is resisted. The person who survives to a very old age has adapted to many, many losses throughout life, often outliving spouse(s), friends, even children. For elders who are active, perhaps just retired, death may deprive them of a long-awaited time to enjoy life. For others who are faced with disability or pain, death may be a welcome relief from the sufferings of this world.

Family's Adaptation to Dying

How do family and beloved others relate to this significant loss? Based on clinical nursing research,

Hampe (1975) identifies eight needs of the spouses of dying persons:

- To be with the dying person
- To be helpful to him
- To have the assurance of his comfort
- To be informed of his condition
- To be informed of his impending death
- To air emotions
- To have comfort and support of other family members
- To have the acceptance and support of professionals

With knowledge of these specific needs of family members, nurses can anticipate their requests and offer the support they need to help the client. Often nurses feel distracted from providing client care when families interrupt; in reality, a small investment in meeting the family's needs allows the family to meet more of the needs of the dying person.

The reactions of grieving family members may parallel or differ drastically from those of the dying person. A wife may show anger, for example, at her husband's denial of his terminal illness; or both may be experiencing depression at the same time. Separate assessments must be made to determine what each person is expressing. Nonparallel feeling states between client and family demand that the nurse be aware of each, meet the needs of each, and help them meet the needs of each other (Fig. 29-3).

After the death of a loved one, survivors typically experience 6 to 12 weeks of acute grief and a period of adaptive grieving lasting 1 to 2 years, as mentioned earlier. The death of someone close is particularly threatening because it reminds us of our own mortality. Indeed, one typical crisis of mid-life occurs after the adult loses both parents and realizes that in the natural order he is next to die. Kalish and Reynolds (1976) interviewed people of various cultures, genders, and ages and discovered that the death of an older person was generally more acceptable and anticipated than death in any other age group. Respondents explained that older people have lived full lives, may be experiencing chronic illnesses and pain, or are nearing the end of their years, and so death is expected.

When younger family members die, survivors may feel robbed of a full lifetime together. Middle-aged persons leave growing families behind to struggle with emotional and economic loss; these families may feel bitter abandonment. Young adults die without establishing themselves in life. With smaller

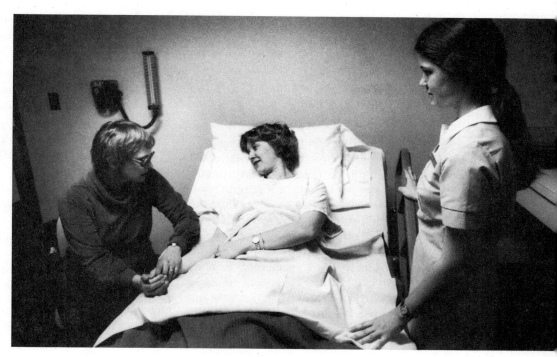

Figure 29-3
The nurse offers family members the support they need
to help the client. *(Photo by Bob Kalmbach)*

families and declining rates of childhood diseases, the loss of one child seems perhaps more tragic now than years ago when families expected to lose several children. These age-related attitudes vary immensely among individuals. In their attempts to understand a relative's death, families will often wish to relive or retell stories about the lost person. This may or may not be acceptable to other friends, relatives, or even health professionals. Often families are afraid others will forget the dead ones they love. Unfortunately, a typical comment of bereaved families is this:

> "Once he died, no one mentioned him any more to me. It was as if I should suffer silently and forget quickly."

This behavior results more from awkward anxiety than insensitivity; nurses need to master the empathy skill necessary to overcome such awkward anxiety and acknowledge the dead person. For example, the nurse might say:

> "It seems that the holidays remind you of your wife."

> or

> "I wonder if seeing these other children reminds you of your son?"

A growing number of resources exist for bereaved family members. Many seek the support of each other, clergy, neighbors, or friends. Others derive assistance from mutual help organizations such as the Widow-to-Widow Program, in which widows who have grieved successfully counsel and support recent widows. Those bereaved family members who seek professional help of therapists and counselors, including nurses, can be assisted to express and resolve their grief. Remember, the losses—anticipated and experienced—are very real, very painful reminders of one's own death.

Nurses' and Other Professionals' Adaptation to Dying

Losing clients can also be considered as a multiple loss situation. As nurses become involved with dying persons and their families, we too experience the grief of losing people about whom we care.

Benoliel (1977) describes five settings in which nurses are most likely to encounter dying and may be ill-prepared to cope with it:

- The intensive care unit, in which people are always "critical," never "dying"

- The emergency room, which is ill-equipped to meet psychosocial needs
- The recovery and postsurgical units, which are oriented to curing
- Chronic care facilities, in which many deaths are expected
- Terminal care programs, in which there is recognition of no curative treatment

If nurses hold the expectations that most clients will live, they may be unable to cope with unexpected client deaths, multiple deaths in a short time span, or waves of staff grief in response to client deaths.

Physicians, nurses, and other professionals, however, well intentioned, often face overwhelming demands on their time that prevent them from dealing with even the obvious grieving of clients, families, and staff. In many situations nurses need more support and sanction for counseling the grieving. Another alternative has been to place mental health personnel or clergy in key locations, such as emergency rooms, to assist the griefstricken (Garfield, 1977).

The question for nurses to consider is one of balancing one's own values with one's capacity to care for the dying. How do you cope with intense emotional interactions daily and still retain the outlook and energy to sustain yourself? With each death, we lose someone; we might identify closely with a client of our age or background, making the loss still more personal. Our own grief, fear, frustration, irrational anger, and depression can easily project onto other personnel. Nurses working with the dying have found strength within themselves and from each other.

Values Clarification

By using values clarification, a self-awareness process, nurses can assess their own strengths and compare views with other nurses (Steele and Harmon, 1979). Several simple values clarification exercises exist to trigger group discussion on dying (Murray and Zentner, 1979; McGrory, 1978; Epstein, 1975). Three brief examples follow:

Example 1. Complete the following lifeline for yourself. The dot represents your birth and the line is your lifeline (Fig. 29-4).

- Extend the line as necessary to represent the length of your lifespan. Place a number on the line representing the age at which you predict your death will occur.
- Place a circled number on the line indicating the age at which ideally you would wish to die. Place an X on the line at your present age.
- Complete the diagram, drawing a symbol representing your concept of death.
- Share and compare lifelines with your colleagues. What concepts do you share? What are your unique values? Can you identify how your values might affect your relationships with dying persons? With other colleagues?

One nursing student wrote the following:

I expect to live well into my nineties because all of my grandparents and two greatgrandparents did and I'm healthier than they were. I'd prefer to die healthy at 85, however; I put my current age down but the X really should be at least ⅓ of the way along the line; I guess I'm further along than I thought. My concept of an afterlife is that of a higher existence in another realm, not back on earth. I think I could become discouraged working with someone who had no concept of anything beyond this life. It might be hard for me to give them hope."

Example 2. In thinking about my own death I would be most afraid of:

- Physical pain
- Loss of control
- Loss of loved ones
- The unknown
- Other

Example 3. If I were able to choose how I would die, I would choose....

Figure 29-4
A personal lifeline

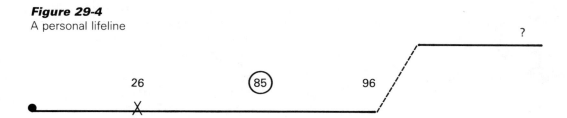

Support Groups/Discussion

Case study discussions provide another alternative for identifying the values of clients, families, and care givers who are experiencing loss.

Although it is important to learn more of one's own values concerning loss and death, support and guidance must be available to the nurse or nursing student during this process. Nurses working in oncology have found that both individually and collectively they experience feelings of guilt, inadequacy, and helplessness (Blake, 1977). These feelings can cause frustration and job dissatisfaction. One way to cope with such overwhelming feelings is to institute a network of mutual support in which nurses help each other to grieve the loss of clients. Formal group discussion, coupled with informal sensitivity and support, have allowed nurses to maintain their caring energies while effectively nursing the dying.

Nursing Process
Applied to the Dying or Grieving Person

With the foregoing concepts of loss, grief, death and dying, the nurse may apply the nursing process to give knowledgeable care to persons experiencing loss.

Grief and Loss

Assessment

Identification of Losses

In assessing someone who is experiencing loss, the nurse strives to gain a holistic picture of the person and his situation. In particular, identifying the current loss and past history of losses is helpful. The client's description of the current loss and its significance to him is required subjective data. Important physical variables to assess include, among others: level of mental alertness; use and effects of any medication including alcohol; and patterns of sleeping, eating, and activity indicative of depression. Developmental achievements, social supports, economic concerns, and patterns of interaction with others provide clues to the person's psychosocial adaptation.

Although these data would often be compiled into a problem-oriented record (POR) system, McGrory (1978) warns that such a system emphasizes the negative aspects of adaptation, especially for a dying person. Instead she advocates a strength-oriented nursing record (SONR) to facilitate a well model approach. Such an assessment would identify, record, and strengthen the person's abilities rather than disabilities. McGrory feels that this approach is essential to the continued hope for the dying and their care givers.

Data Analysis and Loss Statements

In the data analysis step of the nursing process, identifying the actual, potential, or perceived loss may be preferable to listing "problems" for grief-stricken clients. Examples of loss statements include those below:

- Potential loss of self-esteem due to anticipated retirement
- Body image alterations after mastectomy
- Appetite and weight loss due to unresolved grief

Such statements of the loss and apparent cause do not unfairly label the client with a psychiatric diagnosis such as "depressive reaction" or "obsession with recent widowhood," when the person is likely to be experiencing adaptive grieving.

Therapeutic Care

Goals and Goal Statements

In the planning of care, realistic goals preferably are set by the client, but very often grieving or dying clients are unable to be future oriented. Therefore, it becomes a nursing responsibility to monitor readiness and progress toward realistic and very short-term goals. Examples of goal statements include these:

- Client will express the impact of retirement on his life.
- Client will view mastectomy scar; will resume self-care in bathing, dressing, and other ADL.

These represent positive statements of progress for individuals with various losses.

Nursing Interventions

In situations of potential loss, nurses will be providing **anticipatory guidance** or psychosocial support and problem solving prior to the expected loss or crises. Specific examples of anticipatory guidance include the following:

- Preretirement counseling
- Genetic counseling
- Preoperative teaching

Anticipatory guidance allows the griever to prepare, to test out solutions, to share feelings, and to build hope before immersion into an acute grief reaction.

During the grieving process, grief work is facilitated by the factors listed above under Assisting People to Grieve. For nurses, a very typical response is the need to "do something for the grieving client" such as bringing comfort items or repositioning the person. Two skills, being with the person and active listening while providing care, are essential. Many basic needs such as food, drink, and rest, safety, and privacy can be anticipated and met before the client feels angry or helpless.

An open relationship that acknowledges the loss(es), avoids reinforcing denial or anger, and allows expression of feelings, becomes the basis for effective grieving. Small choices can be provided as the griever is ready; to dictate advice or mandate any one approach to grief work robs the client of self-control. It is advisable to allow privacy and dignity for clients and families during grief work to evoke and expect expression of feelings in an open relationship. One key intervention to maintain a well model approach is to identify and reinforce adaptive coping. Any significant family members or others can assist the griever if their own needs for information and support are met.

Evaluation

Determining any individual's progress through the grieving process poses a dilemma of professional judgment. With such varied norms inherent in the grief process, the nurse must exercise caution not to stigmatize or unfairly judge the person who is dealing with lingering grief. The person should be evaluated against the very specific short-term goals set in the nursing process.

As the nurse reassesses the grieving person, the following are indications of long-range progress:

- Decreased preoccupation with the loss
- Ability to assume future-oriented thinking and planning
- Return to pre-loss responsibilities
- Resumption of pleasurable activities without guilt
- Establishment of new relationships or goals

Conclusion

Loss, a universal stressor throughout life, produces a variety of grief reactions determined by the type of loss, cultural norms, and amount of available support. The grieving person's experiences of acute grief and adaptive grief are outlined. Several theoretical constructs of the grief process and stages of grieving provide a framework for examining client and family reactions. Nurses and other care givers experience many of the same grief reactions and feelings as the bereaved persons they help. In order to assist nurses as care givers to the grieving, this chapter presents several factors that facilitate grief work and several that interrupt the process. Dying is explored as a multiple loss situation; dying clients and their families lose many things at once. As a unifying approach, the nursing process provides a structure for meeting the needs of grieving persons.

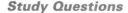

Study Questions

1. In this chapter, the concepts of grief and loss were purposefully emphasized over those of death and dying. Explain the rationale for this emphasis.

2. How can loss be a growth-producing experience?

3. Explain how loss is both universal and uniquely personal.

4. Nurses need help coping with loss just as clients do. Explain.

5. Mr. W., a 45-year-old construction foreman, died unexpectedly of

a massive heart attack while on the job. He had not had any previous history of heart trouble. You are with Mrs. W. in the emergency room when Dr. Jones breaks the shocking news. How might you intervene to assist her?

6. The members of Mrs. S.'s family are in disagreement about whether she should be told of her impending death. How might a nurse intervene to help them resolve the conflict?

7. "Loss" has been presented as a synthesis concept. Helping persons to cope with loss utilizes the other major concepts of the book, *i.e.,* person, adaptation, health, nursing process, communication, and professionalism. Illustrate this synthesis with an example of your choice.

Glossary

Adaptive grief: A resolution of loss that frees up energy previously bound to the loss.

Anticipatory grief: The grief that begins before the loss occurs, once its inevitability is known.

Anticipatory guidance: Psychosocial support and problem solving offered in anticipation of a crisis or loss.

Ethnocentricity: The tendency to judge one's own cultural norms as superior.

Grief: A universal, normal, and developmental adaptive process in reaction to loss.

Hospice: A philosophy and program both of active relief of distress and of personal involvement of the dying with family and care givers.

Loss: The absence or perceived absence of something once possessed.

Morbid grief: A state of chronic unresolved grief.

Object loss: The loss of anyone or anything previously possessed.

Potential losses: Losses perceived as likely to occur in the future.

Reactive grief: The grief that occurs after a loss is sustained.

Secondary gain: The social and psychosocial uses a client may make of symptoms, for example, gaining sympathy, psychological support, financial advantages, or special treatment by virtue of being labeled "ill."

Symbolic losses: Intangible attributes lost such as pride, status, innocence, honesty, or privacy.

Tangible or **real losses:** The absence of valued people or objects that were once present.

Bibliography

Annas G: Rights of the terminally ill patient. J Nurs Adm 4:40–44, March-April, 1974

Benoliel J: Nurses and the human experience of dying. In Feifel H (ed): New Meanings of Death, pp 123–142. New York, McGraw-Hill, 1977

Blake S: Working together to live with dying. Nurs '77 7:64D–N, 1977

Bluebond-Langner M: Meanings of death in children. In Feifel H (ed): New Meanings of Death, pp 47–66. New York, McGraw-Hill, 1977

Burnside I: Multiple loss in the aged: Implications for nursing care. Gerontologist 13:157–162, Summer, 1973

Davitz L, Sameshima Y, Davitz J et al: Suffering as viewed in six different cultures. Am J Nurs 76:1296–1297, August, 1976

Engel G: Grief and grieving. Am J Nurs 64:93–98, September, 1964

Epstein C: Nursing the Dying Patient. Reston, VA, Reston, 1975

Garfield C: Impact of death on the health care professional. In Feifel H (ed): New Meanings of Death, pp 143–151. New York, McGraw-Hill, 1977

Glaser B, Strauss A: Awareness of Dying. Chicago, Aldine, 1965

Hampe S: Needs of grieving spouses in the hospital setting. Nurs Res 24:113–120, March-April, 1975

Hodge J: Help your patients to mourn better. Med Times 99:53–64, 1971

Joe J, Gallerito C, Pino J et al: Cultural health traditions: American Indian perspective. In Branch M, Paxton P (eds): Providing Safe Nursing Care for Ethnic People of Color, pp 81–98. New York, Appleton-Century-Crofts, 1976

Kalish R, Reynolds D: Death and Ethnicity: A Psychocultural Investigation. Los Angeles, University of Southern California Press, 1976

Kastenbaum R: Is death a life crisis? In Datan N, Ginsberg L (eds): Life-Span Developmental Psychology: Normative Life Crises, pp 19–50. New York, Academic Press, 1975

Kastenbaum R: Death and development through the lifespan. In Feifel H (ed): New Meanings of Death, pp 17–45. New York, McGraw-Hill, 1977

Kowalsky E: Grief: A lost life-style. Am J Nurs 78:418–420, March, 1978

Kübler–Ross E: On Death and Dying. New York, Macmillan, 1969

Lindemann E: Symptomatology and management of acute grief. Am J Psychiatry 101:141–148, September 1944

McGrory A: A Well-Model Approach to Care of the Dying Client. New York, McGraw-Hill, 1978

Moustakas C: Loneliness. Englewood Cliffs, Prentice-Hall, 1961

Murray R, Zentner J: Death: The last developmental stage. In Murray R, Zentner J (eds): Nursing Assessment and Health Promotion through the Lifespan, pp 409–438. Englewood Cliffs, NJ, Prentice-Hall, 1979

Nagy M: The child's view of death. In Feifel H (ed): The Meaning of Death, pp 79–98. New York, McGraw-Hill, 1959

Peretz D: Development, object relationship, and loss. In Schoenberg B et al (eds): Loss and Grief: Psychosocial Management in Medical Practice, pp 3–19. New York, Columbia University Press, 1970

Peretz D: Reaction to loss. In Schoenberg B, Carr AC, Peretz D, Kutscher AH (eds): Loss and Grief: Psychosocial Management in Medical Practice, pp 20–35. New York, Columbia University Press, 1970

Saunders C: Dying they live: St. Christopher's Hospice. In Feifel H (ed): New Meanings of Death, pp 153–179. New York, McGraw-Hill, 1977

Schneidman ES: Death work and stages of dying. In Schneidman ES (ed): Death: Current Perspectives, pp 443–451. Palo Alto, CA, Mayfield Publishers, 1976

Schulz R, Alderman D: Clinical research and the 'stages of dying.' Omega 5:137–144, Summer 1974

Steele SM, Harmon VM: Values Clarification in Nursing. New York, Appleton-Century-Crofts, 1979

Thaler OF: Grief and depression. Nurs Forum 5, No. 2:9–22, 1966

Weissman AD: The psychiatrist and the inexorable. In Feifel H (ed): New Meanings of Death, pp 107–122. New York, McGraw-Hill, 1977

Williams JC: Allaying Common Fears in Dealing with Death and Dying. Jenkintown, PA, Intermed Communications, 1976

Wilson HS, Kneisel CR: Psychiatric Nursing. Menlo Park, CA, Addison-Wesley, 1979

The Person Experiencing Surgery: A Synthesis

Mary L. Hunter and Ann Z. Kruszewski

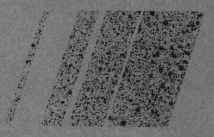

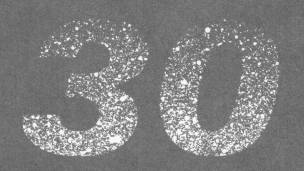

30

The needs of persons hospitalized for surgery provide the student with an opportunity to apply concepts described throughout this book. The holistic health model, nursing process, and the principles of self-care can promote adaptation for those experiencing surgery. The holistic health approach purports that the person is a constitutional whole with mutually dependent parts that are systematically coordinated. Interaction of the parts results in a unique individual.

Surgery is a physical experience because it is performed on a part of the body. The body adapts in various ways in order to heal itself following surgery. If the body is to make a successful adaptation, the mind and spirit need to function at an optimal level. The person needs to experience a sense of hopefulness, a high level of self-esteem, and an ability to use coping strategies that promote adaptation and healing. Surgery often alters one's self-concept, at least temporarily. Nurses need to consider all these issues carefully and facilitate a positive surgical experience for their clients. This chapter assists students to synthesize information already learned and to provide nursing care of the person undergoing surgery. Table 30-1 lists the concepts and subconcepts that you will apply when providing surgical nursing care.

Factors that Affect Adaptation to Surgery

Anxiety

Research studies have indicated that most people awaiting surgery experience some degree of anxiety, whether or not they have had surgery in the past. Generally the following concerns are expressed:

- Finances
- Loss of job
- Concern for dependent family members
- Disruption of present and life plans
- The unknown
- Pain
- Change or destruction of body image
- Loss of control of life (Carnevali, 1966, pp. 1536–1538)

Mild anxiety can be useful to helping one cope with fears, but too much anxiety can be detrimental. For example, stress and anxiety can affect the person's physical status at the time of surgery, influencing the autonomic neural mechanisms and increasing the potential for shock. Nursing research has often demonstrated that stress and anxiety can be significantly reduced if a comprehensive preoperative plan is followed. Such a plan should include the following:

- Assessing the psychological and sociocultural statuses and problem solving when needed.

- Assessing physical statuses to provide baseline data for postoperative evaluation.
- Providing a description of pre- and postoperative activities to the person.
- Offering an opportunity for the person to practice activities in which he will be expected to participate, in order to promote a satisfactory recovery, *i.e.*, activities such as coughing and deep breathing exercises, leg exercises, turning, getting out of bed, ambulation.
- Providing a description of the plan for control of postoperative pain and nausea and explaining how the person can participate in assessing these problems, including what medications are available, and indicating when to ask for medication.
- Including the family and other significant persons in the plan of care.
- Explaining hospital policies about times when the family can visit and where they should wait during surgery.

Because some people become more anxious when they are given information, the nurse should assess each individual in order to provide the appropriate kind and amount of information. However, some parts of a teaching plan, such as postoperative activities, are essential even if they do increase anxiety. Nonetheless, the nurse must remain alert to anxiety states in the client and provide the supportive help needed by listening and providing additional information. Studies indicate that persons receiving a comprehensive care plan have less difficulty with postoperative vomiting and use fewer postoperative

Table 30-1
Concepts and Subconcepts of Person-Centered Nursing Care

Concepts	Subconcepts
Person	Holism
	Systems theory
	Basic needs
	View of self
	Psychosocial development
	Cognitive development
	Self-care
Health and adaptation	Stress
	Crisis
	Coping
	Loss and grief
	Aging
Health-care delivery	Systems
	Consumerism
	Preventive health care
	Nurse advocacy
	Variables that influence health
Professionalism	Responsibility and accountability
	Independent, dependent, and interdependent functions
	Legal implications
	Practice options
Communication	Helping relationship
	Empathy
Nursing process	Psychological status
	Physical statuses
	Culture
	Sexuality
Learning–teaching	Health education
	Level of knowledge
	Level of comprehension
	Learner readiness

pain medications (Dumas and Leonard, 1963; Healy, 1968).

In an unpublished study by Hunter and Britton (1973), some interesting examples of preoperative anxiety were demonstrated. As you read about them, consider the principles of communication from Chapter 13. The study was conducted by giving the Gottschalk anxiety test the night before surgery to 45 subjects about to undergo abdominal hysterectomy. The test consists of the following elements:

- Asking the subject to tell the nurse a short (5-minute) story about an incident in her life. The incident may be recent or past, happy or sad.

- Using the available scoring guide to determine the amount of anxiety the subject has expressed (Gottschalk, 1961).

This test was carried out on all the subjects in the study. The degree of anxiety expressed varied greatly but in each case at least some anxiety was demonstrated. Four stories that were particularly significant are described here. The first two women were cheerful and displayed no overt signs of anxiety, whereas the third and fourth expressed anxiety openly.

Example 1 ☐ Mrs. T., a 45-year-old woman who was married and the mother of four teenagers, described their house fire, which had occurred 2 years previously. Her most significant comment was, ''A great deal of destruction had been done to the inside of the house, but the outside remained unmarred. In fact, the ordinary passerby wouldn't even notice that the house had been damaged.'' ☐

The researchers found this story significant when considering the similarities between the house and the body which was about to undergo internal ''destruction'' that would be essentially hidden from others. A fear of altered body image is suggested by this story.

Example 2 ☐ Mrs. N.'s story expressed pleasure and excitement as she began telling the nurse about her trip to Yugoslavia. However, she then described the night she could not find lodging. Darkness descended, and she realized that driving on the unlit mountain roads was unsafe. She had been warned about bandits in lonely places and she feared attack. Finally she found a campground and rented a camper. However it did not lock and she remained frightened until morning. ☐

This story can be interpreted as reflecting several concerns felt by people about to undergo surgery. The darkness descending could indicate fear of the unknown, while the difficulty in driving safely on mountain roads suggests anxiety over loss of control. Mrs. N.'s comments about fear of attack may be related to concern over an altered body image. Although the two stories suggest emotions that are normal and appropriate for the circumstances, it is nevertheless significant that the women chose these particular incidents to tell the nurse on the evening prior to surgery.

Example 3 ☐ The third woman, Mrs. J., felt severe emotional stress at the time of her surgery. Several weeks earlier, a neighbor of hers had died following surgery for a brain tumor. The woman had been in good health until the symptoms appeared, just prior to the surgery. She died several days after surgery without regaining consciousness. Mrs. J. stated that she knew her own situation was very different and she need not fear the same experience. However, she was so worried about what would happen to her children if she should die that she could not think rationally about it. She also worried about remaining unconscious and thus out of control following surgery. ☐

Although Mrs. J.'s anxiety was severe, she was able to express her concerns. The nurse helped her use her strengths to cope with the anxiety, by drawing upon her awareness that there were differences between her operation and that of her neighbor. Her condition was a benign fibroid tumor of the uterus. She had been examined carefully on several occasions by a physician familiar with her situation. Because her problem was not near the brain, the possibility of coma following surgery was remote. Although Mrs. J. had been aware of these facts she described relief when the discussion with the nurse validated her observations.

Because Mrs. J. was extremely anxious about what would become of her children should she die, the nurse decided to explore this concern with her without alluding to death. She simply asked Mrs. J. how she had planned for her children's care during her hospitalization. As Mrs. J. talked calmly about this, she also realized that these provisions could continue should her illness become severe. After this realization, she began to relax and was no longer teary-eyed. She said she would be able to read a little now, which would keep her ''imagination from running away.''

Example 4 ☐ Mrs. L., age 38, when given the Gottschalk instructions, began to cry and stated, ''I can't think about anything except how much I'm going to vomit after this surgery tomorrow.'' When asked why she feared this, Mrs. L. replied that when she had undergone a tonsillectomy as a child, she had vomited following surgery. The nurse recalled her own experience when she had been hospitalized at the age of 7. The little girl next to her had experienced severe vomiting following surgery. Since then the nurse had learned that vomiting does not always occur after surgery. The nurse informed Mrs. L. that the refinement of anesthetic agents and administration techniques over the years had decreased the incidence of vomiting considerably. She also pointed out that the child's fears might have contributed to the postoperative vomiting. The nurse then described the preoperative care plan that would teach Mrs. L. what to expect on the day of surgery and during the postoperative period. She explained that learning about pre- and postoperative care was known to decrease the incidence of vomiting. She also informed Mrs. L. that at times nausea and vomiting does follow surgery, but it usually lasts for a brief period of several hours and is generally relieved by antiemetic drugs that the doctor would order for her. □

The primary technique in the nurse's approach to Mrs. J. was to focus on reality and then to explore the facts with her. The nurse was fairly passive, simply supporting Mrs. J.'s strengths and validating the ideas she expressed. In the situation of Mrs. L., the nurse was more active, because the woman's comments indicated that she needed information. In both cases the nurse accepted the person's feelings even though her own knowledge indicated that these fears were exaggerated. She encouraged the two women to express their feelings and explore them further. The nurse also used a similar childhood experience to help her understand Mrs. L.'s emotional state.

All four women described did well following surgery. Although asking them to participate in the Gottschalk anxiety test was not planned as an intervention, giving them an opportunity to air some of their concerns through the symbolic use of a story may have had a therapeutic effect.

Mental Status

The ability to understand explanations about the surgical procedure and to understand the nurse's descriptions of pre- and postoperative activities depends partly on the person's ability to grasp information. Remembering Piaget, the nurse will want to assess his ability to think concretely or formally. This will influence the approach and principles of learning and teaching one decides to use. A consideration of Maslow and Erikson will help us be aware of how basic need satisfaction and developmental levels assist or deter understanding. These aspects, together with the level of anxiety, have an important effect on the person's ability to adapt to the surgical experience.

Spiritual Component

People who have a comfortable religious or philosophical approach to life are often able to attach meaning to illness and surgery. As with a high level of anxiety, those who feel hostile or bitter about life or who view it with a sense of despair may do poorly following surgery. A sense of hopelessness and feelings of giving up could be life threatening. The will

to live may well be the most important aspect in recovery and rehabilitation. Chapter 29 on grief and loss describes some of these ideas.

Physical Status

Although all physical statuses can affect the person undergoing surgery, there are several important areas that should be highlighted. A person who is properly nourished and hydrated is better able to withstand the postoperative period of altered nutrition. Those who are underweight have less reserve and less physical strength than those who are at a more ideal weight. They also may have more difficulty ambulating after surgery and find that the healing process takes longer. Overweight persons, on the other hand, are more prone to respiratory, circulatory, and wound healing complications.

Constipation prior to surgery may contribute to an even greater alteration in bowel elimination after surgery, as a result of a typical postoperative decrease in gastrointestinal motility due to anesthesia, immobility, and psychological stress. Persons who have had prior urinary tract infections may have continued difficulty, especially if a catheter is necessary.

Persons with a history of thrombophlebitis or with vascular insufficiency are prone to recurring problems. Those with any sort of respiratory insufficiency or distress will need special attention during and following surgery to prevent complications such as pneumonia and atelectasis. The heavy smoker is also prone to these difficulties. Anyone with an altered respiratory status prior to surgery may undergo pulmonary function studies to determine actual lung capacity and may be encouraged to begin coughing and deep breathing exercises in preparation for surgery.

Preoperative Phase

Assessment

Assessment should be carried out in all the areas mentioned in the preceding discussion. An understanding of the person's psychological and spiritual strengths and needs will provide the necessary information for problem solving. Baseline information about the physiological statuses helps the nurse to know what is normal for this particular person and to be prepared for possible problems or complications following surgery.

Temperature, pulse, respiration, and blood pressure are usually checked. Other sources of pertinent information include height and weight, strength of peripheral pulses, respiratory sounds, and quality and rhythm of the pulse. For baseline data the nurse should also review diagnostic studies that were done preoperatively, such as x-ray examinations, pulmonary function studies, electrocardiograms, and blood tests for red and white cell count, hemoglobin, hematocrit, blood glucose, blood gases, and electrolytes. This information makes the nurse aware of changes that occur postoperatively.

Nursing Interventions

Teaching

As indicated earlier, preoperative teaching should cover a wide range of topics, including a description of pre- and postoperative activities such as coughing and deep breathing exercise, leg exercises, turning routine, and ambulation schedule; a description of the plan for controlling pain; and an explanation of hospital policies concerning visiting schedules (Fig. 30-1). Further information may be obtained by referring to the nursing procedures manual for instructions on postoperative activities.

Proper Identification of the Person

Identification procedures vary according to the hospital, but most institutions require wrist bands and name tags fastened to gowns and O.R. caps. You may know the person well, but others may not. Careful

attention to identification could prevent a tragic error.

Preoperative Medications

The medications prescribed preoperatively will depend on the person's particular problem and the preference of the surgeon and anesthesiologist. In general, a narcotic such as morphine sulfate or demerol and an anticholinergic agent such as atropine are combined and administered. Sometimes a mild tranquilizer such as diazepam (Valium) is given. More recently, cimetidine has been used in some hospitals to decrease gastrointestinal secretions and the possibility of gastrointestinal bleeding.

The purposes of preoperative medications are as follows:

- To promote muscle relaxation
- To provide a sense of well-being
- To decrease the amount of anesthesia needed
- To decrease respiratory and gastric secretions
- To inhibit vagal stimulation of the right atrium of the heart by anesthetic agents, which could cause a decrease in heart rate. Atropine acts as a parasympathetic inhibitor and helps maintain an adequate heart rate.

Informed Consent

Until about 15 years ago the consent form was used primarily to give permission to the surgeon and anesthesiologist to do whatever they felt necessary

Figure 30-1
Preoperative teaching involves providing an opportunity for the client to practice postoperative activities such as coughing exercises.

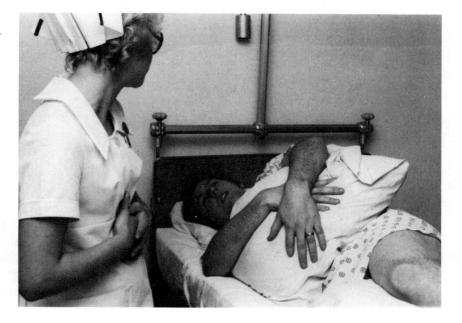

for the person's welfare. However, the consumer movement has worked to bring about changes in the purpose of the consent form. It is no longer just a permission slip but an informed consent that limits the activities of the surgeon and the anesthesiologist or nurse anesthetist to those stated on the form. A major purpose of the informed consent is to offer an opportunity for the person to learn about the benefits and risks of the proposed surgery, consider alternatives, and participate in a safe and informed decision. From a legal perspective the informed consent reminds us that it is the person's right to receive information and participate in decision making. Other purposes of the informed consent include protection of the physicians and the hospital involved. Figure 30-2 is an example of an informed consent form.

The surgeon is provided some latitude through the informed consent to make changes in the procedure. After the surgical area is exposed, the surgeon may find that it is necessary to alter the procedure to save the person's life or to prevent additional surgery in the very near future. The planned procedure, then, can be altered to a reasonable degree. Because it is not possible to develop guidelines for every possible contingency that might arise, these decisions are often difficult for the surgeon to make.

Although it is the surgeon's responsibility to provide the information to the person and obtain the written consent, the nurse, as a patient advocate, must be certain that the consent has been signed before sending the person to the operating room. Moreover, the nurse will want to assess the person's understanding and readiness to proceed with the surgery. Sometimes persons express thoughts to the nurse that they hesitate to mention to the physician. In one such instance, a young woman about to have a hysterectomy expressed to the student nurse her reluctance to undergo the procedure. She made these comments just as the student was about to administer the preoperative medications. The student withheld the medications, informed her instructor, and together they notified the surgeon. He came to talk to the woman and subsequently canceled the surgery, stating that he would not do it until she was ready.

If the preoperative medications are given prior to the actual signing, the legality of the signature may be questioned. If the consent has not been signed, the nurse withholds the medications and notifies the operating room and the surgeon. Table 30-2 lists those who may sign and witness the informed consent.

Other Preoperative Safety Considerations

- Skin—The person should shower before going to surgery. In addition, a skin scrub and shave to the surgical area are done by the nurse or a technician assigned to this task. Both of these

---

Table 30-2
Signers and Witnesses of Informed Consent

Who signs after full information?	Persons 17 or over
	Emancipated minors
	Parents or guardians of persons under 17
	Next of kin if person is unconscious or incompetent
	Court order if no one is available
	Surgeon proceeds without permission if emergency and no one is available to sign
Who witnesses?	Physician
	Nurse only witnesses that person signing is who he says. Nurses do not give medical information regarding procedure.

Informed Consent

Date: _____
Time: _____ A.M.
                                       P.M.

1. I request and authorize the staff of the University Hospital and such doctors and/or assistants as may be assigned to further diagnose or treat the condition(s) which appear indicated by diagnostic studies already performed. The condition(s) which appear indicated are as follows: _____
_____
(Please use layman's terms)*

2. The procedures deemed necessary to diagnose or treat my conditions have been explained to me by Dr. _____, who has also explained the nature of the condition(s) to me. I understand the nature of the procedures summarized below and request and authorize the performance of such procedures. _____
_____
                                                                                        *

3. It has also been explained to me that before, during, and following the procedure described above, unforeseen conditions may be revealed or develop that make an extension of such procedures or different procedures necessary or advisable. I therefore request and authorize that such procedures be performed as are necessary or advisable in the exercise of professional judgment.

4. I have been informed and understand that there are certain risks and consequences associated with the procedures described in paragraph 2. The risks may be: _____
_____
                                                                                        *

5. I also have been informed and understand that in the performance of any surgical procedure and in the administering of anesthesia there are other risks such as severe loss of blood, infection, cardiac arrest, *etc.,* even death.

6. I also have been informed and understand that the practice of medicine, surgery, and dentistry is not an exact science and acknowledge that no guarantees or promises have been or can be made to me concerning the results of the procedures performed.

7. I consent to the photographing, filming, recording, or televising of the procedure to be performed, including appropriate portions of my body for medical, scientific, research, or educational purposes, provided my identity is not revealed by the pictures or by the texts accompanying them.

8. I have been informed and understand that medical and surgical procedures require the cooperation and services of nurses, technicians, assistants, and other personnel and request and authorize such personnel to undertake this service and care.

_____	Witness _____
Signature of patient (If patient is a minor or unable to sign, parent or guardian should sign)	Date

REQUEST AND CONSENT TO ANESTHESIA

Patient: _____   Reg. No. _____
Time: _____ A.M.   Date: _____
                                         P.M.

I have been informed by Dr. _____ and understand that anesthetics will be used in connection with the described procedures and consent to the administration of such general or local anesthetics as may be considered necessary or advisable with the exception of _____
                                                                          (State "none" if none)

_____	Witness _____
Signature of patient (If patient is a minor or unable to sign, parent or guardian should sign)	Date

* If insufficient space, use reverse side.
Note: Any part(s) not applicable or not consented to by patient should be crossed out and initialed by patient.

Figure 30-2
Informed consent: an example (University of Michigan Medical Center Request and Consent to Operation, Radiological Procedures, Anesthesia, or other procedures)

measures are designed to reduce the bacterial count on the surgical area of the body.

- Removal of eyeglasses, contact lenses, dentures, prostheses, hairpieces, and hairpins—These items might become dislodged during surgery and cause trauma to the person. Moreover, they are sometimes lost and cause additional expense when they must be replaced.

- Removal of nail polish and makeup—Clear skin and nails permit members of the operating team to assess important color changes.

Needs of the Family

Although family members have usually been considered the significant people in the person's life, current life-styles have introduced other meaningful relationships. Friends or partners of the opposite or same sex are now often considered family or extended family. Assess the meaning of these relationships to your client and learn in what way he wants others involved in his care.

The person undergoing surgery may be the nurse's primary concern; however, attention to family members is also essential. They too need information and reassurance. It is often helpful to have family members present at the preoperative teaching sessions. The family needs to know what they can expect after the surgery and how they will be able to help the person. Providing this information reduces anxiety for all concerned.

Family members often fear the death of their loved one, even when the possibility of such an outcome is unlikely. If death is a possibility, a sensitive and concerned nurse can employ communication skills in empathizing with family members and helping them adapt to this expectation. Establishing a trusting relationship between yourself and family members, assessing their needs, and providing them with information are all helpful interventions.

Postsurgical Preparation

Immediately after the person is taken to the operating room, the nurse should prepare for his return by anticipating the following needs:

Safety Needs
- Check the mechanics of the bed and side rails for proper functioning.
- Order special equipment such as suction machines, oxygen, or medications that the person will need upon return.

Warmth and Comfort Needs
- Because persons undergoing surgery frequently experience postoperative chills, even in warm weather, extra bath blankets and socks should be readily available.
- Add drawsheets and plastic undersheets to the middle section and the head of the bed. If drainage or vomiting occurs, the sheets can be changed with minimal discomfort to the person.
- See that disposable pads are available to be placed under wound areas. These will also decrease the number of times the person must be moved for linen changes.

Fluid Needs
- An intravenous pole, emesis basin, tissues, and mouth care supplies should be at the bedside.
- Check stock supplies to see that there is an adequate amount of intravenous fluid available.

Intraoperative Phase

Because a person experiencing surgery is unable to help himself and is therefore vulnerable to physical and psychological injury, it is especially important that holistic care be provided at this time.

Psychological Needs

Prior to the administration of anesthesia and during a surgical procedure under local or spinal anesthesia, the person will be conscious and subject to special fears and concerns, especially if he is aware of comments and facial expressions made by the operating team. He may also be aware of physical changes such as lowering of his blood pressure. Even if these changes are not severe enough to be of concern, they may be uncomfortable and frightening. The nurse should be aware that unpleasant or frightening sensations occur and be on hand to alleviate concerns.

Some investigators have speculated that persons under anesthesia can actually hear and understand conversation, although they may not consciously remember it. Whether persons do poorly or well following surgery could be a reflection of hopeless or hopeful attitudes expressed by surgical team members.

Safety Needs

Two important aspects of safety in the operating room are the maintenance of asepsis and the correct positioning of the person on the operating table. Usually, aseptic technique is carefully observed. All members of the professional team are expected to maintain sterile technique and report any breaks they commit or observe. However, it is the responsibility of the nurse in charge of the operating room to provide overall supervision for this very important concern.

There are a number of standard positions for placing patients on the operating table, each of which provides access to a particular surgical area. In addition to the proper position, other positioning considerations include strapping the person to keep his entire body as well as the extremities properly aligned and in place. Strapping should be secure but must not impede circulation or cause nerve damage. Even with careful positioning, shifting frequently occurs during the procedure, and team members can sometimes lean on the extremities or other parts of the body. To protect the person properly, the nurse must remain alert to these possibilities and check positioning frequently.

Physiological Needs

Although the anesthesiologist (physician) or anesthetist (registered nurse) is responsible for monitoring vital signs, color changes, and intake and output of the person under anesthesia, the nurse is also expected to monitor these parameters as part of providing total person-focused care in the operating room.

Role of the Nurse in the Operating Room

The personnel in the operating room function as a team to meet the person's needs. Members of the team include the surgeon and the surgical assistants, who may be other surgeons or medical students, the anesthesiologist or nurse anesthetist, the nurse in charge of the operating room, and the scrub nurse or technician. Because it is essential that team members focus attention on the physical needs of the person undergoing surgery, it is often difficult to provide holistic care in the operating room. Students will want to observe how well all human needs are attended to in the operating room and consider ways for improving this aspect of nursing care. Being aware of the intraoperative experience will also help students understand better the reasons for postoperative pain and discomfort.

The nurse is the one team member who is concerned with the total needs of the person. As client advocates, it is our responsibility to ensure that these needs are met. This is particularly critical because the person is often unconscious and unable to control the events in the operating room. The nurse will also want to consider the meaning of the surgery for the person. He may be expecting or hoping for pain relief, improvement of functional ability, or a cure for a life-threatening disease. Operating room nurses will be able to communicate certain information about expected outcomes to those nurses involved in postoperative care.

Postoperative Phase

Following the surgical procedure, the person will be taken to the recovery room for a period of hours, until his vital signs are stable and he is awake and responding well. In certain situations, the person may be returned to his preoperative unit when physically stable even though he is not alert. In some instances he may spend a period of time in an intensive care unit if he warrants particular observation and care. There has also been an increase in surgical procedures done on an outpatient basis or with a very limited hospital stay. However, all surgical patients require some special immediate postoperative observation.

The remainder of this discussion identifies common postoperative problems and complications and suggests nursing interventions that help prevent difficulty and facilitate adaptation to the surgical experience. You will not find new problems in this section. They have all been examined in earlier chapters. Our purpose is to help you synthesize material that you have already learned and apply it to a person with special needs. Consult nursing process chapters earlier in this text for more complete discussions of the problems.

First, let us consider the concept of stress and adaptation. In the preoperative period, anxiety about surgery serves as a psychological stressor. In the postoperative period, it is the physiological stress of surgery that warrants the greatest attention, although psychological considerations are still present. Of the number of stressors associated with surgery, there are four that really precipitate most of the others:

Table 30-3
Problems and Associated Stressors Experienced by Persons Following Surgery

Problem	Associated Stressors
Wound healing	Overweight
	Old age
	Poor nutrition
Negative nitrogen balance	Poor preoperative nutrition
	Effects of stress response
	Inadequate calorie intake postoperatively
Abdominal distention	Anesthesia
	Surgical trauma
	Immobility
	Decreased peristalsis
Vomiting	Anesthesia
	Diminished peristalsis
	Fear
Thirst and dry mouth	Anticholinergic drugs
	NPO
	Dehydration
	Mouth breathing
Urinary retention	Lower abdominal surgery
	Anesthesia
	Anxiety
Urinary tract infection	Urinary retention
	Bladder catheterization
	History of urinary tract infection
Constipation	Immobility
	Narcotic analgesics
	History of constipation
Pain	Surgical incision
	Abdominal distention
	Urinary retention
	Thrombophlebitis
	Positioning during surgery

anesthesia, surgical trauma, postoperative immobility, and psychological factors. Internal stressors that affect the postoperative course include any nutritional, circulatory, and respiratory deficits, age, self-concept, and so forth. How well the person adapts to the surgical experience depends on the severity of these stressors and his coping strengths. Table 30-3 lists common postoperative problems and associated stressors.

When the person undergoes surgery, a phenom-

Problem	*Associated Stressors*
Altered sleep patterns	Postoperative medication
	Pain
	Postoperative activities
Shock and hemorrhage	Surgical trauma
Venous stasis	Immobility
	Stress response
	Previous venous problems
Increased respiratory secretions	Anesthesia
	Immobility
Diminished ventilation	Advanced age
	Overweight
	Narcotic analgesics
	Abdominal or thoracic incision
	Preoperative respiratory status
	Preoperative smoker
Hypovolemia	Blood loss
	NPO
	Postoperative drainage
	Age
Hypervolemia	Preoperative cardiac and renal status
	Stress response
	IV therapy
Anxiety, grief response	Perceptions of body image changes
	Fear of unknown
Elevated temperature	Surgical trauma
	Infection: bladder, wound, respiratory
	Inadequate fluid intake

enon called the *stress response* results. The stress response elicits the general adaptation syndrome (GAS), which includes an increase in the adrenal hormones aldosterone, cortisol, epinephrine, and norepinephrine; and an increase in the antidiuretic hormone (ADH). These hormones have an effect on the person's postoperative recovery rate. The original research on the stress response was the work of Hans Selye, as discussed in Chapter 6. Table 30-4 is a diagram of the stress response.

Table 30-4
Stress Response

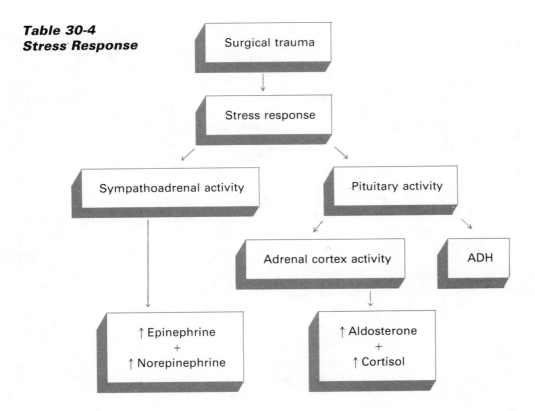

Functional Areas and Common Problems

Skin

Because the skin is the body's first line of defense against bacteria, surgical trauma to the skin can increase the potential for postoperative infection. An increase in cortisol levels associated with the stress response inhibits the steps of inflammation and may decrease antibody production as well. This can decrease the body's ability to resist infection.

Certain persons are at risk for developing other wound healing problems. Wound infections often occur in obese persons because adipose tissue is less resistant to infection. **Dehiscence,** or the separation of the wound, may also occur in obese persons. Persons who are poorly nourished may not have the calories and nutrients necessary for the development of new skin cells. The elderly person may also take longer to heal because of circulatory changes.

Nutrition

A negative nitrogen balance may occur following surgery, as a result of inadequate caloric intake associated with the cessation of oral intake from the midnight before surgery and for several days afterward. The intravenous fluids which are provided usually supply only 600 to 800 calories, and no protein, per 24 hours. Early oral feedings, which often consist of clear liquids, supply minimal calories and protein. Inadequate nutrition, together with an increase in the adrenal hormones from the stress response, causes an increase in protein catabolism to meet energy needs. This results in a negative nitrogen balance and some muscle wasting. Usually this is a transient situation, with the major effect being fatigue. However, prolonged negative nitrogen balance can cause more severe muscle wasting, increased chance of infection, delayed wound healing, and a delayed postoperative rehabilitation.

Gastrointestinal Motility

Peristalsis is decreased during surgery owing to the effects of anesthesia, manipulation of the bowel if the surgery is in the abdominal area, postoperative immobility, and the effects of psychological stress. As a result of the decreased peristalsis, flatus builds and causes abdominal distention and cramping.

Immediate postoperative vomiting may be associated with anesthesia. However, later vomiting may occur as a result of gastric juices accumulating when peristalsis is diminished or absent. Vomiting also occurs more frequently when the anxiety level is high.

Normally peristalsis returns within a few days following surgery. However, if lack of peristalsis persists the state is known as **paralytic ileus,** in which case a nasogastric tube may need to be inserted and attached to suction to remove the accumulated gastric juices. Ileus lengthens the time before oral nutrition may be resumed.

Fluid Balance

Following surgery people frequently complain of a dry mouth and thirst, usually as a consequence of preoperative anticholinergic drugs and the combined effect of taking no oral fluids for a while and breathing through the mouth. If there is a nasogastric tube present, this also contributes to a dry mouth. More serious causes of thirst are inadequate fluid intake and hypovolemia.

The secretion of increased ADH and aldosterone in response to the stress of surgery results in the retention of sodium and water in the body. This is an adaptive mechanism to maintain proper fluid and electrolyte balance during the total surgical experience. However, it can contribute to fluid overload in susceptible persons, namely those with cardiac and renal problems.

Elimination

Urinary retention occurs most commonly following surgery in the lower abdominal area or the lower urinary tract. It may also occur after spinal cord surgery. Retention may be due to the effects of both general and spinal anesthesia, urethral obstruction from clots or swelling, or anxiety related to inability to void.

Urinary tract infection may also occur following surgery and is commonly caused by urinary retention or the indwelling catheter, which is frequently inserted during surgery.

Constipation associated with a decrease in peristalsis is not unusual following surgery. It is more likely to occur if the person has had preoperative constipation difficulties. Narcotic analgesics taken for postoperative pain are implicated in constipation, along with postoperative immobility and decreased peristalsis.

Respiration

Prolonged periods of immobility, such as those spent on the operating table and in the recovery room, can cause an increase in respiratory secretions and a pooling of secretions in the lungs. Anesthesia paralyzes the cilia in the respiratory tract, severely compromising the ability of the person to clear his airway.

Pain caused by abdominal and thoracic incisions during coughing and deep breathing results in a poor breathing effort and diminished alveolar ventilation. Narcotic analgesics may also depress the respiratory rate. The pooling of secretions may cause atelectasis or pneumonia.

Circulation

Immobility and previous venous problems may combine to cause **venous stasis** or pooling of blood in the lower extremities. Increased catecholamines from the stress response increase clotting tendencies. This can result in thrombophlebitis if intervention does not occur.

Shock and hemorrhage can occur in the intra- and early postoperative periods but usually do not occur later if the person is properly assessed throughout the postoperative period (see Chap. 23).

Rest and Comfort

Pain. Because incisional pain is common postoperatively, nurses usually assume that this is the reason the person asks for pain medication. However, there are other causes of pain, and careful assessment is crucial in order not to miss a serious or life-threatening situation. For example, pain may be due to a dressing or cast that is constricting circulation; it could be due to urinary retention, abdominal distention with cramping, calf pain from thrombophlebitis, or chest pain from pneumonia or pulmonary emboli. Back, shoulder, neck, and some leg pain may be associated with positioning in the operating room.

Sleep. The hypnotic effect of narcotics may cause sleep disturbances. Immediately following surgery, people may nap during the day and be restless at night. This disrupts usual sleep patterns and causes an increase in the feelings of fatigue. Pain and postoperative treatments such as dressing changes or respiratory therapy also interfere with sleep.

Psychological Status

Preoperative problems not associated with surgery may seem even more stressful when pain and fatigue occur following surgery. Pathology reports usually take a few days to arrive, and this contributes to feelings of stress. Alterations in self-concept and body image may be temporary if the surgery is not extreme and if the person will soon be able to resume his former activities. However, a more severe psychological response may result if there is a definite change in life-style.

Assessment

The following observations should be made frequently by the nurse in the first 24 to 48 hours following surgery. Exact schedules for checking depend on the severity of the surgical trauma and the person's ability to cope. After the immediate postoperative state, these observations are made less frequently until the person is discharged from the hospital.

Vital Signs. The immediate concern is possible shock, related to hypovolemia from blood or fluid loss, or a decrease in total peripheral resistance. The body's increased cortisol secretion in response to stress helps maintain vasoconstriction and a stable blood pressure. Blood pressure and other vital signs may alter in response to pain; narcotic analgesics can lower blood pressure and depress the respiratory center. A slight temperature elevation, up to 37.8°C (99.8°F), is normal during the first day or two after surgery. Following that period, a temperature elevation could indicate an infection of the respiratory tract, the bladder, or the wound.

Wound. Check for signs and symptoms of inflammation such as erythema, warmth, or unusual pain.

Observe the amount and character of the drainage and the approximation of wound edges.

Intake and Output. The voiding pattern is especially important in the early postoperative stage. If a catheter is in place, output can be carefully monitored. It should be from 30 ml to 50 ml/hr. When a catheter is not used, the time and amount of the first void is measured and recorded. Depending on the type of surgery and the person's condition, the first void should occur from 4 to 12 hours after surgery. If the person does not void, this could indicate urinary retention. However, low urinary output may also mean dehydration and shock. Other output that should be measured and recorded includes that collected from special drains or tubing attached to suction, an approximation of drainage on dressings (weigh dressings before application and after removal), and vomitus. Intake is measured and recorded, whether intravenous or oral, for several days following surgery.

Comfort. Careful assessment to determine whether pain is from surgical trauma or other possible sources is essential. Assessment of former and current sleep patterns helps in planning for proper rest.

Respiratory Assessment. Pre- and postoperative respiratory assessment helps the nurse distinguish normal from abnormal sounds. Assessment before and after coughing and deep breathing can also help to determine whether these exercises are effective.

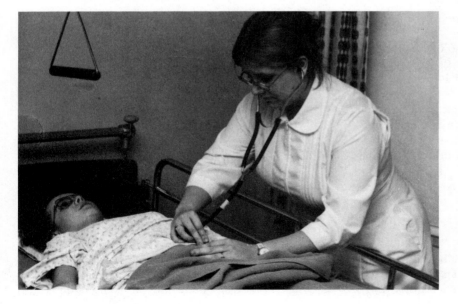

Figure 30-3
The nurse assesses bowel sounds postoperatively to determine resumption of peristalsis.

Abdominal Assessment. As with respiratory status, the abdomen should be assessed preoperatively as well as after surgery so that comparisons can be made. Listening for bowel sounds can help the nurse determine when the person is ready to eat (Fig. 30-3). Although in many hospitals physicians make this decision, if the nurse has complete data, professional collaboration can occur.

Nursing Interventions

The following interventions suggest the common approach to the postoperative person. Nurses need to vary these according to the specific needs of their clients.

- *Turning and positioning*—These measures increase comfort and ventilation and decrease pooled respiratory secretions. If the person is unable to move freely or ambulate early in the postoperative state, these measures are also essential for maintaining intact skin.
- *Leg exercises* increase venous return and prevent the pooling of blood in the lower extremities.
- *Ambulation* improves respiratory ventilation, increases venous return, helps increase peristalsis,

and decreases abdominal flatus. It also contributes to feelings of self-esteem as the person begins to regain strength and resume former activities (Fig. 30-4).

- *Mouth care and fluids* decrease thirst, prevent oral infection, and maintain proper fluid balance. Mouth care also increases comfort and adds to a sense of well-being.
- *Coughing and deep breathing*—Exercises of this type decrease respiratory secretions and increase lung ventilation and oxygenation of body tissues.
- *Comfort measures*—Positioning, massage, mouth care, medication for pain, and a plan for rest and activity to promote exercise and sleep are essential interventions. Inclusion of family members in these interventions is often helpful.
- *Nutrition*—As soon as the person can resume oral intake, the nurse helps him plan to include an increased amount of protein and vitamin C in his diet. This promotes positive nitrogen balance and encourages wound healing. Persons who cannot eat within a few days following surgery are supported by intravenous nutrition.

Figure 30-4 ·
Postoperative ambulation improves respiratory, circulatory, and gastrointestinal function *(Photo by Bob Kalmbach)*

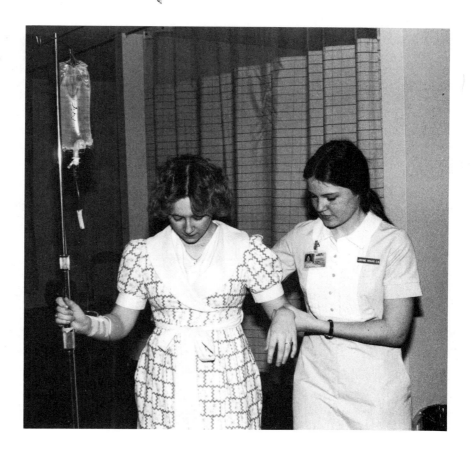

If the inability to eat persists, hyperalimentation may be instituted.

- *Wound care*—An uncomplicated wound may be washed with soap and water as soon as the dressing is removed. The person may bathe or shower when his mobility status is stable. The student is referred to the nursing procedures manual for instructions on reinforcing oozing dressings, wound irrigation and dressing change for problem wounds, and the care of special wound drains inserted during surgery.

- *Psychological interventions*—Encouraging the person to participate in his own care as soon as he is able contributes to feelings of increased self-esteem and positive expectations. Assisting the person to look at or assimilate any alterations caused by surgery and to discuss feelings with the nurse and family members contributes to the promotion of a positive body image.

- *Discharge planning* should begin in the early stages of hospitalization. Plans for discharge and continued rehabilitation may be fairly simple when postoperative recovery is satisfactory. However, when wound care or equipment such as oxygen or suction machines must be attended to at home, special planning is required. The person and his family can be referred to the community health nurse who will plan follow-up care and evaluate progress.

Conclusion

The person in the preoperative, intraoperative, and postoperative phases of surgery has special needs. Surgery is a stressor that affects all systems: physical, psychosocial, and spiritual. Each of these systems must be attended to so that all can function optimally. In order to give holistic care during the surgical experience, nurses can synthesize and apply the person-centered concepts presented throughout this text.

Preoperatively, nurses collect data about physical, psychosocial, and spiritual functioning to identify immediate needs and potential postoperative problems. Because anxiety about surgery is common, emotional support as well as preoperative teaching are important considerations. Additional interventions include properly identifying the person, administering preoperative medications, validating that informed consent has been obtained, and ensuring safety.

During the intraoperative phase the individual is often in an altered state of consciousness and is more vulnerable to physical and psychological injury. Nurses are responsible for maintaining the safety of their clients, as well as ensuring that their physiological and psychological needs are met. Because the unconscious person is unable to help himself, he is reliant on the nurse's ability to identify and meet his needs.

Postoperatively the person is at risk for many physical and psychological problems. Many of those problems can be avoided with preventive nursing care. Nurses assist clients to mobilize internal resources to cope with the stressors associated with surgery. From the preoperative through the postoperative phases, the client is helped to participate in his care to his fullest ability. Well-planned nursing care not only stresses the holistic view but also emphasizes prevention throughout the surgical experience.

Study Questions

1. Refer to Table 30-1. Apply all of these concepts and subconcepts to the person experiencing surgery.

2. Identify at least one potential problem in each of the psychosocial and physical systems (all statuses) of the person that can result in a postoperative problem.

3. List the purposes of preoperative medications.

4. Describe the purposes of the informed consent. How has the consumer movement and the role of the nurse as a client advocate affected a person's consent to have surgery?

5. Describe observations the nurse should make when providing care to the person during the intraoperative phase.

6. Discuss the stress response. In what ways can it affect a person's postoperative course?

7. Develop a care plan for the person in the postoperative phase.

Glossary

Dehiscence: The separation of a wound.

Paralytic Ileus: A state in which intestinal peristalsis is diminished or absent.

Venous Stasis: A pooling of blood in the veins of the lower extremities.

Bibliography

Andrew JM: Recovery from surgery, with and without preparatory instruction for three coping styles. J Pers Soc Psychol 15, No. 3:223–226, July 1970

Carnevali D: Preoperative anxiety. Am J Nurs 66, No. 7:1536–1538, July 1966

Croushort TM: Postoperative assessment: The key to avoiding the most common nursing mistakes. Nurs 79 9, No. 4:47–51, Apr 1979

Dumas R, Leonard RE: The effect of nursing on the incidence of postoperative vomiting. Nurs Res 12:12–15, Winter 1963

Dziurbeijko MM, Larkin JC: Including the family in preoperative teaching. Am J Nurs 78, No. 11:1892–1894, Nov 1978

Ennis CE, Andrassy RJ et al: Nutritional management of the surgical patient. AORN J 31, No. 7:1217–1224, June 1980

Fehlau MT: Applying the nursing process to patient care in the operating room. Nurs Clin North Am 10, No. 4:617–623, Dec 1975

Gottschalk LA: Comparative Psycholinguistic Analysis of Two Psychotherapeutic Interviews. New York, International Universities Press, 1961

Gottschalk LA: The Measurement of Psychological States Through the Content Analysis of Verbal Behavior. Berkeley, University of California Press, 1969

Graham LE, Conley EM: Evaluation of anxiety and fear in adult surgical patients. Nurs Res 20:113–122, Mar–Apr 1971

Gruendemann BJ: The impact of surgery on body image. Nurs Clin North Am 10, No. 4:635–643, Dec 1975

Healy K: Does preoperative instruction make a difference? Am J Nurs 68, No. 1:62–67, 1462–1467, Jan 1968

Hunter ML, Britton AS: The Value of a Preoperative Printed Teaching Tool for Abdominal Hysterectomy Patients. Unpublished Master's Thesis, The University of Michigan, 1973

Koehler JS: Perioperative nursing can be cost effective. AORN J 32, No. 6:1068, 1072, 1074, Dec 1980

Levine D, Fiedler JP: Fear, facts and fantasies about preoperative and postoperative care. Nurs Outlook 58:26–28, Feb 1970

Lindeman CA, VanAerman B: Nursing intervention with the presurgical patient—The effect of structured and unstructured teaching. Nurs Res 20:319–332, July–Aug 1971

Mehaffy NL: Assessment and communication for continuity of care for the surgical patient. Nurs Clin North Am 10, No. 4:625–633, Dec 1975

Methany N: Preoperative fluid balance assessment. AORN J 33, No. 1:51–56, Jan 1981

Mezzanotte EJ: Group instructions in preparation for surgery. Am J Nurs 70:89–91, Jan 1970

————: Nursing grand rounds: Postoperative complications. How to help the patient when everything goes wrong. Nurs 81 11, No. 3:50–53, 1981

————: Proposed recommended practices for documentation of perioperative nursing care. AORN J 33, No. 2:261–263, Feb 1981

Robbins JA, Mushlin AI: Preoperative evaluation of the healthy patient. Med Clin North Am 63, No. 4:1145–1156, Nov 1979

Rockwell DA, Pepitone–Rockwell F: The emotional impact of surgery and the value of informed consent. Med Clin North Am 63, No. 6:1341–1351, Nov 1979

Vander AJ, Sherman JN, Luciano DS: Human Physiology: The Mechanisms of Body Function, 3rd ed. New York, McGraw-Hill, 1980

Voshall B: The effects of preoperative teaching on postoperative pain. Top Clin Nurs 2:39–43, Apr 1980

Wells–Mackie JJ: Clinical assessment and priority setting. Nurs Clin North Am 16, No. 1:3–12, Mar 1981

Wittstock NJ: Preoperative evaluation and physical assessment of the patient. Am Assoc Nurs Anest 49, No. 2:197–206, Apr 1981

Wolfe BM, Phillips GJ, Hodges RE: Evaluation and management of nutritional status before surgery. Med Clin North Am 63, No. 6:1257–1269, Nov 1979

Appendixes
and Index

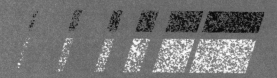

Appendix A
Person Assessment Guide

The purpose of the Person Assessment is to present a data collection guide that is oriented to the whole person in situations of wellness as well as in situations in which the individual is not functioning at his or her optimal level. Inasmuch as the person is more than the sum of biological, psychological, or sociocultural parts, an assessment provides the opportunity to learn the strengths and functional abilities of the individual to cope with daily living.

The Person Assessment is a tool that can be used in a variety of settings and with clients throughout the life span. Likewise, this tool is meant to be used by all nurses, from those just beginning their practice to those with considerable professional experience. The tool is lengthy because it describes assessment data for any client the nurse might see. However, it is not expected that the entire tool would be used with a single client; instead, the areas that are relevant to the client's needs or particular situation would be assessed. For instance, the nurse would postpone discussion of food habits if the person was on a limited-intake diet, until a more normal intake was resumed.

When a nurse first meets a client, the person's overall appearance, as well as signs of anxiety, comfort, pain, difficulty in breathing or mobility, and other significant data are noted. The nurse is also sensitive to the client's response to the explanation of the interview's purpose and estimates his readiness to be interviewed. This consideration facilitates adaptation of the interview to the client's tolerance. For example, if the client were having difficulty breathing or were in pain, the nurse would limit the time of the interview and assess only priority needs until the client was more comfortable.

Once the interview is initiated, data collection may begin within any of the areas of the Person Assessment. For instance, if the client states he is seeking help for pain, the nurse might decide to assess "Rest and Comfort" first. Or the nurse might decide to begin with "Sociocultural Data" when interviewing a well elderly person, as a means of getting to know him better. Wherever assessment is initiated, the following ground rules will be helpful:

1 Begin assessing in the area which the client is most comfortable discussing or around the area of expressed need. Often these are the same, but not always.

2 Interview the client before doing physical assessment, if possible, because trust should be established by talking with the client before touching him. Also, important clues that indicate areas of physical assessment to be performed may be obtained by talking with the client.

3 Continue to assess the client's tolerance throughout the assessment and postpone data collection if he shows discomfort. The client will give verbal or nonverbal cues when he becomes tired or uncomfortable.

The Person Assessment is meant to be flexible and it can be adapted to identify the client's needs in the way in which he is most comfortable. Remember that the purpose of an assessment is to provide the basis for quality care while meeting the needs of the person. The nurse's style of data collection should facilitate, not impede, this goal.

Finally, the person should be considered in the context of the systems of which he is a part. Thus, a holistic assessment of the person involves collecting data about the environment and the family's or significant others' perceptions of the person's needs.

Person Assessment

Date of assessment _____   Age _____

Date of admission _____   Race _____
  if hospitalized or
  current date of en-   Sex _____
  try into health-
  care agency   Current diagnosis _____

Surgery (if any) _____

Part I

I. Sociocultural Data

A. Immediate family

Who lives in client's household? Names? Ages?
What family matters concern client most at this time?
What are client's responsibilities within the household?
Who in the family could assume or share client's responsibilities?

B. Social support

From among client's family, friends, pets, colleagues, helping professionals, community, etc.:
(a) Where does client turn for help in matters of daily living?
(b) Where does client turn in times of difficulty?
(c) What assistance does client receive from these sources?
(d) What other sources of support does client rely upon?

C. Financial resources

1. Occupations (past and present)

Places of employment?
Occupational responsibilities? Hours per week?
How does client's health affect job performance?

2. Other sources of income

What do other members of family contribute?

3. Health insurance

Is client confident about protection?
Concerned about coverage?
What is impact of health-care costs on financial resources?

D. History

1. Ethnic background

Does client identify with a particular ethnic group? European? African? Asian? Other?

2. Birthplace
3. Relocations
4. Education

Formal? Informal?

5. Language(s) spoken/ language barrier

Language most frequently spoken?
Language used for thinking?
Does client need interpreter?

E. Beliefs

1. Life goals

Plans for future?
Attitude toward present situation?
Attitude toward past?

2. Religion	Does client actively participate in an organized religion?
	Does client have spiritual resources?
3. Cultural attitudes and values	Habits; customs; beliefs; values concerning birth, life, death, health, illness, orientation toward time, health-care systems and providers?
	Importance of privacy, etiquette, respect for elders, sex roles, family roles, work ethic?
	Taboos on sexual matters, body parts, special surgery, dead relatives, fears of the unknown? Sanctions on emotional display, religious expression, responses to illness and death?
4. Concepts of health and illness	How does client explain illness?
	Germ theory?
	Cause and effect? Evil spirits?
	Imbalance of heat and cold (yin and yang)?
	Disequilibrium between man and nature?
	Does client view illness as a disruption of his daily life?
	Does client ignore minor discomforts?
	Does client connect good health with success, ability to work and fulfill roles, reward from God, balance with nature?
	Does client adhere to a folk medicine system? African? Asian? European? Folk-religious?
	Does client rely upon lay healers? American Indian medicine men? Mexican-American curanderos? Chinese herbalists? Hougans? Spiritualist? Black-American ministers? Christian Science healers?

II. Life-Style
(other life-style factors are considered elsewhere)

A. Daily routine	
1. At home or at work	What is a typical schedule for client's day? Has client's health caused a change in this schedule?
2. In other settings	
3. In the hospital	
B. Recreational activities	Indoors? Outdoors?
C. Risk taking	
1. Exposure to toxins, disease, violence	Chemicals? Contagious diseases? VD? Unwanted pregnancy? Rape? Other physical abuse?
2. Driving habits	Does client use seatbelts?
	Does client use excessive speed?
	Does client drive while intoxicated?
3. Number of hours spent working	
4. Substance abuse	Drugs? Alcohol?
5. Sexual risk taking	VD exposure; unwanted pregnancy?
D. Current life changes	How has health status affected client's life-style?

III. Environment

A. Neighborhood	
1. Type	Residential? Commercial? Farming? Urban? Rural? Suburban?
2. Health features	Is the neighborhood subject to air or noise pollution?
	What is the quality of water?
	What provisions are made for the disposal of garbage and waste?

3. Available services	How accessible are stores, banks, churches, schools, recreational facilities, health-care facilities? What modes of transportation are available to client?

B. Living space

1. Type of dwelling	Apartment? House? Extended-care facility? Other? Permanent?
2. Length of residence	
3. General state of repair	
4. Facilities	Does client's dwelling contain a bathroom, cooking facilities, laundry facilities? Essential furniture? Does client's dwelling provide adequate privacy, heat, lighting?
5. Layout	Number, size, and arrangement of rooms? Stairways? Recreational and work areas? Does layout suit client's health status?
6. Stimuli	Sights? Sounds? Smells? Personal possessions displayed?
7. Health and safety	Poisons? Unsafe toys? Traffic? Child-Proof devices? Obstacles? Slippery surfaces? What safety devices are in use as required by client's age, mobility, sensory deficits, *etc.?* Combustibles? Electrical hazards? Emergency telephone numbers posted? Disaster procedures posted? First-aid supplies? Smoke detectors? Fire extinguishers? Adequate railings, bars, gates? Security devices? Locks, Lights? Alarms?

C. Hospital setting

1. Safety factors	What safety devices are in use? (See health and safety features above, B.7.)
2. Infection control	What infection control precautions are in use?
3. Arrangement	Does arrangement suit client's preference and needs?
4. Stimuli	Patterns of activity, light, noise, color? Signs of sensory deprivation or overload?
5. Personal preferences	Is the arrangement of client's personal belongings, family pictures, *etc.,* in accord with his preferences?

IV. Developmental Level

Resolution of age-appropriate developmental tasks.

V. Psychological Data

A. Mental capacity
(including cognition/ thinking)

1. Level of consciousness	What are client's eye movement, motor, and speech responses to stimuli? What stimuli elicited these responses?
2. Orientation	Record client's statement of where he is, who he is, and what time it is.
3. Attention span and ability to concentrate	How long can client attend to any given topic?

4. Ability to grasp and handle information

Is client able to discuss, restate, or use information?

5. Ability to handle abstractions

To what extent does client require concrete demonstration or example in order to grasp abstract ideas?

6. Memory: short- and long-term

How accurate and complete is client's recall of the distant past, the past week, the past few hours?

B. Ability to communicate

1. Speech patterns

Does client lisp, stammer, or stutter?

Does the amount, pace, clarity, or tone of client's speech affect his ability to communicate?

Does client have any physical or neurological speech impediments? Missing speech organs? Laryngectomy?

Aphasia?

Do client's individual needs dictate adjustment by the interviewer in the tempo of conversation, use of eye or body contact, mention of particular subjects, style of explanation, or norms of confidentiality?

2. Vocabulary

Does client use simple, nontechnical language or a more complex terminology?

3. Nonverbal behavior

What is client's body posture (body relaxed, rigid)?

How facially expressive is client?

What distinctive gestures does client use?

What is client's general nonverbal response to interviewer?

Is nonverbal behavior consistent with verbal message?

C. Affective behavior

Does client display frequent changes of mood?

How does client express feelings and emotions?

Is emotion appropriate to situation?

D. Self-image concept

What does client identify as his strengths and needs?

E. Adaptive (operant/voluntary) behavior

1. Current stressors

What does client perceive as sources of stress in his life?

2. Coping skills

How does client deal with stress?

What evidence indicates use of defense mechanisms?

3. Patterns of decision making

How does client arrive at decisions?

4. Self sufficiency

How much does client rely upon others for help in making decisions? How confident is client of his decisions once they have been made? Internal strengths? External resources?

Part II

I. Health History

A. Overall health

Client's one-word description of overall health.

B. Past illness, hospitalizations, and surgeries

Significant illnesses, hospitalizations, surgeries, accidents, dates.

C. Current concern

1. Development of concern

Description of client's current concern and its history.

Description of symptoms associated with current concern (if any) including: location (in body), quality, quantity, chronology, setting, aggravating or alleviating factors, associated manifestations.

2. Current therapy

Hospitalization and date, surgery and date, diet, treatments, occupational or physical therapy, other therapy professionally or self-prescribed.

3. Understanding of current health status or problems and therapy

Client's description of health needs or problems and therapy.

Client's perceptions of implications of health status for life-style.

Client's expectations from therapy.

Client's expectations from health-care agency (length of stay, tests, treatments, services).

Client's expectations of nurses or agency staff.

D. Allergies

List of allergies (food, drug, skin, respiratory, *etc.*)

Description of allergic response and current treatment.

E. Medication

1. At home

Name (including prescription and nonprescription drugs), dosage, frequency and time taken, reason, client's understanding of drug.

2. In hospital

Name, dosage, frequency and time taken, reason, client's understanding of drug.

3. Dependency

F. Health maintenance

1. Self-care

Routines for self-examinations, dental habits, exercise and relaxation, diet, hygiene.

2. Professional care

Routines for physical exams, dental care, eye exams, immunizations.

II. Rest and Comfort

A. Sleep

1. Pattern

Amount, time, periods of activity, naps, dreams, disturbances, effects of illness.

2. Environment

Bed, pillows and covers, ventilation, light and noise, effect of change in environment.

3. Aids

Bedtime routine.

Medication.

4. Client's beliefs about sleep

B. Pain

1. Subjective data

Quality, location, rhythm, duration, precipitating factors, meaning to client, client's coping mechanisms, effect on client's life-style.

2. Objective data

Voice patterns.

Physiological signs.

Reaction to environment.

Psychological response.

III. Mobility

A. General movement

Method of mobility (ambulation, wheelchair, stretcher), coordination, ease, general abilities (turning, positioning, transferring).

B. Gait

Coordination, stability, balance, aids (cane, crutches, walkers).

C. Endurance

Amount and type of activity tolerated.

D. Tone, mass, strength	Characteristics of all muscle groups, changes due to health problems.
E. Posture or alignment	Description (slumped, erect, stooped), ability to attain alignment, supportive devices necessary.
F. Condition of joints	Range of motion, swelling, nodules, contractures.
G. Handedness	
H. Deformity or abnormal innervation	Paralysis, paresis, amputation (location, prosthetic devices).
I. Activities of daily living	Normal routine; ability to perform bathing, grooming, dressing, dental care, toileting, cooking, eating, household repairs, cleaning, laundry, shopping; problems encountered with performing daily activities.

IV. Special Senses

A. Vision

1. Acuity	Ability to distinguish objects or print at specified distance.
2. Field	Lateral, horizontal, vertical.
3. Pupils	Equal, reacting.
4. Defects	Myopia, hyperopia, presbyopia, astigmatism, color blindness, diminished night vision, blindness.
5. Corrective or prosthetic devices	Glasses, contact lens, artificial eye.

B. Hearing

1. Acuity	Ability to identify inaudible whisper, audible whisper, spoken voice at specified distance.
2. Dependence on sight	
3. Defects	Conductive, sensorineural, mixed, one ear, both ears, complete, partial.
4. Supportive devices	Hearing aids.

C. Smell

1. Acuity	Ability to discriminate odors.
2. Unusual sensations	

D. Taste

1. Acuity	Ability to discriminate sweet, sour, salty, bitter.
2. Unusual sensations	Lack, aftertaste, metallic taste, other.

E. Touch

1. Acuity	Ability to distinguish sharp, dull, light and firm touch, heat, cold, pain in proportion to stimulus. Ability to discriminate common objects with eyes closed.
2. Unusual sensations	Paresthesia, anesthesia, hyperesthesia.

V. Nutrition

A. Height, weight, body build
  1. Obesity
  2. Emaciation
  3. Cachexia

B. Patterns of weight gain and loss	Amount and time period
1. Planned or un-planned	
2. Emotional factors that alter eating habits	Overeating or undereating to meet emotional needs.
C. Patterns of daily food intake	Typical daily recording of meals and snacks.
D. Appetite	
E. Risk-taking behavior	*E.g.*, alcohol, cholesterol, "junk food," high sodium.
F. Level of nutritional knowledge	
G. Oral cavity	Assess color, integrity, salivary flow for all oral structures.
1. Lips	Complete fusion, evidence of paralysis.
2. Gums and oral mucosa	Presence of bleeding, swelling, vascular spots, white plaque.
3. Tongue	Presence of papillae, size, symmetry, state of hydration (presence of furrows), evidence of paralysis (limited or assymetrical movement).
4. Teeth	State of repair, dentures (full or partial, fit, style, effectiveness).
5. Soft palate	Movement (equal elevation of both sides).
H. Abdomen	
1. Inspection	Contour (flat, concave, lateral borders slightly curved, flanks bulging, abdominal distention [exact location], protrusion of umbilicus, ascites). Movement (outward movement of abdominal wall with respiration, pulsation, peristaltic waves).
2. Auscultation	Characteristics of bowel sounds in all four quadrants (rate, pitch). Borborygmus (location). Hypermotility (rate, pitch; in diarrhea, in bowel obstruction [periods of hypermotility followed by periods of silence]). Friction rub (over enlarged organs). Bruits (over areas of vascular obstruction).
3. Palpation (light)	Location of boundaries (xiphoid process, costal margins, iliac crests). Presence of pain on palpation, ballottement (rebound tenderness). Resistance (location). Rigidity.
4. Percussion	Tympany Areas of dullness, presence of fluid.
I. Altered methods of feeding	
1. Nasogastric tube	
2. Gastrostomy tube	
3. Intravenous tube	

VI. Sexuality

A. Expression	Ability to give and receive affection.
B. Self-concept	Self-esteem or regard, self-acceptance, ideal self.

C. **Threats to self-con-cept**   Internal, external.

D. **Relationships**
  1. Needs   Ability to fulfill sexual needs.
  2. Partners   Sex, number.
  3. Effects of illness or hospitalization on   Needs, functional ability, relationships, roles.

E. **Reproduction**
  1. Menstrual history   Age of menarche, pattern of menses, abnormalities, menopause (age, associated factors).
  2. Fertility history   Number of pregnancies, live births.
  Use of contraception (knowledge, availability, preference, attitudes, male or female responsibility).

F. **Surgical intervention**   Organ removal, circumcision, vasectomy, tubal ligation.

G. **Physical assessment of secondary sex characteristics**
  1. Hair growth   Male or female distribution of facial, axillary, pubic hair.
  2. Breast   Female—masses, discharge, lesions.
  Male—gynecomastia.
  3. Genitalia   Lesions, discharge, history of infection.

VII. *Integument*

A. **Skin**
  1. Color   General pigmentation, deviations from normal (pallor, cyanosis, jaundice, erythema, ecchymosis, purpura, petechiae).
  2. Temperature   General (warm, cool, clammy), comparison of body parts.
  3. Turgor
  4. Texture   Smooth, rough, calloused, scaly, wrinkles, corns, dry scars.
  5. Odor   Description, control measures used.
  6. Integrity   Presence of injury or wound, size, location, appearance, drainage (type, amount, consistency), infecting organisms, dressings (drainage, integrity).
  7. Type, extent, or distribution.

B. **Hair**
  1. Head   Baldness, condition, cleanliness.
  2. Body   Distribution, shaving pattern.

C. **Nails**
  1. Color
  2. Condition   Integrity, length, cleanliness, ingrown nails, hangnails, infected cuticle, flexibility.

VIII. *Fluid and Electrolytes*

A. **Patterns of intake and output**   Amount/24 hr, source (oral, IV, urine, liquid stools, excessive perspiration, wound drainage, vomiting, nasogastric drainage, ileostomy).

B. Indirect signs

1. Hydration — Thirst, weight (changes over several days), turgor, condition of mouth (dry, moist, furrowed tongue), edema.
2. Venous state — Distended, flattened, filling time.
3. Level of consciousness
4. Muscle tonus — Decreased muscle tone, tetany, carpopedal spasm, Chvostek's sign.

C. Laboratory values — Na^+; K^+, CO_2 combining power (HCO_3^-), Cl^-, Ca^{++}, serum pH, Hgb, urine specific gravity and pH.

IX. Circulation

A. General observations

1. General color — Pallor, cyanosis.
2. Obvious pulsations

B. Interview

1. Fatigue and weakness — Amount, type of activity causing fatigue.
2. Shortness of breath — Amount, type of activity causing dyspnea.
3. Pain in legs — Type of activity or distance walked that brings on pain.
4. Pain in chest — Quality, location, radiation.
5. Behavior changes — Decreased attention span, memory lapses, confusion.
6. Indications of edema — Tightness of rings, shoes.

C. Physical assessment

1. Vital signs
   a. Blood pressure — Site, lying and standing values, range.
   b. Pulse — Site, rate, rhythm, quality, range.
2. Extremities
   a. Local skin color — Pallor, cyanosis, rubor.
   b. Skin temperature — Temperature along limb, comparison of bilateral limbs.
   c. Skin integrity — Location, extent of ulcer(s).
   d. Nails — Thickening.
   e. Hair distribution — Sparseness or absence, comparison of bilateral limbs.
   f. Capillary filling
   g. Peripheral arterial pulses — Amplitude, bilateral comparison.
   h. Edema — Location and extent (use tape measure).
3. Neck
   a. Carotid pulse — Quality, left *vs* right.
   b. Jugular vein distention — Presence or absence.
4. Precordium
   a. Visible cardiac impulses
   b. Auscultation — Rate, rhythm, extra sounds, pulse deficit.

X. *Temperature*

**A. Subjective feelings
of warmth or cold**

B. Body temperature
    1. History of elevated   When noted, duration, range.
         temperature
    2. Present tempera-   Site (oral, rectal, axillary), range.
         ture

C. Perspiration   Amount, pattern (day, night, intermittent).

D. Methods of temper-   Medication, hypothermia mattress, sponge baths.
    ature control

XI. *Respiration*

A. Interview
    1. Dyspnea   Amount, type of activity causing dyspnea.
    2. Fatigue   Amount, type of activity causing fatigue.
    3. Cough   Quality (dry, moist, hacking, croupy), onset, duration, time of day most
                 evident.
    4. Sputum produc-   Color, amount, odor, consistency.
         tion
    5. Smoking   Years smoking, packs per day.
    6. Painful respiration

B. Physical assessment
    1. Inspection
        a. Respiratory
           rate, rhythm,
           depth
        b. Cyanosis
        c. Muscles used   Accessory muscle use, retractions.
           for breathing
        d. Posture that fa-
           cilitates breath-
           ing
        e. Clubbing
        f. Changes in   Barrel chest, kyphosis, scoliosis.
           chest contour
    2. Palpation
        a. Chest expan-   General, comparison of left *vs* right side, upper *vs* lower chest.
           sion
        b. Areas of
           tenderness
        c. Tactile fremitus   Areas of increased or decreased fremitus.
    3. Percussion   Resonant, dull, hyperresonant.
    4. Auscultation
        a. Intensity of   Areas of diminished intensity.
           breath sounds
        b. Adventitious   Rales, rhonchi, friction rub (location)
           sounds

    C. Laboratory values and pO_2, pCO_2, chest x-ray, pulmonary function tests.
       diagnostic tests

XII. Elimination

  A. Urinary
    1. Voiding pattern   Diuresis, oliguria, nocturia
    2. History of urinary
       tract diseases
    3. Characteristics of   Sterility, color, clarity, urinary pH, protein, blood, glucose, ketones,
       urine   specific gravity.
    4. Altered urinary   Urinary incontinence, urinary retention, inflammation or infection of
       functioning   the lower urinary tract, use of a catheter.

  B. Bowel
    1. Defecation pat-
       tern
    2. Characteristics of   Color, consistency and form, odor.
       normal stool
    3. Altered bowel   Diarrhea, constipation, flatus, fecal impaction, anal incontinence.
       functioning
    4. Artificial opening   Colostomy, ileostomy.
       for bowel diversion

This version of the person assessment represents the thoughts and efforts of many faculty members who taught in the Fundamentals Area over several years. Nursing assessment of the physiologic statuses is credited to R. Faye McCain and her graduate students of the 1960s at Michigan. Additionally the authors specifically acknowledge Marguerite B. Harms for labeling the concept of person assessment and also including life-style data and developmental tasks. The authors, however, assume full responsibility for this particular adaptation of earlier tools.

Appendix B
Person Assessment and Nursing Care Plan for Mrs. R.

Data Base

I. Demographic Data

A.	**Age**	55
B.	**Sex**	Female
C.	**Race**	Caucasian
D.	**Surgery**	Total abdominal hysterectomy with bilateral salpingo-oophorectomy
E.	**Current concern**	Possible diagnosis of cancer; underwent emergency appendectomy while vacationing in Alabama 6 weeks ago; questionable mass observed on right ovary, possible cancer; returned home for further surgery; has been very distressed while waiting for additional surgery.

II. Sociocultural Data

A.	**Family**	Married with 2 children Son age 30, unmarried, MD in Calif. Daughter, age 29, unmarried, nurse in Detroit
B.	**Social support system**	States very close to husband and confides in him; loves him very much. Dog and cat keep her company during the day.
C.	**Insurance**	Blue Cross–Blue Shield
D.	**Religion**	Belief in God and Jesus; states she prays more often now because she is very anxious about surgery and possible outcome.
E.	**Values**	Values privacy greatly; states, "I'm not a grouch or anything; I just don't like all these people around all the time." States her current room, a ward, lacks privacy.

III. Developmental Tasks

A. Intimacy *vs* isolation

Husband (see sociocultural data); enjoyed her children but with them grown can spend more time with husband; states they make decisions together; he was with her immediately before and after surgery; visits for long periods every day.

B. Generativity *vs* stagnation

Speaks of children in a positive manner and is proud of their independent achievements; expresses strong desire that they will marry and have children. States she does not feel her age but is aware of hair, skin, and energy changes. Belief in God (see sociocultural data).

IV. Psychological Data

A. Orientation

To time, place, person; postop, groggy but oriented

B. Memory

Able to recall past and recent events

C. Pupils

Equal, react to light and accommodation

D. Communication

Speaks with clear tones and diction; articulates well. Postop, speaks with decreased pace.

E. Vocabulary

Able to understand some technical language but prefers common terms. States, "Those doctors use big medical terms. I know what they're talking about because I've heard them so often, but I wish they would just talk normal."

F. Nonverbal behaviors

Preop, body posture relaxed, smiled frequently. Became distressed when speaking of surgery as demonstrated by facial grimaces, wringing of hands, and erect body position.

G. Stressors

Possible cancer (see demographic data): "It has been terrible living with half the story. I wish they would tell me all or nothing!"

H. Strengths

Feels accomplishment in her roles as wife, mother and homemaker. Was able to accept help from nurse by learning from preop teaching and using it postop to promote a recovery. States she knows using the information will help her regain independence more quickly.

V. Motor Status

A. Degree of self-sufficiency

Preop, ADL by self; postop, needs assistance with bathing, mouth care, moving (first day only).

B. Medical restrictions

Ambulation q.i.d. with assistance (first day postop)

C. Musculoskeletal

Has decreased endurance, coordination, and stability related to postop state. All joints mobile; displays active FRJM. Right handed.

VI. Respiratory Status

A. History

No cough or dyspnea; smoked 1½ packs/day for 30 years. Does not feel like smoking immediately postop.

B. Physical assessment

Facial skin and lip color pale. Decreased chest expansion and shallow respirations related to incisional pain, "It hurts even to breathe." Splints incision and does coughing and deep breathing well when assisted by nurse; no mucus produced. Lungs clear on auscultation.

VII. Nutritional Status

A. Ht

5′4″; Wt: 122 lb.

B. Appetite

1. For past 6 weeks has had diminished appetite and did not enjoy meals, related to anxiety about possible cancer.
2. Postop: Appetite returning; states, "A banana milkshake would taste good!"

C. Diet

General, prior to surgery; postop, NPO until noon of first day, then ice chips to clear liquid diet for supper. Returned to general by supper on 2nd day.

D. Oral cavity

Lips dry, pink; gums and oral mucosa pink with a somewhat diminished salivary flow; tongue covered with thin, white coating; teeth all present, in good repair.

E. Abdomen

No bowel sounds heard immediately after surgery; bowel sounds heard in all four quadrants by afternoon of first postop day. Surgical wound dry and intact.

VIII. Rest and Comfort

A. Sleep

States sleep has been altered past 6 weeks related to worry; difficulty falling and remaining asleep, waking frequently during the night. Prior to concerns, slept 7–8 hr without interruption. Requested sleeping pill the evening prior to surgery. Postop, slept well first night; awakened at intervals second night.

B. Pain
1. Subjective data

Postop, dull, continuous over lower right and left quadrants of abdomen associated with surgical wound; intensified by movement, coughing, and deep breathing (see respiratory status). Emotional distress related to dependency on nurses because of surgery and pain; states she is grateful for assistance but very much wishes to regain independence.

2. Objective data

Slow speech, facial grimaces, perspiration during movement; shallow respirations.

Nursing Care Plan for Mrs. R.

Strengths	Problem	Expected Outcomes	Interventions
Finds comfort in religious faith	1. Emotional discomfort related to:	Person will verbalize decreased anxiety and greater comfort re: possible Dx.	Spend time with her even when she does not talk.
High self-esteem related to success in marriage and child raising	a. Possible diagnosis (Dx) of cancer		Provide quiet companionship.
Able to identify presence and source of anxiety			Help her vent feelings re: possible Dx.
Favorable resolution of developmental tasks			Listen carefully to facilitate development of trusting relationship.
			Acknowledge and reinforce all positive growth-oriented behavior.
Has strong desire to recover from surgery and become independent again	b. Invasion of personal space and privacy	Verbalize increased comfort and increased personal space.	Employ comfort measures such as backrubs as she desires.
Able to accept help			Remove any clutter from the environment.
Able to learn from and use health information			Use curtains around bed for privacy.
			Approach quietly and ask permission to sit down or provide care.
			Place in a single room as soon as possible.
Strong family support system: able to give and receive love and support from family	2. Pain related to surgical procedure.	Verbalize greater comfort and a decreased perception of pain.	Explain the usual course of surgical incisional pain.
Well oriented; good memory			Teach appropriate ways to get out of bed and to splint wound while coughing; assist with these activities as needed. Continue to assess pain on a regular schedule (q 3 hr) and plan with her for administration of medication.
Appropriate Ht and Wt proportion			Provide backrubs as she desires.
	3. Altered respiratory status related to:	Maintain clear lungs on auscultation	Assist with coughing and deep breathing q 1–2 while awake and q 3–4 hr during sleep hours. Acknowledge and support distaste for postop smoking for at least 1 week.
	a. Potential increase in bronchial secretions related to anesthesia		
	b. Decreased mobility	Gradually increase mobility from a few steps to regular hall	Assist with ambulation q.i.d. until able to proceed without assistance.

Strengths	Problem	Expected Outcomes	Interventions
		ambulation over the next few days	Help her walk a little farther each time.
	c. Narcotic medications	Use narcotic medications for 1½ days following surgery and then progress to oral analgesics with minimal narcotic.	Explain possibility of drowsiness, dizziness, and shallow respirations accompanying pain medications.
			Advise caution when moving in bed; suggest use of siderails for a while following injection.

	4. Potential injury related to:
	  a. Decreased endurance and stability
	  b. Narcotic medications
		Remain safe and free from injury following surgery.	See interventions related to ambulation and medications: problem 3.

	5. Potential decrease in self-esteem related to:
	  a. Altered body image
	  b. Increased dependency
		Continue to verbalize a high level of self-esteem	Acknowledge and support strengths and help her to view these as useful for coping. Assist her to view herself as a total person rather than focusing on limitations.

			Assist both person and husband to express their feelings to each other.
			Acknowledge her increasing endurance and independence.
	6. Decreased sleep related to anxiety	Verbalize greater comfort and a more restful sleep before discharge	See interventions: problems 3 and 5.
			Provide a slowing of activities and a restful environment for 1–2 hr prior to bedtime.
			Plan periods of rest and activity during day.
			Provide sufficient covers and proper ventilation.
			Group nursing activities for minimal disturbance during sleeping hours.
	7. Dry oral cavity	Demonstrate adequate salivary flow before discharge	Assist with mouth care q 4 hr (toothbrushing), offer lemon–glycerine swabs or mouthwash as needed.

From data and care plan ideas contributed by Lori A. Wissman, Class of 1982, University of Michigan

Index

Numerals followed by an *f* indicate a figure; *t* following a page number indicates tabular material.

abdomen
   assessment of, 387–388, 389t
   boundaries of, 388
abdominal pressure, effect of urinary output, 416
abdominal thrust, use in clearing airway obstruction, 520
abrasion, of skin, 324, 345
absolutistic position, toward sexuality, 597, 607
absorption
   of food, 381, 409
   through skin, 324–325
abstract ideas, mental capacity and, 279–280
accidental crisis, 86, 92
accommodation, to reality, 44–45, 47
accountability, 152–154, 160, 165
acholic stool, 429, 438
acid, definition of, 447, 467
acid–base balance, 447–448
acid–base imbalances, 458, 458f. *See also* acidosis and alkalosis
acidosis
   metabolic, 458–459, 458f, 459t, 467
   respiratory, 460–461, 462f, 462t, 468
acting out behavior, 603–604
active listening, 213, 221
active transport, of electrolytes, 446, 467
activities of daily living, 360, 368–369, 370t, 377
activity theory, of aging, 98, 102
acute pain, 527–528, 537–538
adaptation, 79–94
   assisting with, 87–91, 89f
   concept in person-centered care, 9
   definition of, 44–45, 47, 79, 91
   to dying, 649–653
   in elderly persons, 96–103
     to functional changes, 99–101
     theories of, 98
   to environment, 312
   in nursing, 81–83
   process of, 83–86
   to surgery, 661–664

theories of, 79–83, 80t
adaptive coping, 84–85, 87f, 88f, 89
adaptive grief, 643–648, 655
adjustment
   definition of, 258, 268
   emotional, 258–260, 259t
   to environmental change, 67–68
adolescents
   adaptation to dying, 650
   cognitive development, 45
   developmental tasks in, 41t
   health problems of, 117–118t
   sex education for, 606
   sexuality development of, 596–597
adulthood
   developmental tasks in, 41t–42t
   sexuality development in, 597–600
adults. *See also* elderly persons
   adaptation to dying, 650
   health problems of, 117t–118t
adventitious sounds, in chest, 507t, 508, 522
advocacy, 200
advocates, nurses as, 137–138, 139t
affect, 254, 261, 268, 280, 292
affective learning objectives, 626–627, 632
affirmative action, 166, 171
age. *See also* infancy, childhood, adolescents, adults
   effect on sleep, 550
   sensory function and, 299
agencies, health-care, 120–121, 120t, 121f
aggregation phase, in nursing process, 241, 242t, 245
aging, 96–103. *See also* elderly persons
   adaptation to functional changes, 99–101
   developmental tasks of, 98–99
   health problems and, 118t
   integumentary status and, 329
   mental status and, 273
   myths about, 97–98
   physical changes and, 99–101